Atlas of Endoscopic Ultrasonography

Atlas of Endoscopic Ultrasonography

SECOND EDITION

EDITED BY

Frank Gress, MD
Professor of Medicine
Icahn School of Medicine
Division of Gastroenterology and Hepatology
Mount Sinai Hospital
New York, USA

Thomas Savides, MD
Professor of Clinical Medicine
Division of Gastroenterology
University of California
San Diego, California, USA

Brenna Casey, MD
Assistant Professor of Medicine
Division of Gastroenterology
Massachusetts General Hospital
Harvard Medical School
Boston, Massachusetts, USA

Everson L. A. Artifon, MD
Associate Professor of Surgery
Department of Surgery
University of São Paulo
São Paulo, Brazil

WILEY Blackwell

This edition first published 2022

Edition History
Blackwell Publishing Ltd (1e, 2012)

Registered Offices
John Wiley & Sons, Inc., 111 River Street, Hoboken, NJ 07030, USA
John Wiley & Sons Ltd, The Atrium, Southern Gate, Chichester, West Sussex, PO19 8SQ, UK

Editorial Office
9600 Garsington Road, Oxford, OX4 2DQ, UK

For details of our global editorial offices, customer services, and more information about Wiley products visit us at www.wiley.com.

Wiley also publishes its books in a variety of electronic formats and by print-on-demand. Some content that appears in standard print versions of this book may not be available in other formats.

Library of Congress Cataloging-in-Publication Data

Names: Gress, Frank G., editor. | Savides, Thomas J., editor. | Casey, Brenna, editor. | Artifon, Everson L. A., editor.
Title: Atlas of endoscopic ultrasonography / edited by Frank G. Gress, Thomas John Savides, Brenna Casey, Everson L. A. Artifon.
Description: Second edition. | Hoboken, NJ : Wiley-Blackwell, 2022. | Includes bibliographical references and index.
Identifiers: LCCN 2021015783 (print) | LCCN 2021015784 (ebook) | ISBN 9781119523000 (hardback) | ISBN 9781119523093 (adobe pdf) | ISBN 9781119523031 (epub)
Subjects: MESH: Endoscopy, Digestive System | Digestive System Diseases–diagnostic imaging | Digestive System–diagnostic imaging | Ultrasonography | Atlas
Classification: LCC RC801 (print) | LCC RC801 (ebook) | NLM WI 17 | DDC 616.3/07545–dc23
LC record available at https://lccn.loc.gov/2021015783
LC ebook record available at https://lccn.loc.gov/2021015784

Cover Design: Wiley
Cover Images: Courtesy of Dalton Chaves, Courtesy of Anthony Teoh, Courtesy of Cynthia Behling, Courtesy of David L. Diehl, MD, Courtesy of Wilson Kwong, Courtesy of Spencer Cheng, Courtesy of Julio Iglesias Garcia, Courtesy of Toltech

Set in 9/12pt Meridien by Straive, Pondicherry, India

Printed and bound by CPI Group (UK) Ltd, Croydon, CR0 4YY
C9781119523000_121224

Contents

Contributors, vii

Preface, xi

About the Companion Website, xii

Part 1 Normal EUS Anatomy, 1

1 Normal Human Anatomy, 3
John C. Deutsch

2 Esophagus: Radial and Linear, 10
James L. Wise and John C. Deutsch

3 Normal Mediastinal Anatomy by EUS and EBUS, 14
Juan Corral, Sebastian Fernandez-Bussy, and Michael B. Wallace

4 Stomach: Radial and Linear, 19
Joo Ha Hwang

5 Bile Duct: Radial and Linear, 22
Kapil Gupta

6 EUS of the Normal Pancreas, 25
Richard A. Erickson and James T. Sing, Jr.

7 Liver, Spleen, and Kidneys: Radial and Linear, 30
Nalini M. Guda and Marc F. Catalano

8 Anatomy of the Anorectum: Radial and Linear, 33
Christoph F. Dietrich

Part 2 Upper and Lower GI EUS, 37

9 Esophageal Cancer, 39
Armen Eskandari and Syed M. Abbas Fehmi

10 EUS for Achalasia, 46
Michael Chang

11 Malignant Mediastinal Lesions, 49
M. Babitha Reddy, David H. Robbins, and Mohamad A. Eloubeidi

12 Benign Mediastinal Lesions, 51
M. Babitha Reddy, David H. Robbins, and Mohamad A. Eloubeidi

13 Gastric Cancer, 53
Douglas O. Faigel and Sarah A. Rodriguez

14 Gastric and Esophageal Subepithelial Masses, 58
Muhammad Tahir and Andrew J. Bain

15 Anorectal Neoplasia, 67
Manoop S. Bhutani and Everson L.A. Artifon

16 Anal Sphincter Disease: Fecal Incontinence and Fistulas, 72
Raymond S. Tang and Thomas J. Savides

17 Endometriosis, 78
José Celso Ardengh, Juan Pablo Román Serrano, Samuel Galante Romanini, Juliana Silveira Lima de Castro, and Isabela Trindade Torres

18 Vascular Anomalies and Abnormalities, 88
John C. Deutsch

Part 3 Pancreatico-biliary, 93

19 Duodenal and Ampullary Neoplasia, 95
Brenna Casey and Kumar Krishnan

20 Biliary Tract Pathology, 98
Brenna Casey and Kumar Krishnan

21 Gallbladder Pathology, 101
Sam Yoselevitz and Ann Marie Joyce

22 Pancreatic Adenocarcinoma, 104
Douglas G. Adler

23 Pancreatic Malignancy (Non-adenocarcinoma), 108
Larissa Fujii-Lau, Michael J. Levy, and Suresh T. Chari

24 Autoimmune Pancreatitis, 113
Larissa Fujii-Lau, Michael J. Levy, and Suresh T. Chari

25 Pancreatic Cystic Lesions: The Role of EUS, 117
William R. Brugge

26 Intraductal Papillary Mucinous Neoplasms: The Role of EUS, 121
William R. Brugge

27 Chronic Pancreatitis, 125
David G. Forcione

28 Liver Pathology, 130
Indraneel Chakrabarty and Ann Marie Joyce

Part 4 How to Section, 135

29 How to Interpret EUS-FNA Cytology, 137
Cynthia Behling

30 How to do Mediastinal FNA, 146
Sammy Ho

31 How to do Pancreatic Mass FNA, 150
Yunseok Namn and Jonathan M. Buscaglia

32 How to do Pancreatic Cyst FNA, 155
Ahmad Najdat Bazarbashi and Linda S. Lee

33 How to do Pancreatic Pseudocyst Drainage, 160
Shyam Varadarajulu and Vinay Dhir

34 How to do EUS-guided Pancreatic Cyst Chemoablation, 165
Matthew T. Moyer and John M. DeWitt

35 How to do Celiac Plexus Block, 173
Sam M. Serouya and Adam J. Goodman

36 How to Place Fiducials for Radiation Therapy, 176
Antonio R. Cheesman, Satish Nagula, and Christopher J. DiMaio

37 How to Inject Chemotherapeutic Agents, 179
V. Raman Muthusamy and Kenneth J. Chang

38 How to do EUS-guided Pelvic Abscess Drainage, 182
Shyam Varadarajulu and Sandeep Lakhtakia

39 How to do Doppler Probe EUS for Bleeding, 186
Richard C.K. Wong

40 How to do Endoscopic Ultrasound-guided Portal Pressure Gradient Measurement, 194
Rintaro Hashimoto and Kenneth J. Chang

41 How to do Endoscopic Ultrasound-guided Liver Biopsy, 197
David L. Diehl

42 How to do EUS-guided Treatment of Gastric Varices, 202
Dalton Marques Chaves and Filipe Tomishige Chaves

43 How to do EUS-guided Arterial Embolization, 205
Marc Barthet and Jean-Michel Gonzalez

44 How to do EUS-guided Radiofrequency Ablation of Pancreatic Neuroendocrine Tumors, 209
Marc Barthet, Mohamed Gasmi, and Jean-Michel Gonzalez

45 How to do EUS Pancreatic Duct Access and Drainage, 214
Alberto Larghi, Mihai Rimbaş, and Mauricio K. Minata

46 How to do EUS Gallbladder Drainage, 220
Shannon Melissa Chan and Anthony Yuen Bun Teoh

47 How to do an EUS-guided Gastrojejunostomy, 226
Sohini Sameera and Michel Kahaleh

48 How to do EUS Elastography, 229
Julio Iglesias-Garcia, Jose Lariño-Noia, Daniel de la Iglesia-García, and J. Enrique Dominguez-Muñoz

49 How to do Contrast-enhanced EUS, 237
Yasunobu Yamashita and Masayuki Kitano

50 How to do EUS-guided Ablation of Pancreatic Neurendocrine Tumors, 248
Sabrina Gloria Giulia Testoni, Gemma Rossi, Livia Archibugi, and Paolo Giorgio Arcidiacono, 248

51 How to do EUS-guided Needle Confocal Laser Endomicroscopy of Pancreatic Cysts, 254
Prashant Bhenswala and Frank G. Gress

52 How to use ex vivo Models in Teaching Therapeutic Endoscopic Ultrasound, 256
Spencer Cheng, Mauricio K. Minata, Carlos K. Furuya, and Edson Ide

53 How to do Endoscopic Necrosectomy, 265
Wilson T. Kwong

54 How to Perform Pancreatic Mass Fine Needle Biopsy, 270
Ahmad Najdat Bazarbashi and Linda S. Lee

55 How to Perform Endoscopic Ultrasound-directed Transgastric Endoscopic Retrograde Cholangiopancreatography (EDGE), 274
M. Phillip Fejleh and Wilson T. Kwong

Index, 278

Contributors

Douglas G. Adler, MD, FACG, FASGE
Peak Gastroenterology Associates
Colorado Springs, CO, USA

Livia Archibugi, MD
Pancreas Translational and Clinical Research Center
Division of Pancreato-Biliary Endoscopy and Endosonography
San Raffaele Scientific Institute IRCCS
Vita-Salute San Raffaele University
Milan, Italy

Paolo Giorgio Arcidiacono, MD, FASGE
Pancreas Translational and Clinical Research Center
Division of Pancreato-Biliary Endoscopy and Endosonography
San Raffaele Scientific Institute IRCCS
Vita-Salute San Raffaele University
Milan, Italy

José Celso Ardengh, MD, PHD, FASGE
Professor of Surgery and Anatomy
Ribeirão Preto Medical School
University São Paulo, Ribeirão Preto
São Paulo, Brazil
Head in the Endoscopy Service Hospital 9 de Julho
Sao Paulo, Brazil

Everson L.A. Artifon, MD, MBA, PhD, FASGE
Associate Professor of Surgery
Department of Surgery
University of Sao Paulo
Sao Paulo, Brazil
Ana Costa Hospital
Santos, Brazil

Andrew J. Bain, MD
Roswell Park Comprehensive Cancer Center
Buffalo, NY, USA

Marc Barthet, MD, PHD
Head of Gastroenterology Department
Digestive endoscopy and gastroenterology department
North Hospital, Marseille, France

Ahmad Najdat Bazarbashi, MD
Division of Gastroenterology, Hepatology and Endoscopy
Brigham and Women's Hospital
Harvard Medical School
Boston, MA, USA

Cynthia Behling, MD, PHD
Pacific Rim Pathology Group
Sharp Memorial Hospital
San Diego, CA, USA

Prashant Bhenswala, MD, MSCR
Department of Medicine
Mount Sinai South Nassau Hospital
Oceanside, NY, USA

Manoop S. Bhutani, MD, FASGE, FACG, FACP, AGAF
Professor of Medicine, Experimental Diagnostic Imaging and Biomedical Engineering
Director, Endoscopic Research and Development
University of Texas MD Anderson Cancer Center
Houston, TX, USA

Brenna Casey, MD, FASGE
Interventional Gastroenterology
Director of Interventional Endoscopy
Massachusetts General Hospital
Harvard Medical School
Boston, MA, USA

William R. Brugge, MD
Director, Gastrointestinal Endoscopy
Massachusetts General Hospital
Professor of Medicine
Harvard Medical School
Boston, MA, USA

Jonathan M. Buscaglia, MD
Director of Advanced Endoscopy
Assistant Professor of Medicine
Stony Brook University Hospital
Renaissance School of Medicine at Stony Brook University
Stony Brook, NY, USA

Marc F. Catalano, MD
Clinical Associate Professor of Medicine
Medical College of Wisconsin
Pancreatobiliary Services
St. Luke's Medical Center
Milwaukee, WI, USA

Indraneel Chakrabarty, MD, MA
Clinical Associate of Medicine
Tufts University School of Medicine
Division of Gastroenterology
Lahey Clinic Medical Center
Burlington, MA, USA

Shannon Melissa Chan, MBCHB, FRCSEd, FHKAM (SURGERY)
Department of Surgery
Prince of Wales Hospital
The Chinese University of Hong Kong
Shatin, Hong Kong

Kenneth J. Chang, MD
Professor of Clinical Medicine
Division Chief, Gastroenterology
University of California
Irvine, CA, USA

Michael Chang, MD
Assistant Professor
Department of Medicine
University of California San Diego
La Jolla, CA, USA

Suresh T. Chari, MD
MD Anderson Cancer Hospital
Houston, TX, USA

Dalton Marques Chaves
Gastrointestinal Endoscopy Unit
University of Sao Paulo
Sao Paulo-Brazil

Filipe Tomishige Chaves
Gastrointestinal Endoscopy Unit
University of Sao Paulo
Sao Paulo-Brazil

Antonio R. Cheesman, MD
Division of Gastroenterology
Icahn School of Medicine at Mount Sinai
New York, NY, USA

Spencer Cheng, MD, PHD
Department of Gastroenterology
Gastrointestinal Endoscopy Unit
University of São Paulo
São Paulo, Brazil

Juan Corral, MD
Division of Gastroenterology and Hepatology
Mayo Clinic College of Medicine
Jacksonville, FL, USA

Juliana Silveira Lima de Castro, MD
Staff of Endoscopy Service
Hospital Nove de Julho
Sao Paulo, Brazil

Daniel de la Iglesia-García, MD
Department of Gastroenterology and Hepatology
Health Research Institute
University Hospital of Santiago de Compostela
Santiago de Compostela, Spain

John C. Deutsch, MD
Essentia Health Care Systems
Duluth, MN, USA

John M. DeWitt, MD, FACG, FACP, FASGE
Associate Professor of Medicine
Co-Director, Endoscopic Ultrasound Clinical Program
Division of Gastroenterology and Hepatology
Indiana University Medical Center
Indianapolis, IN, USA

J. Enrique Dominguez-Muñoz, MD, PHD
Department of Gastroenterology and Hepatology
Health Research Institute
University Hospital of Santiago de Compostela
Santiago de Compostela, Spain

Vinay Dhir, MD, DNB
Director Clinical Research and Chief of Endosonography
Institute of Advanced Endoscopy
Mumbai, India

David L. Diehl, MD, FASGE
Professor of Medicine
Geisinger Medical Center and Geisinger Commonwealth School of Medicine
Danville, PA, USA

Christoph F. Dietrich, MD
Professor, Second Department of Internal Medicine
Caritas-Krankenhaus
Bad Mergentheim, Germany

Christopher J. DiMaio, MD
Director of Therapeutic Endoscopy
Icahn School of Medicine at Mount Sinai
New York, NY, USA

Mohamad A. Eloubeidi, MD, MHS, FASGE, FACP, FACG, AGAF
Professor of Medicine
American University of Beirut School of Medicine
Beirut, Lebanon

Richard A. Erickson, MD, FACP, FACG, AGAF
Director, Division of Gastroenterology
Scott and White Clinic and Hospital
Professor of Medicine
Texas A&M Health Science Center
Temple, TX, USA

Armen Eskandari, MD
Division of Gastroenterology and Hepatology
University of California San Diego
La Jolla, CA, USA

Douglas O. Faigel, MD, FACG, FASGE, AGAF
Professor of Medicine
Mayo Clinic College of Medicine
Scottsdale, AZ, USA

Syed M. Abbas Fehmi, MD
Clinical Assistant Professor of Medicine
Division of Gastroenterology and Hepatology
University of California San Diego
La Jolla, CA, USA

M. Phillip Fejleh, MD
Division of Gastroenterology
University of California San Diego Health Sciences
La Jolla, CA, USA

Sebastian Fernandez-Bussy, MD
Division of Pulmonary Medicine and Critical Care
Mayo Clinic College of Medicine
Jacksonville, FL, USA

David G. Forcione, MD
Associate Director of Interventional Endoscopy
Massachusetts General Hospital
Harvard Medical School
Boston, MA, USA

Larissa Fujii-Lau, MD
University of Hawaii
Honolulu, HI, USA

Carlos K. Furuya JR., PHD, MD
Assistant Professor of Medicine
Department of Gastroenterology
Gastrointestinal Endoscopy Unit
University of São Paulo
São Paulo, Brazil

Mohamed Gasmi, MD
Digestive endoscopy and gastroenterology department
North Hospital, Marseille, France

Jean-Michel Gonzalez, MD, PHD
Head of Endoscopy Unit
Digestive endoscopy and gastroenterology department
North Hospital, Marseille, France

Adam J. Goodman, MD
Associate Professor of Medicine
NYU Langone Health
New York, NY, USA

Frank G. Gress, MD, MBA
Department of Medicine
Division of Gastroenterology and Hepatology
Icahn School of Medicine at Mount Sinai and Mount Sinai South Nassau Hospital
Oceanside, NY, USA

Nalini M. Guda, MD, FASGE
Clinical Associate Professor of Medicine
University of Wisconsin, School of Medicine and Public Health
Pancreatobiliary Services
St. Luke's Medical Center
Milwaukee, WI, USA

Kapil Gupta, MD, MPH
Associate Director, Pancreatic and Biliary Diseases
Interventional Endoscopy
Division of Gastroenterology
Cedars-Sinai Medical Center
Los Angeles, CA, USA

Rintaro Hashimoto, MD, PHD
Department of Gastroenterology
University of California
Irvine, CA, USA

Sammy Ho, MD
Assistant Professor of Medicine
Director of Pancreaticobiliary Services and Endoscopic Ultrasound
Division of Gastroenterology
Montefiore Medical Center/AECOM
Bronx, NY, USA

Joo Ha Hwang, MD, PHD
Stanford University
Palo Alto, CA, USA

Edson Ide, PHD, MD
Department of Gastroenterology
Gastrointestinal Endoscopy Unit
University of São Paulo
São Paulo, Brazil

Julio Iglesias-Garcia, MD, PHD
Department of Gastroenterology and Hepatology
Health Research Institute
University Hospital of Santiago de Compostela
Santiago de Compostela, Spain

Ann Marie Joyce, MD
Assistant Professor of Medicine
Tufts University School of Medicine
Burlington, MA, USA

Michel Kahaleh, MD, AGAF, FACG, FASGE
Distinguished Professor of Medicine
Clinical Director of Gastroenterology
Chief of Endoscopy
Director Pancreas Program
Rutgers Robert Wood Johnson Medical School
New Brunswick, NJ, USA

Masayuki Kitano, MD, PHD
Second Department of Internal Medicine
Wakayama Medical University
Wakayama, Japan

Kumar Krishnan, MD
Interventional Endoscopy
Harvard Medical School
Massachusetts General Hospital
Boston, MA, USA

Wilson T. Kwong, MD, MS
Assistant Professor of Medicine
Division of Gastroenterology
University of California San Diego Health Sciences
La Jolla, CA, USA

Sandeep Lakhtakia, MD, MNAMS, DM
Consultant
Asian Institute of Gastroenterology
Hyderabad, India

Alberto Larghi, MD, PHD
Digestive Endoscopy Unit
Fondazione Policlinico A. Gemelli IRCCS
Rome, Italy

Jose Lariño-Noia, MD
Department of Gastroenterology and Hepatology
Health Research Institute
University Hospital of Santiago de Compostela
Santiago de Compostela, Spain

Linda S. Lee, MD
Division of Gastroenterology, Hepatology and Endoscopy
Brigham and Women's Hospital
Harvard Medical School
Boston, MA, USA

Michael J. Levy, MD
Consultant
Mayo Clinic
Rochester, MN, USA

Mauricio K. Minata, MSC, MD
Digestive Endoscopy Unit
University of São Paulo
SP, Brazil

Matthew T. Moyer, MD, MS, FASGE
Associate Professor of Medicine
Division of Gastroenterology and Hepatology
Penn State Hershey Medical Center
Hershey, PA, USA

V. Raman Muthusamy, MD, FACG, FASGE
Director, Gastroenterology Fellowship Program
Health Sciences Associate Clinical Professor of Medicine
Division of Gastroenterology
Department of Medicine
University of California
Irvine, CA, USA

Satish Nagula, MD
Director of Endoscopic Ultrasound
Icahn School of Medicine at Mount Sinai
New York, NY, USA

Yunseok Namn, MD
Stony Brook University Hospital
Renaissance School of Medicine at Stony Brook University
Stony Brook, NY, USA

M. Babitha Reddy, DO, MPH
Gastroenterology Fellow
Lenox Hill Hospital
New York, NY, USA

Mihai Rimbaș, MD, PHD
Department of Gastroenterology
Colentina Clinical Hospital;
Internal Medicine Department
Carol Davila University of Medicine
Bucharest, Romania

David H. Robbins, MD, MSC
Associate Director
Lenox Hill Hospital
New York, NY, USA

Sarah A. Rodriguez, MD
Assistant Professor of Medicine
Oregon Health and Science University
Portland, OR, USA

Samuel Galante Romanini, MD
Staff of Endoscopy Service
Hospital Nove de Julho
Sao Paulo, Brazil

Gemma Rossi, MD
Pancreas Translational and Clinical Research Center
Division of Pancreato-Biliary Endoscopy and Endosonography
San Raffaele Scientific Institute IRCCS
Vita-Salute San Raffaele University
Milan, Italy

Sohini Sameera, MD
Rutgers Robert Wood Johnson Medical School
New Brunswick, NJ, USA

Thomas J. Savides, MD
Division of Gastroenterology
University of California San Diego
La Jolla, CA, USA

Sam M. Serouya, MD
Assistant Professor of Medicine
NYU Langone Grossman School of Medicine
New York, NY, USA

Juan Pablo Román Serrano, MD
Staff of Endoscopy Service
Hospital Nove de Julho
Sao Paulo, Brazil

James T. Sing JR., DO, FACG, AGAF
Assistant Professor of Medicine
Texas A&M University Health Science Center
Director, Endoscopy
Department of Medicine
Scott and White Clinic and Hospital
Texas A&M University Health Science Center
Temple, TX, USA

Muhammad Tahir, MD
Roswell Park Comprehensive Cancer Center
Buffalo, NY, USA

Raymond S. Tang, MD
Clinical Professional Consultant
Institute of Digestive Disease
The Chinese University of Hong Kong
Prince of Wales Hospital
Shatin, New Territories
Hong Kong, China

Anthony Yuen Bun Teoh, MBCHB, FRCSED, FHKAM (SURGERY)
Department of Surgery
Prince of Wales Hospital
The Chinese University of Hong Kong
Shatin, Hong Kong

Sabrina Gloria Giulia Testoni, MD
Pancreato-Biliary Endoscopy and Endosonography Division
Pancreas Translational and Clinical Research Center
San Raffaele Scientific Institute IRCCS
Vita-Salute San Raffaele University
Milan, Italy

Isabela Trindade Torres, MD
Staff of Endoscopy Service
Hospital Nove de Julho
Sao Paulo, Brazil

Shyam Varadarajulu, MD
Director of Endoscopy
University of Alabama at Birmingham School of Medicine
Birmingham, AL, USA

Michael B. Wallace, MD, MPH
Division of Gastroenterology and Hepatology
Mayo Clinic College of Medicine
Jacksonville, FL, USA

James L. Wise, MD
Essentia Health Care Systems
Duluth, MN, USA

Richard C.K. Wong, MD, FASGE, FACG, AGAF, FACP
Professor of Medicine
Case Western Reserve University;
Medical Director, Digestive Health Institute Endoscopy Unit
University Hospitals Case Medical Center
Cleveland, OH, USA

Yasunobu Yamashita, MD, PHD
Second Department of Internal Medicine
Wakayama Medical University
Wakayama, Japan

Sam Yoselevitz, MD
Clinical Associate of Medicine
Tufts University School of Medicine
Burlington, MA, USA

Preface

Learning to perform and interpret endoscopic ultrasound (EUS) requires both didactic learning and repetitive exposure to images usually accomplished through procedural volume. We provided detailed aspects of the didactic portion of learning in the Gress and Savides textbook *Endoscopic Ultrasonography*. We then created the Gress, Savides, Bounds and Deutsch *Atlas of Endoscopic Ultrasonography* to provide aspiring endosonographers access to numerous images and videos to assist them with improving their pattern recognition of pathologic conditions.

In this second edition of the Atlas, we are grateful that the renowned Brazilian endoscopist Everson Artifon has joined our team, along with our previous editor Brenna Casey who has continued with the Atlas. Our previous editor, John Deutsch, has retired and fortunately his timeless and superb chapters related to learning EUS anatomy are retained.

In this edition, we are excited to have expanded our international panel of world class endosonographers as contributing authors to provide a variety of styles and approaches to EUS. Our authors include some of the "first-generation" pioneers of endoscopic ultrasound as well as the next generation of interventional EUS pioneers who are improving the imaging abilities of new and enhanced EUS technology and expanding the breadth of interventional techniques. We are especially pleased to offer many new sections on "How to do" aspects of interventional and therapeutic EUS procedures.

We hope this Atlas will appeal to a wide spectrum of endosonographers, from those who are beginning their training to those who are looking to expand their horizons with therapeutic techniques.

Finally, we want to thank our families, colleagues, editors, authors, and especially Jenny Seward from our publisher, Wiley, for all their support without whom this Atlas could not be possible.

Frank Gress MD
Thomas Savides MD

About the Companion Website

This book is accompanied by a companion website:

www.wiley.com/go/gress/atlas

- Videos showing procedures described in the book.

(All videos are referenced in the text at the end of each chapter.)

- All figures from the book available for downloading

1 Normal EUS Anatomy

1 Normal Human Anatomy

John C. Deutsch
Essentia Health Care Systems, Duluth, MN, USA

Introduction

The Visible Human Project at the University of Colorado has generated large volumes of human anatomy data. The original information is captured by slowly abrading away frozen human cadavers in a transaxial manner and capturing the anatomy by digital imaging. The digital data is compiled and then over the years is manipulated by scientists at the University's Center for Human Simulation to allow access to identified cross-sections in any plane as well as to models which can be lifted from the data set. Details regarding the Visible Human Project and its applications to gastroenterology and endosonography have been previously described.

This atlas is fortunate to be able to use the interactive anatomy resources developed by Vic Spitzer, Karl Reinig, David Rubenstein, and others to create movies that help explain what takes place during endoscopic ultrasound (EUS) evaluations. Since EUS is a "real-time" examination, it seems reasonable to present this section primarily as "real-time" videos. The videos can be viewed over and over, allowing endosonographers to look not only at the highlighted structures, but also at structures they might visualize during EUS that are not specifically identified on the selected video.

This chapter uses the terms "radial array orientation" to describe planar anatomy which would be found perpendicular to a line going through the digestive tract (as would be generated by a radial array echoendoscope, Figure 1.1) and "linear array orientation" for planar anatomy generated parallel to a line going through the digestive tract (as would be generated by a linear array echoendoscope, Figure 1.2).

Normal EUS anatomy from the esophagus

Radial array orientation (Video 1.1)

Video 1.1 starts with Visible Human Models of the left atrium (purple), trachea and bronchi (light blue), aorta and pulmonary arteries (red), vena cava (dark blue), and the esophagus (brown). A plane is shown passing through the esophagus. This plane contains the transaxial cross-sectional anatomy images which then follow, starting in the oropharynx and going caudally. The upper esophageal sphincter (UES) is identified. As the images proceed distally, the trachea and esophagus can be followed to a point where the brachiocephalic left carotid and left subclavian arteries are evident just above the aortic arch. Below the aortic arch is the aortopulmonary window. The azygos arch can be seen exiting the superior vena cava (SVC). This occurs just above the tracheal bifurcation. The esophagus (labeled as "E") is surrounded by the descending aorta, the vertebrae, and the trachea. The thoracic duct (not labeled) is visible between the aorta and vertebrae, inferior to the esophagus. Going distally, the pulmonary artery becomes prominent. The region between the right mainstem bronchus (RMB) and left mainstem bronchus (LMB) is the subcarinal space. The video progresses to a level where the left atrium surrounds the superior aspect of the esophagus and then the video ends as the esophagus passes the gastroesophageal junction.

An image plane cross-section taken from a radial array orientation at the level of the subcarinal space is shown in Figure 1.3.

Linear array orientation (Video 1.2)

Video 1.2 starts with the same models as above (the left atrium [purple], trachea and bronchi [light blue], aorta and

Atlas of Endoscopic Ultrasonography, Second Edition. Edited by Frank Gress, Thomas Savides, Brenna Casey, and Everson L. A. Artifon.

Companion website: www.wiley.com/go/gress/atlas

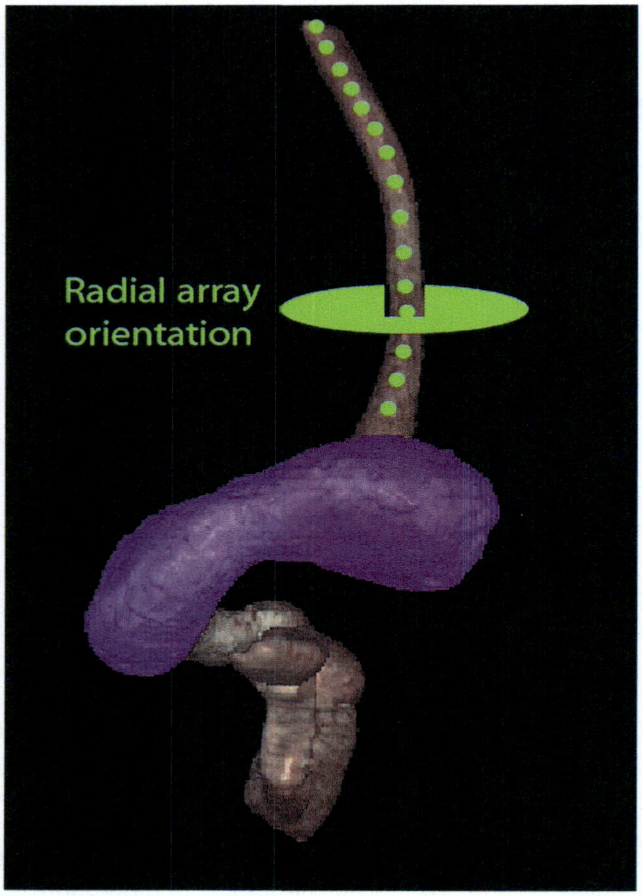

Figure 1.1 Visible Human Mocel of esophagus, stomach, and duodenum. The green circle shows a p ane perpendicular to the axis and is similar to a plane developed during radial array endosonography.

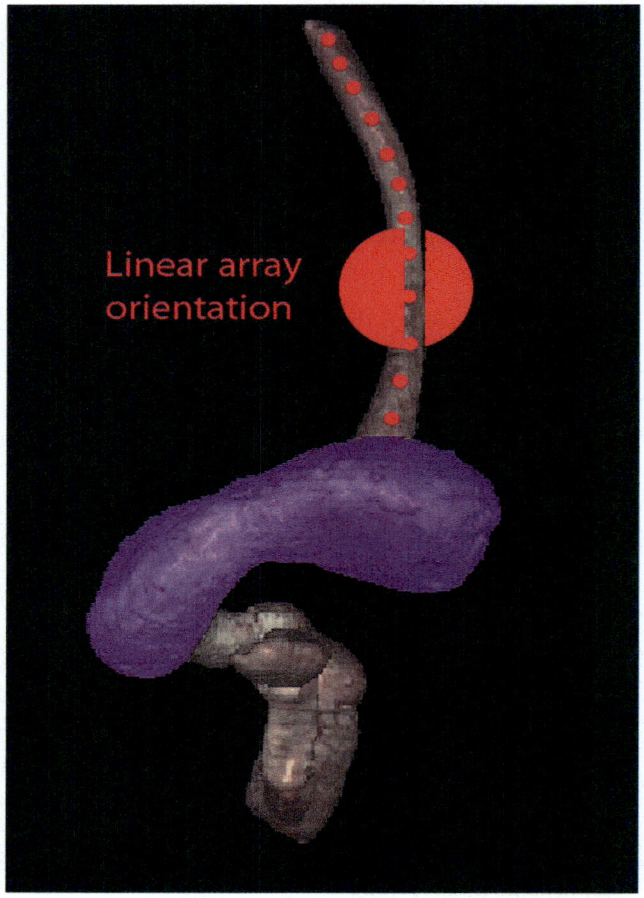

Figure 1.2 Visible Human Model of esophagus, stomach, and duodenum. The red circle shows a plane parallel to the axis and is similar to a plane developed during linear array endosonography.

pulmonary arteries [red], vena cava [dark blue], and the esophagus [brown]). The plane shows potential ways that cross-sectional anatomy can be generated. The video then shows a sagittal image with the descending aorta inferior to the esophagus, much as what is done during linear array EUS. In this orientation the pulmonary artery (PA) and left atrium are superior. The image plane is rotated to bring the left atrium and pulmonary artery to the inferior side of the esophagus. The models are then shown again, and the plane is moved in the caudal and cephalad directions, much as during EUS.

Normal EUS anatomy from the stomach

Radial array orientation (Video 1.3)

Endoscopic ultrasound of the stomach differs from EUS at other sites since the stomach does not constrain the endoscope tightly. It is important to follow anatomical structures (such as in a station apprcach) to avoid getting lost.

The video shows models of the stomach, esophagus, duodenum, gallbladder, pancreas (brown), the aorta, splenic

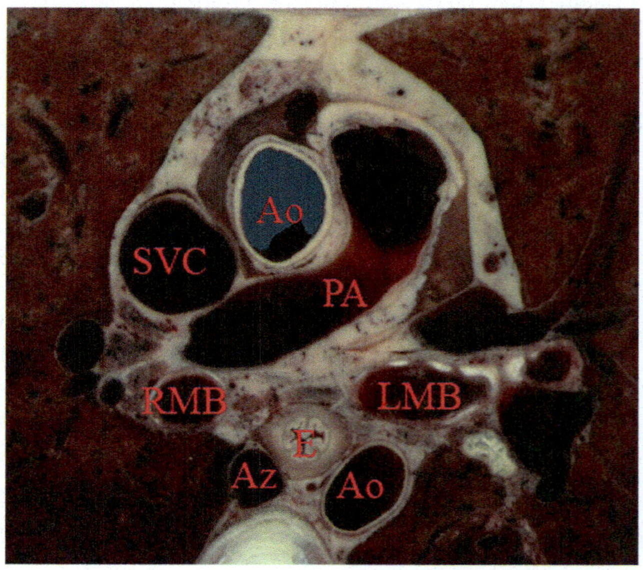

Figure 1.3 Transaxial cross-section of digital anatomy taken at the level of the subcarinal space. Ao, aorta (both ascending, superior in the image, and descending, inferior in the image, are shown); Az, azygos vein; PA, pulmonary artery; RMB and LMB, right and left mainstem bronchi; SVC, superior vena cava.

artery, hepatic artery and left gastric artery (red), adrenal glands (pink), and splenic, superior mesenteric veins (dark blue) as viewed from behind. A plane is passed that is similar to the image plane generated during radial array EUS. The resultant cross-sectional anatomy starts at the level of the gastroesophageal junction, with the aorta and inferior vena cava (IVC) labeled. The aorta (which is collapsed) is followed, which brings the pancreas and left adrenal gland into view. The first artery that comes off the aorta in the abdomen is the celiac artery. There is a trifurcation into the splenic, hepatic, and left gastric arteries (LGA), although the LGA is generally smaller and difficult to see. It is shown in the video at the "x" just before the bifurcation into the celiac and hepatic arteries as identified.

The superior mesenteric artery (SMA) comes off the aorta just distal to the celiac artery. Various endoscope maneuvers can be used to bring the portal confluence into view, and then the splenic vein can be used as a guide to visualize the pancreas body, left adrenal, kidney, and spleen. The diaphragm can be easily imaged between the kidney and the vertebrae.

Linear array orientation (Video 1.4)

The linear array exam also follows the aorta to the stomach, but, as shown Video 1.4, the image plane across the pancreas is generally obtained through a sweeping motion. The first major gastric landmark is the origin of the celiac artery and SMA from the aorta (Figure 1.4). The superior mesenteric vein (SMV), portal vein, and splenic vein can be used as guides to go back and forth across the pancreas and in the process, the left adrenal, kidney, and spleen can be seen. The splenic artery runs roughly parallel to the splenic vein, but is generally tortuous.

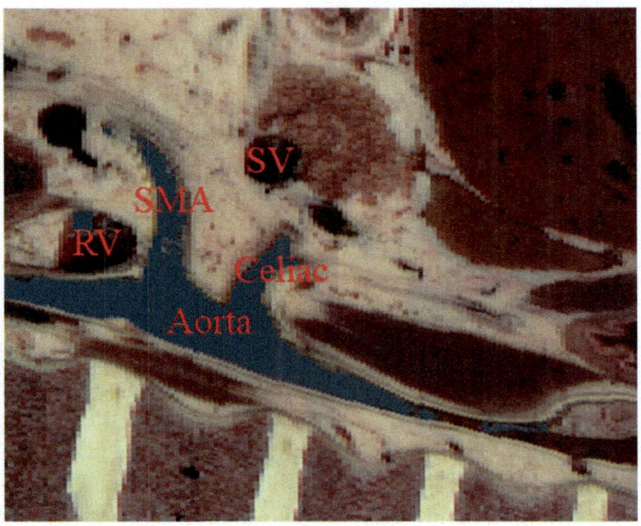

Figure 1.4 Sagittal cross-section of digital anatomy at the level of the gastroesophageal junction, similar to a view seen during linear array endoscopic ultrasound (EUS). The celiac and superior mesenteric arteries (SMA) are shown at their insertion into the aorta. The renal vein (RV) is shown adjacent to the SMA and the splenic vein is shown adjacent to the pancreas.

Normal EUS anatomy from the duodenum

Radial array orientation (Video 1.5)

The radial array EUS examination through the duodenum follows a constrained path, but the endoscope can be rotated to put various structures into the inferior aspect of the image plane, as shown in the models of the duodenum, pancreas (brown), portal and superior mesenteric veins (blue), aorta (red), and SMA (silver). There are many structures of interest in a rather small area, and most of the images obtained are from the posterior view, with the liver to the right and the pancreas to the left of the image screen. After leaving the pylorus, the pancreas can be oriented with the tail pointed either to the left or inferiorly, and the splenic vein runs in the same direction as the pancreas. Going through the duodenal bulb, the gastroduodenal artery (GDA) often appears. Without Doppler, the GDA can be confused with the common bile duct (CBD) since these structures are nearly parallel in orientation and are very close to each other. As the apex of the duodenal bulb is reached, the image plane captures a longitudinal view of the CBD and the portal vein. As the descending duodenum is reached, the bile duct is seen in cross-section and the IVC comes into view. As the third part of the duodenum is reached, the image plane rotates in such a way as to give a longitudinal cut through the IVC and then passes underneath the junction of the SMA with the aorta. Branches of the SMV can be found and the renal vein is visible in the "armpit" formed at the insertion of the SMA into the aorta. A special area is then highlighted in Video 1.5. Models show how the gastroduodenal artery and the hepatic artery (in red) relate to the CBD (in orange).

Figure 1.5 shows a model with an image plane and Figure 1.6 shows the resultant planar anatomy, which forms the stack sign – a phenomenon in which the portal vein, CBD, and main pancreatic duct are captured in the same field.

Linear array orientation (Video 1.6)

The linear array exam of the duodenum is an excellent way to see the CBD and pancreatic head. The anatomy is difficult to understand since the endoscope image is tipped into the C-sweep of the duodenum, and then the image plane is swept in various angles, resulting in a cross-sectioning of the CBD and pancreatic duct (PD). The image planes employed can be appreciated from observing the models in the video. The cross-sections obtained can be positioned to first give a longitudinal view of the CBD and both longitudinal views and cross-sections of the portal vein and SMV.

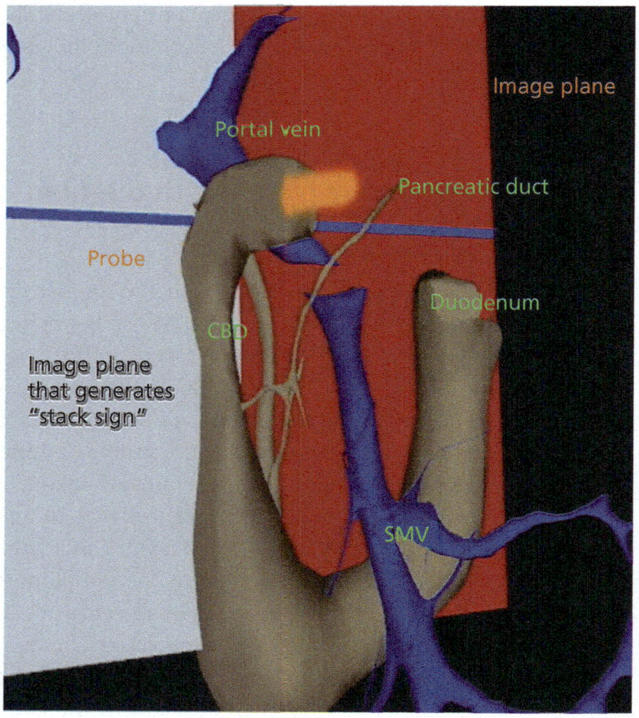

Figure 1.5 Visible Human Model of an image plane that is in the location in which radial array endoscopic ultrasound (EUS) generates the "stack sign", in which the portal vein, common bile duct (CBD), and pancreatic duct are in the same field. A probe in orange is shown going into the proximal duodenum. The superior mesenteric vein (SMV) is also shown.

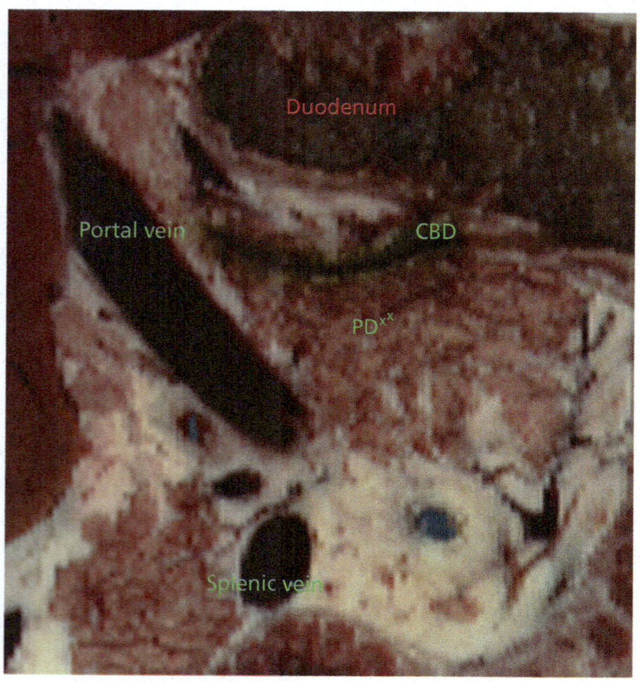

Figure 1.6 The cross-sectional anatomy within the plane shown in Figure 1.3. The common bile duct (CBD), pancreatic duct (PD), and portal vein are all in the same field ("stack sign").

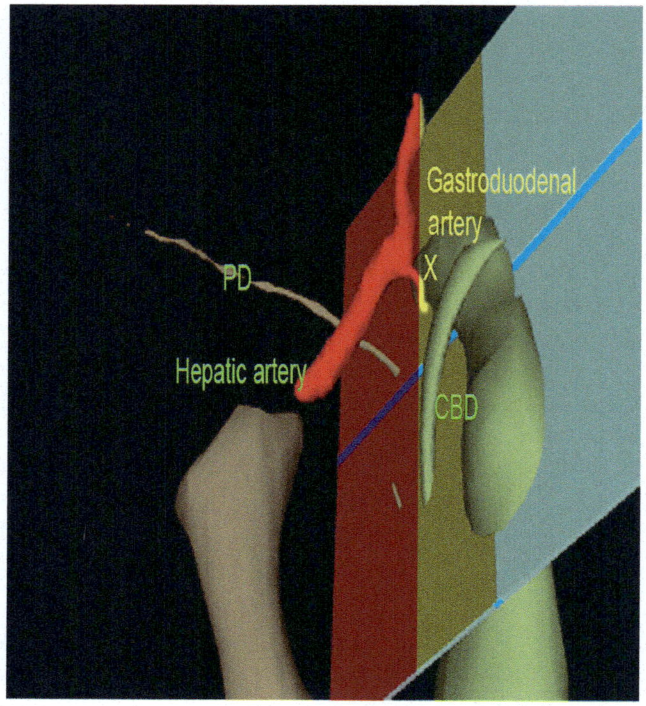

Figure 1.7 Visible Human Model with a plane that is in a location similar to what can be generated during linear array endoscopic ultrasound (EUS), showing the relative position of the gastroduodenal artery, pancreatic duct (PD), hepatic artery, and common bile duct (CBD).

As seen in the first part of Video 1.6, if the endoscope is in the second part of the duodenum, the bile duct goes to the ampulla away from the transducer and the liver is towards the transducer. If the endoscope is in the duodenal bulb, as shown in the second part of the video, the liver is away from the transducer.

The GDA drapes over the portal vein and can be found most readily using Doppler. Figure 1.7 shows a model and Figure 1.8 the resultant cross-section where the GDA can be found.

Normal EUS anatomy from the rectum

Radial array orientation, male (Video 1.7)

Video 1.7 shows models of various male pelvic structures, starting with the rectum and sigmoid colon, the aorta, and the iliac arteries with internal and external branches. The SMA is included to show the anterior direction of the models. The prostate, bladder, coccyx, and sacrum are added sequentially. A second set of models is then shown which contains the rectum, sigmoid colon, prostate, bladder, coccyx, sacrum, external iliac arteries (red), veins (blue), as well as three-dimensional models of the internal and external anal sphincters. The sphincters and sigmoid colon are then removed.

Planar anatomy in the radial array orientation from the male rectum is then shown, starting distally and moving proximally. The anal sphincters are labeled, followed by the

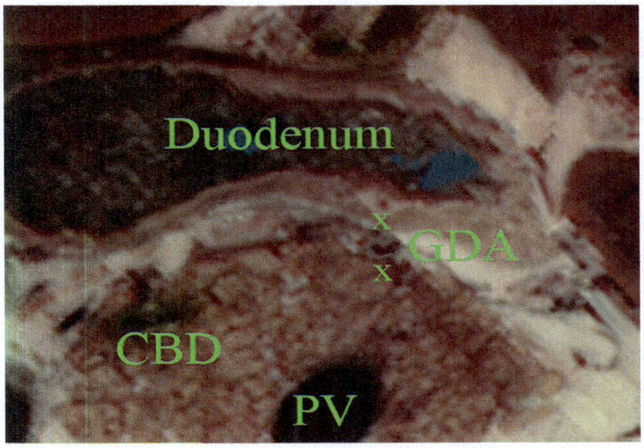

Figure 1.8 Cross-sectional anatomy generated within the plane shown in Figure 1.5. The gastroduodenal artery (GDA) and common bile duct (CBD) are shown with the pancreatic head. The portal vein (PV) is shown near the portal confluence.

prostate, urethra, levator ani, and coccyx. The sacrum and seminal vesicles are then shown, followed by the right internal iliac artery.

Radial array orientation, female (Video 1.8)

Video 1.8 starts distally at the end of the anal canal. The internal and external sphincters are shown, and residual stool is present in the rectum. Moving proximally, the vagina and urethra are shown, followed by the cervix and bladder.

Linear array orientation, male (Video 1.9)

Video 1.9 starts with a sagittal plane through the pelvis with the body facing the left. The prostate, rectum, anal canal, and bladder are identified. The plane is rotated, and the seminal vesicles and internal anal sphincter are labeled. The coccyx and sacrum are apparent at the start and end of the video but are unlabeled.

Linear array orientation, female (Video 1.10)

Video 1.10 starts with a sagittal plane through the pelvis with the body facing the left and slightly face down. The anal canal, rectum, uterus, and bladder are identified. Stool is present in the rectal vault. The plane is rotated, and towards the end of the video the internal anal sphincter (IS) and external anal sphincter (ES) are identified.

Vascular videos

Arterial (Video 1.11)

Video 1.11 shows models of some of the main arteries that are visualized during endosonography. A close-up view shows the celiac artery with its branches (hepatic, splenic, and left gastric arteries). The gastroduodenal and pancreaticoduodenal arteries are shown coming off the hepatic artery. The internal and external iliac arteries are then identified, followed by identification of the arteries associated with the aortic arch (left subclavian, left carotid, brachiocephalic) and the branches of the brachiocephalic (right subclavian and right carotid). Various organs are then placed in the model starting with the esophagus, then pancreas, stomach, and duodenum.

Venous (Video 1.12)

Some of the major veins visualized during endosonography are shown. At first, the vena cava and right atrium are identified, after which, the renal veins and azygos veins are added. The portal system with the portal vein, SMV, splenic vein, and inferior mesenteric vein (not labeled) are placed in blue. The systemic veins are then colored and removed. The pancreas is placed on the portal vein and its branches, showing how the head runs parallel to the SMV and the tail runs parallel to the splenic vein.

Endobronchial ultrasound anatomy (Video 1.13)

Extratracheal anatomy is similar to extraesophageal anatomy and many of the structures seen in the extratracheal spaces are the same as what is seen in the extraesophageal spaces. The endoluminal views of the trachea are oriented so that the membranous trachea is inferior and is splayed wider than the cartilaginous trachea at the level of the carina, putting the right mainstem bronchus (RMB) to the right and the left mainstem bronchus (LMB) to the left (Figure 1.9). As one goes right the bronchus immediately branches superiorly towards the right upper lobe (RUL), and continues straight as bronchus intermedius (BI) (Figure 1.10), which then branches towards the right middle lobe (RML) and right lower lobe (RLL) of the lung (Figure 1.11).

Going left from the carina, one goes down the relatively long left mainstem bronchus until it branches towards the left upper lobe (LUL) and left lower lobe (LLL) of the lung (Figure 1.12). An overview of the bronchial tree is shown in Figure 1.13.

Video 1.13 starts with the cervical trachea. All images are in a linear array orientation as endobronchial ultrasound (EBUS) is exclusively linear. The esophagus is inferior and the brachiocephalic artery and vein are superior. The video begins with rotation of the image plane. The superior part of the plane moves left and the inferior part moves right. This moves the esophagus out of view and brings the left subclavian artery and left carotid artery into the inferior part of the image. Eventually, the esophagus is seen in the superior part of the image and, with continued motion, the esophagus again appears inferior to the trachea. At this point, the image plane moves caudally to the carina. The right pulmonary artery, brachiocephalic artery (BA), and left brachiocephalic vein (LBV) are labeled. The plane is again rotated to splay the right (RMB) and left (LMB) mainstem bronchi apart. The plane is then moved to better visualize the right mainstem bronchus, showing the branch to the right upper lobe (RUL), the azygos arch (AzArch), the bronchus intermedius (BI).

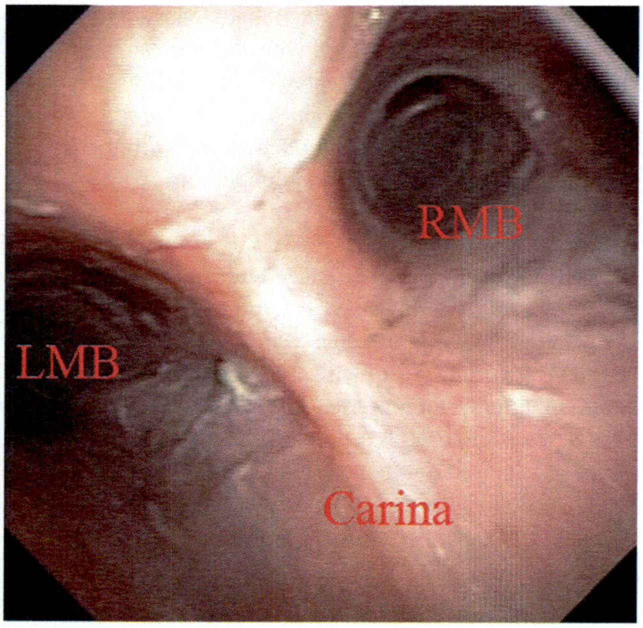

Figure 1.9 Endobronchial view of the carina, showing the right (RMB) and left (LMB) mainstem bronchi.

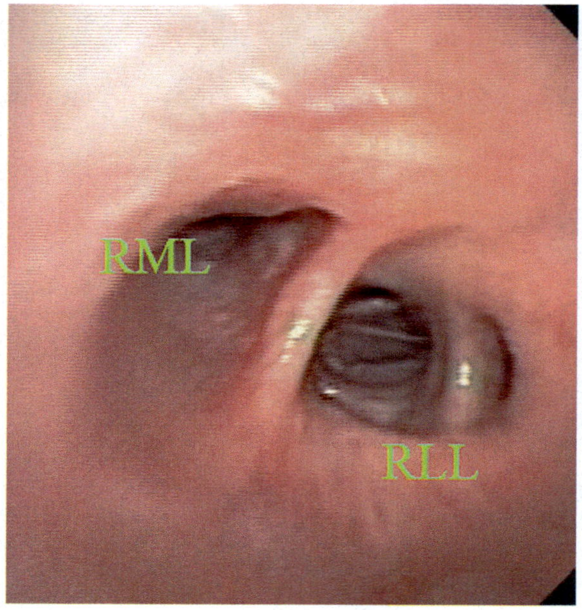

Figure 1.11 Endobronchial view of the bifurcation of the bronchus intermedius towards the right middle lobe (RML) and the right lower lobe (RLL).

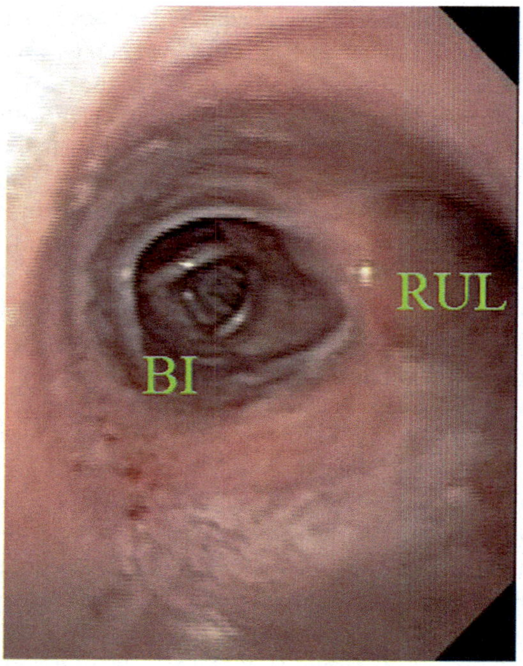

Figure 1.10 Endobronchial view of the first branch of the right mainstem bronchus towards the right upper lobe (RUL) and the bronchus intermedius (BI).

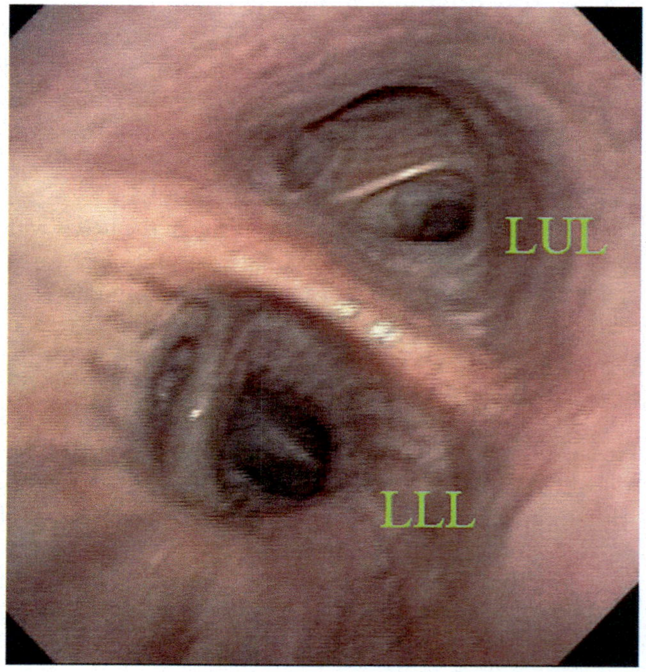

Figure 1.12 Endobronchial view of bifurcation of the left mainstem bronchus towards the left upper lobe (LUL) and left lower lobe (LLL).

This same plane shows the relation of the aortic arch (AoArch) and left pulmonary artery to the left mainstem bronchus (LMB). As the plane goes down the right mainstem bronchus/bronchus intermedius (RMB) towards its next bifurcation, the azygos arch (AzAr), right pulmonary artery (RPA), and right pulmonary vein (RPV) are shown.

The plane is brought back to the carina to visualize the left mainstem bronchus (LMB), and the azygos arch (AzAr), aortic arch (AoAr), left pulmonary artery (LPA), and vein (LPV) are identified. The branching to the left upper lobe (LUL) and left lower lobe (LLL) are shown, and the aorta (Ao) and left pulmonary artery are labeled.

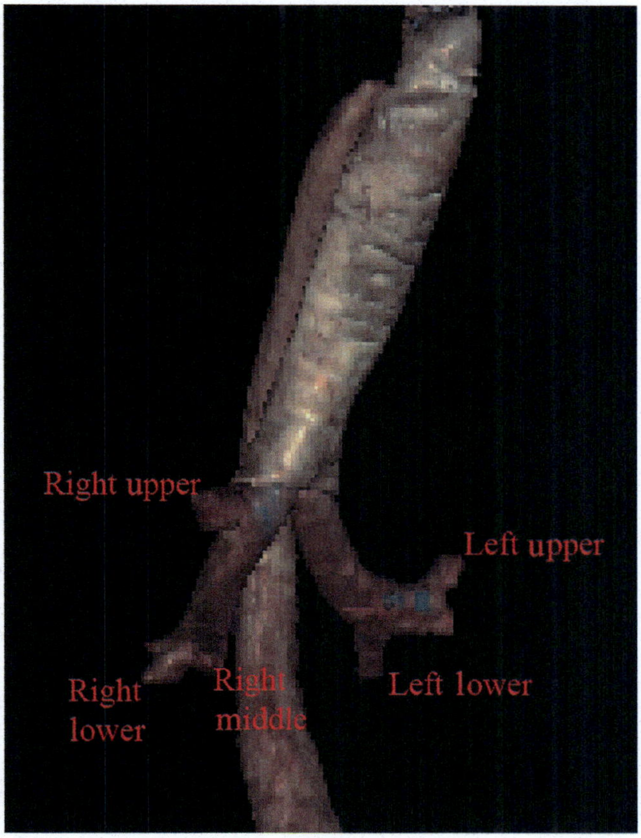

Figure 1.13 A Visible Human Model of the bronchial tree.

Chapter video clips

Video 1.1 Esophageal-related models and cross-sectional anatomy: radial orientation.

Video 1.2 Esophageal-related models and cross-sectional anatomy: linear orientation.

Video 1.3 Gastric-related models and cross-sectional anatomy: radial orientation.

Video 1.4 Gastric-related models and cross-sectional anatomy: linear orientation.

Video 1.5 Duodenal-related models and cross-sectional anatomy: radial orientation.

Video 1.6 Duodenal-related models and cross-sectional anatomy: linear orientation.

Video 1.7 Male rectum-related models and cross-sectional anatomy: radial orientation.

Video 1.8 Male rectum-related cross-sectional anatomy: linear orientation.

Video 1.9 Female rectum-related cross-sectional anatomy: radial orientation.

Video 1.10 Female rectum-related cross-sectional anatomy: linear orientation.

Video 1.11 Arterial models.

Video 1.12 Venous models.

Video 1.13 Bronchial anatomy in a linear orientation.

2 Esophagus: Radial and Linear

James L. Wise and John C. Deutsch
Essentia Health Care Systems, Duluth, MN, USA

Layers of the esophageal wall

Staging the depth of involvement of tumors and the layer of origin of subepithelial masses is an important component of competency in endoscopic ultrasonography (EUS). An intimate knowledge of the normal layers of the esophageal wall is critical for this to be done accurately. The wall of the esophagus has four readily appreciable layers by EUS using standard operating frequencies (5–12 MHz). The layers are seen in concentric, alternating rings of hyperechoic and hypoechoic structures emanating out distally from the tip of the endoscope. Starting with the layers closest to the scope tip, they are as follows:

- Interface echo between the superficial mucosa and water (hyperechoic).
- Deep mucosa (hypoechoic).
- Submucosa plus the acoustic interface between the submucosa and muscularis propria (hyperechoic).
- Muscularis propria minus the acoustic interface between the submucosa and muscularis propria (hypoechoic).

If a higher resolution frequency probe is used, greater number of layers could be visualized as detailed in Chapter 4. The esophagus lacks an obvious fifth layer as there is no serosa.

In our opinion, visualization and discernment of the layers of the esophageal wall is usually best accomplished using radial compared to linear instruments.

Figure 2.1 shows the esophageal walls using radial and linear instruments. To help separate the layers, these images include a muscularis mucosae leiomyoma that was subsequently resected. Images show subepithelial hypoechoic lesion in echolayer II as well as in the other defined layers of the esophageal wall.

Normal radial extraesophageal anatomy

(Video 2.1)

Standard examination of the esophagus and mediastinum begins with advancing the radial instrument to the gastroesophageal (GE) junction at or near the squamocolumnar junction. At this level the aorta is seen as an anechoic circular structure in the 5 o'clock position. The descending aorta is kept in this position as all radial mediastinal imaging will then correlate quite nicely with cross-sectional imaging. Other structures visible at the level of the GE junction are the inferior vena cava (IVC) seen between 7 and 9 o'clock and the liver between 6 o'clock and 12 o'clock surrounding the IVC (Figure 2.2).

As the scope is withdrawn, the vena cava moves clockwise and superiorly into the right atrium. The spine soon comes into view adjacent to the descending aorta at 6 o'clock.

Further withdrawal upward to usually around 30–35 cm reveals the anechoic chamber of the left atrium in the 12 o'clock position (Figure 2.3). With this field, relatively slight movement of the scope will reveal the mitral valve (Figure 2.4), aortic root, and the aortic valve (Figure 2.5). In the inferior portion of the field the descending aorta, the spine, the thoracic duct, and a relatively prominent azygos vein can be seen.

As the scope is withdrawn the bronchi come together at the carina. At or just proximal to this level the azygos arch (Figure 2.6) can be identified traveling superiorly and laterally into the superior vena cava. This is also the area of the aortopulmonary (AP) window at approximately 2 o'clock.

The endoscope can be pushed down from here or pulled up slightly from the position of the left atrium to reach the subcarinal space. Of interest in the subcarinal space are the right and left mainstem bronchi seen emanating out as ribbed-like

Atlas of Endoscopic Ultrasonography, Second Edition. Edited by Frank Gress, Thomas Savides, Brenna Casey, and Everson L. A. Artifon.

Companion website: www.wiley.com/go/gress/atlas

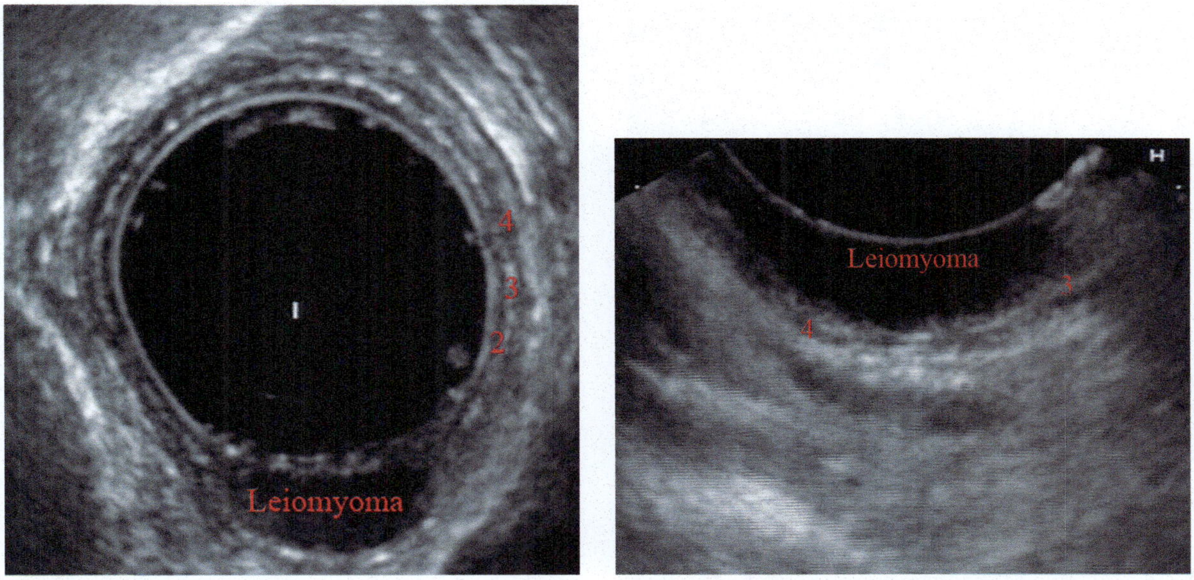

(a) (b)

Figure 2.1 (a) Radial array image of esophageal wall with small echolayer II leiomyoma. (b) Linear array image of esophageal wall with small echolayer II leiomyoma.

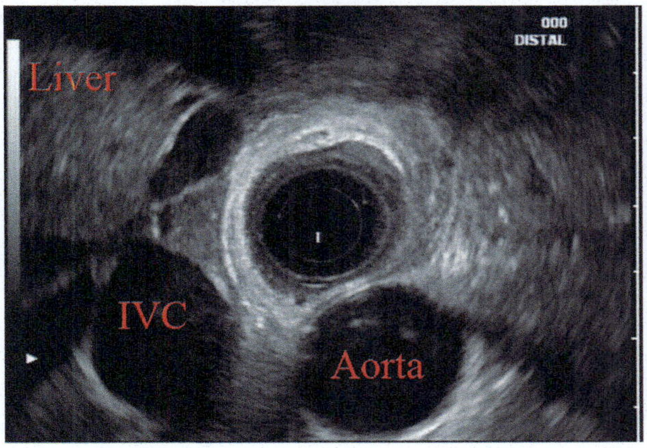

Figure 2.2 Radial array image at gastroesophageal (GE) junction. IVC, inferior vena cava.

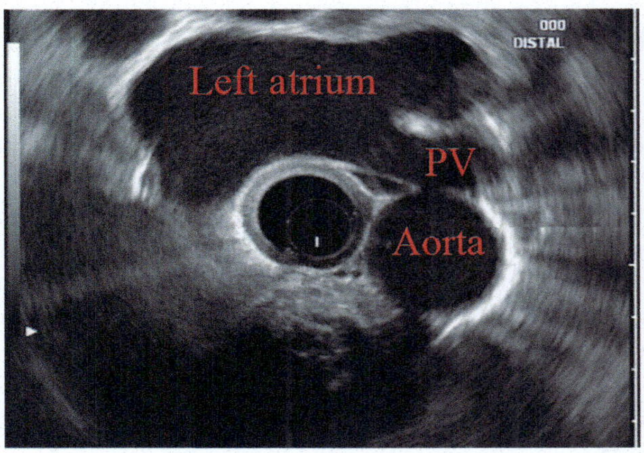

Figure 2.3 Radial array image at the level of the left atrium. PV, pulmonary vein.

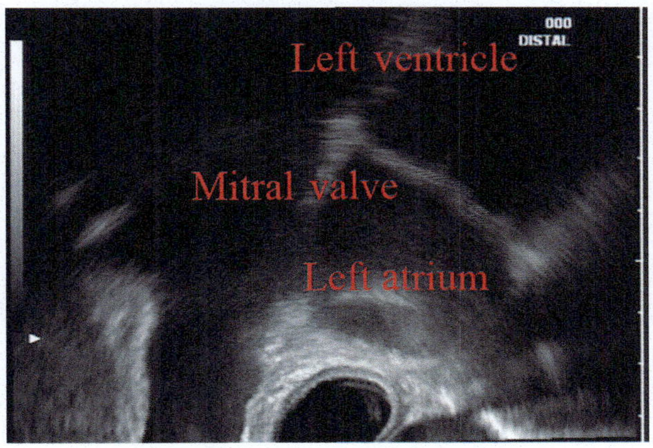

Figure 2.4 Radial array image at the level of the mitral valve.

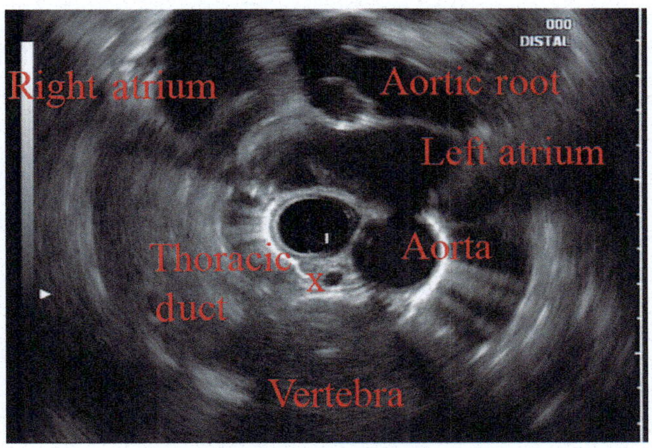

Figure 2.5 Radial array image at the level of the aortic root.

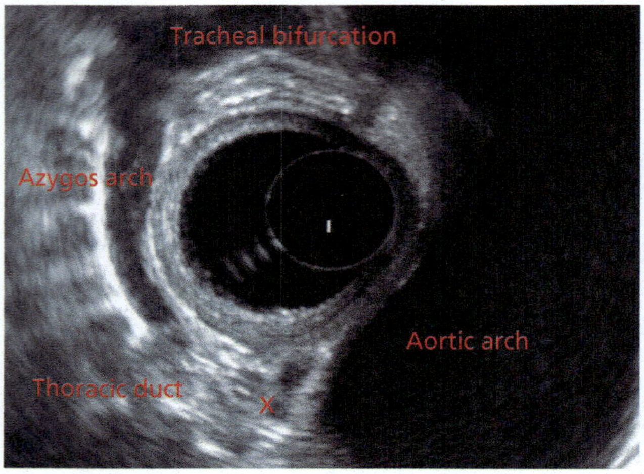

Figure 2.6 Radial array image at the level of the azygos arch.

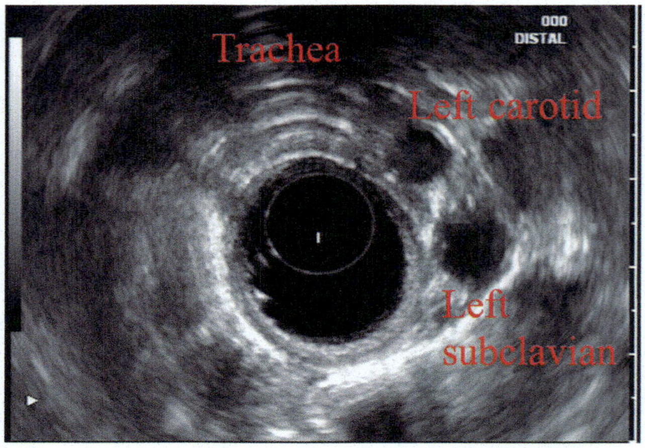

Figure 2.8 Radial array image at the level of the left carotid and subclavian arteries.

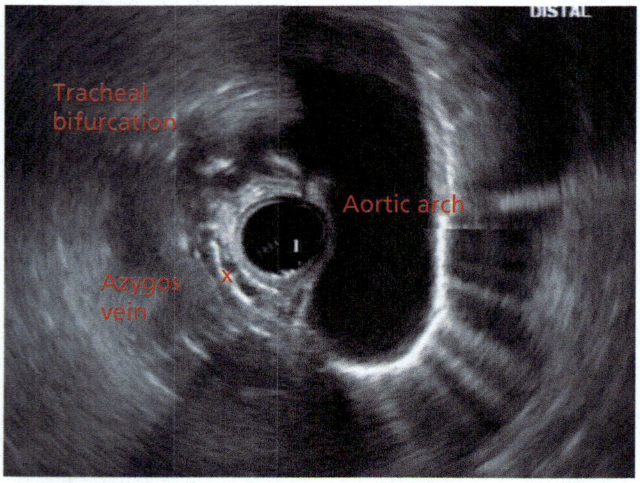

Figure 2.7 Radial array image at the mid aortic arch.

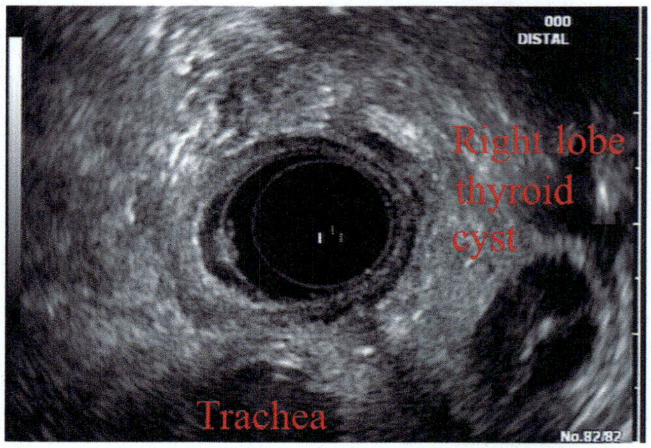

Figure 2.9 Radial array image at the level of the thyroid.

air-filled structures. As many have suggested, these can be imagined to have the appearance of two headlights.

More proximally from the area at the AP window the aorta elongates and forms the aortic arch (Figure 2.7). This usually creates a semicircle on the entire right side of the image correlating to the left-sided arch. However, with usual orientation the aorta should not cross the midline. The left carotid and left subclavian artery can easily be seen to leave the aortic arch as small round structures on the right side of the image (Figure 2.8). The brachiocephalic artery can sometimes be seen as well superior to the carotid on the right. As the scope is withdrawn the thyroid comes into view. For example, on the right of Figure 2.9 a prominent thyroid can be seen with a cystic structure within it.

Normal linear thoracic anatomy

The linear scope is advanced to the GE junction by following the descending aorta from the level of the arch downward (Figure 2.10). In order to follow this path, the scope is usually torqued clockwise 90–180 degrees and, as the aorta is followed down, the scope is gently rotated counterclockwise to stay on the aorta. As seen in Video 2.2, the thyroid is visualized briefly and the scope is then advanced to the level of the GE junction.

The origin of the celiac artery (Figure 2.11) is identified and then the scope can be withdrawn. This is the standard reference point for the beginning of the exam during withdrawal. Examination of the extraesophageal and thoracic structures is more time consuming than the radial approach as this echoendoscope's narrow focal point has to be torqued back a further 180 degrees to cover the same field of examination. This is done by withdrawing the scope at increments with constant back and forth torque.

As the scope is withdrawn 3–5 cm back from the GE junction, the scope will need to be rotated 180 degrees off the aorta to see the left atrium and cardiac structures. The cardiac structure can be discerned quite readily using the linear scope. The mitral valve is just adjacent to the aortic root,

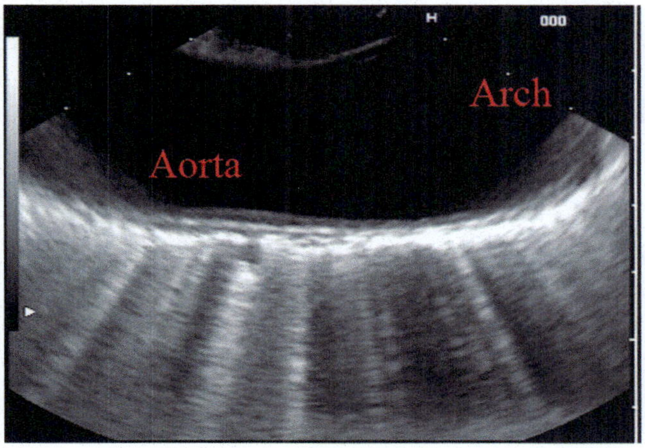

Figure 2.10 Linear array image at the mid aorta.

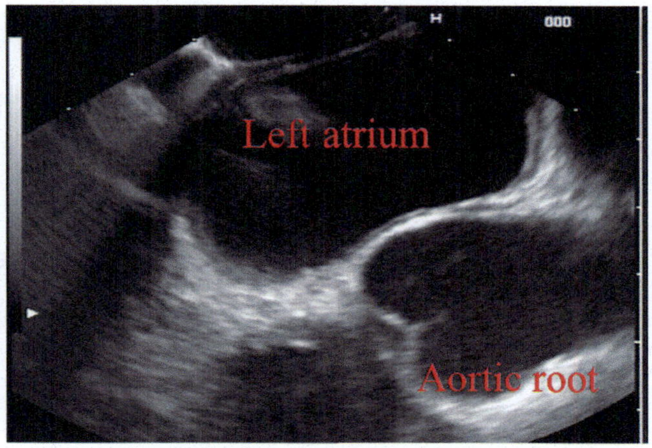

Figure 2.12 Linear array image at the aortic root.

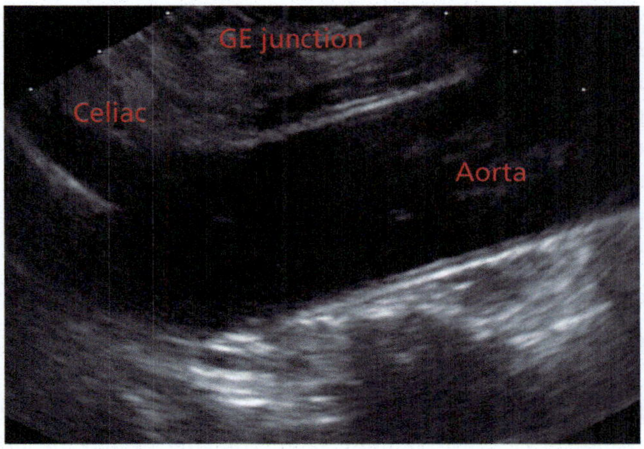

Figure 2.11 Linear array image at the level of the celiac artery.

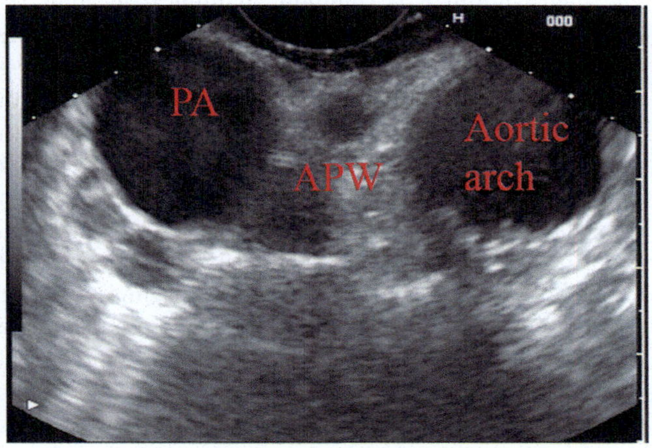

Figure 2.13 Linear array image at the aortopulmonary window (APW). PA, pulmonary artery.

which is just at clockwise rotation from the mitral valve. The aortic valve can be visualized at various angles with appropriate endoscopic manipulation given its position relative to the esophagus (Figure 2.12).

Withdrawing from the level of the left atrium by 1–2 cm reveals the subcarinal space. This is the area between the pulmonary artery and the left atrium. The bifurcation of the trachea by definition occurs at this level as well.

The AP window is just proximal to this area by several centimeters' orientation and is slightly clockwise torque from the subcarinal space. The space between the aortic arch and the pulmonary artery make up this region. This is below the level of the aortic arch by a few centimeters. There is a small node seen on the image which could be readily sampled via endoscopic ultrasound-guided fine needle aspiration (EUS-FNA) (Figure 2.13).

The azygos arch is also visualized around this area, just at or slightly below the aortic arch. The azygos vein can be followed distally along the spine, as in the accompanying Video 2.2. Occasionally intercostal veins are visible.

Chapter video clips

Video 2.1 Radial array examination of the extraesophageal spaces.

Video 2.2 Linear array examination of the extraesophageal spaces.

3 Normal Mediastinal Anatomy by EUS and EBUS

Juan Corral[1], Sebastian Fernandez-Bussy[2], and Michael B. Wallace[1]

[1] Division of Gastroenterology and Hepatology, Mayo Clinic College of Medicine, Jacksonville, FL, USA

[2] Division of Pulmonary Medicine and Critical Care, Mayo Clinic College of Medicine, Jacksonville, FL, USA

Introduction

The mediastinum is a common anatomical location for lymph node (LN) metastases in lung cancer as well as many other malignant and inflammatory conditions. The presence and specific location of mediastinal LN metastases in non-small cell lung cancer (NSCLC) dictates therapy with surgery for localized disease, combination therapy when contralateral LNs are involved, and palliative therapy when contralateral LNs and metastases are encountered. Unfortunately, cross-sectional imaging with computed tomography (CT), magnetic resonance imaging (MRI), or positron emission tomography (PET) alone is not adequate to confirm a diagnosis; thus, a tissue sample is preferred. Recently, it has been suggested that the use of endoscopic ultrasound-guided fine needle aspiration (EUS-FNA) associated with endobronchial ultrasound-guided transbronchial fine needle aspiration (EBUS-TBNA) can adequately sample LNs in the mediastinum, avoiding the need for a futile surgery.

The purpose of this chapter is to provide the basic anatomical information as well as technical maneuvers used to investigate the mediastinum successfully.

Anatomical definitions

The LNs in the mediastinum were classified in different stations based on surgical and anatomical landmarks for the purpose of staging lung cancer but this schema is now widely used in other chest diseases (Figure 3.1). The LNs with their respective stations and corresponding anatomical locations are described in Table 3.1.

EUS-FNA is usually best suited to sample LNs adjacent to the esophagus which runs posterior to the trachea. Because of ultrasound artifacts created by the air-filled trachea, lesions immediately anterior to the trachea are not well seen. EUS-accessible stations include 2L, 2R, 4L, 4R, 5, 7, 8, 9, and, sometimes depending on the size, station 6. On the other hand, EBUS-TBNA can target LNs either anterior or lateral to the trachea to the level of the carina, and alongside the left and right bronchial tree including stations 2L, 2R, 4L, 4R, 7, 10, and 11. Although both procedures overlap in stations 2 L/R, 4 L/R, and 7, in other stations they are complementary, and in combination allow nearly complete mediastinal access.

Equipment

Radial and curvilinear array echoendoscopes are available (Figure 3.2), with scanning radius ranging from 270–360 degrees for radial to 100–180 degrees for the linear echoendoscope. These scopes have standard accessory channels (2.0–2.8 mm) and larger accessory channels (3.7 mm) capable of delivering needles and other therapeutic devices such as a 10 French (Fr) plastic stent.

EUS can use several types of needles: 19 gauge (G), 22 G, and 25 G for FNA, as well as Tru-cut needles for core biopsy. The needle is occluded with a stylet during passage through the gastrointestinal tract wall and bronchial wall to minimize contamination from passage through those structures.

EBUS equipment comprises a curvilinear array echoendoscope with an outer diameter of 6.7 mm and a biopsy channel of 2 mm. The ultrasonic frequency is 7.5 MHz with a penetration depth of 4–5 cm, making it well suited for FNA of LNs and lung masses through the trachea and bronchi. A 22 G needle is used to perform TBNA in the same manner as in EUS. Both systems have integrated oblique-viewing optics to guide intubation and limited inspection.

Atlas of Endoscopic Ultrasonography, Second Edition. Edited by Frank Gress, Thomas Savides, Brenna Casey, and Everson L. A. Artifon.

Companion website: www.wiley.com/go/gress/atlas

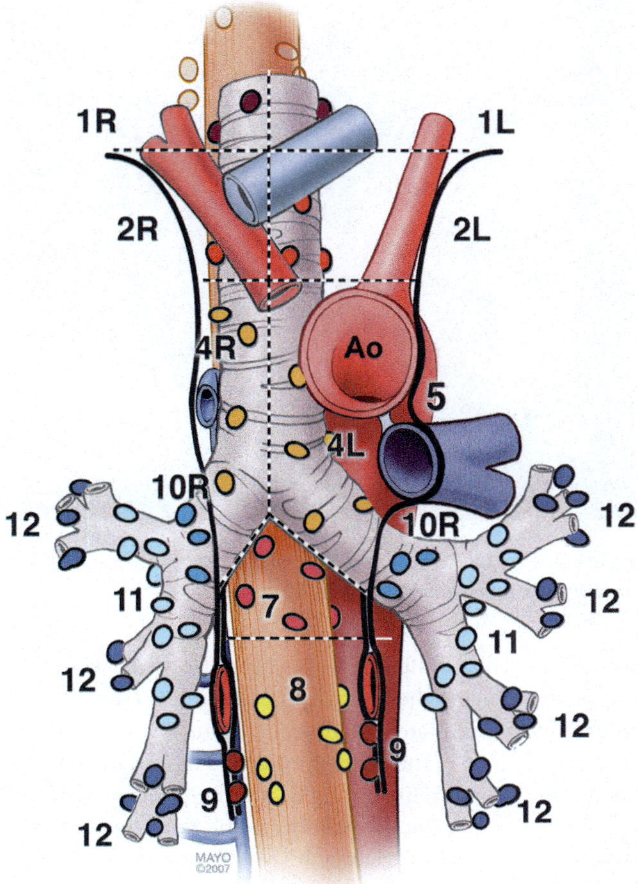

Figure 3.1 Mediastinal lymph node stations.

Table 3.1 Mediastinal lymph node stations with their anatomical correlations.

Level	Anatomical correlation
Superior mediastinal lymph nodes	
1	Highest mediastinal
2	Upper paratracheal
3	Prevascular and retrotracheal
4	Lower paratracheal (including azygos nodes)
Aortic lymph nodes	
5	Aortopulmonary (AP) window or subaortic
6	Para-aortic (ascending aorta and phrenic)
Inferior mediastinal lymph nodes	
7	Subcarinal
8	Paraesophageal (below carina)
9	Pulmonary ligament
N1 lymph nodes	
10	Hilar
11	Interlobar
12	Lobar
13	Segmental
14	Subsegmental

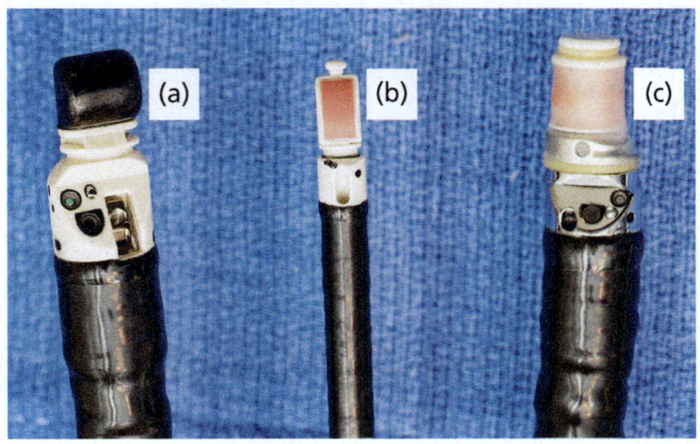

Figure 3.2 Types of echoendoscopes: (a) linear probe; (b) endobronchial probe; (c) radial probe.

Endoscopic ultrasound technique

The initial examination can be performed with either the radial or linear array echoendoscope; however, the linear scope is required to perform FNA. Given the obvious efficiencies, we prefer to use a single linear echoendoscope for both imaging and FNA.

Linear scanning

The balloon should be deflated or inflated only slightly to provide good acoustic coupling with the tissue. The mediastinum is imaged by first finding the descending aorta starting at the cardia. The examination can be performed by rotating 360 degrees from the cardia, then withdrawing the shaft 4–5 cm and performing another rotation. Alternatively, one can survey from the cardia to the cervix, then rotating 90 degrees and repeating the maneuver until the whole mediastinum is examined. It is useful to use the following five stations as described by Deprez (Videos 3.1.1–3.1.3). For radial examination, see Video 3.2.

Inferior posterior mediastinum

The descending aorta is a large echo-poor longitudinal structure on linear array with a bright deep wall due to the air interface with the left lung. Clockwise rotation will sequentially image left lung, left pleura, left atrium, right lung, right pleura, azygos vein, and spine. The azygos vein can be localized by rotating approximately 30 degrees counterclockwise from the descending aorta. It is a thin echo-poor structure that can be followed proximally to its union with the superior vena cava. This is the area of LN stations 8 and 9 (Figure 3.3).

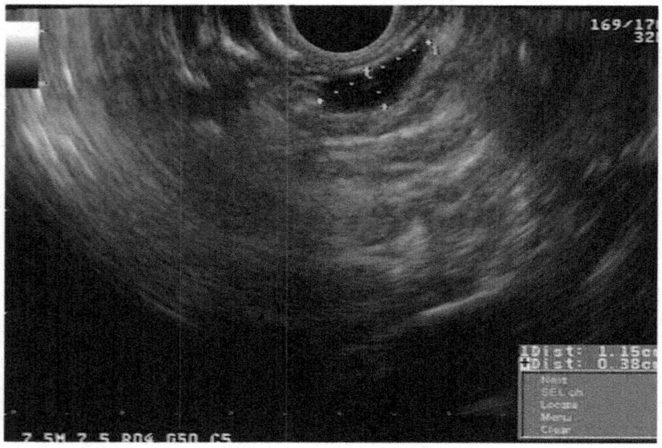

Figure 3.3 Lymph node at station 8 (between calipers).

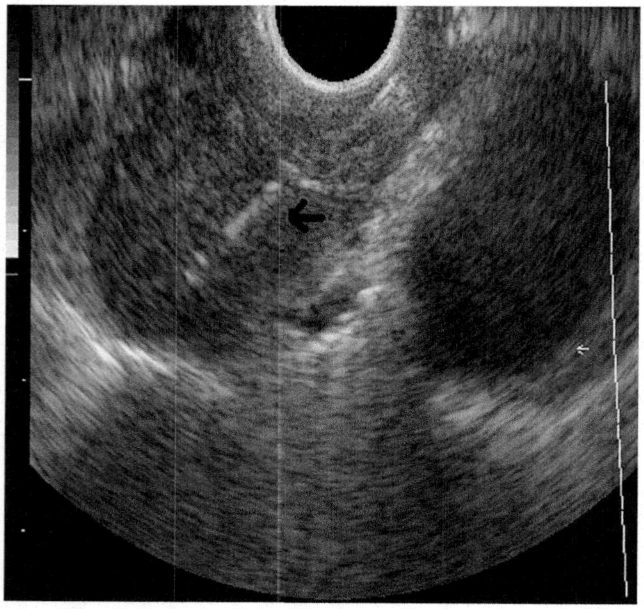

Figure 3.4 Subcarinal station (station 7).

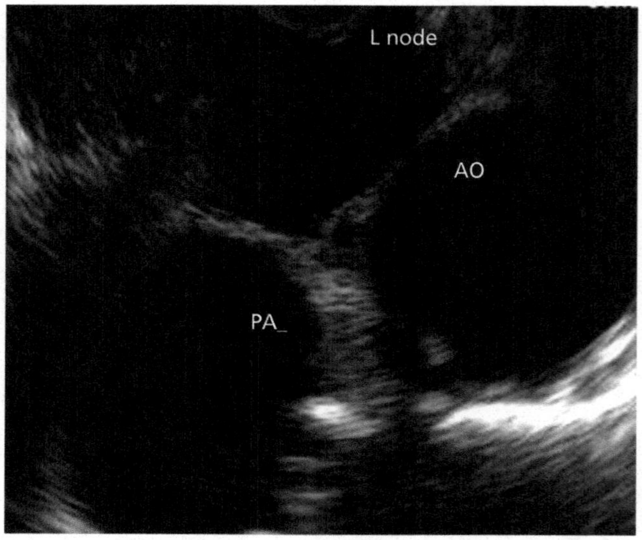

Figure 3.5 Aortopulmonary window station (stations 4L, 5 and 6). AO, aorta; L node; lymph node; PA, pulmonary artery.

Subcarinal area

At approximately 30 cm the subcarinal area is easily recognized by finding the left atrium, a large hypoechoic structure with cardiac motion, and pulling back until it disappears on the left edge of the screen. Then one should have the pulmonary artery in the right portion of the screen (Figure 3.4). Slight movements to the right and left have to be performed to completely interrogate this station. This is the area of LN station 7 (Videos 3.3 and 3.4).

Aortic arch area

The azygos arch is located at 24–25 cm from the incisors. The aortopulmonary (AP) window (station 5) is situated between the aortic arch and the pulmonary artery. The AP window is found by following the aorta cephalad until its arch, rotating clockwise approximately 90 degrees, then advancing 1–2 cm with slight tip up of the echoendoscope. The aorta will be the echo-poor structure on the right and the pulmonary artery will be to the left; the AP window is the space between the two just outside the AP ligament (which is not seen by EUS). The 4L region is immediately medial (close to the esophagus and EUS scope) to the AP window (Figure 3.5). Alternatively, from the subcarinal area, rotating 90 degrees counterclockwise, crossing the left main bronchus and pulling it back 2–3 cm will put you in the same location. Further withdrawal of the echoendoscope with slight rotation will show the origin of the left subclavian artery. Occasionally, the left carotid artery can be seen above the brachiocephalic (innominate) vein.

Cervical area

Between 22 and 24 cm from the incisors, the superior part of the lungs can be imaged along with the trachea, cricoid bone, jugular veins, and carotid arteries.

Thyroid gland

At 17–20 cm from the incisors, the inferior thyroid gland can be imaged as well as cervical LNs, which can be targeted for FNA.

Radial scanning

For radial scanning, one should enter the stomach, inflate the balloon, and pull back the scope until the GE junction. The aorta with be visualized as a large round echo-poor structure. The aorta should be rotated to the 5 o'clock position, and the spine will be at 7 o'clock with the azygos vein in the middle. Then the balloon should be deflated and a slow pull-back is performed observing all the mediastinal areas. It is important to note that, for a complete lung cancer staging with both radial and linear, the celiac axis, the left adrenal, and the left lobe of the liver should be surveyed. This is easily accomplished with a slight tip down on the echoendoscope and and then pushing it into the stomach; the celiac take-off can be seen and the left adrenal can be seen at the 6 to 4 o'clock position with its usual "seagull" appearance. For the liver, one goes to the gastric antrum, aspirates all the air, inflating the balloon, and then tip up with a slow pull-back.

Endobronchial ultrasound

Just like EUS, EBUS can be performed with conscious sedation, deep sedation, or general anesthesia. The tip of the scope is placed under direct visual contact in different positions, starting from the segmental bronchi to the trachea usually scanning 90–120 degrees every 0.5–1 cm. The diameter of the EBUS scope (6–7 mm) precludes passage beyond the second or third airway generation. EBUS-TBNA is performed under the same principles as EUS-FNA. As mentioned before, this technique is particularly useful for LN stations 2, 4, 7, 10, and 11 (Figure 3.6). The upper and middle third of the esophagus can be visualized from the upper and lower trachea respectively Currently, we have different sizes of needle available, including 19, 21, 22, and 25 G.

EBUS anatomical landmarks

It is important to note that all right tracheal lymph node stations are found from the left lateral border of the trachea to the right aspect of the trachea.

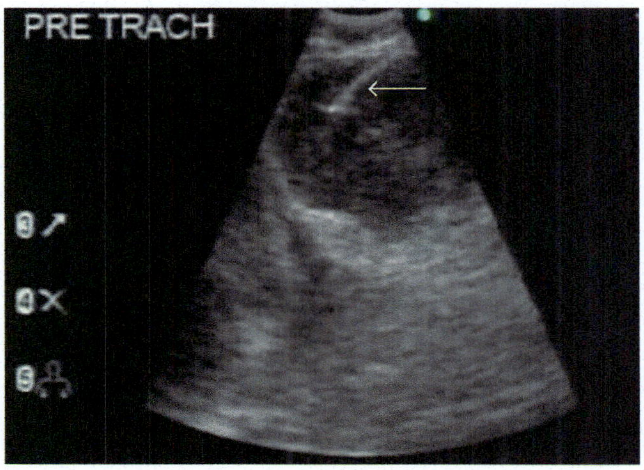

Figure 3.6 Endobronchial ultrasound (EBUS) images of common mediastinal stations (4L, 7 and 11L). The esophagus and vertebral bodies can be visualized posteriorly from the upper and lower trachea.

- Right upper paratracheal nodes (station 2R): the upper border is the apex of the right lung, the lower border is the intersection of the innominate vein with the trachea. This station is usually found facing the scope to the right lateral wall of the trachea, at 3 o'clock, at the level of the fifth tracheal cartilage.
- Left upper paratracheal nodes (station 2L): the upper border is the apex of the left lung, the lower border is the superior limit of the aortic arch. This station is usually found facing the scope to the left lateral wall of the trachea, at 9 o'clock, at the level of the fifth tracheal cartilage.
- Right lower paratracheal nodes (station 4R): the upper border is the innominate vein, the lower border is the azygos vein. This station is usually found just proximal to the main carina, between 12 and 3 o'clock.
- Left lower paratracheal nodes (station 4L): the upper border is the superior limit of the aortic arch, the lower border is superior limit of the left pulmonary artery. This station is usually found at the level of the main carina, left lateral wall of the trachea, at 9 o 'clock. The view of the AP window is very similar to that seen by the EUS scope with the aortic arch on the right and pulmonary artery on the left.
- Subcarinal nodes (station 7): the upper border is the main carina, the inferior border is the superior limit of the left lower lobe take-off on the left side, and the inferior limit of the bronchus intermedius on the right side. This station is found at the medial wall of the left mainstem bronchus or the medial wall of the right mainstem bronchus and bronchus intermedius.
- Right hilar nodes (station 10R): the upper boder is the azygos vein, the lower border is the interlobar region. This station is usually found just proximal to the right upper lobe take-off, facing to the anterior and lateral airway wall.
- Left hilar nodes (station 10L): the upper border is the pulmonary artery, the lower border is the interlobar region. EBUS scope should be faced just proximal to the left upper lobe, at 11 o'clock.
- Right interlobar superior nodes (station 11Rs): the upper limit is the right upper lobe bronchus, the lower limit is the distal bronchus intermedius. This station should be found at the lateral wall of the airway, between 2 and 4 o'clock.
- Right interlobar inferior nodes (11Ri): lymph nodes are between the right middle lobe and the right lower lobe. EBUS scope should be placed just proximal to the right lower lobe bronchus, facing laterally.
- Left interlobar nodes (station 11L): the upper limit is the left upper lobe bronchus, the lower limit is the left lower lobe bronchus. Place EBUS scope at the left lower lobe take-off, facing anterior and lateral.
- Right/left lobar nodes (station 12R/L): any lymph nodes adjacent to the lobar bronchi.

Complications and safety

EUS-FNA and EBUS-TBNA are highly safe procedures in experienced hands, with a complication rate of 0.8%. A major safety precaution with FNA is to visualize the entire length of the needle and to use color Doppler to avoid any blood vessels in the needle path.

Conclusions

EUS-FNA and EBUS-TBNA are complementary procedures with a high degree of sensitivity and specificity for diagnosing and staging benign and malignant diseases of the chest. Careful attention to technique must be applied to prevent the omission of important clinical information.

Chapter video clips

Video 3.1.1 Normal mediastinal anatomy by linear EUS: vascular anatomy. Source: Hitachi.

Video 3.1.2 Normal mediastinal anatomy by linear EUS: right and left atrium and AP window. Source: Aloka.

Video 3.1.3 Normal mediastinal anatomy by linear EUS: aorta, heart and great vessels. Source: Hitachi.

Video 3.2 Normal mediastinal anatomy by radial EUS.

Video 3.3 Paratracheal and subcarinal lymph node evaluation by EBUS. Source: Hitachi.

Video 3.4 Subcarinal lymph node (station 7) as seen by EBUS with performance of FNA.

4 Stomach: Radial and Linear

Joo Ha Hwang
Stanford University, Palo Alto, CA, USA

Endoscopic ultrasound (EUS) examination of the stomach is often performed to evaluate subepithelial lesions, staging of mucosa-associated lymphoid tumor (MALT) lymphomas, staging of gastric cancer, and evaluation of thickened gastric folds. Examination can be performed using mechanically scanning or electronic array echoendoscopes, or with ultrasound catheter probes.

The basic technique for performing EUS imaging of the gastric wall initially requires clearing the gastric lumen of any mucus or debris. The lumen should be thoroughly irrigated with water and suctioned. If there are excessive amounts of bubbles in the gastric lumen, a small amount of simethicone can be added to the irrigating water and suctioned. Once the gastric lumen has been cleared the gastric lumen should be decompressed and then filled with clean water. Ideally, degassed water should be used to fill the gastric lumen; however, this is often not available and clean water typically is sufficient. However, efforts should be made to minimize the presence of bubbles within the water as this will degrade the image quality. It is important to make sure that all air is aspirated from areas where imaging is to be performed. When filling the gastric lumen with the patient on their left side, the fundus and body will fill preferentially due to gravity. If the area of interest is in the antral wall, positioning the patient on their right side may be necessary to safely fill the gastric lumen with water for imaging. Filling of the gastric lumen with water places the patient at risk of aspiration; therefore, precautions should be taken to protect against an aspiration event.

After aspirating the air out of the lumen and distending the gastric lumen with water, the gastric wall can be surveyed with a radial scanning echoendoscope by starting the exam with the ultrasound probe in the antrum and slowly withdrawing the probe (Figure 4.1). If only a focal area needs to be examined, the use of a water-filled balloon can be used, especially for evaluating non-mucosal lesions such as subepithelial tumors. However, the use of a water-filled balloon creates an additional interface echo that impacts the image quality at the balloon–mucosa interface. Therefore, a water-filled balloon should not be used to provide acoustic coupling to mucosal lesions.

It is also important to perform imaging within the focal region of the transducer. The mechanical radial scanning echoendoscopes and catheter probes have a fixed natural focus where the best image resolution is obtained. The focal distance can easily be determined by adjusting the distance of the transducer from the gastric wall. The best resolution will be seen when the area of interest is at the focus of the imaging transducer. Electronic array echoendoscopes (radial and curvilinear) have the ability to electronically adjust the location of the focal region; therefore, when imaging the gastric wall, the focal region should be adjusted accordingly.

For imaging superficial lesions, the use of a catheter probe through a double-channel endoscope allows for visual guidance of probe placement. The use of a double-channel endoscope allows for one channel to be used for the ultrasound catheter probe and the other channel to be used for injecting water into the gastric lumen and suctioning water and air from the gastric lumen. Ultrasound catheter probes are available in frequencies of 12, 20, and 30 MHz. The image resolution increases with increasing frequency; however, penetration (depth of imaging) decreases as frequency increases.

The stomach has a well-developed five-layered wall structure (Video 4.1). This is easily visualized when water is placed in the lumen. The second layer is often prominent because of the relatively thick columnar mucosa and glands (Figure 4.2). The fourth layer is often thicker in the distal stomach compared to the proximal stomach. The fifth layer generally corresponds to surrounding structures and perigastric fat as the serosa is too thin to be resolved with endoscopic ultrasound. EUS imaging of the gastrointestinal (GI) tract wall typically exhibits five layers; however, seven or nine layers can be resolved if imaging is performed at higher

Atlas of Endoscopic Ultrasonography, Second Edition. Edited by Frank Gress, Thomas Savides, Brenna Casey, and Everson L. A. Artifon.

Companion website: www.wiley.com/go/gress/atlas

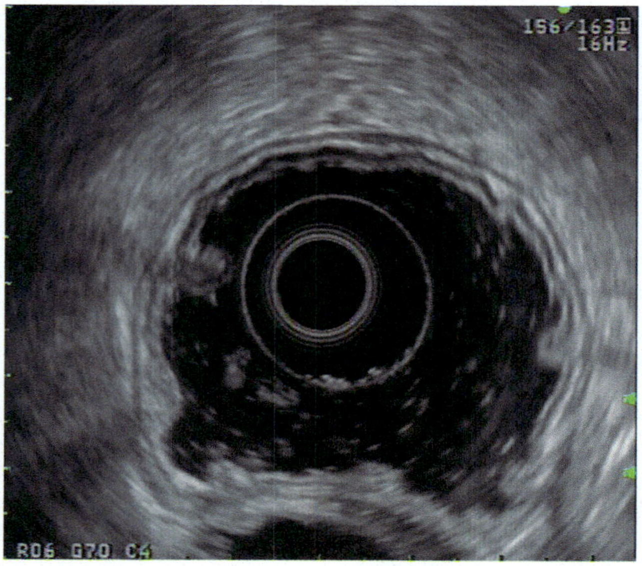

Figure 4.1 Circumferential image of the gastric wall after filling and distending the gastric lumen with water. Image is taken with an electronic radial array echoendoscope at 5 MHz.

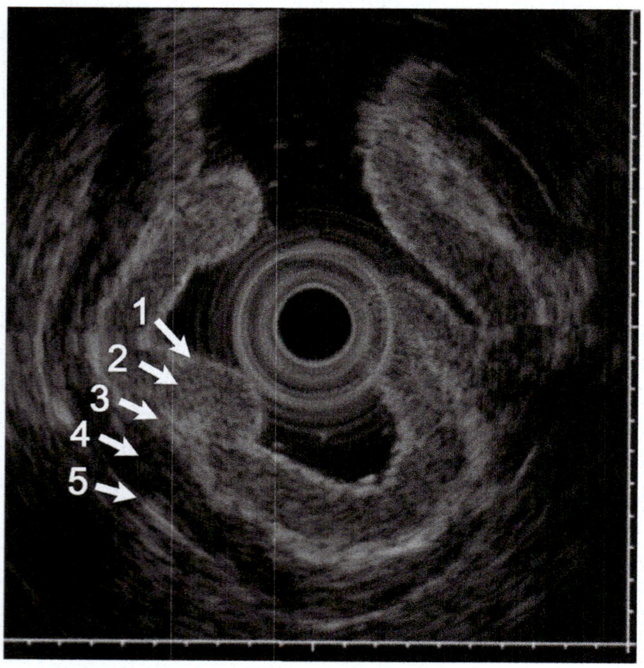

Figure 4.2 Five-layer structure of the gastric wall demonstrating a relatively thick mucosal layer (layers I and II). Image is taken with a 20 MHz catheter probe.

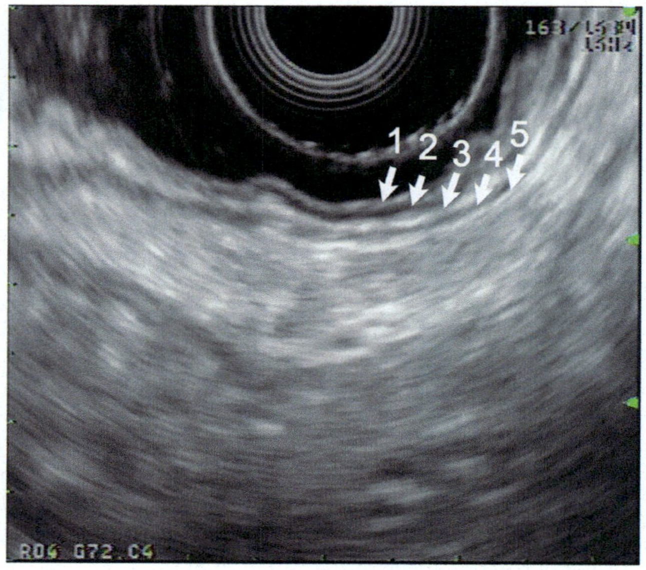

Figure 4.3 Five-layer structure of the gastric wall obtained with an electronic radial array echoendoscope at 5 MHz.

frequencies depending on the region of the GI tract being examined. Initial interpretation of the EUS images assumed direct correspondence of the layers seen on EUS to those seen on histology. It was presumed that the first echogenic layer represented the mucosa, the second echolucent layer the muscularis mucosae, the third echogenic layer the submucosa, the fourth echolucent layer the muscularis propria, and the fifth echogenic layer the serosa and subserosal fat. However, it was later proven that this was an incorrect interpretation of the EUS images of the GI tract wall. In fact, it was demonstrated that the five layers seen on EUS imaging correspond to the following (Figures 4.2 and 4.3).

1. Interface echo between the superficial mucosa and water (hyperechoic).
2. Deep mucosa (hypoechoic).
3. Submucosa plus the acoustic interface between the submucosa and muscularis propria (hyperechoic).
4. Muscularis propria minus the acoustic interface between the submucosa and muscularis propria (hypoechoic).
5. Serosa and subserosal fat (hyperechoic).

If a high-frequency (10 MHz or greater) transducer is used, seven or nine layers can potentially be identified on EUS imaging. These nine layers correspond to the following (Figure 4.4).

1. Epithelial interface (hyperechoic).
2. Epithelium (hypoechoic).
3. Lamina propria plus the acoustic interface between the lamina propria and the muscularis mucosae (hyperechoic).
4. Muscularis mucosae minus the acoustic interface between the lamina propria and muscularis mucosae (hypoechoic).
5. Submucosa plus the acoustic interface between the submucosa and inner muscularis propria (hyperechoic).
6. Inner muscularis propria minus interface between the submucosa and inner muscularis propria (hypoechoic).
7. Fibrous tissue band separating the inner and outer muscularis propria layers (hyperechoic).
8. Outer muscularis propria (hypoechoic).
9. Serosa and subserosal fat (hyperechoic).

An important aspect of EUS imaging in the stomach is to maintain orientation of the imaging plane to avoid tangential

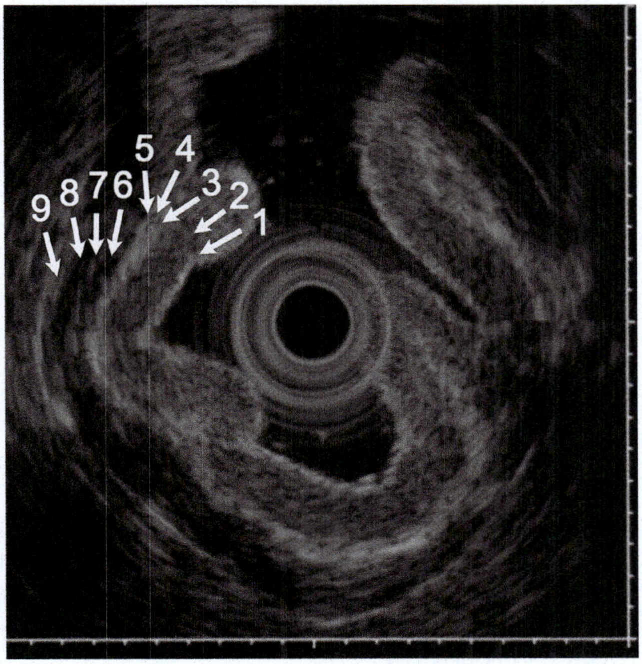

Figure 4.4 Nine-layer structure of the gastric wall obtained with a 20 MHz catheter probe. The image is the same as Figure 4.2 except additional layers are identified.

imaging, especially when evaluating mucosal lesions. Tangential imaging can result in overstaging of lesions.

In conclusion, the only available *in vivo* method for examining the full thickness of the GI wall, beyond the mucosal surface, is EUS. It provides gastroenterologists with a valuable diagnostic tool to assess pathology in the GI tract to help guide clinical management of the patient. Selection of the correct transducer and using good technique are important in obtaining high-quality images. When imaging the wall of the GI tract, the method of acoustic coupling is critical. Without good acoustic coupling to the mucosal surface, high-quality images cannot be obtained. The highest frequency available should be used to image the wall of the GI tract since deep penetration is not necessary unless imaging a large tumor arising from the wall. Using a higher frequency transducer will result in better resolution and allow for better identification of the layers involved. Lower frequencies may be required to identify the size of a mass and if there is involvement with any adjacent structures (T-staging), and to assess nodal involvement (N-staging).

Chapter video clip

Video 4.1 Layers of the gastric wall. Source: Aloka.

5 Bile Duct: Radial and Linear

Kapil Gupta
Cedars-Sinai Medical Center, Los Angeles, CA, USA

Normal bile duct anatomy

Endoscopic ultrasound provides excellent imaging of the biliary tree and gallbladder. Using radial and linear echoendoscope, visualization of the bile duct is performed from two main stations: from the duodenal bulb and from the second portion of the duodenum. The gallbladder is usually seen from the duodenal bulb or the antrum of the stomach. As the entire biliary tree can be visualized only using linear echoendoscope, more endosonographers are primarily using linear echoendoscope for evaluating bile duct anatomy.

Normal anatomy of the bile duct and gallbladder with radial echoendoscope

The echoendoscope is advanced through the pylorus into the duodenal bulb. To achieve this, the scope is usually in a long position along the greater curvature. The big wheel is then turned downwards and the scope is either turned slightly clockwise or the small wheel rotated slightly to the right to deflect the tip of the echoendoscope towards the apex of the duodenal bulb and impacted there. To achieve a stable position the balloon can be inflated, which helps in maintaining the tip of the scope in the bulb.

Here, with slight right and left movement, the liver is oriented at 12 o'clock. In this position the portal vein and the common bile duct can be visualized as two parallel tubular structures to the left of the transducer (Figure 5.1). With slight right rotation the bile duct can be followed towards the head of the pancreas into the ampulla where a thin pancreatic duct can be visualized below the bile duct (Figure 5.2). With left rotation or slight counterclockwise rotation the bile duct can be followed upwards into the liver (Video 5.1).

The gallbladder is usually visualized along the under surface of the liver (Figure 5.3) and with slight rotation, withdrawing, and pushing the echoendoscope the entire gallbladder can be visualized (Video 5.1).

To visualize the bile duct from the second portion of the duodenum, the transducer is placed along the ampulla and with slight movement the bile duct and the pancreatic duct can be visualized as two round anechoic structures (Figure 5.4) (Video 5.1).

Normal anatomy of the bile duct and gallbladder with linear echoendoscope

The bile duct is visualized with a linear echoendoscope from either the duodenal bulb or the second portion of the duodenum. The transducer of the echoendoscope is advanced across the pylorus. Once in the bulb the balloon can be filled slightly with water to maintain a stable position. Initially the tip of the echoendoscope is impacted at the apex of the bulb; to achieve this, the big wheel is turned downwards. With slightly counterclockwise torque and turning the big wheel down further the bile duct is visualized as a round structure, right in the center of the field (Figure 5.5). The cut section of the visualized bile duct is in the region of the common bile duct or the common hepatic duct. In this view the portal vein is usually visualized below the bile duct, and also the inferior vena cava (IVC) can be seen to the right of the field (Figure 5.5). The common hepatic artery can also be visualized coursing in between the bile duct and the portal vein towards the left of the bile duct. From this view the inward impacted position of the tip of the transducer is maintained. By rotating the transducer in a counterclockwise manner the bile duct is followed towards the hilum into the liver and the bifurcation at the porta hepatis can be visualized. Cystic duct take-off can also be visualized by tracing the bile duct.

Undoing the counterclockwise rotation, and rotating the scope to the right, the transducer is rotated to follow the bile

Atlas of Endoscopic Ultrasonography, Second Edition. Edited by Frank Gress, Thomas Savides, Brenna Casey, and Everson L. A. Artifon.

Companion website: www.wiley.com/go/gress/atlas

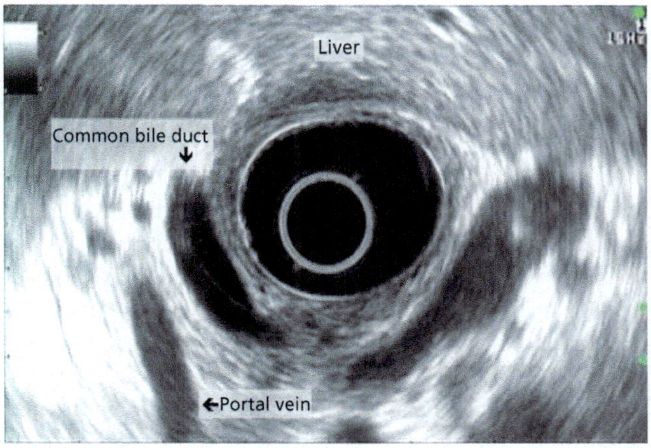

Figure 5.1 Bile duct as visualized from the duodenal bulb (radial echoendoscope).

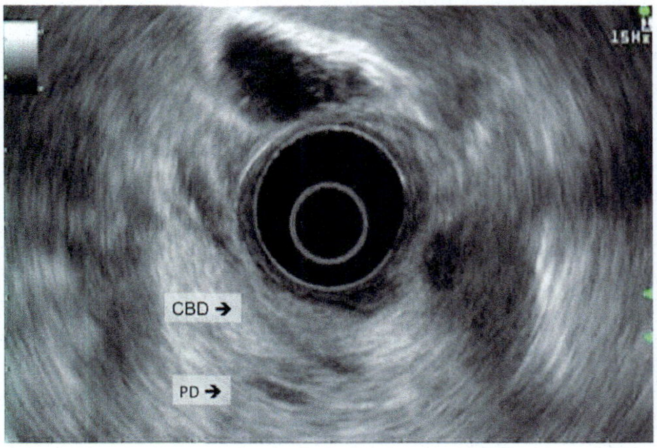

Figure 5.2 Bile duct followed towards the head of the pancreas from the duodenal bulb (radial echoendoscope). CBD, common bile duct; PD, pancreatic duct.

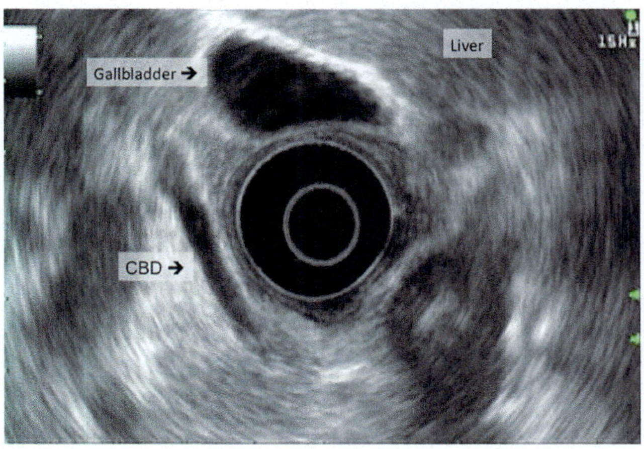

Figure 5.3 Gallbladder from the duodenal bulb (radial echoendoscope). CBD, common bile duct.

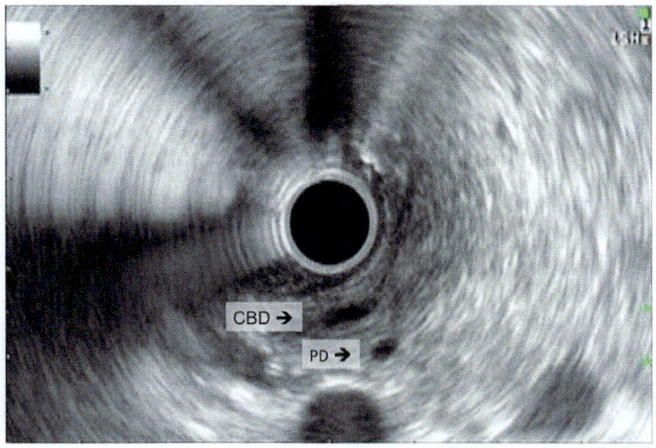

Figure 5.4 Bile duct and pancreatic duct from the second portion of the duodenum (radial echoendoscope). CBD, common bile duct; PD, pancreatic duct.

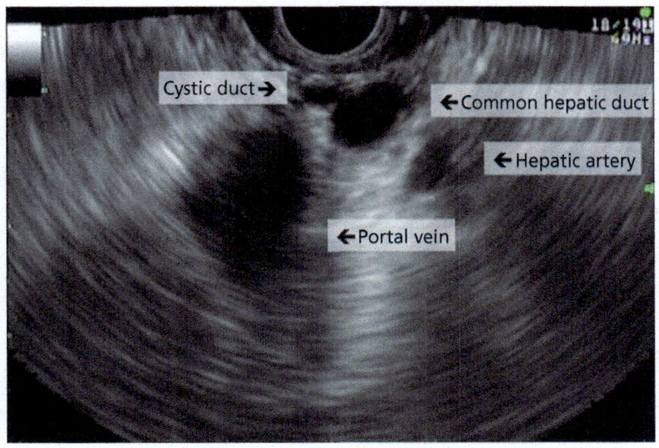

Figure 5.5 Common hepatic duct and cystic duct as visualized from the duodenal bulb (linear echoendoscope).

duct in the intrapancreatic portion towards the papilla. With this maneuver the entire bile duct can be followed. In most of the instances the bile duct can be traced downstream all the way to the point where it joins the pancreatic duct into the ampulla. Just below the bile duct, in the intrapancreatic portion, the pancreatic duct can be visualized (Video 5.1).

For visualizing the gallbladder the transducer is impacted in the bulb and the big wheel is turned up and the scope rotated counterclockwise so the transducer now faces the undersurface of the liver; by turning the small wheel to the right and left the gallbladder can be seen in the subhepatic region. Moving the big wheel up and down, and turning the small wheel right and left, the entire gallbladder can usually be scanned. Sometimes the scope is slightly withdrawn to visualize the entire gallbladder (Video 5.1).

Care should be taken when advancing the echoendoscope into the second portion. By slight inward push, turning the big wheel down and the small wheel to the right, the scope tip usually points in the axis of the second portion of the

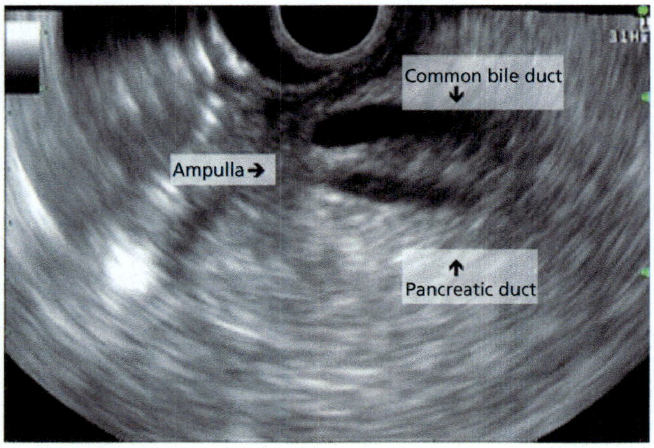

Figure 5.6 Bile duct and pancreatic duct from the second portion of the duodenum (linear echoendoscope).

duodenum. Carefully moving the big wheel up and down the scope tip falls into the second portion of the duodenum. At this point the small wheel is kept turned towards the right and the scope is reduced to a short position to align the transducer along the papilla.

The transducer is kept in close apposition with the major papilla. With slight right and left torque while withdrawing the scope, the bile duct is visualized as a long tubular structure closer to the duodenal wall, and deep to it lays the pancreatic duct (Figure 5.6). The bile duct can then be followed towards the liver with continued slow withdrawal of the scope and slight right and left torque. Usually the bile duct can be followed to the common hepatic duct portion when the scope tends to slip back into the stomach; to prevent this scope is again pushed inwards with counterclockwise rotation to gain a position similar to one in the duodenal bulb (Video 5.1).

Combining views from both the stations, namely the duodenal bulb and the second portion of the duodenum, the entire biliary tree can be visualized.

Chapter video clip

Video 5.1 Radial and linear array images of the bile duct from the duodenum.

6 EUS of the Normal Pancreas

Richard A. Erickson and James T. Sing, Jr.
Scott and White Clinic and Hospital, and Texas A&M Health Science Center, Temple, TX, USA

Radial examination of the pancreas

In radial examination of the pancreas, the organ is usually first encountered with the instrument in the mid to upper body of the stomach. On entering the stomach, the abdominal aorta can be followed a few centimeters distally to the take-off of the celiac artery. From there, advancing the scope just a few centimeters more distally will result in it crossing the neck/body of the pancreas (Figure 6.1). The confluence of the portal vein (PV) and splenic vein (SV) should appear deep to the pancreas neck with some minor manipulations of the orientation of the echoendoscope tip. The superior mesenteric artery can be seen in cross-section deep to the confluence surrounded by the echogenic fat of the retroperitoneum. The portal/splenic vein confluence has been described as looking like a golf club with the portal vein being the head of the club, the splenic vein the shaft, and the superior mesenteric artery the golf ball (Figure 6.2). By continuing to follow the pancreas and splenic vessels towards the patient's left and slightly withdrawing the echoendoscope, the tail of the pancreas is imaged (Figure 6.3). Following the splenic vessels to the left will lead to the hilum of the spleen, which is an important landmark as it marks the leftward limit of the tail of the pancreas. It is important to not forget that the tail of the pancreas may move deep from the stomach wall nestled between the left kidney and spleen (Figure 6.4). If this area is not examined carefully, pancreatic tail lesions can be easily missed. From the confluence of the portal/splenic vein, gently advancing the tip of the echoendoscope forward and angulating the tip of the echoendoscope posterior one can view the pancreatic neck (Figure 6.5). Again, if this area is not examined carefully, pancreatic neck lesions may go unnoticed.

On advancing the echoendoscope deep into the duodenum, the side-by-side cross-sections of the inferior vena cava and abdominal aorta come into view. On withdrawing the echoendoscope from the deep duodenum, the most caudad portion of the ventral pancreas will usually come into view just to the patient's left (counterclockwise) of the abdominal aorta (Figure 6.6). On gentle withdrawal, the ampulla can usually be located by identifying the first visible portions of pancreatic duct in the ventral pancreas (VP) and following the course of the duct by slow withdrawal towards the duodenal wall and ampulla (Figure 6.7). The triangular-shaped ventral pancreas may appear more echolucent than the dorsal pancreas (DP) in about 75% of normal people and should not be mistaken for an echolucent tumor (Figure 6.6). The echolucency of the ventral pancreas can occasionally even be seen in views of the organ through the stomach. Further withdrawal reveals more of the pancreatic head where longitudinal views of the pancreatic duct may occasionally be seen (Figure 6.8). The confluence of the superior mesenteric vein with the portal vein and splenic vein is seen deep to the pancreatic head (Figure 6.9). This is an important view for examining splanchnic venous involvement by pancreatic head malignancies. As the echoendoscope comes around the junction of the second and first portion of the duodenum, small changes in orientation of the tip will result in major shifts in views. Sometimes the best views of the head of the pancreas are obtained when the echoendoscope first enters into the duodenal bulb with the scope in a long position. It is this orientation which most commonly provides a "stack sign" of the common bile duct (CBD) running parallel to the deeper main pancreatic duct (Figure 6.10). A stack sign can be demonstrated in more than 80% of patients with normal pancreatic ductal anatomy. When pancreas divisum exists (3–7% of normal people), a stack sign can only be demonstrated in about one-third of patients. Instead of the absence of a stack sign in pancreas divisum the more specific crossed duct sign may be seen. The crossed duct sign

Atlas of Endoscopic Ultrasonography, Second Edition. Edited by Frank Gress, Thomas Savides, Brenna Casey, and Everson L. A. Artifon.

Companion website: www.wiley.com/go/gress/atlas

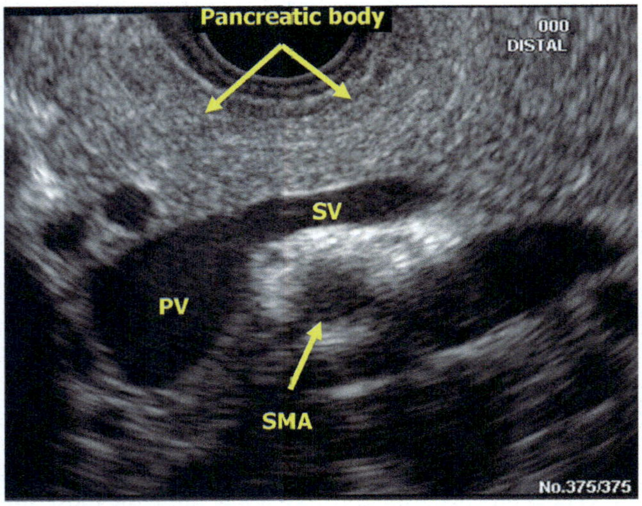

Figure 6.1 Radial EUS: pancreatic body and portal/splenic vein confluence. PV, portal vein; SMA, superior mesenteric artery; SV, splenic vein.

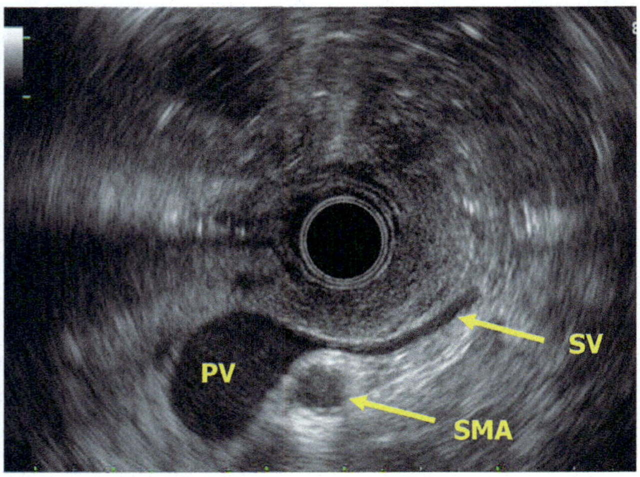

Figure 6.2 Radial EUS: portal/splenic vein confluence. PV, portal vein; SMA, superior mesenteric artery; SV, splenic vein.

results from the CBD being seen in cross-section while the pancreatic duct, draining to the minor ampulla, is seen in longitudinal section.

Linear examination of the pancreas

The linear endosonographic examination of the pancreas through the stomach differs fundamentally from the radial examination in that complete imaging of the pancreas must be provided by rotating the shaft of the scope. Since the retroperitoneal structures are all posterior to the stomach, clockwise (rightward) rotation of the echoendoscope will point the echoendoscope towards the patient's left and counterclockwise (leftward) rotation towards their right side. To find the

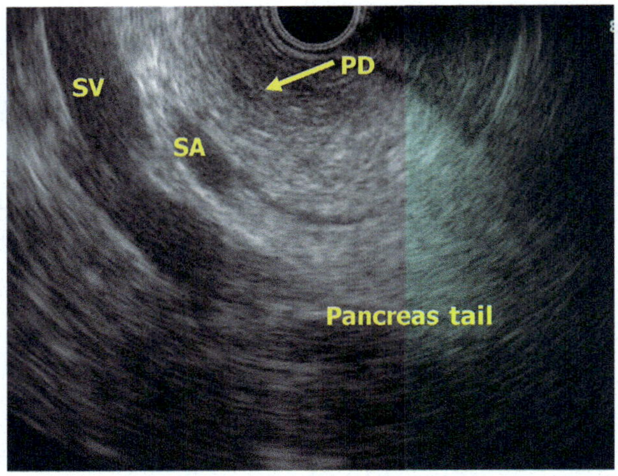

Figure 6.3 Radial EUS: pancreas tail. PD, pancreatic duct; SA, splenic artery; SV, splenic vein.

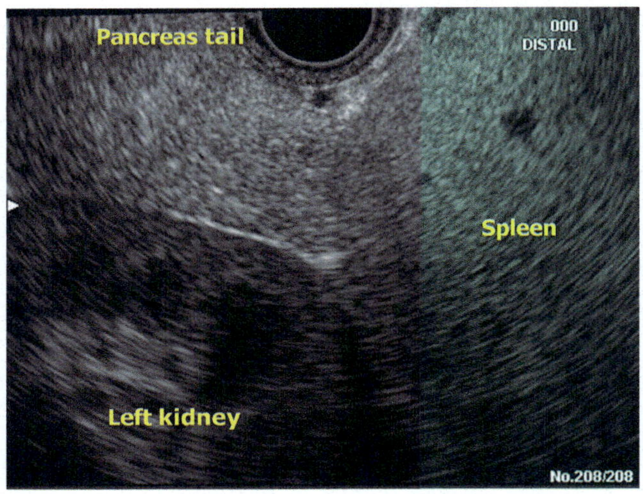

Figure 6.4 Radial EUS: pancreas tail.

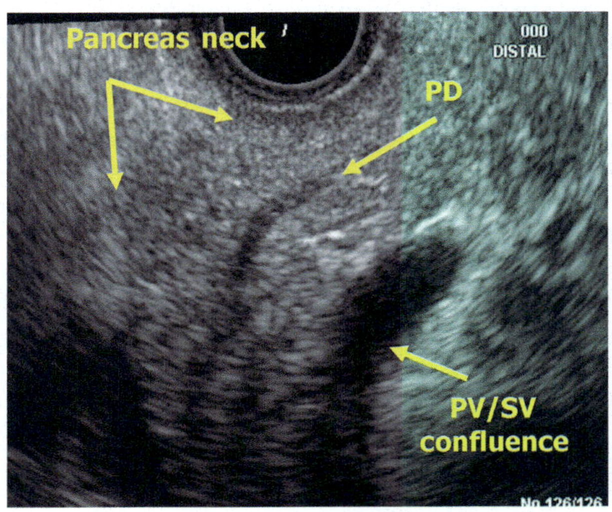

Figure 6.5 Radial EUS: pancreas neck. PD, pancreatic duct; PV, portal vein; SV, splenic vein.

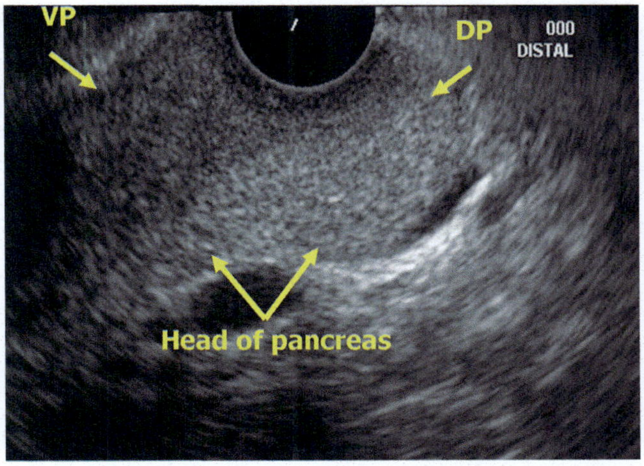

Figure 6.6 Radial EUS: head of pancreas. DP, dorsal pancreas; VP, ventral pancreas.

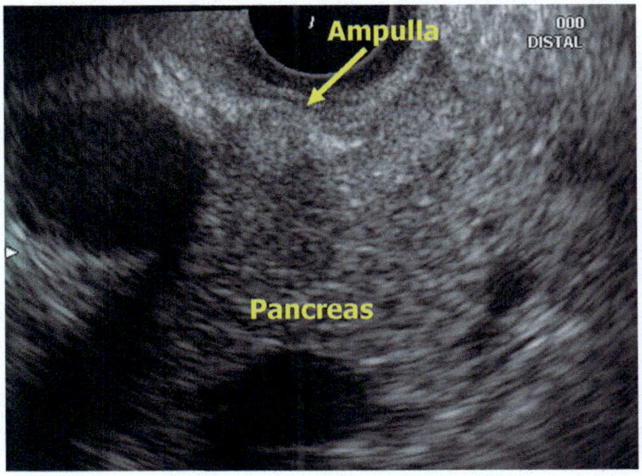

Figure 6.7 Radial EUS: ampulla.

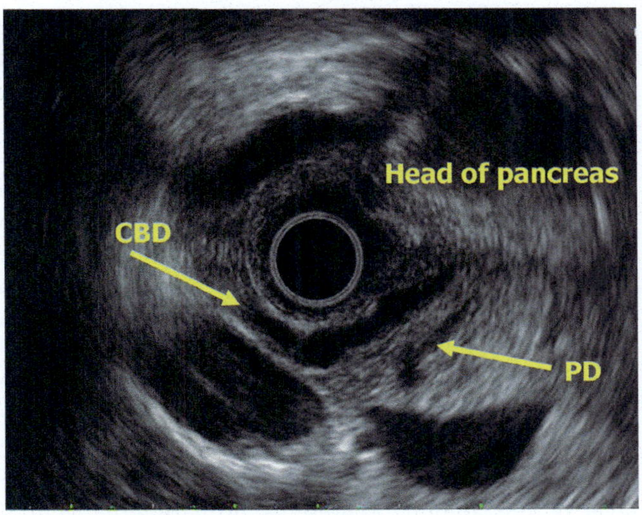

Figure 6.8 Radial EUS: head of pancreas. CBD, common bile duct; PD, pancreatic duct.

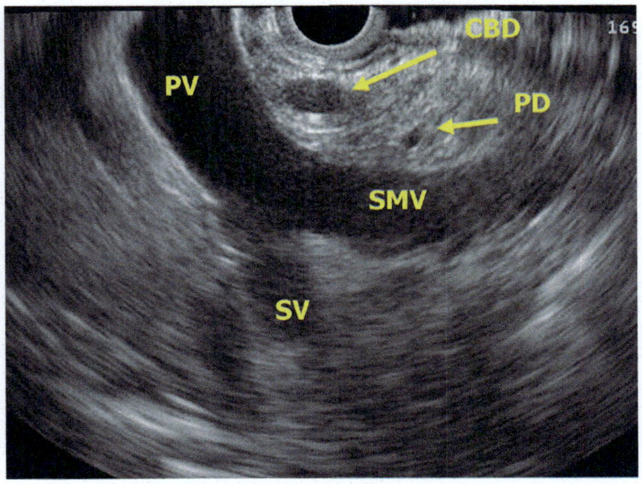

Figure 6.9 Radial EUS: head of pancreas, vasculature. CBD, common bile duct; PD, pancreatic duct; PV, portal vein; SMV, superior mesenteric vein; SV, splenic vein.

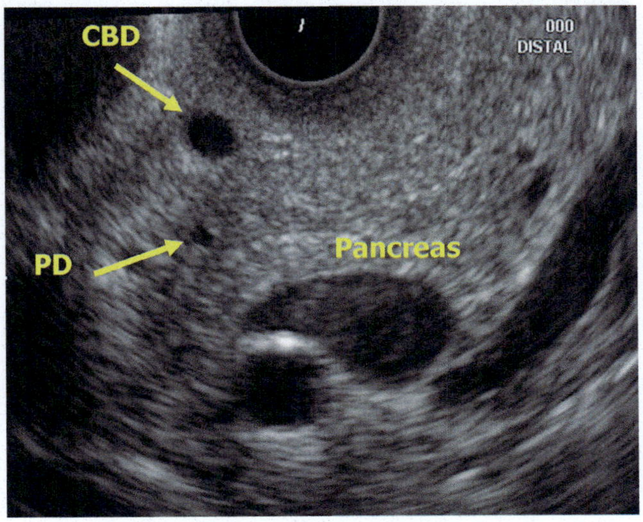

Figure 6.10 Radial EUS: head of pancreas. CBD, common bile duct; PD, pancreatic duct.

pancreas in the stomach, one starts at the abdominal aorta near the gastroesophageal junction and follows its course distally until the take-off of the celiac artery is visible. Usually, the more oblique take-off of the superior mesenteric artery is apparent just distal to this. Further advancement of the instrument distally will find the pancreas neck/body nestled between the "V" of the celiac and superior mesenteric artery. The splenic artery will course tortuously in and out of the pancreas body/tail, but the splenic vein usually has a straight course and is the larger, deeper and more ovoid of the two vessels (Figure 6.11). The pancreas is interrogated sequentially from the neck to the body and tail through the stomach at this level by rotating the echoendoscope to the right (clockwise) with slight withdrawal following the splenic vein and splenic artery as they run into the hilum of the spleen. The

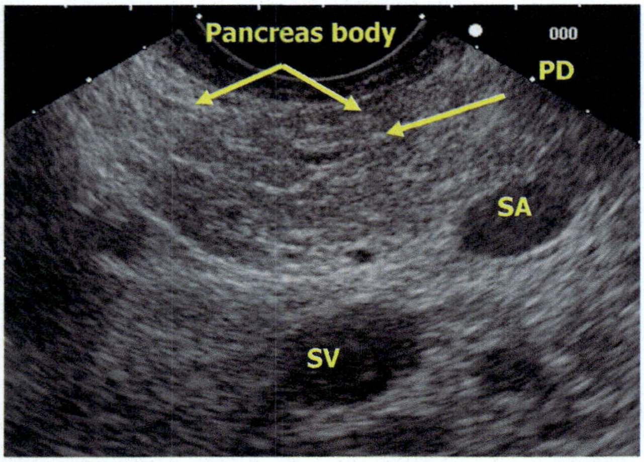

Figure 6.11 Linear EUS: pancreas body. PD, pancreatic duct; SA, splenic artery; SV, splenic vein.

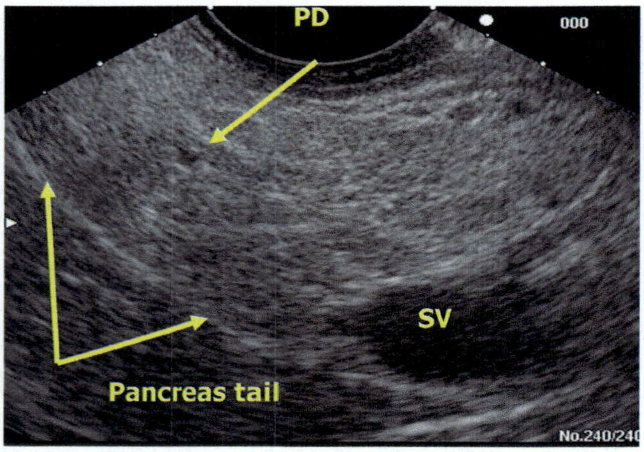

Figure 6.12 Linear EUS: pancreas tail. PD, pancreatic duct; SV, splenic vein.

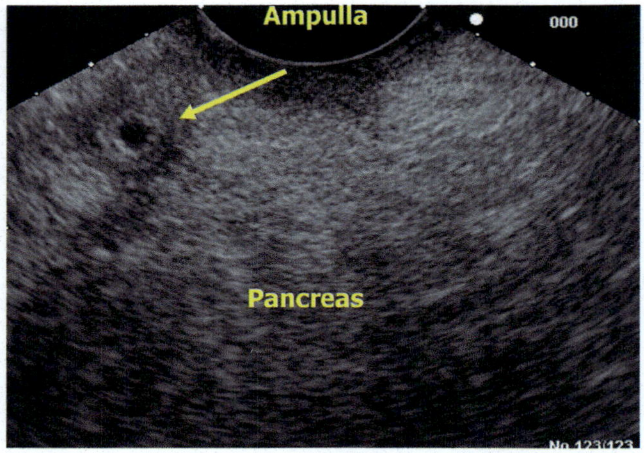

Figure 6.13 Linear EUS: ampulla.

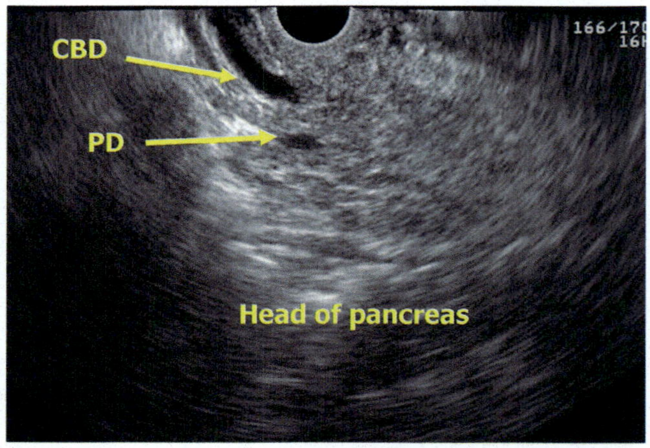

Figure 6.14 Linear EUS: head of pancreas. CBD, common bile duct; PD, pancreatic duct.

pancreas neck, body, and tail will appear be the tissue found between the splenic vein and the posterior gastric wall. The pancreatic duct is usually seen in cross-section through the stomach (Figure 6.12). A normal caliber duct will appear as a small, sometimes difficult to see, echolucent dot in the middle of the pancreatic parenchyma. Rotation to the left at the level of the celiac axis and body of the pancreas brings into view the pancreatic neck with the portal vein confluence deep to it. The splenic vein merges into the confluence from the patient's left and the superior mesenteric vein runs caudad from the portal vein confluence. A little further leftward rotation of the echoendoscope may produce views of the right border of the pancreatic neck looking down towards the pancreatic head. Sometimes, longitudinal views of the pancreatic duct can be obtained from this view.

As with radial endosonography, the linear duodenum presents the endosonographer with the most variability in endosonographic relationships of vessels, ducts, and periduodenal organs. There is a marked transition in the direction of the scope tip and therefore anatomic views between entering the duodenal bulb in a "long position," where the scope tip is pointing cephalad and posterior, and a "short position" when withdrawing from the second portion of the duodenum, where the scope tip is pointing caudad. Generally, we try to start by inserting the linear echoendoscope deep into the second portion of the duodenum. With the echoendoscope in a short position in the second portion of the duodenum, the scope is designed to be facing the medial wall of the duodenum near the region of the ampulla (Figure 6.13). On slightly rotating the scope right or left with very gentle withdrawal, usually the pancreatic duct will be seen first traveling relatively perpendicularly away from the transducer. The CBD will be seen to originate from the ampulla between the duodenal lumen and the pancreatic duct (Figure 6.14). The pancreatic parenchyma seen at the level of the ampulla represents primarily the ventral pancreas. The relative echolucency of the ventral anlage commonly seen by radial endosonography may be less apparent by linear endoscopic ultrasound (EUS). At this level, if vessels are seen deep to the pancreatic head they are usually the superior mesenteric vein and artery. If one inserts the echoendoscope deeper into the third portion of the duodenum, the uncinate portion of the pancreas nestled among the vessels of the mesenteric root may be seen. Because this is a difficult view to get with a radial instrument, this view using a linear instrument is sometimes the only way in which deep uncinate tumors may be seen. From the ampullary region, further gradual withdrawal and rotation to the left (counterclockwise) will follow the course of the tubular structures of the porta hepatis. The pancreatic head will appear as the tissue between the superior mesenteric vein/portal vein and the duodenal wall.

Endosonographic appearance of the normal pancreatic parenchyma

There is considerable variability in the endosonographic appearance of the pancreatic parenchyma. Classically it has a homogeneous, fine, "salt and pepper" appearance with echogenicity similar to the spleen. The ventral anlage is more echolucent because of its different embryologic origin and its lesser content of echogenic fat. In the elderly, the pancreas can get more nodular with courser echogenicity. In obese patients, the pancreas becomes infiltrated with fat and can almost disappear into the retroperitoneal fat. Fortunately, any pathologic pancreatic lesions, such as dilated ducts, cysts, or neoplasms, will be easily visible in the bright background of retroperitoneal fat. Thin patients typically offer particularly detailed imaging of the pancreas.

Chapter video clips

Video 6.1 Linear array EUS head of pancreas.

Video 6.2 Linear array EUS of the pancreas neck to tail.

Video 6.3 Radial array EUS head of pancreas.

Video 6.4 Radial array EUS of the pancreatic neck to tail.

7 Liver, Spleen, and Kidneys: Radial and Linear

Nalini M. Guda[1] and Marc F. Catalano[2]

[1] University of Wisconsin, School of Medicine and Public Health, Pancreatobiliary Services, St. Luke's Medical Center, Milwaukee, WI, USA

[2] Medical College of Wisconsin, Pancreatobiliary Services, St. Luke's Medical Center, Milwaukee, WI, USA

Introduction

This chapter describes the endosonographic features of the major organs of the abdomen: the liver, spleen, kidneys, and adrenal glands. Ultrasound features of the pancreas and bile duct are described elsewhere.

The liver, spleen, kidneys, and adrenal glands (left side) are visualized from the stomach (Videos 7.1 and 7.2).

Liver

Radial endosonography

As the radial probe is advanced through the esophagus into the gastric cardia, the liver is the predominant organ visualized. When positioning the abdominal aorta at the 6 o'clock position, the left lobe of the liver is seen anteriorly and medially to the right (Figure 7.1). The aorta, with a dark hypoechoic band which is the diaphragmatic crux, is seen immediately adjacent to the probe. In this position, near the hiatus, the hepatic veins are seen as anechoic structures, entering the inferior vena cava (IVC). In this position, possibly with left tip deflection, the spleen can be seen on the right of the screen. As the aorta is traced distally, maintaining its 6 o'clock position, the liver may still be seen anteriorly. Vascular structures can be differentiated from ductal structures by a thicker (echogenic) wall and the presence of flow.

When advancing the echoprobe towards the antrum, the gallbladder is often visualized as an oval-shaped anechoic structure. In this position, the porta hepatis can be seen with subtle tip deflection upwards.

Linear endosonography

With the probe at the level of the diaphragmatic hiatus, the longitudinal aorta and celiac artery origin are the most recognizable reference points (Figure 7.2), demonstrated as tubular longitudinal structures. Here, rotation of the probe counterclockwise will bring into view the liver parenchyma and its vascular structures (Figure 7.3).

Advancing the probe at the level of the pylorus and duodenal bulb, clockwise rotation and superior tip deflection brings into view the porta hepatis along with several vascular structures. Use of Doppler can differentiate arterial from venous structures as well as biliary structures.

The entire liver is not visualized by endoscopic ultrasound (EUS). Despite this limitation, it is useful to carefully examine the liver since metastatic processes can be easily identified and biopsied and could lead to a change in clinical staging and management of a suspected tumor.

Spleen

The spleen appears as a homogeneous structure seen between the tail of the pancreas, left kidney, and gastric wall. With a radial scope it is imaged from the gastric cardia. It is similar to liver in echogenicity except that it is devoid of any ducts and vessels (Figure 7.4). It can be easier to follow the splenic vein after visualizing the pancreas from the gastroesophageal (GE) junction. The splenic artery, splenic vein, renal vein, and the left adrenal are usually visualized as well while attempting to scan the spleen. The splenic vein can be easily traced along the inferior aspect of the body and tail of the pancreas; however, the splenic artery is tortuous and it is difficult to follow its course to the celiac trunk. With a linear scope one has to scan inferior to the left kidney and laterally to visualize the spleen (Figure 7.5).

Kidney

Both the right and left kidneys can be visualized by EUS. The left kidney is readily identified from the fundus of the stomach.

Atlas of Endoscopic Ultrasonography, Second Edition. Edited by Frank Gress, Thomas Savides, Brenna Casey, and Everson L. A. Artifon.

Companion website: www.wiley.com/go/gress/atlas

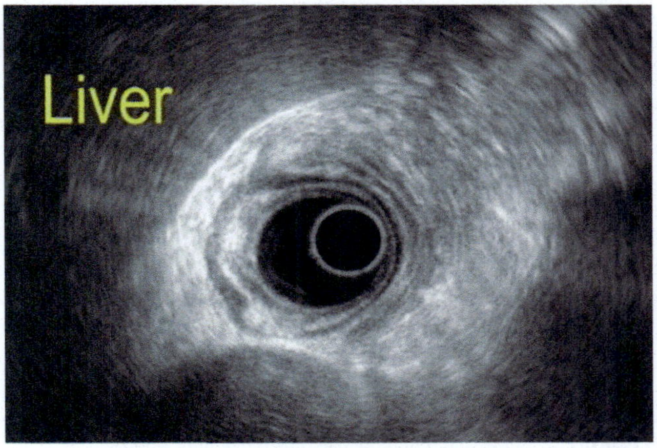

Figure 7.1 Image of the liver scanned by radial ultrasound.

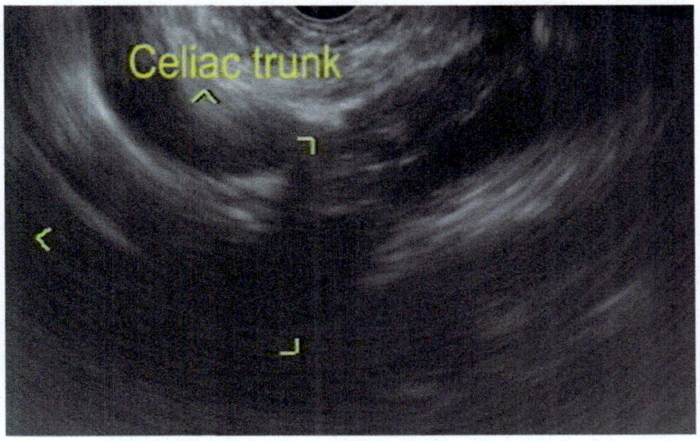

Figure 7.2 Celiac artery imaging by linear ultrasound.

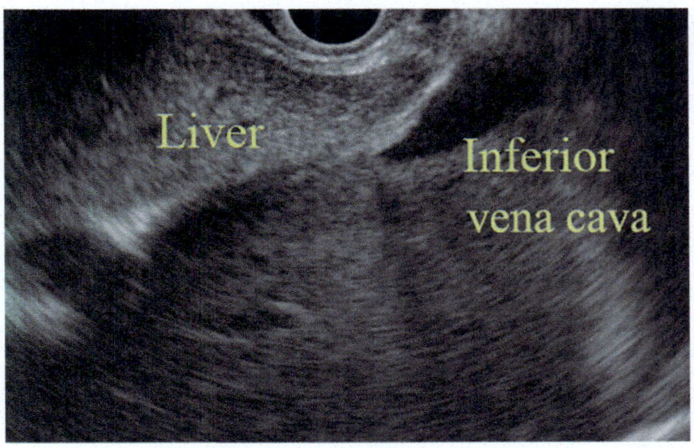

Figure 7.3 Image of liver by linear ultrasound.

It has a complex echogenicity with hypoechoic parenchyma and hypertonic areas within representing the calyceal system.

Radial endosonography

With the echoendoscope in the gastric cardia the left kidney is readily visualized. One can see the calyceal system and the renal vessels (Figure 7.6). To visualize the right kidney the echoscope is placed in the D-3 position. Visualization of the IVC and aorta provide easily identifiable landmarks. Upon slow withdrawal, the image brings into view the right kidney immediately right of the probe along with the right renal vein and artery. As the kidney is traced proximally, lateral deflection of the tip may bring into view the right adrenal gland.

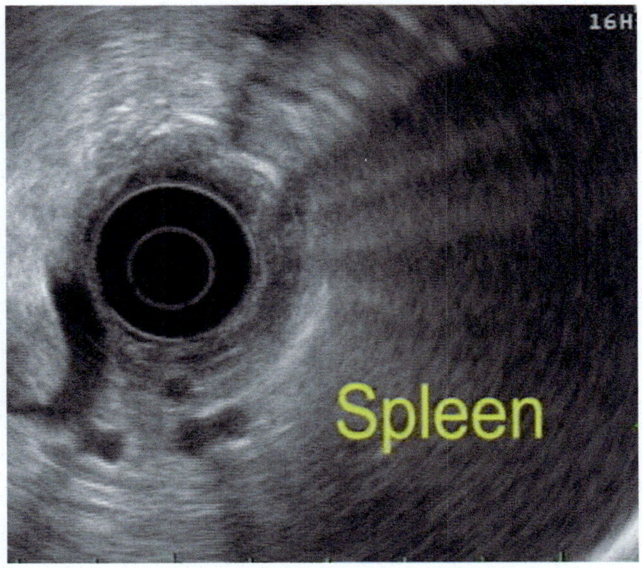

Figure 7.4 Image of spleen by radial ultrasound.

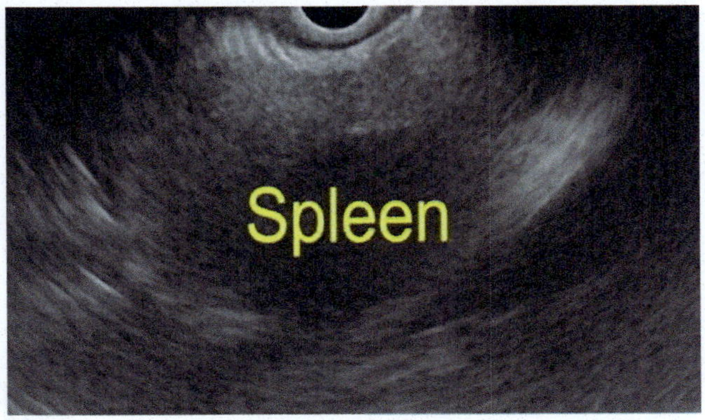

Figure 7.5 Image of spleen by linear ultrasound.

Linear endosonography

With a linear scope one can withdraw the scope in the fundus posteriorly towards the pancreas until the tail is visualized and then push the scope inferiorly to see the left kidney (Figure 7.7). To view the right kidney, the probe is placed just below the level of the papilla and counterclockwise rotation brings into view the right kidney and its vascular structures. Slow withdrawal allows for visualization of the right adrenal glands.

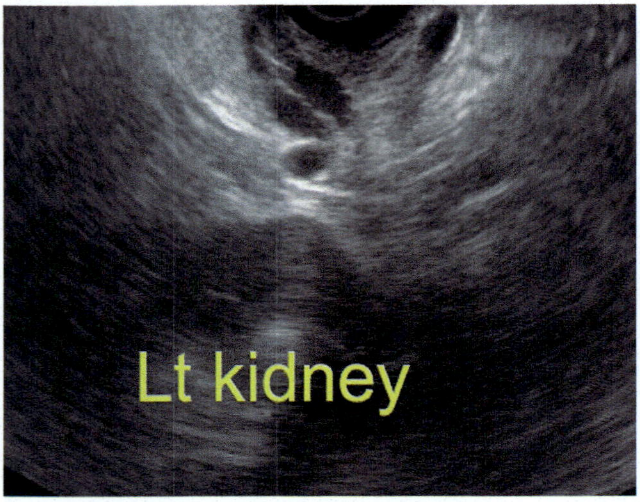

Figure 7.6 Image of left kidney by radial ultrasound.

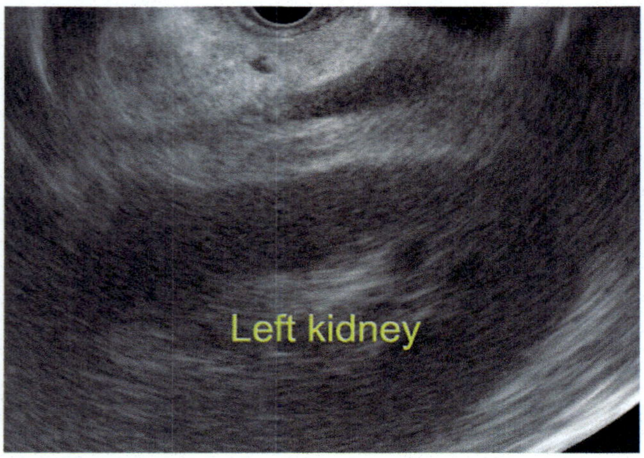

Figure 7.7 Image of left kidney by linear ultrasound.

Adrenal glands

Radial endosonography

With the probe in the gastric fundus, the left adrenal gland can be found immediately proximal to the celiac artery and left of the aorta. It is seen as an echo-poor, thin strip of tissue ("seagull" shaped). The left adrenal gland can also be located by tracing the left kidney cephalad, located medial to the upper pole of the kidney (Figure 7.8).

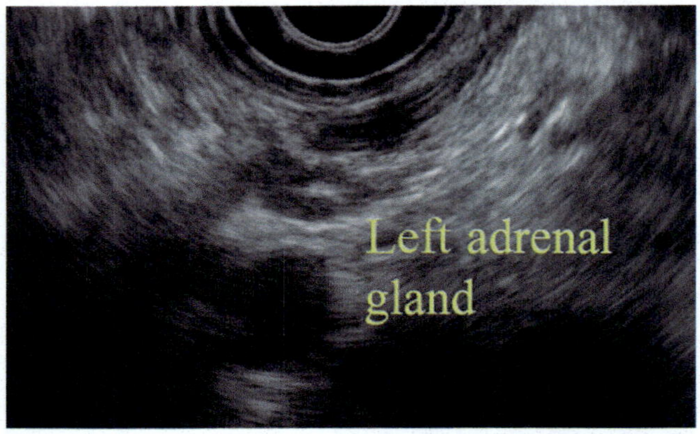

Figure 7.8 Image of left adrenal gland by radial ultrasound.

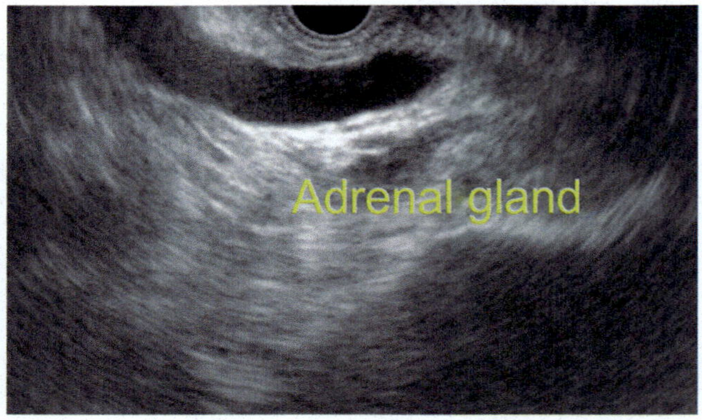

Figure 7.9 Image of left adrenal gland by linear ultrasound.

Linear endosonography

With the probe at the level of the celiac trunk take-off, slight clockwise rotation brings into view the left adrenal gland seen as a thin echo-poor structure (Figure 7.9).

Chapter video clips

Video 7.1 Normal imaging of liver, spleen, kidney, and adrenal by radial ultrasound. Source: Aloka.

Video 7.2 Normal imaging of liver, spleen, kidney, and adrenal by linear ultrasound. Source: Aloka.

8 Anatomy of the Anorectum: Radial and Linear

Christoph F. Dietrich
Caritas-Krankenhaus, Bad Mergentheim, Germany

Introduction

Radial and also longitudinal endorectal ultrasound (ERUS) allows precise imaging of the rectal wall in multiple planes and detailed information about the surrouding structures. The same is true for the generally not well known but effective anorectal ultrasound using a conventional transabdominal transducer technique (perineal ultrasound, PNUS). A transversal section with a 360-degree transducer is most helpful for orientation and therefore for the examination of the anal canal, whereas for examination of more orally located structures (flexible or stiff) radial as well as sector scanners can be used. Sagittal, frontal and transverse, and other variable longitudinal sections have to be considered.

The anatomical relationship between the internal anal sphincter (IAS), external anal sphincter (EAS), levator ani and puborectal muscles, and ischiorectal fossa can be reconstructed by the examiner's anatomical knowledge and his or her aptitude for multidimensional imagination. Reproducible documentation and imaging can be also done using three-dimensional (3D) techniques or real-time 3D technique (also called 4D).

Examination technique

A comprehensive categorization of the anal canal and distal rectum can be achieved by examining at different levels. From a didactic point of view, a step-by-step approach of retracting the transducer to indicate the distance in centimeters from the anocutaneous level seems to be helpful. A pushing forward technique may also be done but is less often used due to reduced reproducibility. Orientation is achieved by identification of the surrounding leading structures (bladder, prostate, vagina, puborectal muscle, etc.) and details are best seen with appropriate focusing and instrument adjustment (Video 8.1).

Retracting the transducer, corresponding sections at 4–6 cm (perirectal tissue, prostate, seminal vesicles, cervix, vagina), at 2–4 cm (IAS, EAS, puborectal muscle), and at a superficial level of 0–2 cm (EAS with continuous fibers radiating into the subcutaneous fat) are visualized.

Orientation

Reporting of the anatomy and findings should always use clock orientation as a reference (i.e. the pubic symphysis is always at the 12 o'clock position).

Normal anatomy

Anatomical remarks

The anal canal is covered by a columnar epithelium below the anal crypts. The mucosa is a transitional cell epithelium and begins at the height of the anal crypts. It can, however, be only inconstantly visualized as a faintly dark layer with scattered echoes of medium echogenicity. The transitional epithelium disappears in the first echo-rich border area depending on the type and frequency of the ultrasound probe. The dentate line and the anorectal crypts are of importance with respect to fistula formation but often cannot be seen mainly due to the compression of the anal canal by the endorectal probe. Normally, the hemorrhoidal plexus is virtually invisible, unless very thin probes are used or thrombosis is present. Important anatomical details are summarized in Table 8.1.

Rectal wall

The rectum can be examined at any level by endoscopic and/or visual orientation. The echogenicity of the various mural layers in the anal canal is similar to that in the gastrointestinal

Atlas of Endoscopic Ultrasonography, Second Edition. Edited by Frank Gress, Thomas Savides, Brenna Casey, and Everson L. A. Artifon.

Companion website: www.wiley.com/go/gress/atlas

tract elsewhere and characterized by different, well-separated bands when imaged from the lumen. Above the transition zone the typical sonographic features of the five (or nine) layered rectal wall are found. The typical five layers comprise the echo-rich borderline between the probe and the mucosa, the echo-poor mucosa, the echo-rich submucosa, the echo-poor muscularis propria, and the echo-rich serosa and the border area to the perirectal fat tissue. Using highly sophisticated equipment up to nine layers can be displayed, including the two parts of the muscularis propria, differentiating the stratum circulare (inner ring layer) and the stratum longitudinale (outer ring layer) separated by a connective tissue-like septum. A further differentiation of the inner layers yields additional layer separation in the mucosa and submucosa. In addition, it is relevant to note that these layer structures are important in staging rectal cancer according to the TNM classification.

Table 8.1 Anatomical structures and abbreviations.

ARUS	Anorectal endosonography (alternative: perineal ultrasound, PNUS)
ERUS	Endorectal endosonography
C	Cutis (skin)
Muc	Mucosa
IAS	Internal anal sphincter. Musculus sphincter ani internus (inner [ring] muscle fibers of the rectum radiating into M. sphincter ani internus)
EAS	External anal sphincter. M. sphincter ani externus
LAM	Levator ani muscle (M. puborectalis, M. ischiococcygeus, M. iliococcygeus, M. pubococcygeus; endosonographic separation of the muscle layer is not always possible)
LM	Longitudinal muscle, M. corrugator ani (longitudinal muscle fibers of the rectum radiating into M. sphincter ani externus)

Level of the prostate or cervix uteri

The standardized approach starts at a level of 4–6 cm above the anocutaneous line (ab ano) by delineating the seminal vesicles, prostate, and urethra in men, whereas at this level the cervix uteri and vagina can be displayed in women, and the urinary bladder in both. The internal iliac vessels cross the rectosigmoid colon just proximal to this region, but definite determination of the edge between the rectum and sigmoid colon is endosonographically still an unsolved problem. The surrounding bones and muscles of the pelvic floor, namely the levator ani muscles (ischiococcygeus, iliococcygeus, and pubococcygeus) including the V-shaped puborectal muscle (Figure 8.1), should be identified since the anal canal ends at this level and the rectum begins. The funnel-like structure of the levator ani muscle separates the extraperitoneal pelvis into an infraperitoneal or pelvirectal and a subcutaneous or ischiorectal space. The lateral border of the pelvic floor corresponds to the M. obturatorius internus with the foramen obturatorium.

External anal sphincter level

The second section at 2–4 cm ab ano shows as a leading structure the prominent EAS as a 5–10 mm broad layer characterized by often concentrically arranged echo-rich and sometimes inhomogeneous series of lines (Video 8.1 and Figure 8.2) depending on the examination technique used (criteria: radial or linear probes, diameter of the probe, transducer frequency, tissue harmonic imaging, focus zone).

The EAS is composed of three more or less separated parts, i.e. the subcutaneous (pars subcutanea), the superficial (pars superficialis), and the deep (pars profunda) components which are confluent with each other. It is of great importance to understand that the shape and configuration of the EAS differs significantly between males and females.

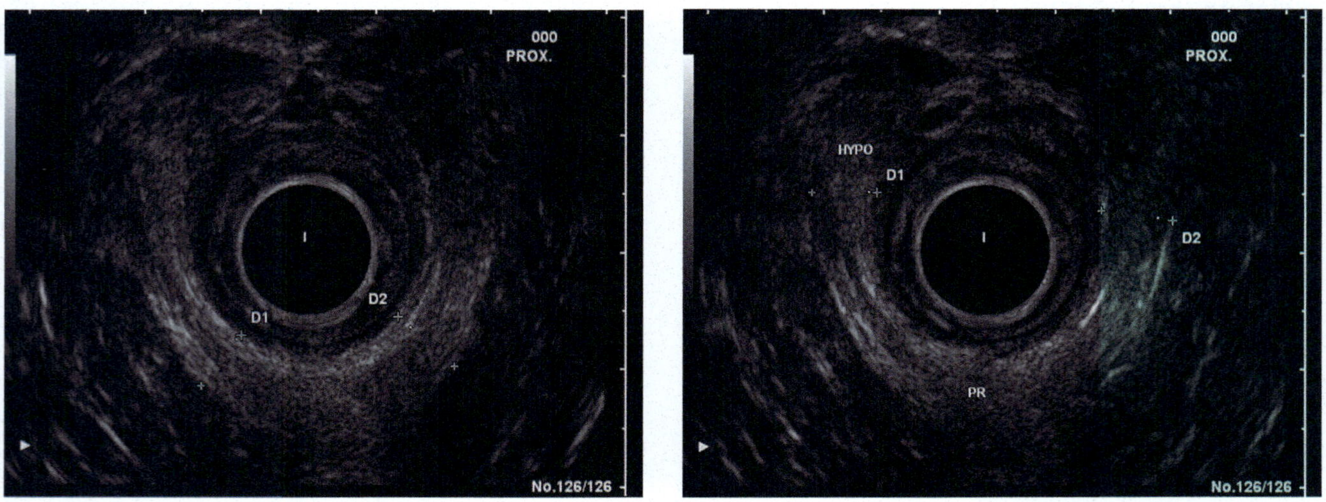

(a) (b)

Figure 8.1 (a) Levator ani muscle with the puborectal part (PR) in between markers. (b) The more distant parts of this muscle often show a more inhomogeneous and hypoechoic appearance (Hypo).

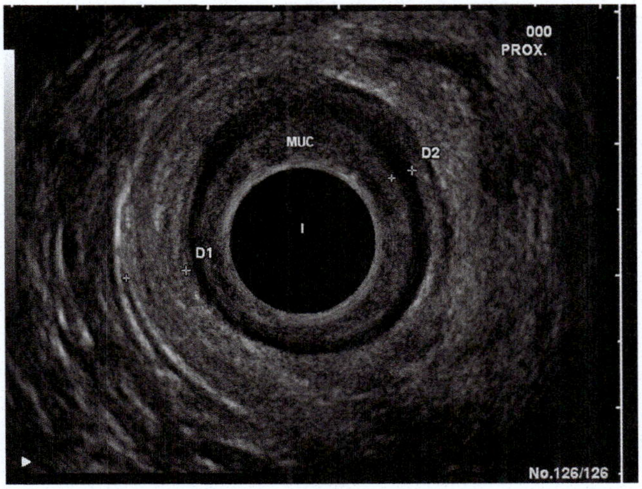

Figure 8.2 Internal anal sphincter (echo-poor) and external anal sphincter (echo-rich). The superficial layer of the anal canal is also indicated (MUC).

The EAS continues into the puborectal muscle (PRM) at the cranial margin of the anal canal, which is of importance for the delineation of ischiorectal and pelvirectal fossae. More orally the muscular structures are no longer vertically imaged so that this part of the muscle yields a weaker and less defined image (Video 8.1). At this level the os coccygeum with the coccygeal ligament can be also delineated. Ventrally this broad muscle layer reaches the inferior part of the pubic bone with inclusion of the urethra and the inferior part of the prostate or the vagina, respectively.

Coming back to gender differences, one has to keep in mind that the anal canal is generally 0.5–1.0 cm longer in males and the three different parts of the EAS are configured cylindrically around the anus, which means that the muscle shape and length is roughly the same ventrally and dorsally. In contrast, the three sections of the EAS are fused to a narrow band ventrally at the level of the pars superficialis in females. The notion of this anatomical difference is of importance in order not to misinterpret normal anatomical findings.

Normal sphincter values are highly dependent on age, sex, and examination technique parameters (Table 8.2). The less pronounced echo-poor IAS can be visualized more distally than the PRM and EAS (see below).

Internal anal sphincter level

The IAS can regularly be seen as a homogeneous echo-poor layer with a thickness of 2–4 mm, without any relevant gender-dependent differences, a little more distally than the EAS (Figure 8.2). The anal mucosa and the IAS muscle are

Table 8.2 Normal sphincter values. This is highly dependent on age, sex, and probe diameter, since the measured thickness depends on the probes used, as an increasing probe diameter will lead to a thinning of the surrounding structures.

M. sphincter ani internus	1.5–4.0 mm
M. sphincter ani externus	5–10 mm

considered the continuation of the inner rectal ring muscle. However, the measured thickness depends on the probes used, as an increasing probe diameter will lead to a thinning of the surrounding structures. The echo texture and thickness of the IAS tend to increase with age. The normal thickness, however, does not exceed 4 mm even in the elderly.

The intersphincteric space with fibers of the corrugator (or longitudinal) muscle as a continuation of the rectal external longitudinal muscle layer is seen endosonographically as a thin echo-poor layer containing echo-rich connective tissue septa representing the border areas of the echo-poor IAS and the first less echogenic layer of the EAS. It can be identified a little above 2 cm from the anocutaneous line. At this level the fossa ischiorectalis, the anococcygeal ligament, and the os coccygeum can be visualized. Additional points of orientation at this level are the radix penis with the ischiocavernosus muscle and the ramus ossis ischii. At this level also the echo-rich border area between the ultrasound probe and the mucosa (or the anal cutis), the echo-poor extremely thin mucosa which often cannot be recognized as a defined layer due to a lacking muscularis and its very thin diameter, and the echo-rich submucosa (and subcutis) can be differentiated leading to the structures of the lowest level.

Cutis and subcutis

The last section shows the cutis, the transitional epithelium, and the subcutis with the transition to the submucosa and more orally the IAS surrounded by the superficial and profound transverse perineal muscle and the fossa ischiorectalis as already described. The submucosa and the subcutaneous connective tissue appear as a homogeneous echogenic layer increasing in thickness from the superior to the inferior margin of the anal canal. The transversus perinei profundus and superficialis muscles and the ischiocavernosus muscle can also be imaged by ERUS.

Chapter video clip

Video 8.1 Radial array EUS of the distal rectum and anal canal in a male subject. Source: Hitachi, Ltd.

2 Upper and Lower GI EUS

9 Esophageal Cancer

Armen Eskandari and Syed M. Abbas Fehmi
Division of Gastroenterology and Hepatology, University of California San Diego, La Jolla, CA, USA

Introduction

In 2018 there were more than 570 000 new cases of esophageal cancer in the world [1]. According to the American Cancer Society, in 2019, 17 650 new cases of esophageal cancer will be diagnosed in the USA with an attributable 16 080 deaths. The incidence of esophageal adenocarcinoma continues to rise in the USA, albeit at a slower rate. In the last 15 years, the role of endoscopic ultrasound (EUS) has evolved in the management of esophageal cancer, with EUS currently essential for accurate locoregional staging and addressing the key management question of operability.

Updated American Joint Committee on Cancer staging guidelines for esophageal cancer 2017 and implications for endosonographers

The eighth edition of the American Joint Committee on Cancer (AJCC)/Union for International Cancer Control (UICC) includes clinical, pathologic and neoadjuvant staging groups to facilitate staging in an increasing number of patients undergoing chemoradiation prior to esophagectomy and in patients who may not undergo esophagectomy at all due to advanced disease (Table 9.1).

The important changes affecting the endosonographer in daily practice include a change in the definition of tumor location from the upper border of the tumor in the seventh edition to the epicenter of the tumor in the eighth edition. The location of the primary tumor is defined by the epicenter of cancer in centimeters from the incisors (cervical esophagus 15 cm to <20 cm; upper thoracic esophagus 20 cm to <25 cm; middle thoracic esophagus 25 cm to <30 cm; and lower esophagus 30–40 cm). In addition, cancers involving the esophagogastric junction (EGJ) whose epicenter is within 2 cm of the cardia are stage grouped similar to lower thoracic esophageal cancer. EGJ tumors with their epicenter located more than 2 cm into the proximal stomach are staged as stomach cancers, as are all cardia cancers not involving the EGJ.

The eighth edition of the TNM classification is shown in Table 9.1. As in the previous edition, stage groupings are separate for squamous cell cancer and adenocarcinoma; however, the criteria for T, N, and M stage designation for the two histologic types is similar.

Role of EUS in staging of esophageal cancer

The locoregional staging of esophageal cancer is most accurately done by EUS when compared to any other imaging modality, including computed tomography (CT), positron emission tomography (PET), or magnetic resonance imaging (MRI). Accurate staging helps predict the prognosis, optimize management strategy, and provides a standard platform for comparison of patients for research purposes.

It is recommended to perform a standard upper endoscopy prior to EUS examination. The endoscopy report should mention the location of the tumor, presence and degree of obstruction, presence of skip lesions, and whether EUS staging was incomplete due to obstruction precluding passage of the echoendoscope. EUS can examine the different wall layers of the esophagus, which forms the basis for its superiority over other imaging modalities.

The reported accuracy of EUS for T staging is 80–90%. Accuracy for distinguishing T3 or T4 disease from T1 or T2 disease is better than distinguishing T1a or T1b from T2 disease. In our practice, the role of EUS in the setting of Barrett's esophagus for Tis lesion (defined as high-grade dysplasia) is to exclude periesophageal lymphadenopathy or a mass. T1 lesions can be divided into T1a or T1b depending on whether tumor is

Atlas of Endoscopic Ultrasonography, Second Edition. Edited by Frank Gress, Thomas Savides, Brenna Casey, and Everson L. A. Artifon.

Companion website: www.wiley.com/go/gress/atlas

Table 9.1 American Joint Committee on Cancer (AJCC) staging of esophageal cancer, 2017 (eighth edition).

TX	Primary tumor cannot be assessed
T0	No evidence of primary tumor
Tis	High-grade dysplasia
T1	Tumor invades the lamina propria, muscularis mucosae, or submucosa
T1a	Tumor invades the lamina propria or muscularis mucosae
T1b	Tumor invades the submucosa
T2	Tumor invades the muscularis propria
T3	Tumor invades the adventitia
T4	Tumor invades adjacent structures
T4a	Resectable tumor invading the pleura, pericardium, diaphragm, azygos vein and peritoneum
T4b	Unresectable tumor invading the other adjacent structures such as aorta, vertebral body, trachea, etc.
NX	Regional lymph nodes cannot be assessed
N0	No regional lymph node metastasis
N1	Metastasis in 1–2 regional lymph nodes
N2	Metastasis in 3–6 regional lymph nodes
N3	Metastasis in 7 or more regional lymph nodes
M0	No distant metastasis
M1	Distant metastasis

limited to mucosa (Figure 9.1) versus submucosal invasion (Figures 9.2 and 9.3). If the tumor is observed to invade the fourth layer (muscularis propria or proper muscle layer), the tumor is classified as T2 (Figures 9.4 and 9.5). When the tumor invades through the muscularis propria into the adventitia, it is classified as a T3 lesion (Figures 9.6 and 9.7, and Video 9.1). The T4 stage has been revised in the updated guidelines. In addition to involvement of pleura, diaphragm, and pericardium, tumors that are found to invade the azygos vein and peritoneum are now also considered T4a and hence potentially resectable (Figure 9.8) Involvement of the aorta, trachea, and vertebral body indicates T4B disease which is considered unresectable (Figure 9.9).

For N staging, EUS has an accuracy of 75–80%. Endoscopic ultrasound-guided fine needle aspiration (EUS-FNA) can improve accuracy, but care must be taken that the needle does not penetrate the area of the tumor in order to prevent false-positive results. The positive predictive value of four subjective endosonographic features of lymph nodes (round, hypoechoic, sharp edges, and size 1 cm or more in short axis) is about 90%. If these are present, there is less need to do FNA. In the 2017 TNM classification, the N component has been subclassified according to the number of regional lymph nodes containing metastasis (N1 indicating metastases in one to two regional nodes; N2 metastases in three to six nodes; and N3 metastases in seven or more). Additionally, celiac lymphadenopathy distant from the primary tumor site is no longer considered distant metastasis in the new classification. M1 disease is now defined as metastasis to non-regional lymph nodes or distant sites. EUS can visualize liver metastases of less than 1 cm or even malignant ascites, and EUS via FNA can provide endoscopic opportunity for providing a tissue diagnosis for either of these findings.

Limitations

It is important to note that edema, cellular infiltration, and neoplastic masses can produce an endosonographic image of a thickened esophageal wall upstaging early disease. EUS is considerably less accurate (40%) for restaging of disease after chemoradiation therapy secondary to the associated fibrosis and inflammation. Recent studies suggest that FNA of even benign-appearing lymph nodes may increase the sensitivity (50% vs. 75%) and specificity (78% vs. 100%) of qualitative EUS [2] in this setting. The sensitivity of EUS in detecting pathologic complete response (ypCR) has been reported from as low as 10% to as high as 96.4% [3,4].

Impact of EUS staging on management

The management for early disease may differ somewhat between institutions, but the treatment outcome for patients is highly stage dependent. Therefore, in most circumstance a multimodal approach to preoperative staging is adopted which includes cross-sectional imaging with CT or hybrid PET/CT. With increasing use of PET/CT, the role of EUS has decreased in some practices. However, a recent study on 279 patients who received upfront PET and were also staged with EUS showed that EUS impacted the management plan in 28.7% of patients including change in radiation field in 22.6%, curability in 1.8%, and lymphadenectomy in 17.2%. Additionally, FNA provided definitive information regarding lymph node status in 7.5% [5]. For early-stage disease, operability is the key question that heavily depends on accurate T staging by EUS. Currently, for Tis or T1a disease in the absence of any lymph nodes, the endoscopic approach is usually the preferred option. Even for T1b disease, endoscopic mucosal resection (EMR) has usually been done to confirm submucosal invasion when endoscopic submucosal dissection (ESD) is not available. The role of ESD is rapidly evolving for early/superficial disease in the USA and is well established outside the USA (e.g. Japan and Europe). A recent practice update from the American Gastroenterology Association recommends consideration of ESD in selected patients with Barrett's esophagus if they have a large or bulky area of nodularity, confirmed or suspicious submucosal invasion, or recurrent dysplasia. In some poor surgical candidates, ESD or other aggressive endoscopic therapy like cryoablation may also be offered. Usually for T2 disease with no obvious lymph node involvement, surgery is done. However, if lymph node involvement is suspected or it is T3 disease, neoadjuvant

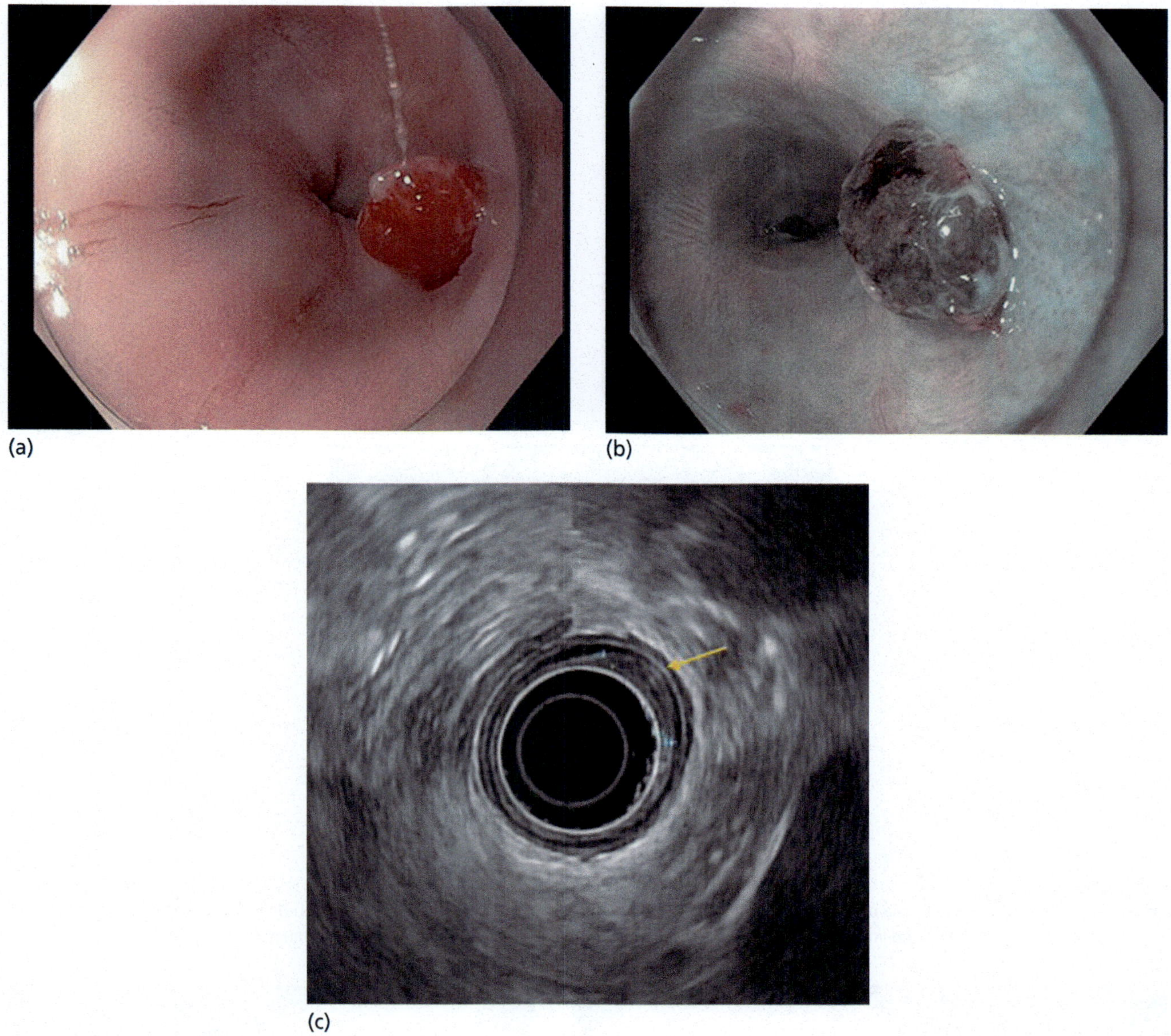

Figure 9.1 Distal esophageal adenocarcinoma shown to be T1a on pathology. (a) White light and (b) narrow band imaging; (c) EUS image shows intact submucosa (yellow arrow).

therapy followed by surgery is usually the preferred option. T4b disease is usually unresectable with no surgical opportunity for cure. The use of neoadjuvant therapy with subsequent surgery is becoming increasingly popular; this in turn poses the difficulty of restaging patients after neoadjuvant therapy. As described earlier, EUS performs poorly in patients who have undergone neoadjuvant therapy.

Technique

The endosonographer must be familiar with the patient's history (specifically the presence and degree of dysphagia) and the impact of EUS findings on management. It is advisable to perform an esophagogastroduodenoscopy (EGD) before EUS to confirm the extent of the lesion (for accurate staging), assess patency of the lumen (hence, the for need of dilation), and report skip lesions. In some centers, surgery is being offered for staging with an initial approach being minimally invasive; in most centers, though, EUS is used. The radial array echoendoscope is most frequently used due to its 360-degree imaging and ease of use. The standard technique is to do multiple pull-backs from the stomach into the proximal esophagus, paying close attention to the wall layers and periesophageal lymph nodes. Effort should be made to evaluate the liver for metastasis. For stenotic tumors not allowing passage of the usual 13-mm tip echoendoscopes, dilation to 15 mm or 45 Fr is usually required. Risks of dilation need to be

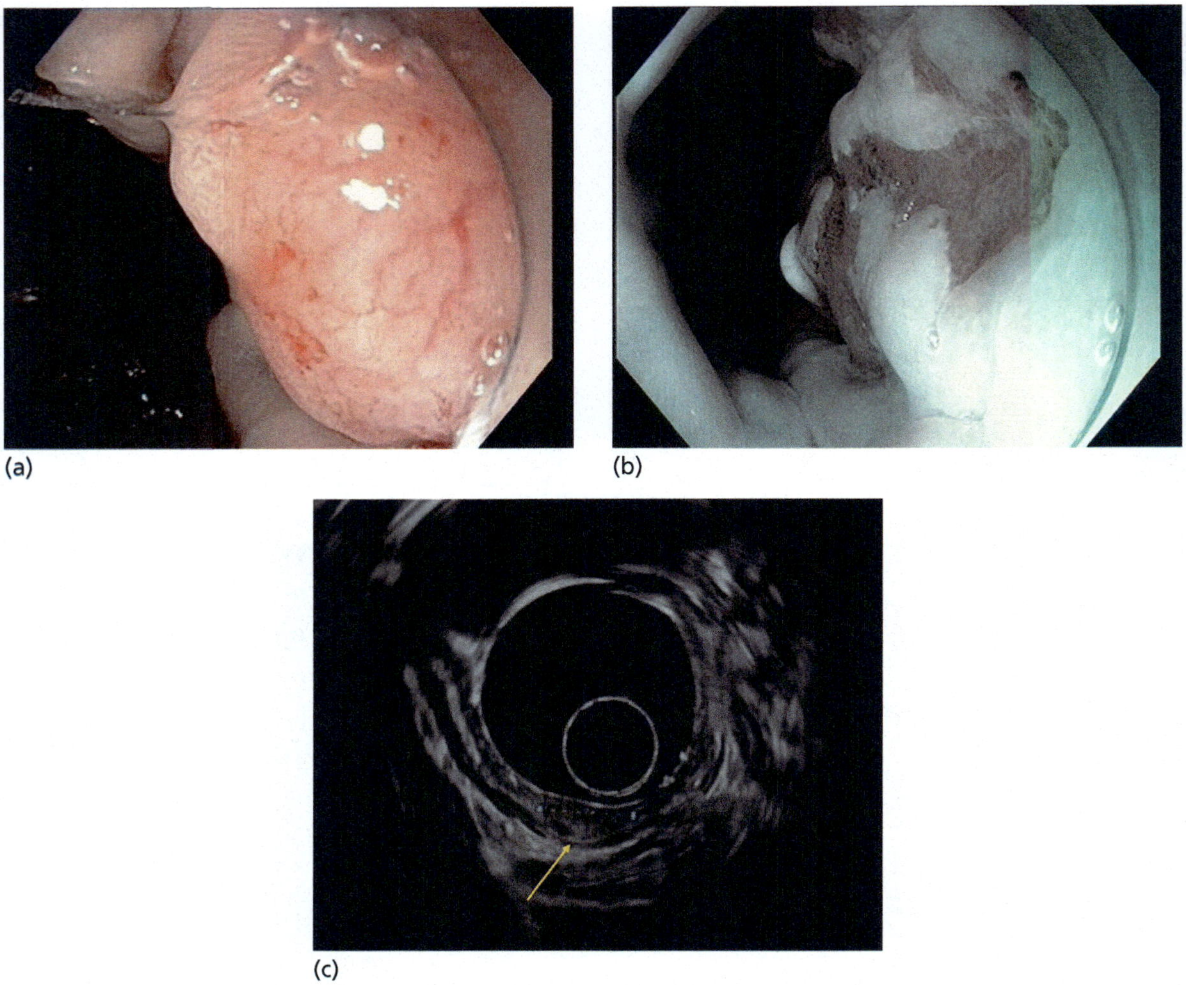

Figure 9.2 T1b adenocarcinoma in a background of Barrett's esophagus at the gastroesophageal junction. (a) High-definition white light image shows irregular pit pattern. (b) Narrow band imaging of the same lesion. (c) EUS image with yellow arrow showing intact muscularis propria.

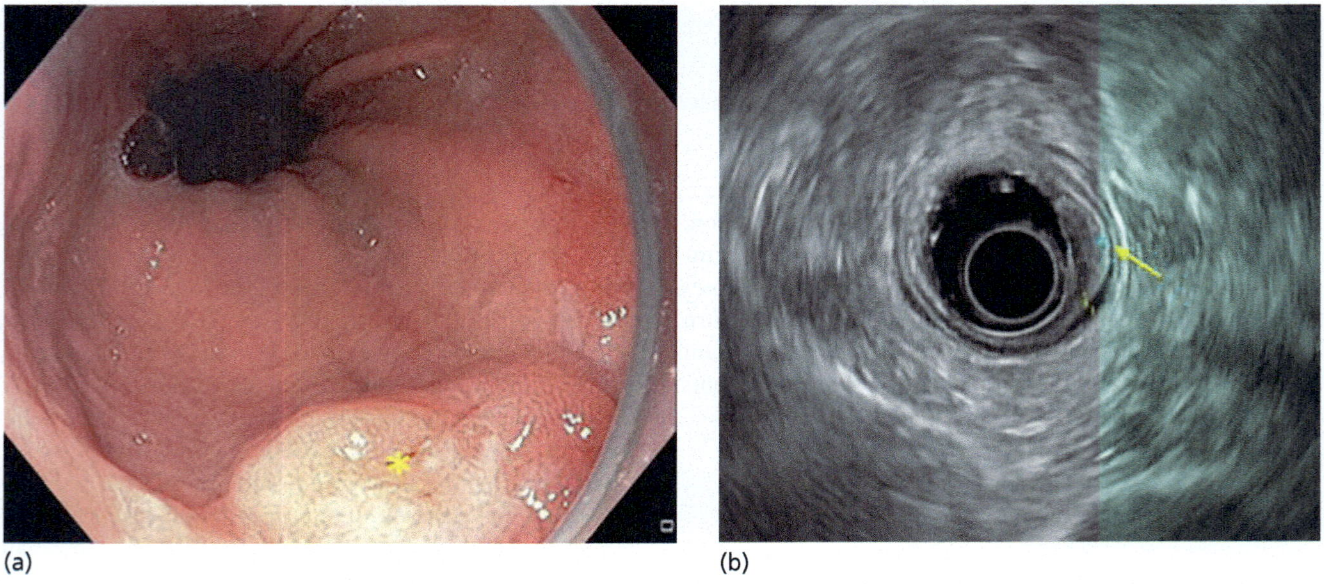

Figure 9.3 (a) T1b adenocarcinoma at the gastroesophageal junction with central depression shown by asterisk. (b) EUS image showing submucosal invasion but no involvement of muscularis propria shown by yellow arrow.

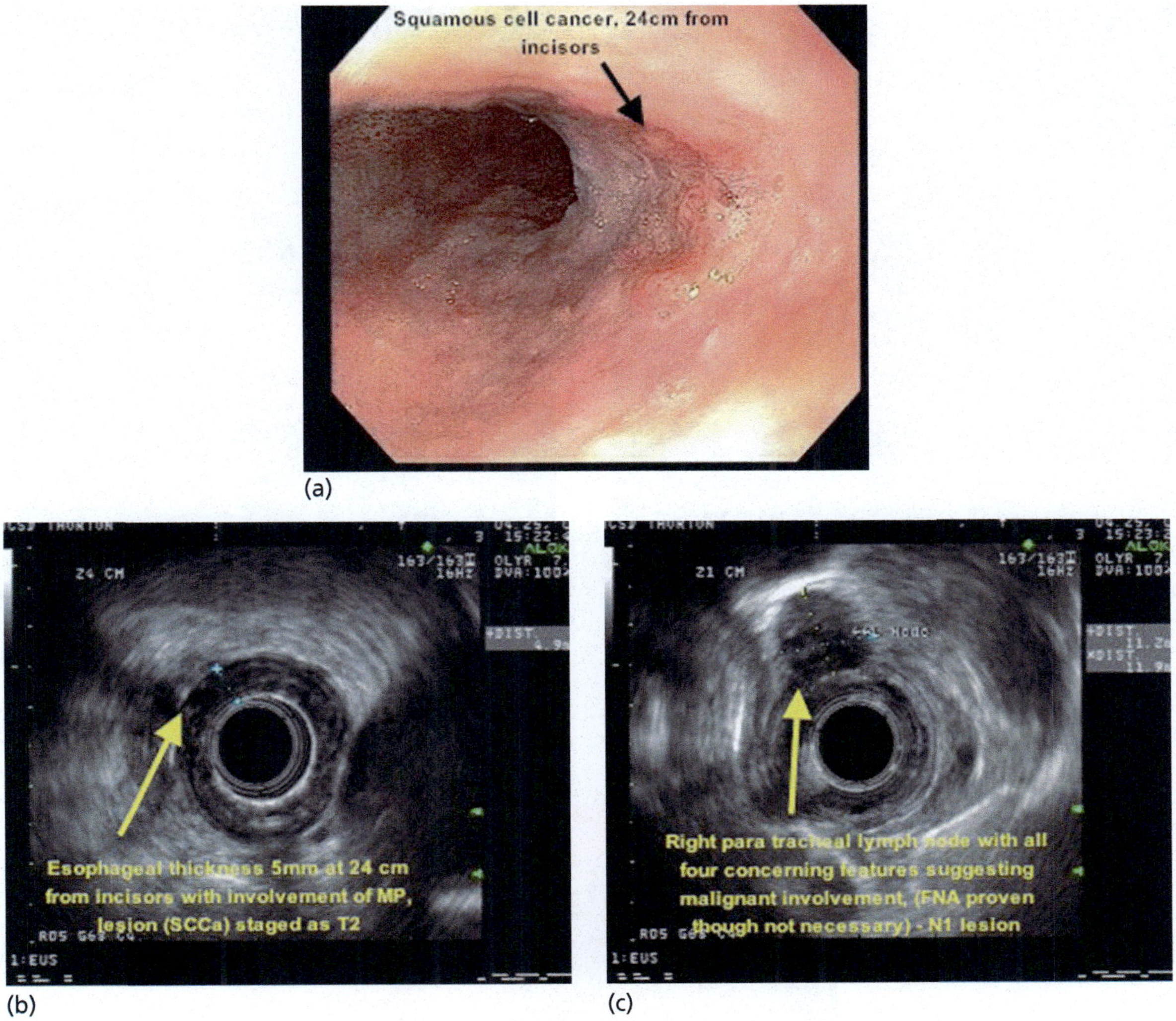

Figure 9.4 (a) T2N1Mx lesion, squamous cell cancer with ulceration 24 cm from incisors shown by yellow arrow. (b) EUS image showing invasion of muscularis propria (MP) but not through the MP, shown by arrow. (c) Malignant-appearing paratracheal lymph node also observed and marked by arrow. This has all four concerning features suggesting malignant involvement (fine needle aspiration [FNA] proven though not necessary). Since a total of two or less lymph nodes are observed during exam, lesion classified as N1 according to the eighth edition of the AJCC classification system.

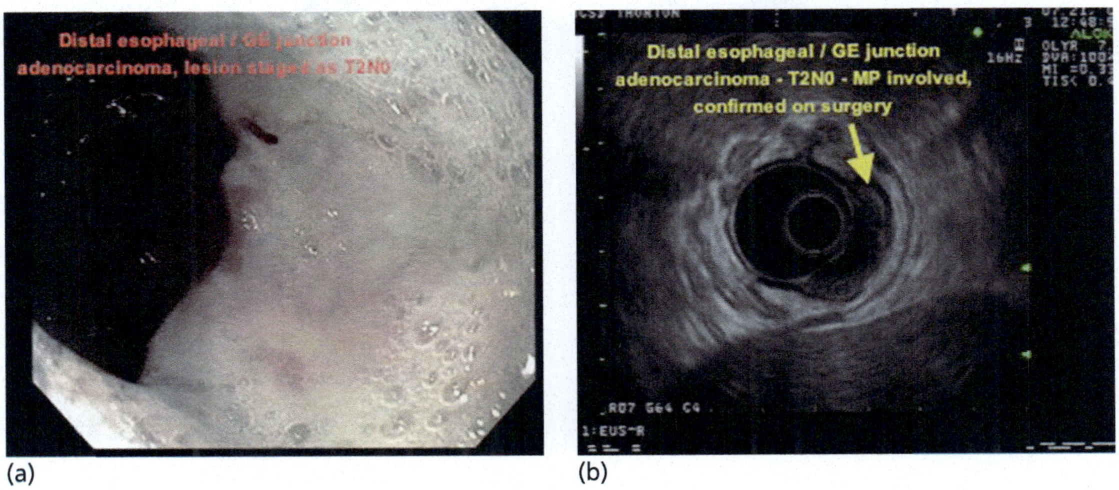

Figure 9.5 (a) T2N0Mx lesion, adenocarcinoma of lower thoracic esophagus involving gastroesophageal (GE) junction, marked by arrow. (b) EUS image showing invasion of muscularis propria (MP) but not through the MP, marked by arrow.

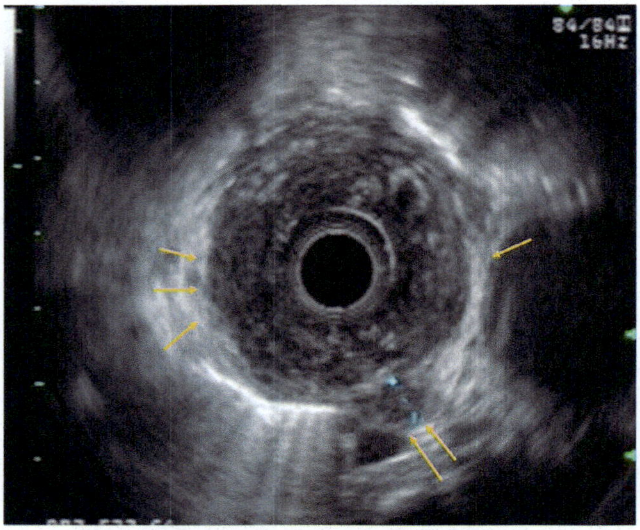

Figure 9.6 T3N3Mx lesion, adenocarcinoma involving the lower thoracic esophagus, lesion invading through the muscularis propria (MP) into the periesophageal fat marked by three arrows. Note malignant-appearing lymph node (LN) marked by double arrows; a total of eight such LNs were observed during the exam, making this an N3 lesion (according to the eighth edition of the AJCC guideline). Note also the intact plane between the lesion and aorta marked by single arrow.

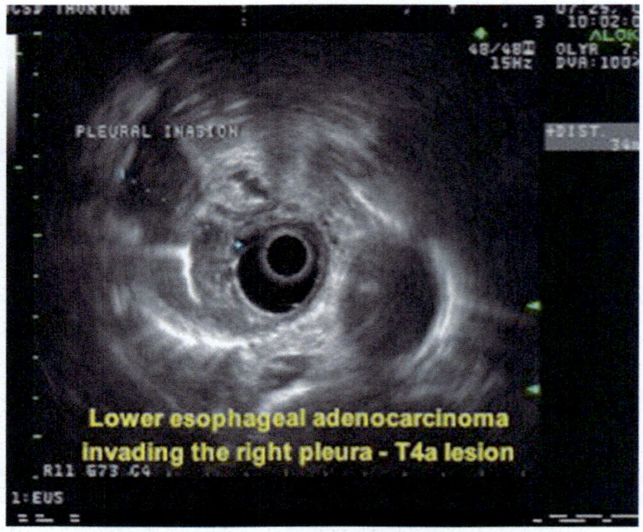

Figure 9.8 T4a lesion, adenocarcinoma in lower thoracic esophagus invading through the muscularis propria and the periesophageal fat into the right pleura (note made of loss of echogenic plane between lesion and right pleura). According to the eighth edition of the AJCC guideline, this is a potentially resectable lesion staged as T4a.

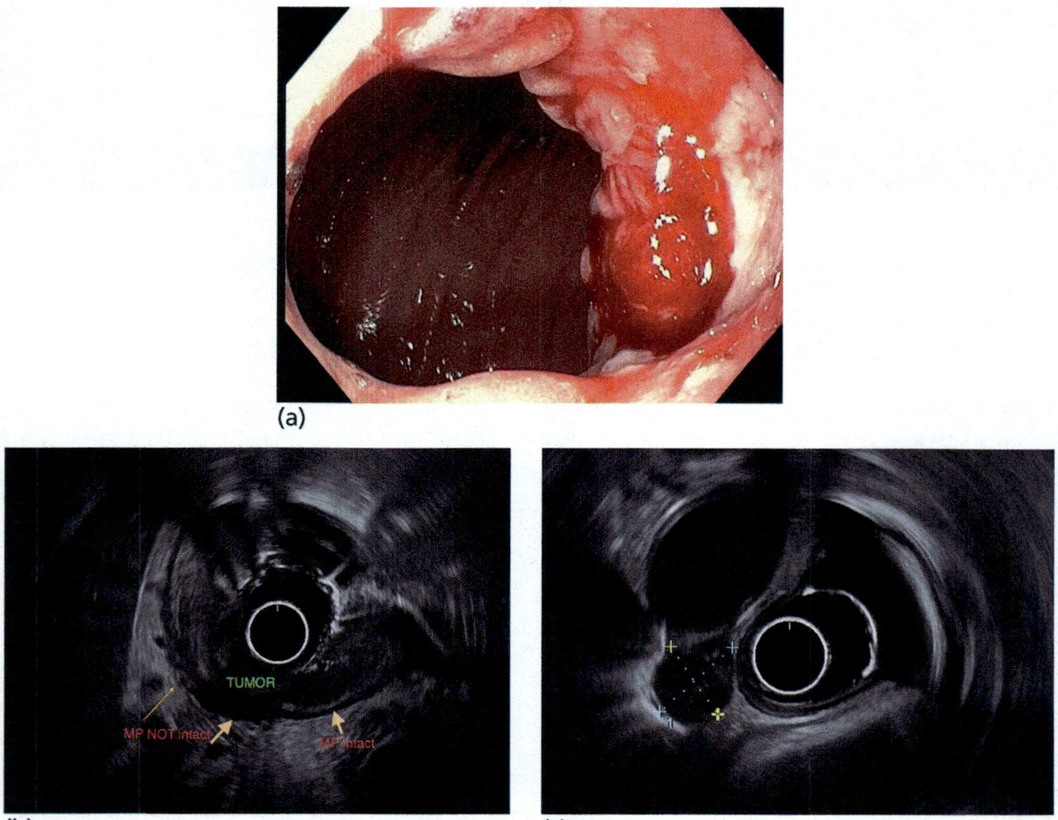

(a) (b) (c)

Figure 9.7 (a) T3N1Mx adenocarcinoma with friable mass at the gastroesophageal junction. (b) EUS image showing lesion invading through the muscularis propria (MP) into the periesophageal fat, marked by arrow. (c) Round, hypoechoic, symmetrical lymph node larger than 10 mm suggestive of malignancy.

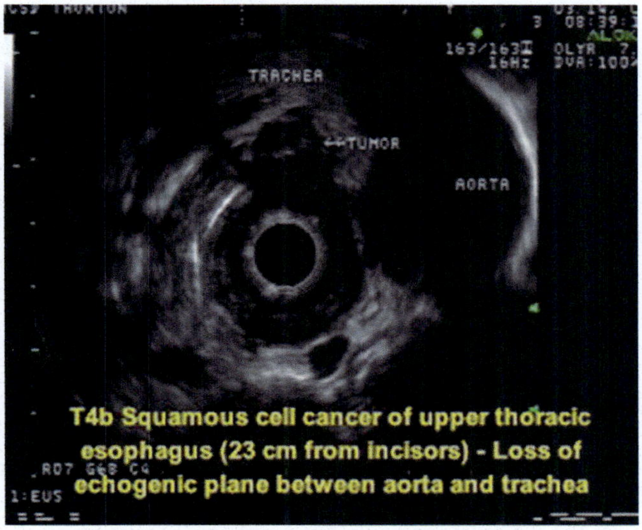

Figure 9.9 T4b lesion, squamous cell cancer in upper thoracic esophagus invading through the muscularis propria and the periesophageal fat into the aorta and trachea (note made of loss of echogenic plane between lesion and the aorta and trachea). According to the eighth edition of the AJCC guideline, this is an unresectable lesion staged as T4b.

weighed against perceived benefits of any additional information gained by passing the endoscope distal to the stenosis. Some strategies include use of thin non-optic probes or endobronchial scopes versus embedding the tip of a regular EUS scope in the proximal aspect of tumor and trying to obtain as much information as possible (T3 lesion or N1). Non-optic probes with high frequency can also be used to distinguish T1a and T1b lesions with high accuracy. However, with newer electronic EUS scopes and improved processors, imaging has improved so that high-frequency probes may not be routinely used. In addition, EMR is being increasingly utilized for better histologic assessment for mucosal versus submucosal involvement. When an obstructing tumor precludes passage of the echoendoscope, the report should mention that the examination may not be accurate.

Chapter video clip

Video 9.1 Esophageal cancer endosonography.

References

1. Bray F, Ferlay J, Soerjomataram I, et al. Global cancer statistics 2018: GLOBOCAN estimates of incidence and mortality worldwide for 36 cancers in 185 countries. *CA Cancer J Clin* 2018;68(6):394–424.
2. van der Bogt RD, van der Wilk GJ, Poley J-W, et al. Endoscopic ultrasound and fine-needle aspiration for the detection of residual nodal disease after neoadjuvant chemoradiotherapy for esophageal cancer. *Endoscopy* 2020;52(3):186–192.
3. de Gouw DJJM, Klarenbeek BR, Driessen M, et al. Detecting pathological complete response in esophageal cancer after neoadjuvant therapy based on imaging techniques: a diagnostic systematic review and meta-analysis. *J Thorac Oncol* 2019; 14(7):1156–1171.
4. van Rossum PSN, Goense L, Meziani J, et al. Endoscopic biopsy and EUS for the detection of pathologic complete response after neoadjuvant chemoradiotherapy in esophageal cancer: a systematic review and meta-analysis. *Gastrointest Endosc* 2016; 83(5):866–879.
5. Hulshoff JB, Mul VEM, de Boer HEM, et al. Impact of endoscopic ultrasonography on ^{18}F-FDG-PET/CT upfront towards patient specific esophageal cancer treatment. *Ann Surg Oncol* 2017;24(7):1828–1834.

10

EUS for Achalasia

Michael Chang
Department of Medicine, University of California San Diego, La Jolla, CA, USA

Introduction

Achalasia is characterized by impaired deglutitive relaxation of the lower esophageal sphincter (LES), considered to be a result of neuronal degeneration in the myenteric plexus and consequently an imbalance between excitatory and inhibitory neurons. Achalasia can present at any age, with a peak incidence between 30 and 60 years, without a racial or gender predilection. The etiology of achalasia is typically idiopathic, but can also be associated with diseases such as Chagas, sarcoidosis, or malignancies.

Clinical presentation and diagnosis

Progressively worsening dysphagia for both liquids and solids is present in over 90% of patients with achalasia. Other symptoms may include chest fullness, heartburn, regurgitation, early satiety, and weight loss.

High-resolution esophageal manometry is the gold standard for diagnosing and classifying achalasia. An elevated median integrated relaxation pressure (IRP) along with absent peristalsis is suggestive of type I achalasia (classic achalasia), or of type II achalasia when accompanied with panesophageal pressurization. In type III achalasia, esophageal contractility will be spastic in the setting of an elevated median IRP. Barium esophagram, a helpful complementary diagnostic test, may demonstrate a dilated esophagus with a classic "bird's beak" appearance in type I or II achalasia. In the case of type III achalasia, corkscrewing in the esophageal body may be seen on barium esophagram. Functional lumen imaging probe is another complementary diagnostic tool in achalasia, in which distensibility at the esophagogastric junction is reduced and contractile response to distension in the esophageal body is abnormal. All patients with a diagnosis of achalasia or suspected achalasia should undergo upper endoscopy to confirm the diagnosis and rule out esophageal malignancy.

Role of EUS in achalasia

Endoscopic ultrasound (EUS) can play an important role in the evaluation of achalasia. EUS can evaluate for malignancy as a cause of symptoms, sample suspicious lesions via a fine needle aspirate, and also finely measure the thickness of the esophageal circular wall layer. EUS measurement of the length and thickness of the esophageal circular wall layer can help to tailor the myotomy length for therapies such as peroral endoscopic myotomy (POEM) or surgical Heller myotomy. In particular, in type III, or spastic, achalasia, the circular muscle layer is often thicker proximal to the LES at varying lengths and benefits from proximally extended myotomy. When using modern EUS endoscopes in conjunction with newer processors and high frequency (10 Hz or higher), EUS imaging of the muscularis propria can easily delineate the circular and longitudinal muscle wall layers. The innermost, hypoechoic muscle wall layer is the circular muscle wall layer and it is separated from the longitudinal, outermost, muscle wall layer by a hyperechoic interface of connective tissue (Figure 10.1). The normal thickness of the circular wall layer of the esophagus is typically 0.3–1 mm (Figure 10.2). In patients with achalasia the thickness of the circular wall layer can vary from 1.5 to 6 mm (Figures 10.3–10.7).

Our approach for evaluating the muscle thickness and length in achalasia is to use a radial echoendoscope to measure the circular muscle wall layer thickness from the gastroesophageal junction and every centimeter proximally

Atlas of Endoscopic Ultrasonography, Second Edition. Edited by Frank Gress, Thomas Savides, Brenna Casey, and Everson L. A. Artifon.

Companion website: www.wiley.com/go/gress/atlas

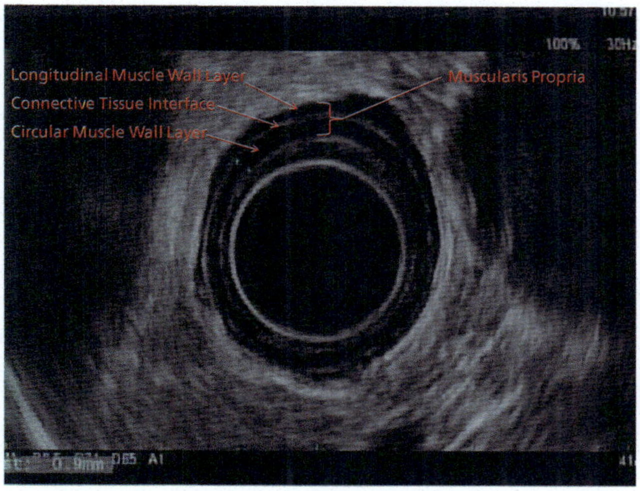

Figure 10.1 The muscularis propria is divided into two layers, the outer longitudinal muscle wall layer and the inner circular muscle wall layer, separated by a connective tissue interface.

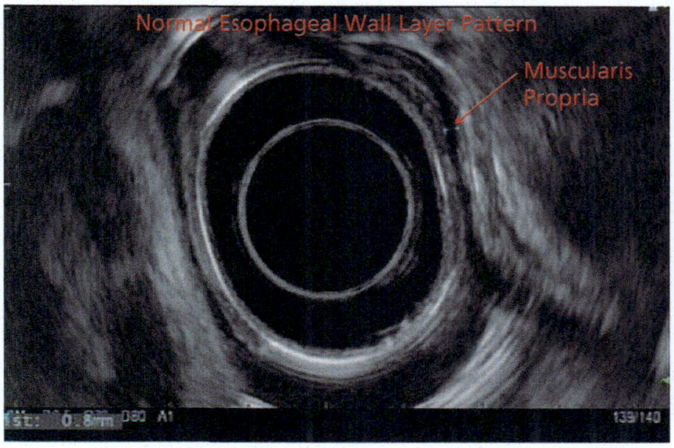

Figure 10.2 Normal esophageal wall layer pattern. Normal thickness of muscularis propria demonstrated here is 0.8 mm.

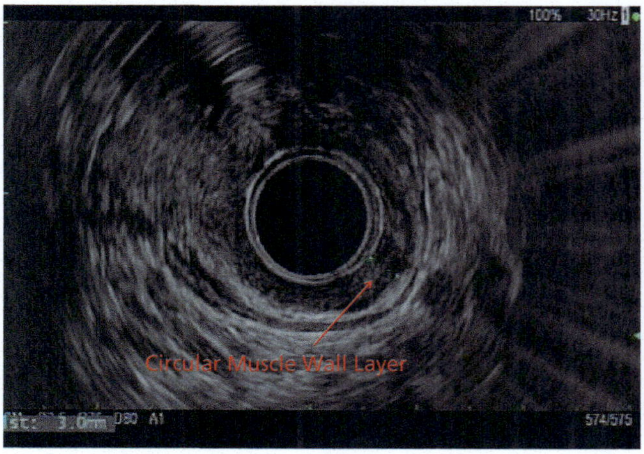

Figure 10.3 Thickening of the circular muscle wall layer to 3 mm in a patient with achalasia.

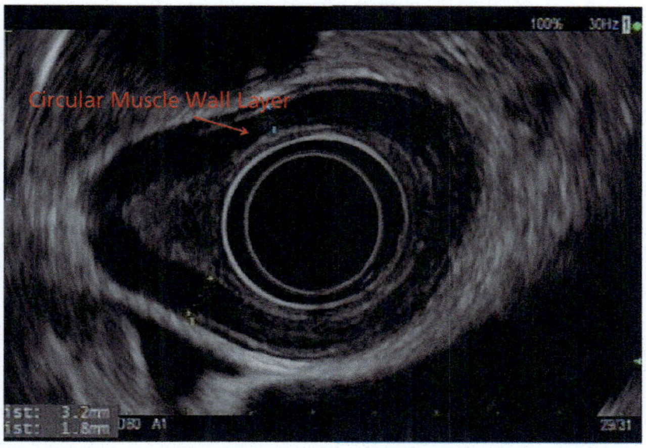

Figure 10.4 Thickening of the circular muscle wall layer to an average of 2.5 mm in a patient with achalasia.

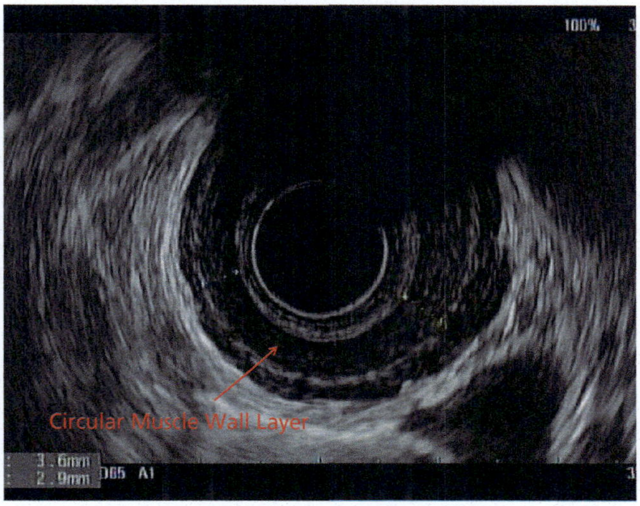

Figure 10.5 Thickening of the circular muscle wall layer to an average of 3.25 mm in a patient with achalasia.

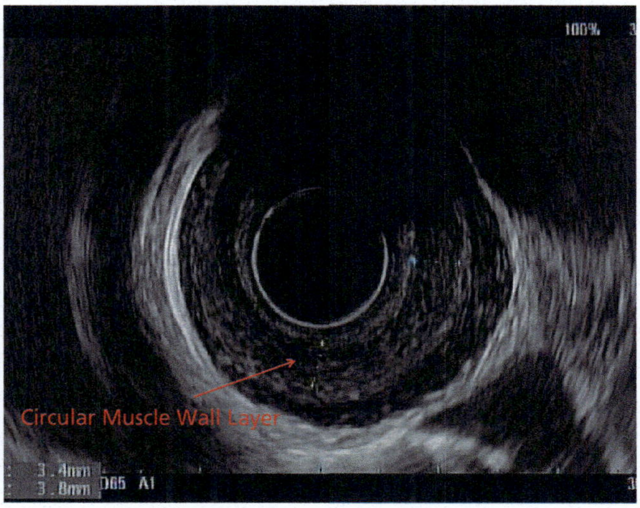

Figure 10.6 Thickening of the circular muscle wall layer to an average of 3.6 mm in a patient with achalasia.

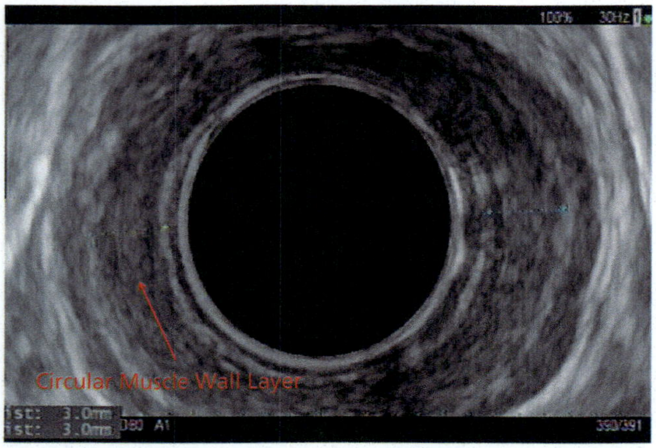

Figure 10.7 Uniform thickening of the circular muscle wall layer to an average of 3 mm in a patient with achalasia.

as measured in distance from the incisors. The measurements continue until the circular wall layer thickness becomes normal or to the level of the upper esophageal sphincter. Some patients with achalasia will have a very dilated esophagus and the thickness of the circular wall layer may appear to vary at a given distance from the incisors (see Figures 10.4–10.6). In such cases we measure two or three sites along the circular wall layer and take the average thickness. Care should be taken to use only the minimal amount of EUS balloon inflation necessary to maintain mucosal contact and the endoscope tip should be kept centrally within the esophageal lumen to minimize overdistending or stretching the esophageal wall layers.

11 Malignant Mediastinal Lesions

M. Babitha Reddy[1], David H. Robbins[1], and Mohamad A. Eloubeidi[2]

[1] Lenox Hill Hospital, New York, NY, USA

[2] American University of Beirut School of Medicine, Beirut, Lebanon

Transesophageal endoscopic ultrasound (EUS) allows imaging of posterior mediastinal lymph nodes, which is where lung cancer as well as other cancers can metastasize. Additionally, large lung tumors abutting the esophagus can be imaged, as can primary posterior mediastinal lung tumors. EUS-guided biopsies can be performed with either transesophageal endoscopic ultrasound-guided fine needle aspiration (EUS-FNA) or endobronchial ultrasound-guided fine needle aspiration (EBUS-FNA).

The EUS characteristics of malignant lymph nodes include short axis diameter greater than 10 mm, round shape, well demarcated, and hypoechoic echotexture. Malignant mediastinal masses are generally greater than 3 cm in short axis diameter.

Staging of lung cancer is based on the American Thoracic Society lymph node map (Figure 11.1). Transesophageal EUS can visualize the paratracheal lymph nodes (station 2), posterior aorto-pulmonic window lymph nodes (station 5),

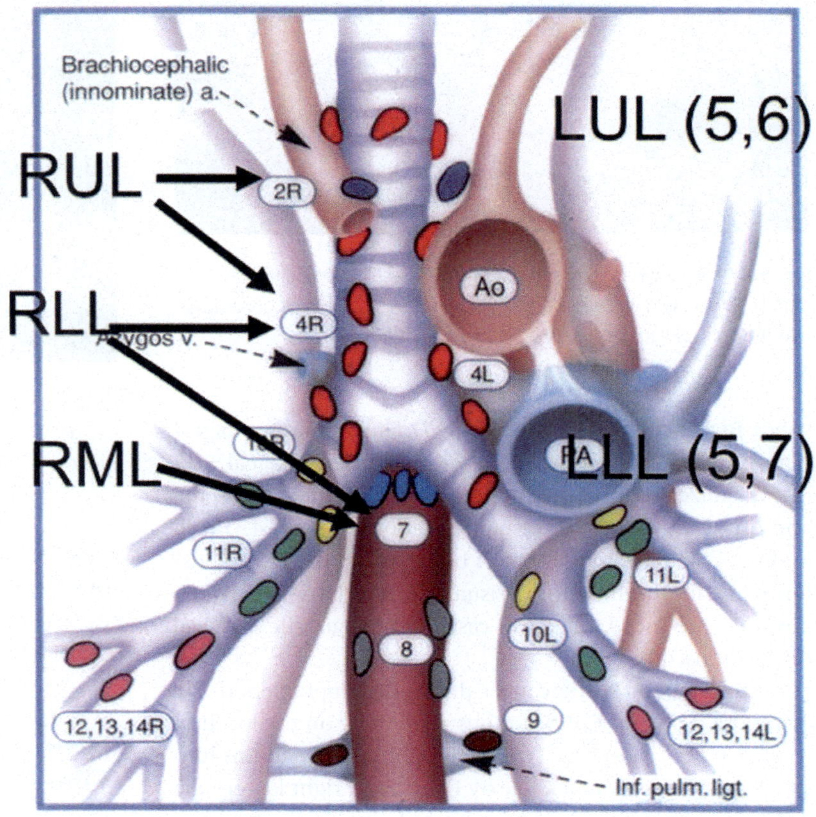

Figure 11.1 American Thoracic Society staging diagram for posterior mediastinal lymph nodes. Note that station 2 is paratracheal lymph nodes, station 5 is aorto-pulmonic window, station 7 is subcarinal, and station 8 is paraesophageal. The superimposed lung locations show the lymphatic drainage of each part of the lung. LLL, left lower lobe; LUL, left upper lobe; RLL, right lower lobe; RML, right middle lobe; RUL, right upper lobe.

Atlas of Endoscopic Ultrasonography, Second Edition. Edited by Frank Gress, Thomas Savides, Brenna Casey, and Everson L. A. Artifon.

Companion website: www.wiley.com/go/gress/atlas

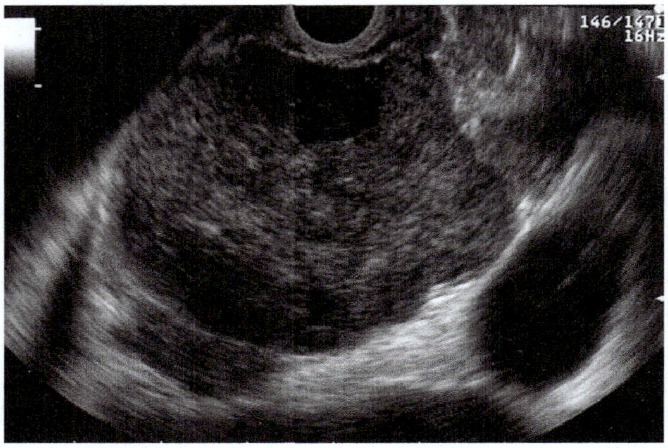

Figure 11.2 Metastatic posterior mediastinal melanoma. Endoscopic ultrasound-guided fine needle aspiration (EUS-FNA) along with immunostains confirmed recurrent metastatic melanoma in the mediastinum.

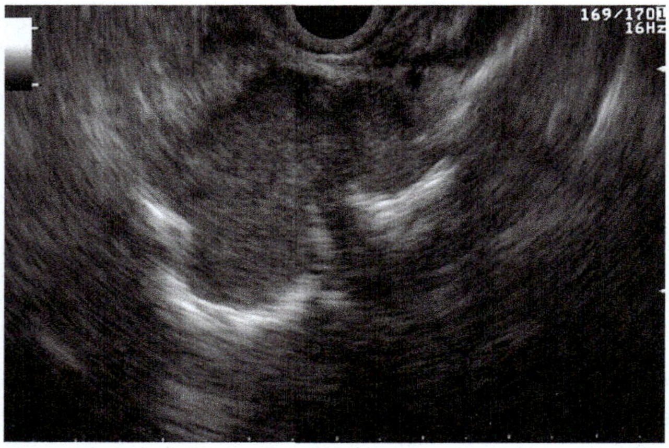

Figure 11.3 Renal cell cancer metastasis. The lesion was identified slightly above the gastroesophageal junction. Endoscopic ultrasound (EUS) was the only non-surgical approach to reach this lesion.

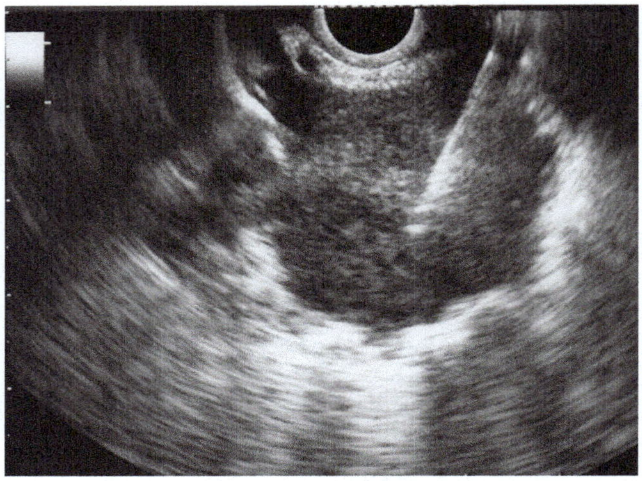

Figure 11.4 Lung cancer mass. Endoscopic ultrasound-guided fine needle aspiration (EUS-FNA) of a centrally located mass confirmed primary non-small cell lung cancer.

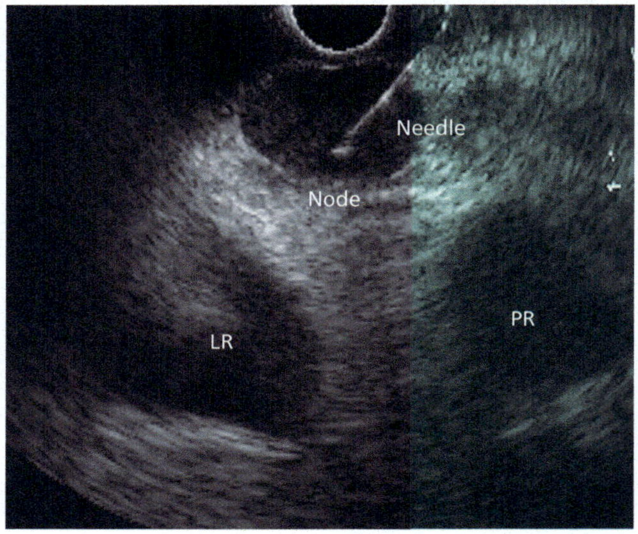

Figure 11.5 Malignant lymph node. The needle is within the rounded, well-demarcated, hypoechoic lymph node. LA, left atrium; PA, pulmonary artery.

subcarinal lymph nodes (station 7), and paraesophageal lymph nodes (station 8). In addition, transesophageal EUS can visualize other sites of metastases such as the left adrenal and the liver. EBUS can visualize stations 1, 2, 3, 4, 7, 10, and 11. Using a combination of both, nearly the entire posterior mediastinum can be visualized and biopsied, which obviates the need in most cases for diagnostic surgical mediastinoscopy.

Intrapulmonary lung cancer drains to lymphadenopathy at various EUS and EBUS stations depending on the location of the cancer (Figure 11.1). The right upper lobe drains into stations 2R and 4R, accessible by EBUS. The right lower lobe drains into stations 4R and 7 accessible by EBUS and EUS, respectively. The right middle lobe drains into station 7 which is accessible by EBUS and EUS. Recent case series demonstrated safety in sampling lymph nodes and intrapulmonary masses at station 6, lateral to the aorta, via the trans-aortic approach. The left upper lobe drains into stations 5 and 6 accessible by EUS and the left lower lobe drains into stations 5 and 7 accessible by EUS and EBUS (Figures 11.2–11.5).

Chapter video clips

Video 11.1 EUS-FNA Tru-cut biopsy of large posterior mediastinal mass.

Video 11.2 EUS-FNA of malignant lymph node in the posterior aortopulmonic window (station 5).

12 Benign Mediastinal Lesions

M. Babitha Reddy[1], David H. Robbins[1], and Mohamad A. Eloubeidi[2]
[1] Lenox Hill Hospital, New York, NY, USA
[2] American University of Beirut School of Medicine, Beirut, Lebanon

Benign mediastinal lymphadenopathy is a common incidental finding during endoscopic ultrasound (EUS) (Figures 12.1–12.5). Benign enlarged mediastinal lymph nodes can be reactive lymph nodes from exposure to a pulmonary infection, or granulomatous lymph nodes from sarcoid, histoplasmosis, or tuberculosis. Echogenic features include a crescent or triangular shape. Sometimes there is a central hyperechoic strand suggestive of a blood vessel. The borders are irregular and the short axis is often less than 1 cm. There are often multiple lymph nodes. It is not uncommon to encounter the benign "draping" subcarinal lymph node, which can be ovoid, intermediate in echogenicity, and up to 2 cm in length.

The most commonly found posterior mediastinal cystic lesions are congenital foregut cysts. These are classified as bronchogenic (defined as cystic lesions located away from the esophageal wall) and neuroenteric (found adherent to the esophageal wall such as an esophageal duplication cyst or a neuroenteric cyst). The malignant potential for duplication cysts is exceedingly low and clinical monitoring without intervention is acceptable. Heterogeneous echogenicity or internal mass is a suspicious finding for malignancy and is an acceptable indication for surgical resection and/or endoscopic sampling. Hyperechoic reflectors within cystic lesions may suggest thick, tenacious debris which can limit tissue

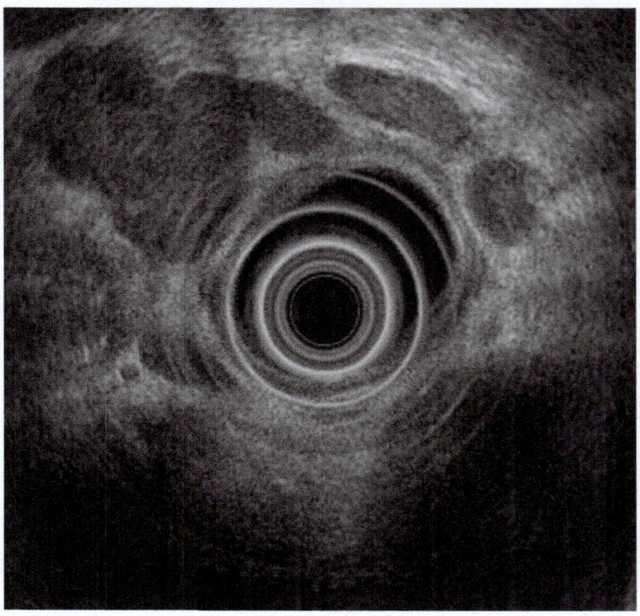

Figure 12.1 Benign subcarinal lymph nodes. Note the oval and triangular-shaped benign-appearing nodes.

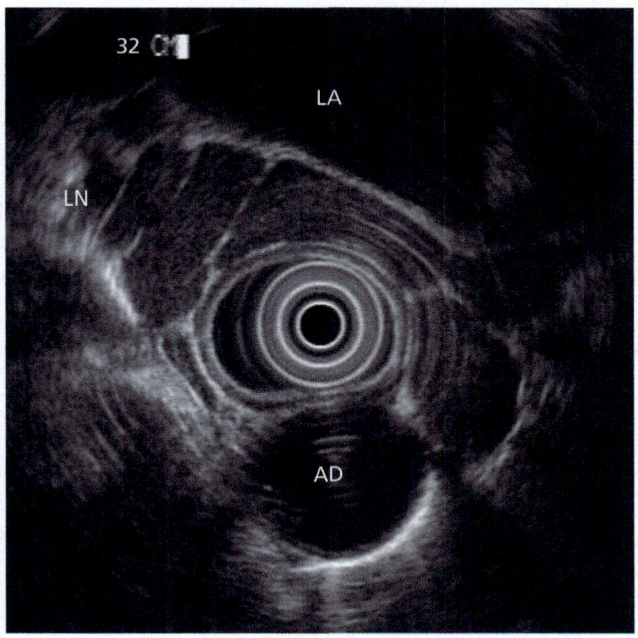

Figure 12.2 Sarcoid lymph nodes. Note the matted together, draping nodes with triangular and rectangular shapes in the subcarinal space. AO, aorta; LA, left atrium.

Atlas of Endoscopic Ultrasonography, Second Edition. Edited by Frank Gress, Thomas Savides, Brenna Casey, and Everson L. A. Artifon.

Companion website: www.wiley.com/go/gress/atlas

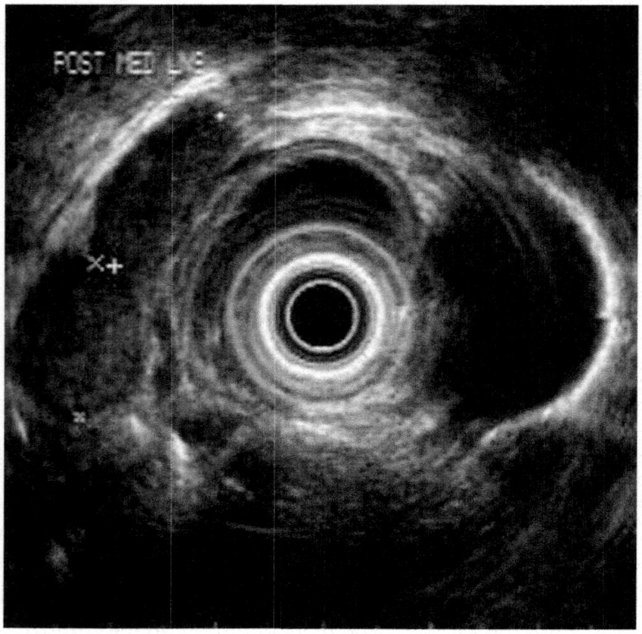

Figure 12.3 Cryptococcal lymph node. These were incidental lymph nodes found in a patient with acquired immunodeficiency syndrome (AIDS). Endoscopic ultrasound-guided fine needle aspiration (EUS-FNA) was important in establishing the diagnosis. Source: courtesy of Thomas Savides, MD.

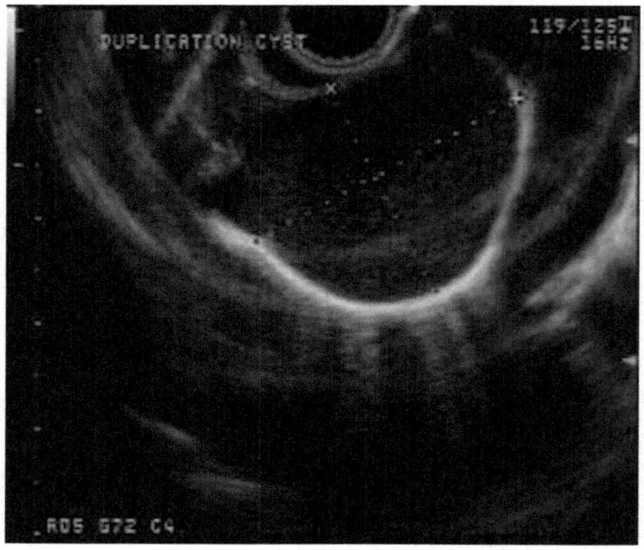

Figure 12.4 Duplication cyst. Note the anechoic appearance with acoustic enhancement of the cyst wall. Source: courtesy of Thomas Savides, MD.

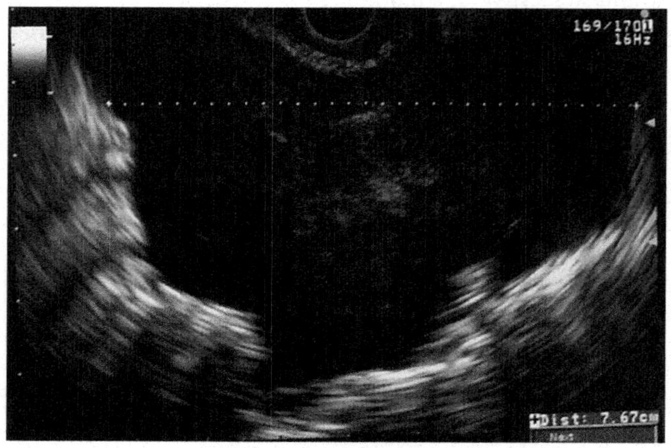

Figure 12.5 Enlarged lymph node due to *Blastocystis hominis* infection. Source: courtesy of John Deutsch, MD.

sampling for cytologic evaluation. In addition, intractable symptoms of chest pain, dyspnea, cough, or dysphagia secondary to an enlarging cystic lesion are other acceptable indications for intervention. The risk of infection and mediastinitis can be significant and therefore endoscopic ultrasound-guided fine needle aspiration (EUS-FNA) should be avoided as much as possible in suspected cysts. If FNA is performed due to uncertainty of the diagnosis, antibiotics should be given prior to and after the exam.

13 Gastric Cancer

Douglas O. Faigel[1] and Sarah A. Rodriguez[2]

[1] Mayo Clinic College of Medicine, Scottsdale, AZ, USA

[2] Oregon Health and Science University, Portland, OR, USA

Endoscopic ultrasound (EUS) is frequently employed for the diagnosis and staging of gastric cancers and lymphomas. This chapter reviews EUS imaging and staging of these malignancies.

The majority of gastric malignancies are adenocarcinomas. They are staged using the American Joint Commission on Cancer Staging TNM Classification (Table 13.1). These cancers may be either of the intestinal or diffuse type. The intestinal type arises from the mucosa and form discrete tumors. They appear as poorly circumscribed hypoechoic lesions which, at the edges, can be seen to be arising from the mucosal layers. T1 lesions are limited to the mucosa (first and second layers) or may penetrate into the submucosa (third layer) (Figure 13.1). There should be a demonstrable, intact, bright layer of submucosa between the lesion and the dark band of the muscularis propria (fourth layer). T2 lesions extend into but not through the muscularis propria (Figure 13.2). Endosonographically, T2 lesions extend through the bright third layer corresponding to where the tumor penetrates through the submucosa into the muscularis propria. However, the interface at the outer margin of the muscularis where it contacts the serosa (fourth and fifth layers) is smooth and undisturbed by the cancer. In T3 lesions the hypoechoic lesion extends completely through the fourth layer, and the serosa (fifth layer), which would otherwise be smooth, is interrupted and clearly invaded (Figure 13.3). Finger-like projections of tumor, termed pseudopodia, may be seen extending into the extragastric space. If the lesion extends into a local organ (e.g. liver, pancreas, spleen, diaphragm) or large vessel (e.g. aorta, celiac axis) it is classified as a T4-stage lesion (Figure 13.4).

Diffuse-type adenocarcinoma (also known as "linitis plastica") are poorly differentiated tumors that infiltrate the stomach wall. Histologically, they consist of single cells or small clusters of cells that contain large mucin vacuoles pushing the nucleus to one side to produce a signet ring appearance. The result of the diffuse infiltration by the cancer cells is a thickened, rigid stomach that has been likened to a leather bottle. Endoscopic ultrasound examination has been found to be exceptionally helpful in evaluating the patient with a suspected infiltrating malignancy. The normal stomach is 3–4 mm in thickness. When an infiltrating cancer is present, the stomach is thickened to greater than 4 mm, and one of two EUS patterns may be seen. In the first, there is complete loss of the normal five-layer pattern, with the markedly thickened wall assuming a homogeneously dark appearance. All layers of the stomach are generally involved and these tumors are stage T3. In the second EUS pattern, the thickened stomach maintains its five-layer pattern, but the muscularis propria (fourth layer) is a prominent, thick, dark band beneath a thickened, bright, third layer (submucosa) (Figure 13.5). Finding either of these patterns should prompt an aggressive search for an infiltrating malignancy. However, this finding is not specific to gastric adenocarcinoma and may be seen in metastatic cancer to the stomach (Figure 13.6) and in gastric lymphoma.

The stomach is the most common site for primary extranodal lymphoma, comprising one-fourth of all extranodal cases and at least half of all primary gastrointestinal (GI) lymphomas. Endoscopically, primary gastric lymphomas usually appear as an exophytic mass, although a more diffuse infiltration can occur, causing a linitis plastica appearance (Figures 13.7 and 13.8). Gastrointestinal lymphomas are staged differently than carcinomas (Table 13.2). Tumors confined to the GI tract are stage IE, and these patients have significantly higher survival rates than those with lymph node involvement or distant spread.

Atlas of Endoscopic Ultrasonography, Second Edition. Edited by Frank Gress, Thomas Savides, Brenna Casey, and Everson L. A. Artifon.

Companion website: www.wiley.com/go/gress/atlas

Table 13.1 American Joint Committee on Cancer (AJCC) Staging: TNM classification for gastric cancer (with permission from AJCC).

Tumor (T) stage	
Tx	Primary tumor cannot be assessed
T0	No evidence of primary tumor
T1s	Carcinoma in situ: intraepithelial tumor without invasion of the lamina propria
T1	Tumor limited to mucosa or submucosa
T2	Tumor invades muscularis propria or subserosa
T2a	Tumor invades muscularis propria
T2b	Tumor invades subserosa
T3	Tumor invades serosa
T4	Tumor invades adjacent structures
Tx	Primary tumor cannot be assessed
Nodal (N) stage	
Nx	Regional lymph nodes cannot be assessed
N0	No regional lymph node metastasis
N1	Metastasis in 1–6 regional lymph nodes
N2	Metastasis in 7–15 regional lymph nodes
N3	Metastasis in more than 15 regional lymph nodes
M: distant metastasis	
Mx	Distant metastasis cannot be assessed
M0	No distant metastasis
M1	Distant metastasis present (e.g. hepatic metastasis, peritoneal dissemination)
Stage grouping	
Stage 0	Tis N0 M0
Stage IA	T1 N0 M0
Stage IB	T1 N1 M0, T2a/b N0 M0
Stage II	T1 N2 M0, T2a/b N1 M0, T3 N0 M0
Stage IIIA	T2a/b N2 M0, T3 N1 M0, T4 N0 M0
Stage IIIB	T3 N2 M0
Stage IV	T1–3 N2 M0, T4 N1–3 M0, or any T, any N, M1

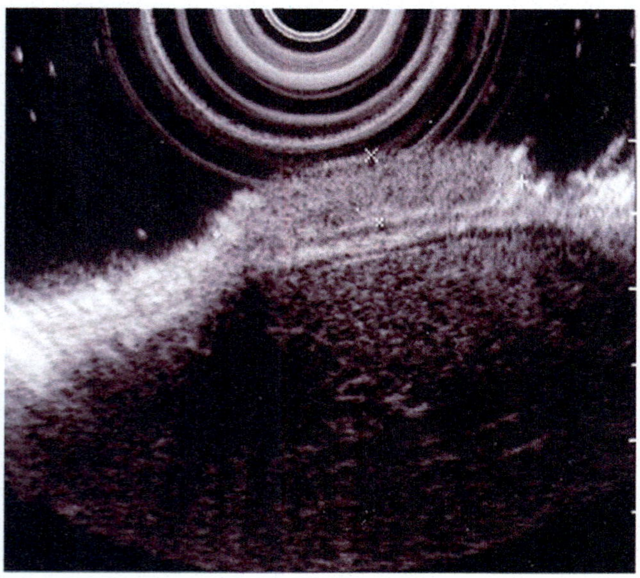

Figure 13.1 T1 gastric cancer. This is a 2.2 × 0.5 cm thick tumor confined to the mucosa without penetration of the muscularis propria.

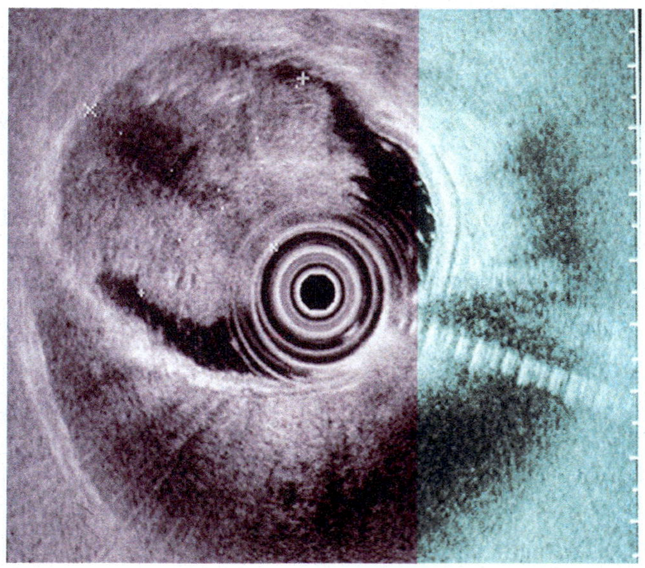

Figure 13.2 T2 gastric cancer. This large 4.2 × 3.6 cm exophytic tumor invades deeply into the gastric wall but does not traverse the serosa. Note the deep margin of the tumor is smooth without deeper pseudopodic extension.

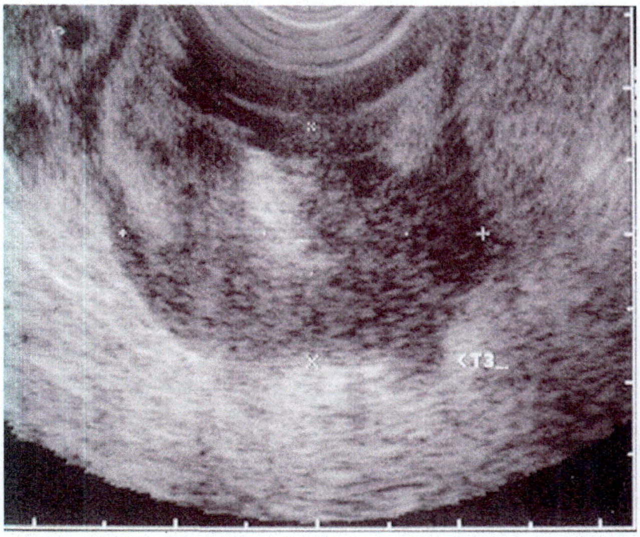

Figure 13.3 T3 gastric cancer. This 2.5 × 1.6 cm tumor invades through all layers of the stomach. A pseudopod of tumor extends through the serosa into the perigastric space (marked by "<T3").

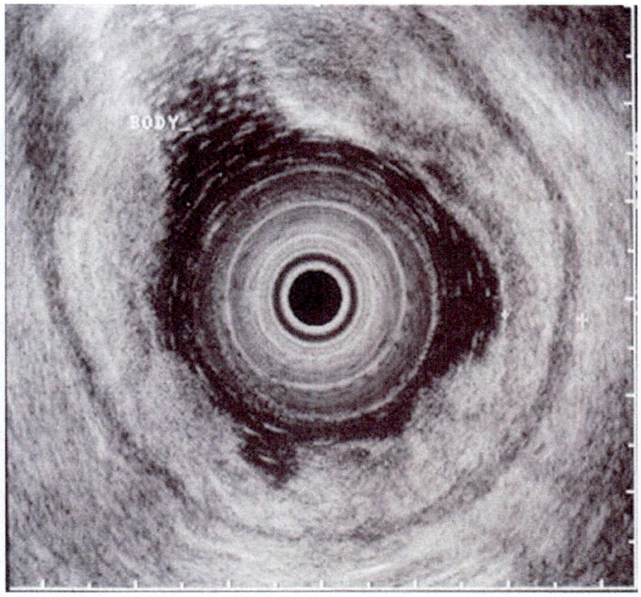

Figure 13.5 Diffuse gastric cancer. The stomach is thickened to 0.8 cm (normal <0.5 cm). The pattern of thickening shows prominence of the bright third layer (submucosa) and dark fourth layer (muscularis propria). This pattern is produced by diffuse infiltration by the signet-ring cell carcinoma.

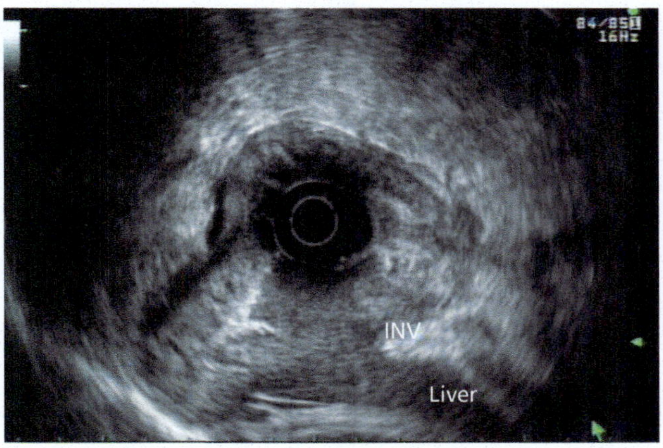

Figure 13.4 T4 gastric cancer. This invasive poorly differentiated cancer invades through the gastric wall to directly involve the adjacent left lobe of the liver. Note the lack of a hyperechoic interface between the gastric tumor and the liver (marked by "INV").

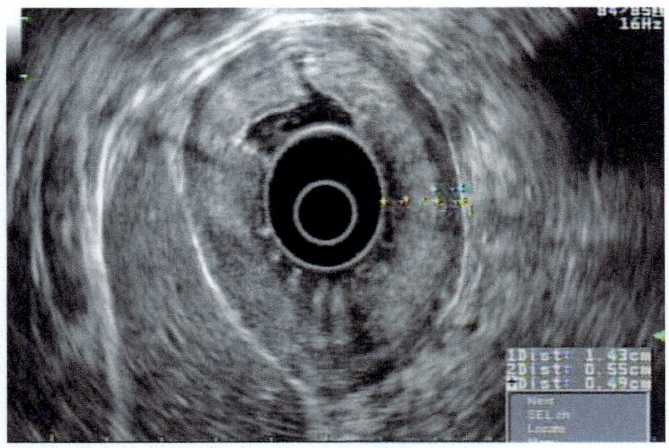

Figure 13.6 Pseudo-linitis plastica. A patient with breast cancer has metastases to the stomach which are infiltrating the wall, giving the appearance of linitis plastica. The five-layer pattern is preserved, but the wall is markedly thickened to 14.3 mm (normal <5 mm) and the submucosa (5.5 mm) and muscularis propria (4.9 mm) are prominently thickened. Source: Gress F, Savides T. *Endoscopic Ultrasonography*, 2nd edn. Oxford: Wiley-Blackwell, 2009.

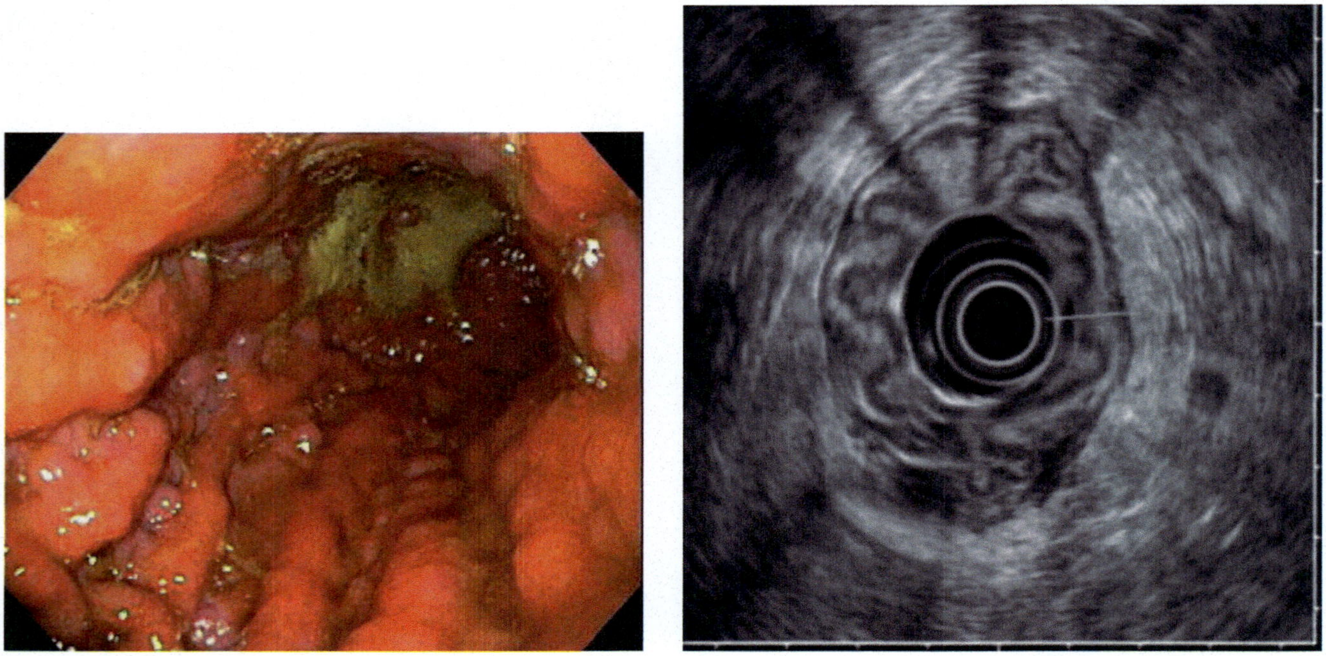

(a) (b)

Figure 13.7 Gastric lymphoma causing a linitis plastica appearance. This patient with a diffusely infiltrating B-cell lymphoma has poorly distensible thickened abnormal-appearing gastric folds on endoscopy (a). On endoscopic ultrasound (b), there is preservation of the five-layer pattern but marked thickening of the gastric wall to 10.9 mm with a thickened muscularis propria to 2.5 mm (normal 1 mm or less).

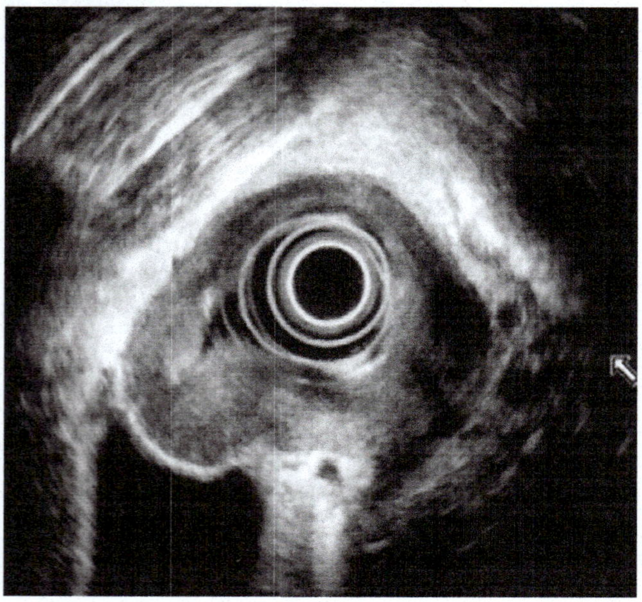

Figure 13.8 Gastric lymphoma. The five-layer wall pattern is obliterated and the gastric wall is markedly thickened. Source: Gress F, Savides T. *Endoscopic Ultrasonography*, 2nd edn. Oxford: Wiley-Blackwell, 2009.

Table 13.2 Ann Arbor staging system for gastrointestinal lymphomas.

Stage	Sites of involvement
IE	Tumor confined to gastrointestinal tract ("E" designates lymphoma outside of lymph nodes)
IIE_1	Tumor with regional nodal involvement
IIE_2	Tumor with extraregional subdiaphragmatic nodal involvement (e.g. para-aortic, iliac)
IIIE	Tumor with nodal involvement on both sides of the diaphragm
IVE	Tumor with extranodal disseminated involvement (e.g. bone marrow, lungs, liver)

Sources: adapted from Carbone PP, Kaplan HS, Musshoff K, et al. Report of the Committee on Hodgkin's Disease Staging Classification. *Cancer Res* 1971;31(11):1860–1861 and Lister TA, Crowther D, Sutcliffe SB, et al. Report of a committee convened to discuss the evaluation and staging of patients with Hodgkin's disease: Cotswolds meeting. *J Clin Oncol* 1989;7(11):1630–1636.

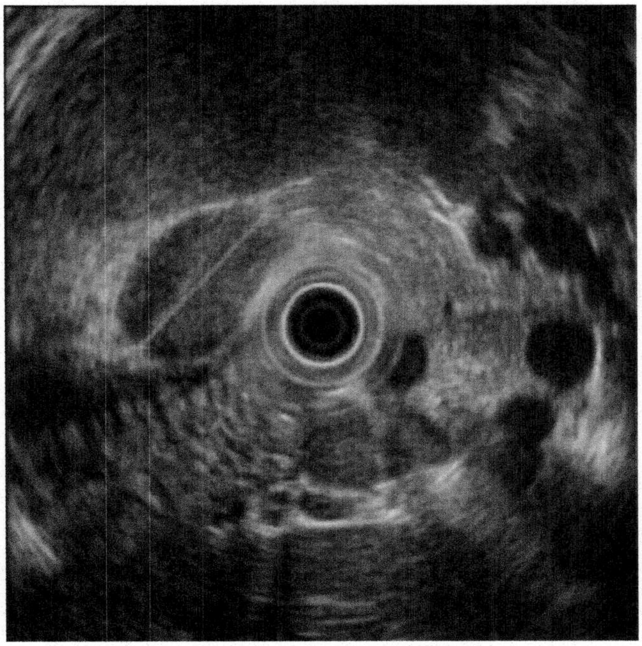

Figure 13.9 Perigastric lymphadenopathy in a patient with primary gastric lymphoma. Note the very large 25.7 × 18.3 mm lymph node. In addition to being large (>1 cm) it has additional malignant features, including a rounded shape with sharp borders, hypoechoic echogenicity, and a homogeneous echotexture.

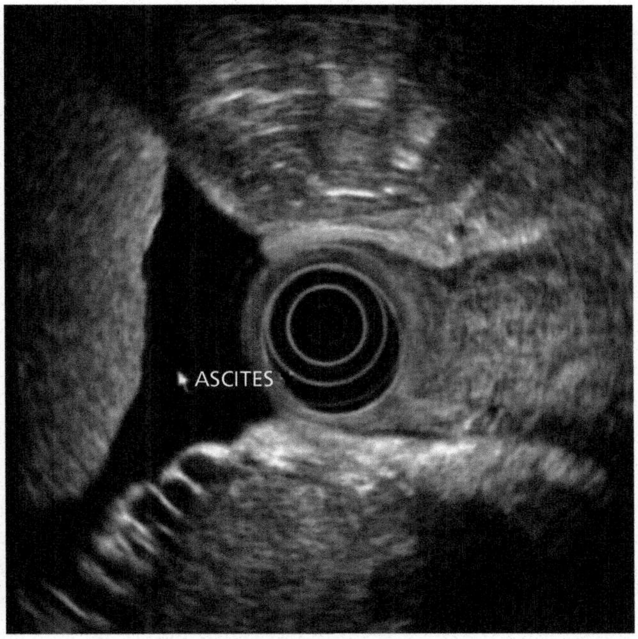

Figure 13.10 Ascites. A large pocket of hypoechoic material is seen next to the liver, located on the left, in a patient with gastric cancer. The ascites was accessed via a 22-gauge needle placed through the duodenum and was positive for malignancy, denoting M1 disease. Source: Gress F, Savides T. *Endoscopic Ultrasonography*, 2nd edn. Oxford: Wiley-Blackwell, 2009.

Endoscopic ultrasound evaluation of suspected gastric malignancies should include a thorough search for metastatic lymph nodes, especially in the perigastric, celiac, and gastrohepatic regions (Figure 13.9). The presence of malignant adenopathy is a poor prognostic sign for both adenocarcinoma and lymphoma and may alter management to primary or adjuvant chemotherapy. The presence of ascites raises the likelihood that there is peritoneal seeding (Figure 13.10). Lymph nodes, liver lesions, and ascites may be sampled via EUS-guided fine needle aspiration (FNA) provided that tumor is not traversed (Figure 13.11).

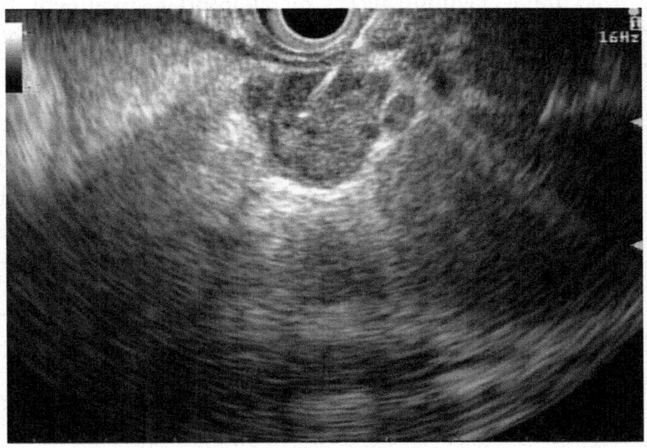

Figure 13.11 Endoscopic ultrasound-guided fine needle aspiration (EUS-FNA) of a perigastric lymph node. This is the same patient as in Figure 13.9 with gastric lymphoma and extensive perigastric lymphadenopathy. The EUS-FNA is performed through a normal-appearing stomach into a malignant-appearing lymph node. Cytology confirmed the presence of lymphoma within the node.

14 Gastric and Esophageal Subepithelial Masses

Muhammad Tahir and Andrew J. Bain
Roswell Park Comprehensive Cancer Center, Buffalo, NY, USA

Introduction

Gastrointestinal subepithelial masses are lesions that lie underneath normal-appearing mucosa. They are usually asymptomatic incidental findings detected during upper endoscopy performed for other reasons. Rarely do subepithelial masses present with symptoms of bleeding or obstruction. The incidence of gastrointestinal subepithelial masses has increased with the widespread use of esophagogastroduodenoscopy (EGD) for various indications. Most esophageal and gastric subepithelial masses are benign; however, some have malignant potential. Therefore, it is important to establish a correct diagnosis and exclude malignancy. Obtaining an accurate diagnosis allows for appropriate treatment of patients with observation/reassurance versus surgical or endoscopic resection. Tissue sampling with standard endoscopic techniques is often unsuccessful in establishing a diagnosis due to inadequate depth of sampling. Endoscopic ultrasonography (EUS) is important in obtaining a diagnosis by virtue of minimally invasive tissue characterization with ultrasound, determination of wall layer of origin (Table 14.1), and by allowing fine needle aspiration (FNA) or fine needle biopsy (FNB) for pathologic diagnosis.

Lipoma

Lipomas are benign growths of mature lipocytes that can be seen in any part of the gastrointestinal tract. Esophageal lipomas are extremely rare, whereas gastric and duodenal lipomas are more common. Endoscopically, lipomas appear as a smooth bulge with normal overlying mucosa with a discernible yellow tint (Figure 14.1a). The *pillow or cushion sign*, whereby a closed forceps is pressed against the mass leaving a slight indentation, is a reasonably specific endoscopic sign for lipomas. On EUS, lipomas are hyperechoic, homogeneous oval masses with smooth margins located in the submucosal layer (Figure 14.1b). Tissue sampling is rarely necessary given the excellent diagnostic accuracy of EUS characterization. If pursued, tunnel biopsies can strip away the superficial mucosa revealing glistening fat located within the submucosal layer (Figure 14.1c). Asymptomatic lipomas generally require no additional surveillance.

Carcinoid tumors

Carcinoid tumors are neuroendocrine tumors with malignant potential. They are most commonly found in the appendix and rectum, but can also be found in the stomach, esophagus, and duodenum. Carcinoid tumors arise from the mucosal layer but can invade into the submucosal layer forming a subepithelial mass. Endoscopically, carcinoids appear as smooth, round, yellowish masses (Figure 14.2a) that can display central erythematous depression or ulceration. On EUS, carcinoids appear hypoechoic or isoechoic, homogeneous with smooth borders, and are usually located in the mucosal/submucosal layer (Figure 14.2b). Unlike most true submucosal tumors, the diagnosis of carcinoids can often be made with standard biopsy forceps. In general, endoscopic resection can be considered for carcinoid tumors of less than 1 cm located within the mucosal or submucosal layer without associated lymphadenopathy. Endoscopically resected carcinoid tumors should be followed periodically with both endoscopy and EUS to assess for local recurrence. Larger tumors should be surgically removed.

Granular cell tumor

Granular cell tumors (GCTs) are generally benign lesions that originate from neural tissue. They are most commonly

Atlas of Endoscopic Ultrasonography, Second Edition. Edited by Frank Gress, Thomas Savides, Brenna Casey, and Everson L. A. Artifon.

Companion website: www.wiley.com/go/gress/atlas

Table 14.1 Endoscopic ultrasound (EUS) characteristics of gastric and esophageal subepithelial masses.

Lesion	Wall layer	EUS features
Lipoma	Submucosa	Hyperechoic, homogeneous, oval
Carcinoid tumor	Mucosa/ submucosa	Hypoechoic/isoechoic, homogeneous
Granular cell tumor	Submucosa	Hypoechoic
Duplication cyst	Submucosa	Anechoic, round, acoustic enhancement
Pancreatic rest	Submucosa/ mucosa	Hypoechoic, heterogeneous, ductal structure
Varices	Submucosa	Anechoic, tubular, Doppler flow
GIST and leiomyoma	Muscularis propria	Hypoechoic
Glomus tumor	Muscularis propria	Hyperechoic/hypoechoic with strong Doppler signal
Gastritis cystica profunda	Submucosa	Heterogeneous, cystic spaces
Extrinsic compression	Outside of wall layers	Lesion dependent

GIST, gastrointestinal stromal cell tumor.

found in the oropharynx and subcutaneous tissue, but can involve any part of the gastrointestinal tract. The most common location in the gastrointestinal tract is the esophagus followed by the stomach and colon. Although multifocal GCTs have been described, they most commonly present as solitary lesions. Endoscopically, they appear as subepithelial masses with normal overlying mucosa displaying a yellowish hue and feel firm and rubbery when palpated with biopsy forceps (Figure 14.3a). On EUS, they appear as hypoechoic lesions with smooth margins located in the mucosal and/or submucosal layer (Figure 14.3b). Endoscopic ultrasound findings that suggest malignancy include invasion through the intestinal wall and increasing size during surveillance. GCTs have a low, but not zero risk of metastasizing, and therefore attempts should be made at resection. Endoscopic mucosal resection (EMR) appears to be an excellent modality for removal of tumors less than 2 cm in diameter (Figure 14.3c–f). Surgery is most appropriate for lesions of greater than 2 cm. Repeat EGD with EUS can be used for surveillance in patients not undergoing resection.

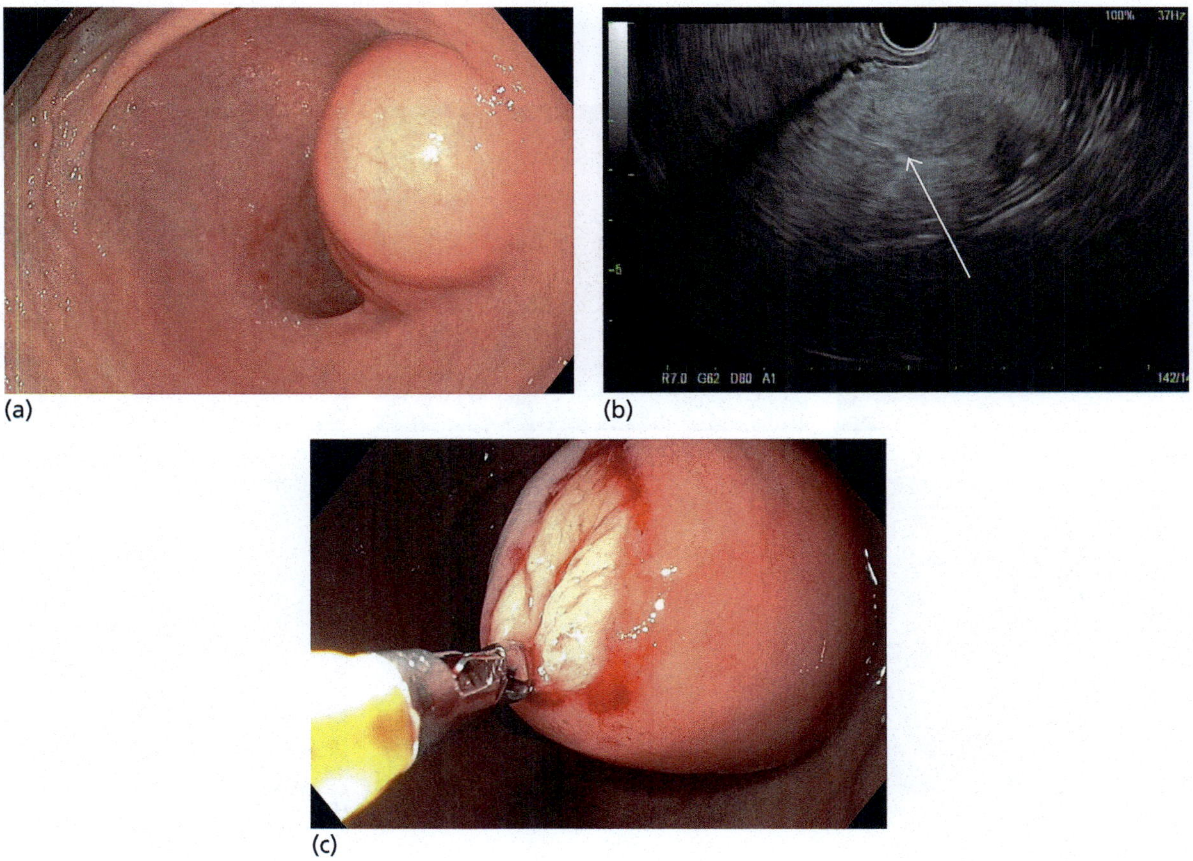

Figure 14.1 Lipoma. (a) Endoscopic view of lipoma with smooth overlying mucosa. (b) EUS showing large hyperechoic gastric mass in the submucosal layer of gastric antrum. (c) Tunnel biopsy showing glistening yellow submucosal fat tissue.

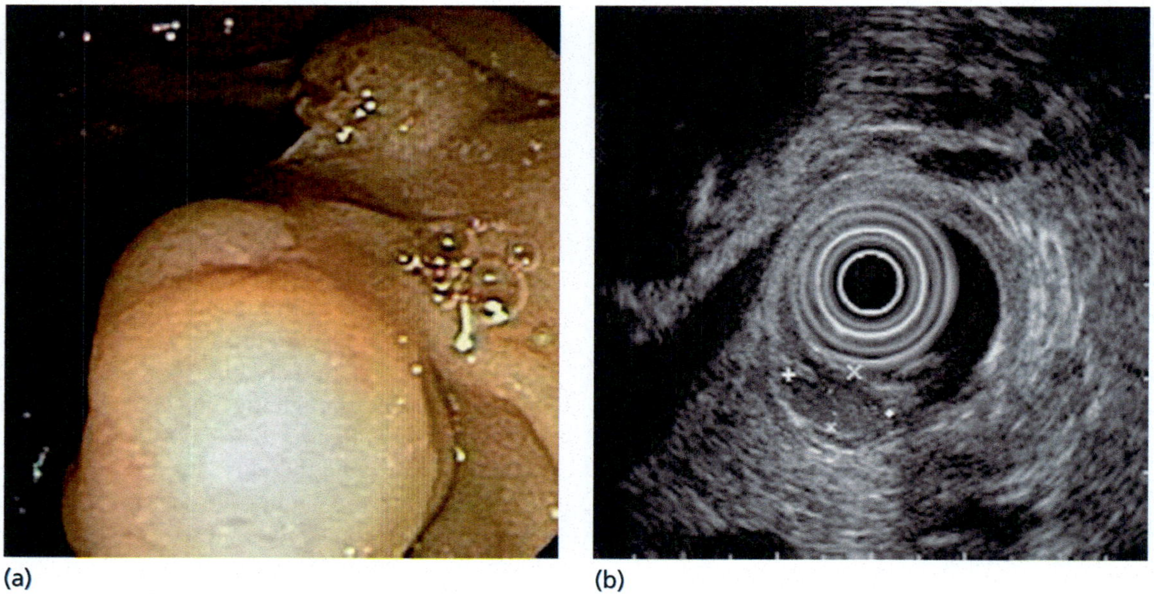

Figure 14.2 Carcinoid tumor. (a) Endoscopic view of a carcinoid tumor. (b) Endosonographic view of a carcinoid tumor which appears as an oval homogeneous, hypoechoic mass located in the submucosa.

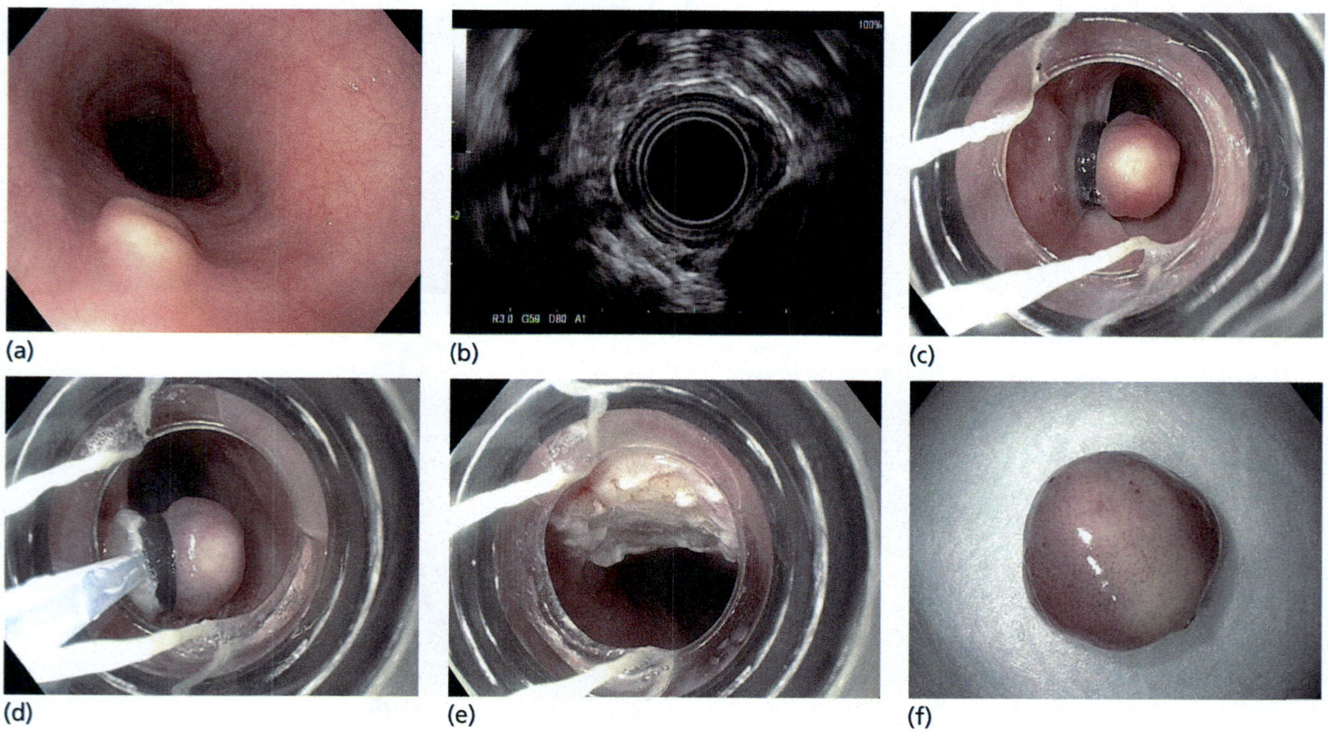

Figure 14.3 Granular cell tumor. (a) Endoscopic view of esophageal granular cell tumor. (b) EUS showing a 6 × 3 mm well-defined hypoechoic mass located within the submucosal layer of the esophageal wall. (c) Band ligation EMR of a granular cell tumor with band in place (d) Band ligation EMR of a granular cell tumor with snare below the band. (e) Granular cell tumor EMR defect. (f) Granular cell tumor EMR specimen.

Duplication cyst

Duplication cysts arise during embryonic development, estimated to occur in 1 in 8000 live births. These cysts can be located anywhere within or adjacent to the luminal gastrointestinal tract and the majority do not communicate with the lumen. They are spherical or tubular, contain mucin, possess a smooth muscle layer, and are lined by the same mucosa as the adjacent bowel. It is not uncommon for esophageal duplication cysts to be multifocal (Figure 14.4a). Duplication cysts are usually asymptomatic, but can result in symptoms due to mass effect, bleeding, or perforation. Duplication cysts rarely have been reported to undergo malignant transformation. Endoscopic ultrasound of duplication cysts usually reveals a round anechoic lesion in the submucosa that has acoustic enhancement (increased through transmission of ultrasound signal which gives a bright appearance on the side distal to the ultrasound transducer, similar to a flashlight effect) (Figure 14.4b). They may have endosonographic findings of echogenic debris which can be mucinous material. The diagnosis can be confirmed with FNA of the fluid, although this is not generally necessary and may unnecessarily expose the patient to risk of cyst infection. The optimal management of asymptomatic cysts is unknown. Periodic EUS surveillance to observe for enlargement may be appropriate. Treatment of symptomatic or enlarging duplication cysts has traditionally been surgical resection.

Pancreatic rest

Pancreatic rest (also known as aberrant pancreas, ectopic pancreas, and heterotopic pancreas) are submucosal tumors consisting of dilated exocrine cells. The majority are 10 mm in diameter, located 1–4 cm from the pylorus in the 6 o'clock endoscopic position in the gastric antrum (Video 14.1). Endoscopically, they appear as submucosal masses with smooth overlying mucosa and may display characteristic central umbilication through which secretions drain (Figure 14.5a). On EUS, pancreatic rests are hypoechoic and/or heterogeneous lesions located in the mucosal/submucosal layer (Figure 14.5b). Occasionally, EUS can visualize a ductal structure traveling upward to the mucosal surface. Asymptomatic pancreatic rests require no further evaluation or treatment; however, those that are symptomatic, enlarging, or in which the diagnosis is in question should be removed endoscopically or surgically. The surgical resection is preferred when muscularis propria is involved.

Varices

Gastroesophageal varices can occur within the submucosal layer (esophageal or gastric varices) or outside the wall as collateral vessels (paraesophageal or paragastric varices) (Figure 14.6a). The EUS appearance is that of tubular anechoic structures that can be traced with the ultrasound probe (Figure 14.6b). Doppler ultrasound allows for easy visualization of varices (14.6c). For detection of esophageal varices, endoscopy is more sensitive than EUS, but for gastric varices EUS is more sensitive than endoscopy.

Gastrointestinal stromal cell tumors and leiomyomas

Spindle cell neoplasms are the most common mesenchymal tumors of the gastrointestinal tract. These include benign leiomyomas, as well as gastrointestinal stromal cell tumors (GISTs)

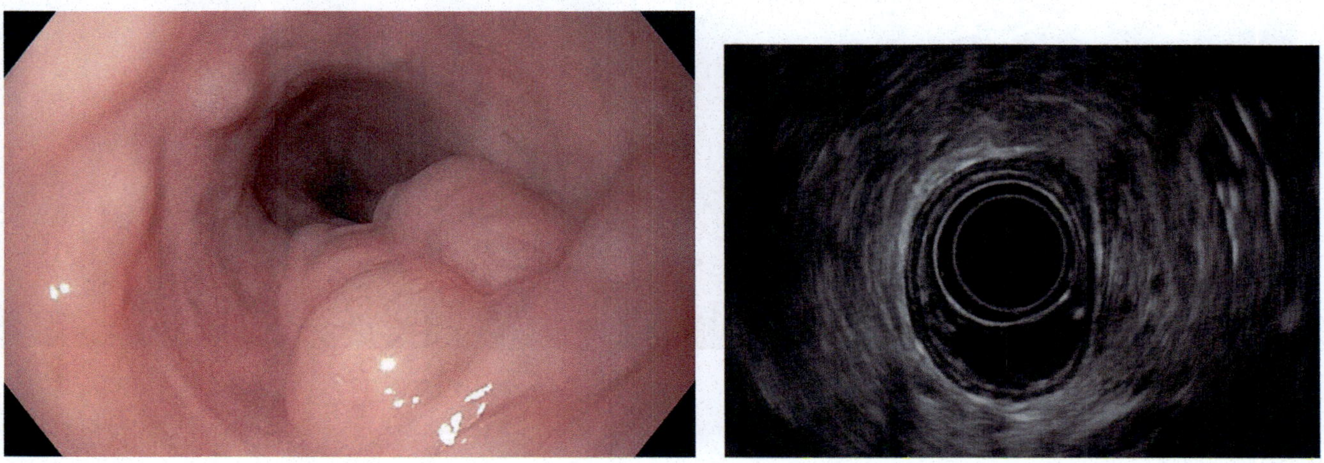

(a) (b)

Figure 14.4 Esophageal duplication cysts. (a) Endoscopic view of several esophageal duplication cysts. (b) EUS showing a 13 × 6 mm anechoic lesion in the submucosal layer of the distal esophageal wall.

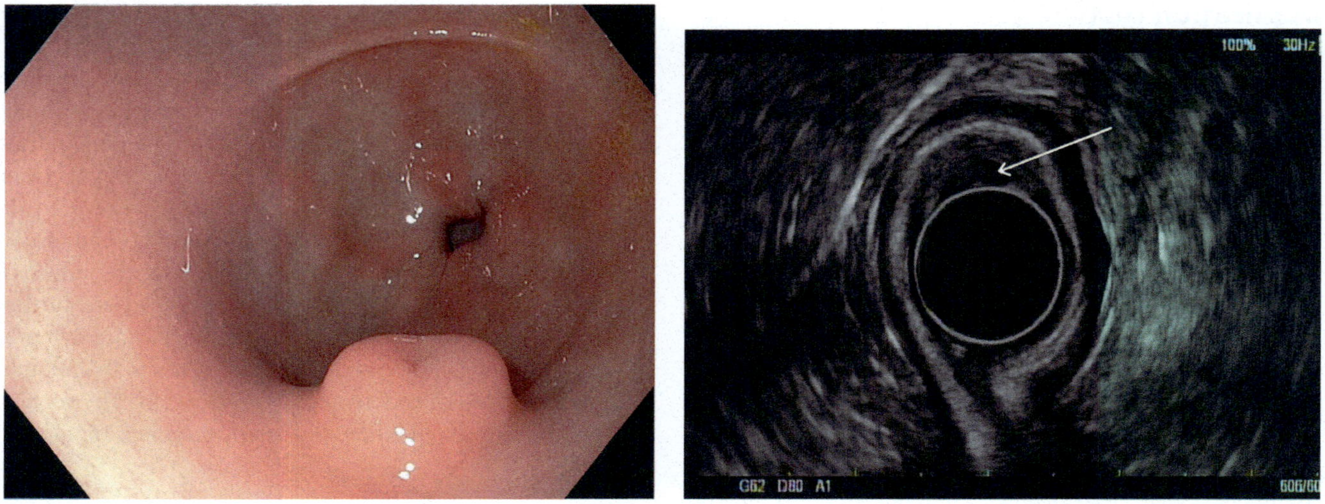

(a) (b)

Figure 14.5 Pancreatic rest. (a) Endoscopic view of a gastric antral pancreatic rest. (b) EUS showed a 9 × 4 mm hypoechoic, heterogeneous mass located within the submucosa of the gastric antrum.

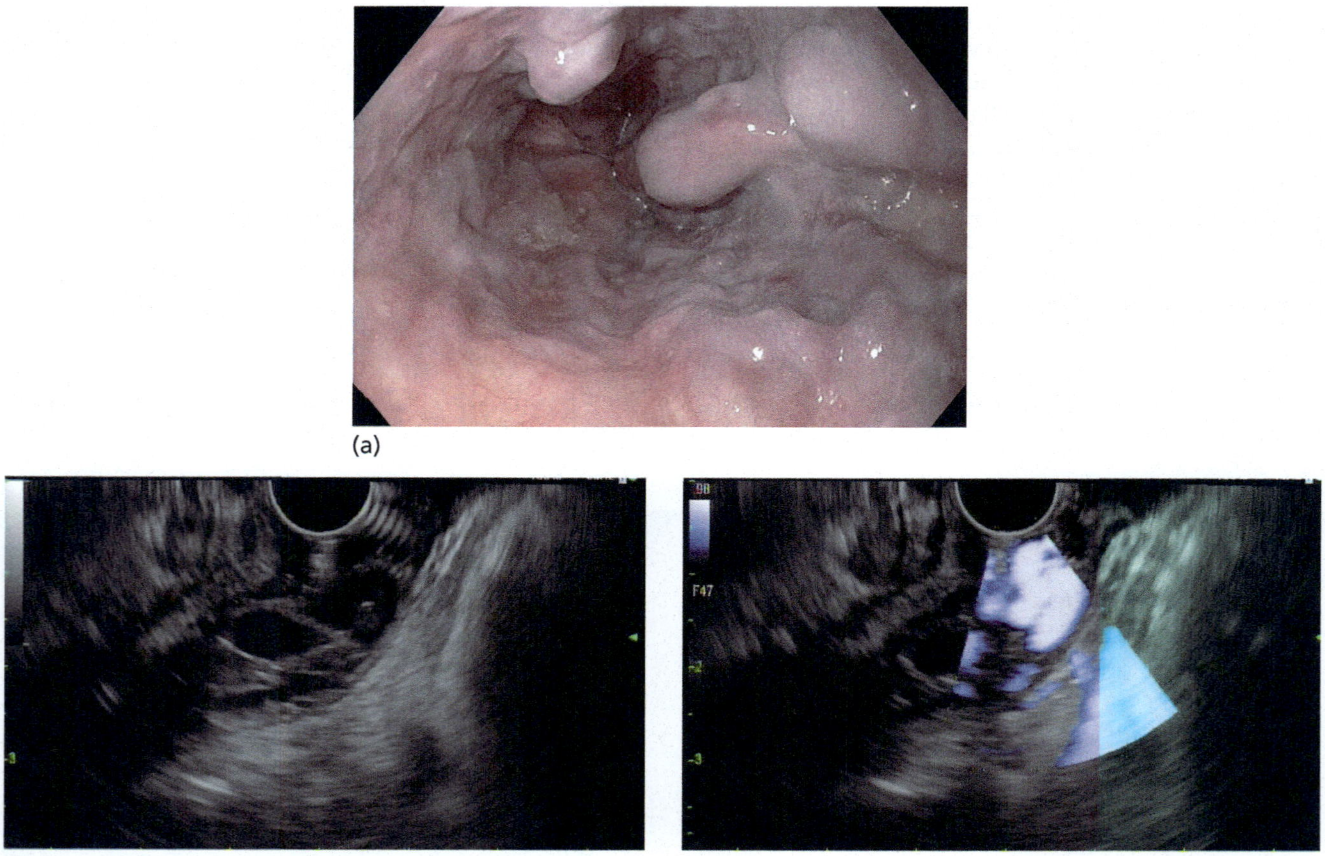

(a) (b) (c)

Figure 14.6 Esophageal varices. (a) Endoscopic view of grade 3 esophageal varices. (b) Esophageal varices on EUS without Doppler. (c) Esophageal varices on EUS with Doppler.

which have some malignant potential. GISTs are thought to originate from the interstitial cells of Cajal. The majority (90%) of GISTs are c-kit positive, which confers a gain of function resulting in cell proliferation and survival. Approximately two-thirds of all GISTs occur in the stomach. Endoscopy reveals a submucosal mass which is often dumbbell-shaped and may have mucosal ulceration (Figure 14.7a). Clinically they may present as the source of upper GI bleeding, or as an incidental finding. The EUS appearance of GISTs is usually a hypoechoic mass that originates from the muscularis propria (Figure 14.7b), although occasionally they can arise from the muscularis mucosa. The EUS features associated with risk of metastases for GISTs include a tumor size greater than 4 cm, irregular extraluminal border, echogenic foci (>3 mm), and cystic spaces (>4 mm). Endoscopic and endosonographic imaging cannot differentiate benign leiomyomas (Figure 14.8) from potentially malignant GISTs. Therefore, EUS-FNA or FNB is commonly performed to obtain tissue for immunohistochemical staining for c-kit. The majority of GISTs are c-kit positive, whereas leiomyomas are c-kit negative. EUS-guided fine needle biopsy with newer core needles often provides sufficient material to comment on the number of mitoses per high power field, which is a marker for metastatic potential. For this reason, EUS-FNB may be preferred over traditional FNA. Surgical resection is the treatment of choice for symptomatic or large GISTs, although tumors smaller than 3 cm without EUS features of malignancy can be followed serially with EUS. Metastastic disease is treated with imatinib, a selective inhibitor of certain tyrosine kinases including c-kit.

Glomus tumor

Glomus tumors are extremely rare mesenchymal tumors composed of modified smooth muscle cells representing a neoplastic counterpart of the perivascular glomus bodies. They are most commonly found in the skin, but can also be found in the gastrointestinal tract, with the gastric antrum representing the most common location. Endoscopically, they appear as subepithelial masses with smooth overlying mucosa (Figure 14.9a). On EUS, they typically originate from the muscularis propria (Figure 14.9b). Glomus tumors can appear hyperechoic or hypoechoic and tend to have internal hyperechoic foci. They also manifest a strong Doppler signal consistent with the vascular nature of these tumors. EUS-FNA immunostaining helps to differentiate glomus tumors from GISTs and carcinoid tumors. Treatment usually is surgical excision.

Gastritis cystica profunda

Gastritis cystica profunda (GCP) is a benign tumor that is usually composed of gastric glands. The pathogenesis is unclear, although ischemia and chronic inflammation are thought to be the most important factors. The most common location is in the body and antrum. The endoscopic appearance varies from prominent gastric folds to a protruding subepithelial mass (Figure 14.10a). On EUS, GCP usually appears as a heterogeneously enhancing lesion with cystic spaces within the submucosal layer (Figure 14.10b).

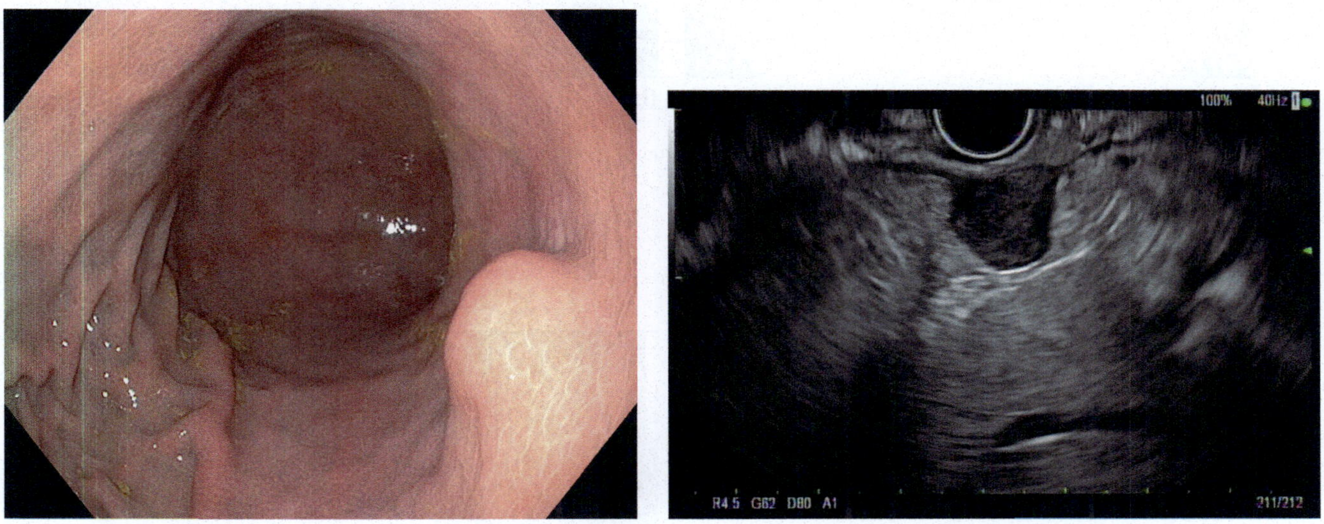

(a) (b)

Figure 14.7 Gastric gastrointestinal stromal tumor (GIST). (a) Endoscopic view of a gastric body GIST. (b) EUS view of a GIST appearing as a 16 × 11 mm hypoechoic well-defined mass originating from the muscularis propria of the gastric body.

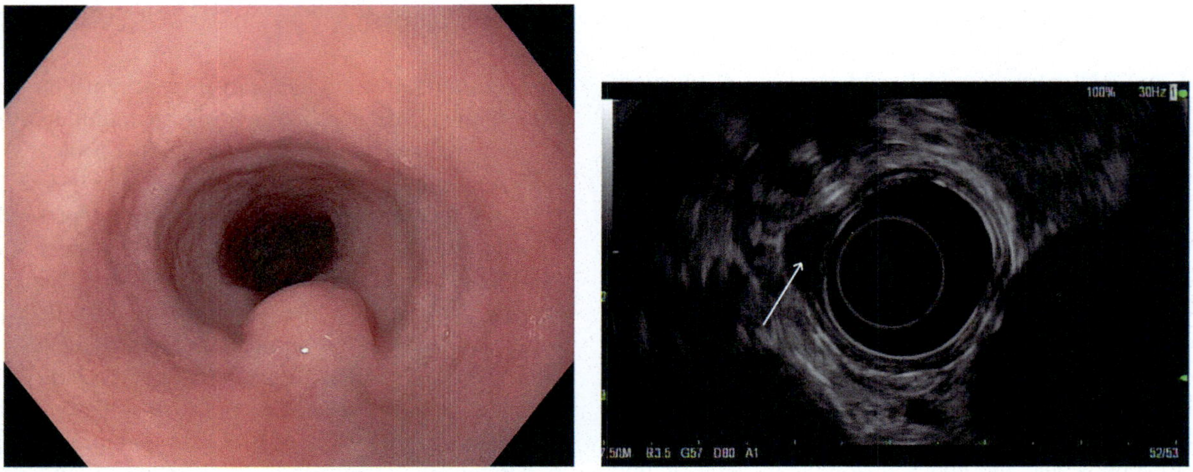

(a) (b)

Figure 14.8 Leiomyoma. (a) Endoscopic view of an esophageal leiomyoma. (b) EUS shows hypoechoic well-defined mass originating from the esophageal muscularis propria.

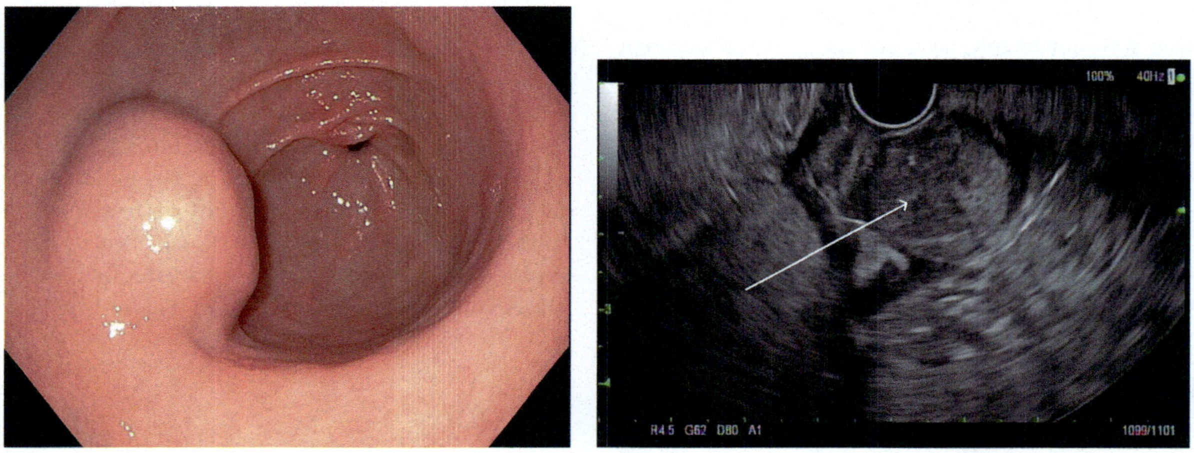

(a) (b)

Figure 14.9 Glomus tumor. (a) Endoscopic view of a gastric antral glomus tumor. (b) EUS showing a 20 × 18 mm isoechoic well-defined mass that appeared to originate from the gastric muscularis propria.

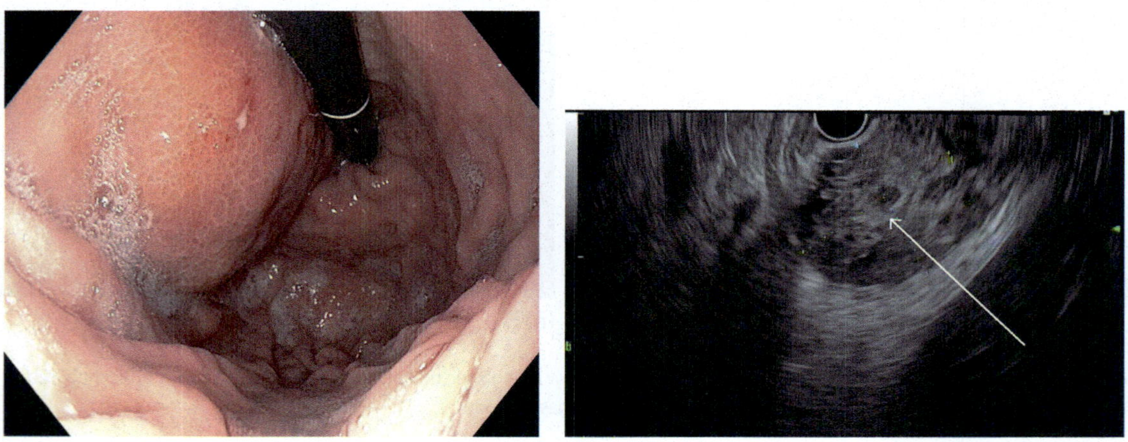

(a) (b)

Figure 14.10 Gastritis cystica profunda (GCP). (a) Endoscopic view showing GCP in the fundus. (b) EUS showing a heterogeneous submucosal mass with cystic spaces.

Extrinsic compression lesions

Normal abdominal organs can cause indentations in the gastrointestinal tract that may mimic a submucosal mass (Figure 14.11). Extrinsic compression can be seen in the esophagus by the aortic arch, left atrium, and spine and in the stomach by the gallbladder (Figure 14.11a), the left lobe of the liver (Figure 14.11b), and splenic vessels (Figure 14.11c). Pathologic compression may occur from malignant lymph nodes or masses in either the stomach or the esophagus. EUS can identify lesions outside the gastrointestinal tract exerting mass effect on the intestinal lumen. Table 14.2 summarizes the different lesions with the corresponding intraluminal location.

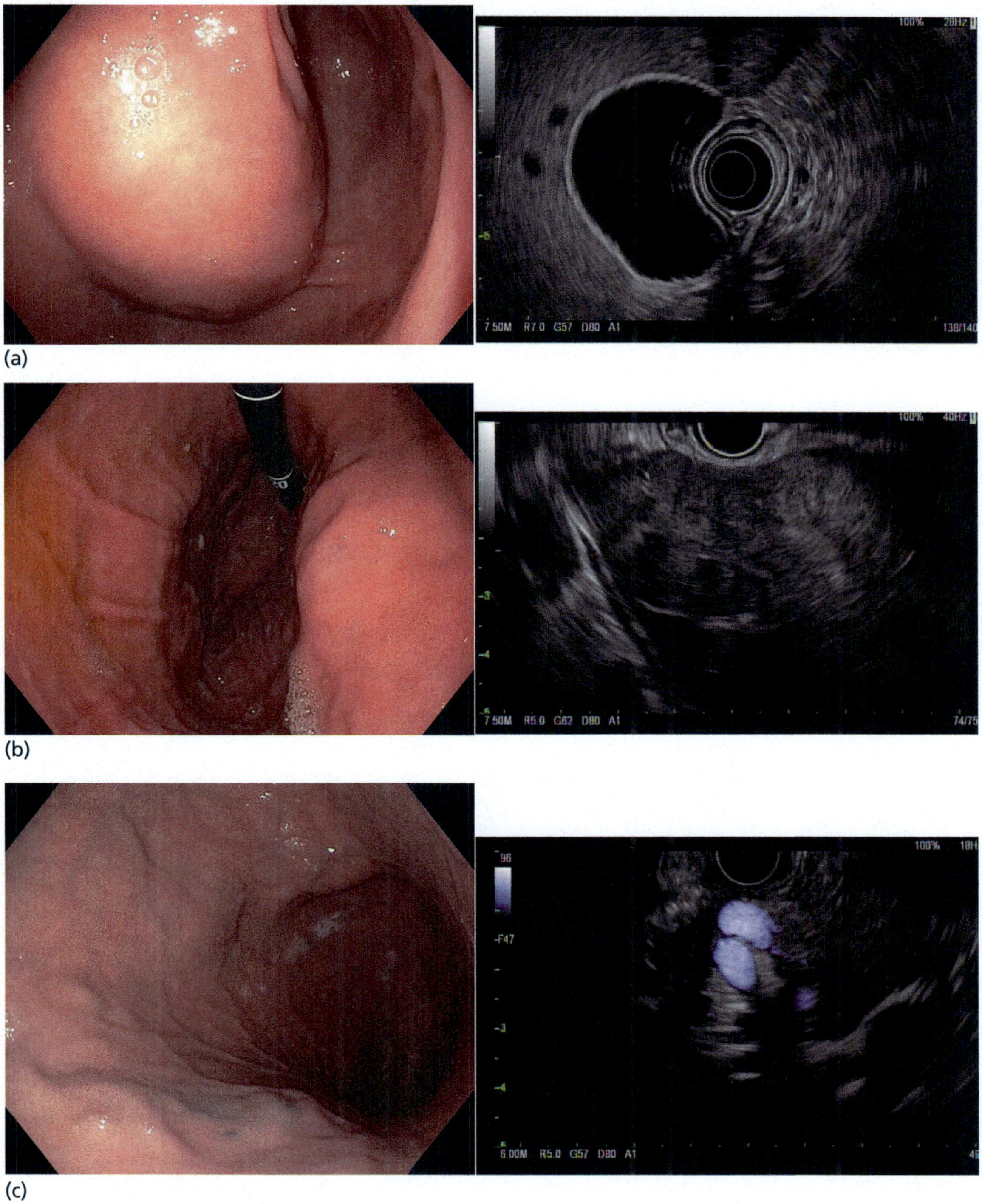

Figure 14.11 Extrinsic compression. (a) Endoscopic and EUS view of extrinsic compression from the gallbladder. (b) Endoscopic and EUS view of extrinsic compression from the left lobe of the liver. (c) Endoscopic and EUS Doppler view of extrinsic compression from the splenic vessels.

Table 14.2 Extrinsic compression of the esophagus and stomach.

Type of extramural lesion	Most common location of intraluminal impression
Aortic arch, dilated left atrium	Esophagus
Mediastinal lymph node and tumors	Esophagus
Gallbladder	Gastric antrum
Left lobe of the liver	Proximal gastric body
Splenic vessels	Proximal gastric body, posterior wall
Pancreatic lesions	Gastric body or antrum, posterior wall

Chapter video clip

Video 14.1 Gastric antral pancreatic rest.

15 Anorectal Neoplasia

Manoop S. Bhutani[1] and Everson L.A. Artifon[2]

[1] University of Texas MD Anderson Cancer Center, Houston, TX, USA

[2] University of São Paulo, São Paulo, Brazil and Ana Costa Hospital, Santos, Brazil

Colorectal cancer staging by EUS

Tumor (T) stage

Malignant colorectal tumors by endoscopic ultrasound (EUS) appear as hypoechoic masses. A tumor that by EUS appears to be limited to the mucosa or the submucosa (first three echo layers) is classified as a T1 lesion by EUS (Figure 15.1). A colorectal carcinoma invading into the muscularis propria (hypoechoic fourth EUS layer) but with an intact outer margin of the muscularis propria and with no penetration completely through the muscularis propria will be a T2 lesion by EUS (Figure 15.2). A T3 lesion by EUS penetrates completely through the rectal wall and all the EUS layers, has irregular outer margins, or has tumorous pseudopodia extending beyond the five echo layers (Figures 15.2b and 15.3). A T4 lesion by EUS is a colorectal cancer that is locally invading into an adjacent organ, e.g. the prostate or vagina.

N stage

Lymph nodes during EUS may be seen as round, oval, or sometimes triangular structures that may be hypoechoic, echogenic, or with mixed echogenicity. In addition, if color Doppler is available on the echoendoscope it may further help in differentiating a vascular structure from a lymph node by observing color flow within a vessel (Figure 15.4). When no lymph nodes are seen during EUS, or if the lymph nodes visualized during EUS are considered reactive and not malignant, the N stage is classified as N0. When lymph nodes visualized during EUS are believed to be malignant, N1 stage by EUS is diagnosed with one to three regional lymph nodes and N2 stage is diagnosed with four or more regional lymph nodes. In rectal cancer, the size cutoff for lymph nodes considered as suspicious for malignant invasion is 5 mm instead of 10 mm. The application of endoscopic ultrasound-guided fine needle aspiration (EUS-FNA) may be used as an adjunct to accurate lymph node assessment during EUS and it has been applied in patients with rectal cancer (Figure 15.5 and Video 15.1). EUS-FNA of lymph nodes is not an option for those in the immediate vicinity of the primary tumor since traversing of the EUS-FNA needle through the primary will lead to false-positive results.

Endoscopic ultrasound for local recurrence of colorectal carcinoma

Local recurrence of colorectal cancer after attempted curative resection occurs in 2.6–32.0% of patients. Endosonography may be useful in the diagnosis of suspected local recurrence when no lesions arising from the mucosa are seen during conventional endoscopy. Endoscopic ultrasound in such cases may reveal hypoechoic areas (or areas of mixed echogenicity) outside the colorectal wall (Figure 15.6). Endosonographic alterations due to the primary surgery need to be kept in mind. The risk of recurrence after surgery for rectal cancer is greatest in the first two years after surgery. Detection of local recurrence in a resectable stage provides an opportunity for repeat surgery with curative intent.

Restaging after chemotherapy and radiation

Neoadjuvant chemoradiation is often utilized for downstaging of a rectal cancer prior to surgical resection. Although EUS is very accurate in T and N staging for rectal cancer prior to initiating any treatment, restaging after chemoradiation is problematic. Inflammation and necrosis after chemoradiation appears hypoechoic and indistinguishable from malignant tissue. This results in the obvious problem of overstaging by EUS after radiation and chemotherapy.

Atlas of Endoscopic Ultrasonography, Second Edition. Edited by Frank Gress, Thomas Savides, Brenna Casey, and Everson L. A. Artifon.

Companion website: www.wiley.com/go/gress/atlas

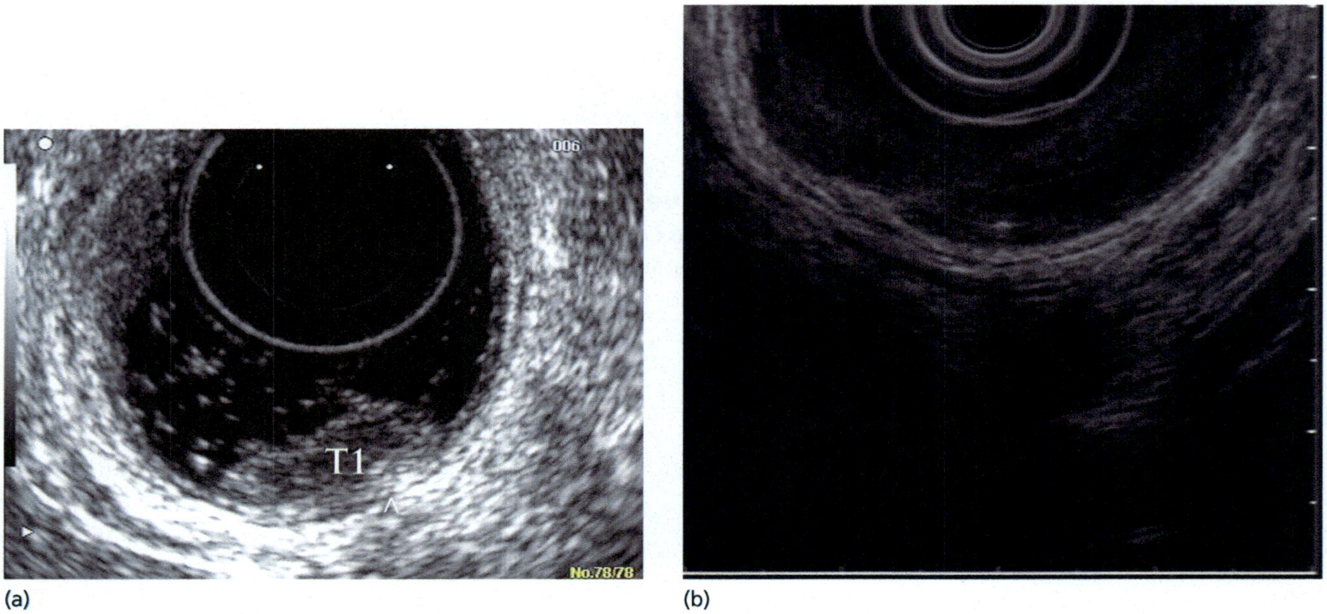

Figure 15.1 (a) A T1 rectal adenocarcinoma (by radial EUS) arising in a villous adenoma with an intact submucosa and muscularis propria (arrowhead) underneath. (b) A larger T1 rectal cancer (compared to Figure 15.1a) arising from the mucosa with an intact submucosa underneath the cancer.

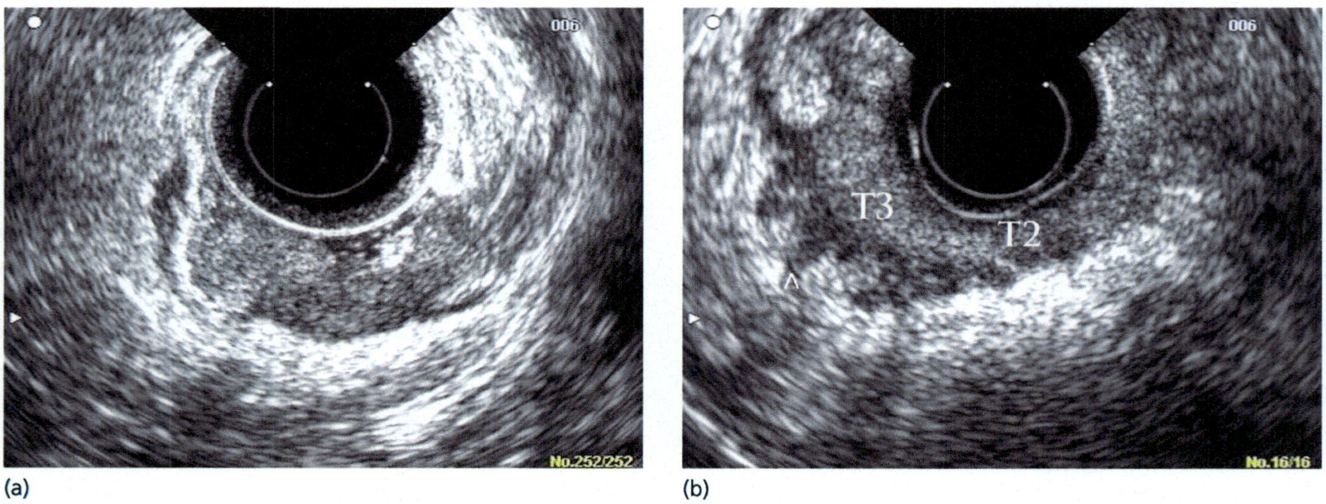

Figure 15.2 (a) A rectal adenocarcinoma that appears to be T2 (penetration into muscularis propria). (b) Radial EUS image of a rectal adenocarcinoma that appears to be T2 (penetration into muscularis propria) in one portion and T3 (penetration through the muscularis propria into perirectal fat as indicated by arrowhead) in another.

Submucosal tumors of the colorectal wall

It is difficult to predict the cause of an endoscopically visible bulge into the gastrointestinal lumen when the overlying mucosa is normal (Figure 15.7a). A lipoma is characterized by a homogeneous echogenic lesion that is contiguous with the third echo layer corresponding with the submucosa. Most lipomas are benign and malignant transformation is a rare phenomenon. Thus, there is controversy about the need for endoscopic removal once a lipoma is diagnosed by EUS. However, EUS would be a prerequisite prior to contemplating endoscopic removal of a lipoma. Endoscopic ultrasound may also help in monitoring this lesion if it is not removed.

A myogenic tumor appears as a hypoechoic mass that is contiguous with the fourth echo layer representing the muscularis propria (Figure 15.7b). The differential diagnosis of a myogenic tumor includes a leiomyoma, leiomyosarcoma, leiomyoblastoma, or a gastrointestinal stromal cell tumor (GIST). A myogenic tumor that is greater than 4 cm in diameter and which has an irregular margin, with cystic or echogenic foci, is more likely to be a malignant lesion. However, there is overlap between benign and malignant myogenic or

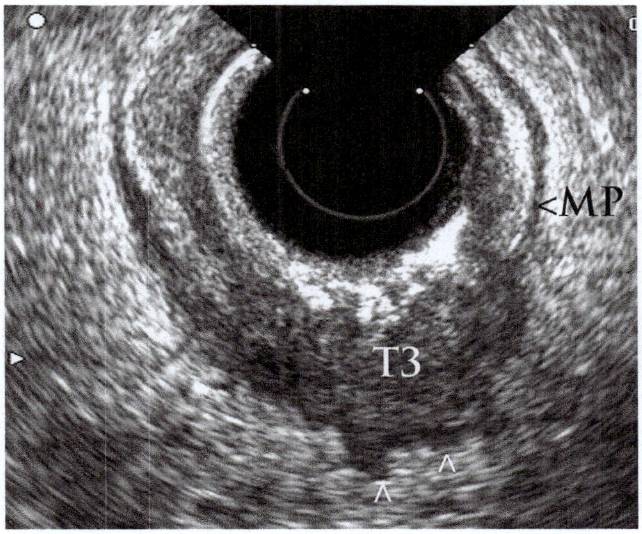

Figure 15.3 Radial EUS of a T3 lesion showing the primary rectal tumor penetrating through the muscularis propria (MP) into perirectal fat (arrowheads).

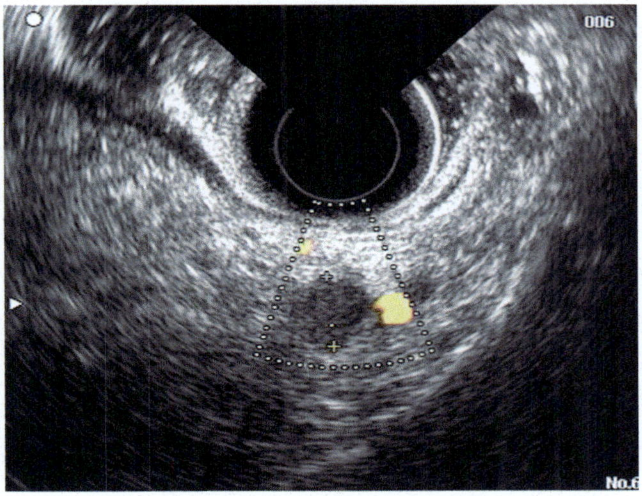

Figure 15.4 Radial EUS of the patient in Figure 15.3 showing a 7-mm round, perirectal, hypoechoic lymph node with no flow on color Doppler with an adjoining vessel nearby with color flow.

GIST lesions, and resection of the entire lesion is the surest way to ensure absence of malignancy. If, however, a decision is made to monitor a myogenic lesion that appears benign, EUS may be useful. Any change in echo features, such as size, echogenicity, margins, or appearance of lymphadenopathy, may then warrant a surgical resection.

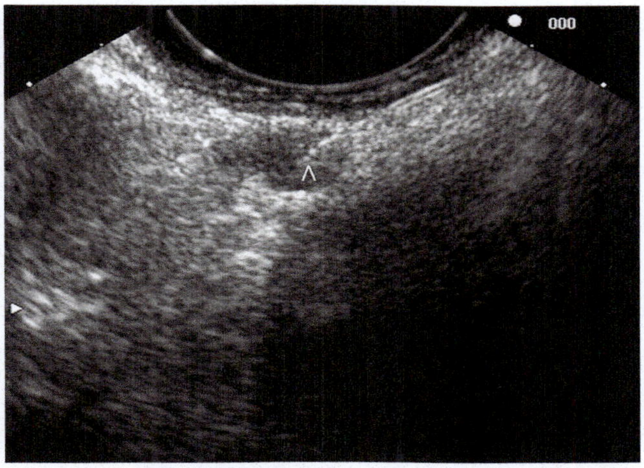

Figure 15.5 EUS-guided fine needle aspiration of a perirectal lymph node. The tip of the needle is within the lymph node (arrowhead).

Carcinoid tumors of the rectum are not uncommon. They generally appear as a firm, small, submucosal nodule (Figure 15.8a). By EUS a rectal carcinoid appears as a hypoechoic mass arising from the second echo layer and sometimes compressing or extending to the submucosa (Figure 15.8b).

Colonic lymphangiomas can also produce a submucosal compression. By endosonography they appear as multiple anechoic (cystic) lesions with echogenic septations located within the third echo layer corresponding with the submucosa. These lesions are generally benign and are left alone unless they cause symptoms such as bleeding, intestinal obstruction, or intussusception. The endosonographic image of a rectal lesion–colitis cystic profunda is similar to echo features of colonic lymphangiomas. There have also been isolated case reports of endosonography in colonic pneumatosis cystoides intestinalis and polypoid prolapsing mucosal folds associated with colonic diverticular disease. Recurrence of colorectal carcinoma, malignant lymphoma, and appendiceal mucocele may also cause submucosal elevation in the colorectum.

Chapter video clip

Video 15.1 Linear EUS-guided transrectal FNA of an oval perirectal lymph node in a patient with rectal cancer. Source: Hitachi.

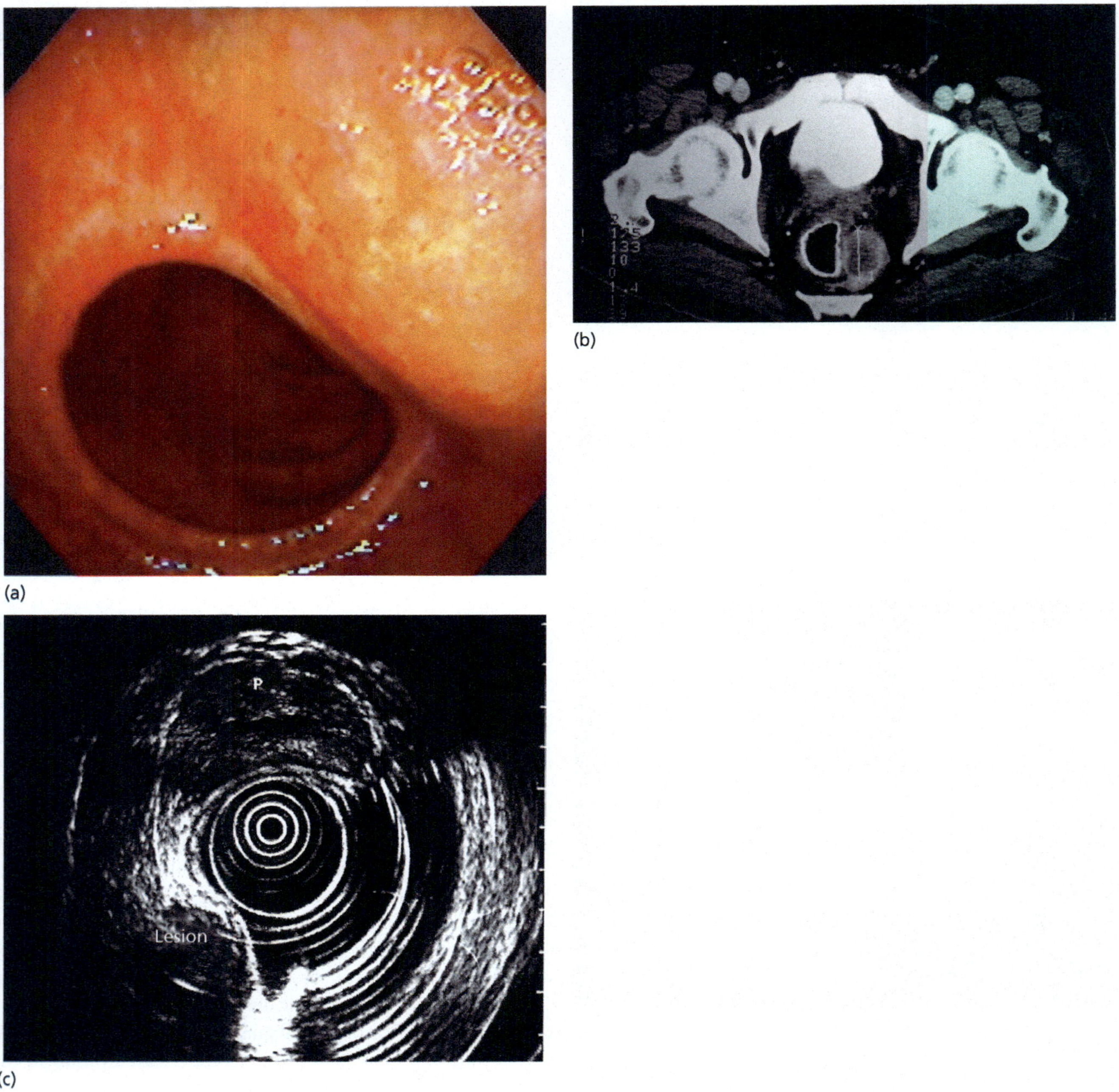

Figure 15.6 Recurrent rectal cancer. During surveillance colonoscopy in a patient post-sigmoidectomy for colorectal cancer, a bulge was noted at the anastomosis (a). A computed tomography (CT) scan examination (b) and EUS (c) revealed tumor recurrence at the anastomosis, with involvement of the muscularis propria and submucosa.

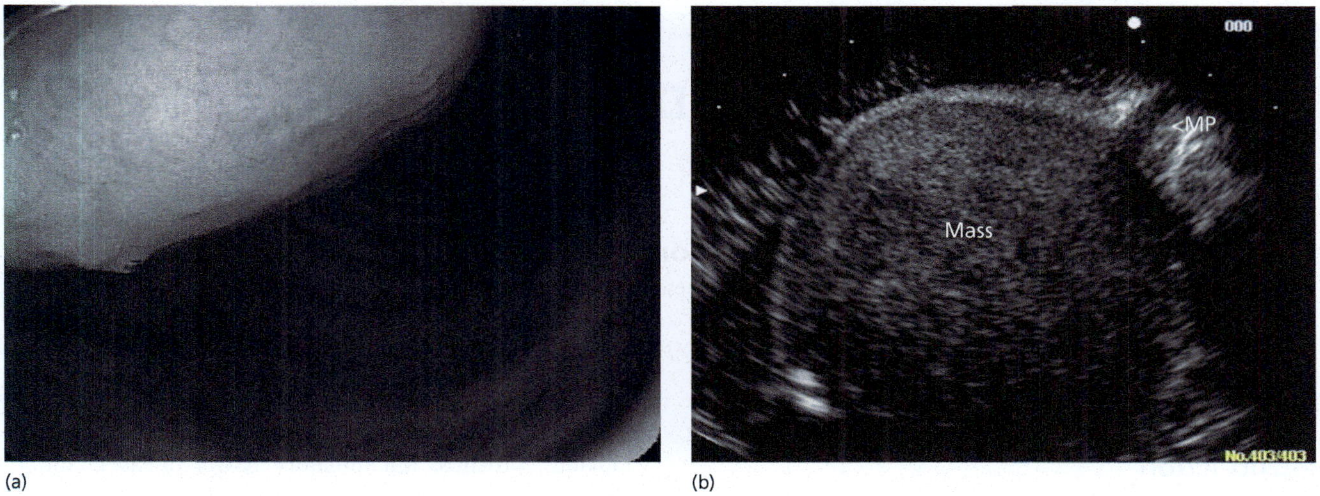

Figure 15.7 (a) A subepithelial bulge in the rectum from a large intramural subepithelial mass. (b) EUS of the mass in Figure 15.7a shows it to be a hypoechoic mass that is contiguous with the muscularis propria. EUS-guided fine needle aspiration revealed it to be a gastrointestinal stromal cell tumor.

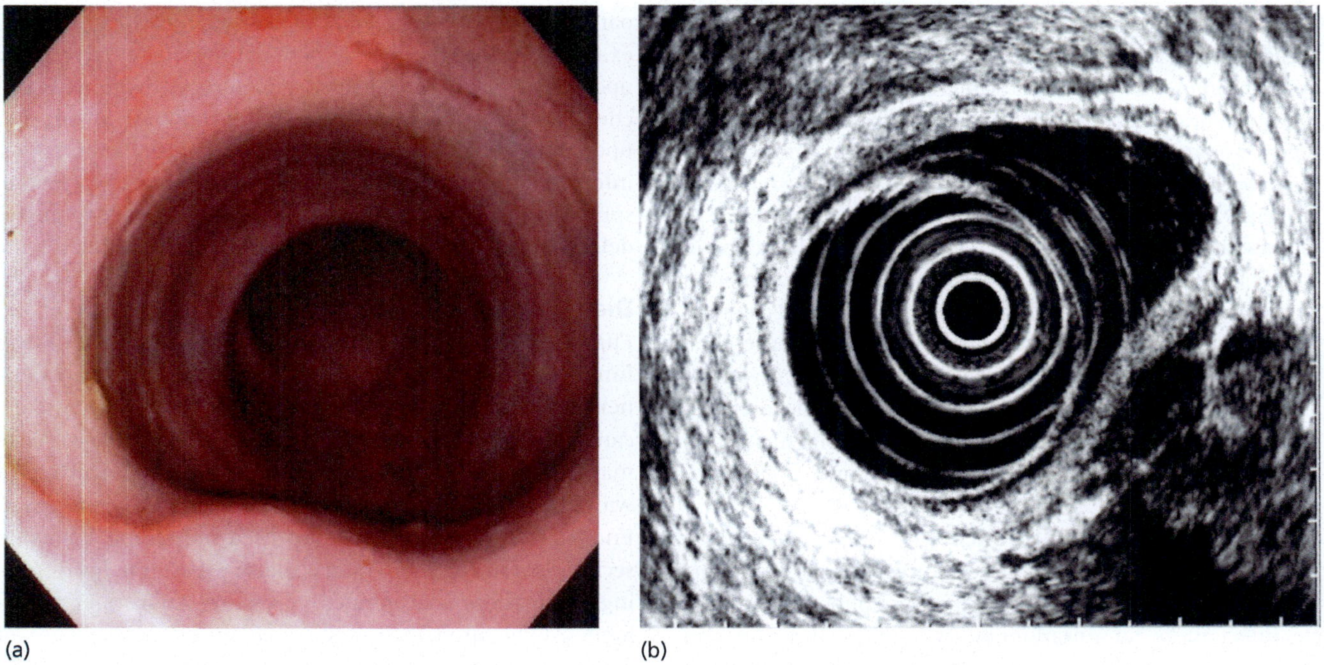

Figure 15.8 Rectal carcinoid. (a) A rectal bulge was noted during routine colonoscopy. (b) EUS showed a hypoechoic lesion in posterior rectum, with involvement of the submucosa and muscularis propria. Histopathological examination was diagnostic of a carcinoid tumor.

16 Anal Sphincter Disease: Fecal Incontinence and Fistulas

Raymond S. Tang[1] and Thomas J. Savides[2]

[1] Institute of Digestive Disease, The Chinese University of Hong Kong and Prince of Wales Hospital, Shatin, New Territories, Hong Kong, China

[2] Division of Gastroenterology, University of California San Diego, La Jolla, CA, USA

Introduction

Endoanal ultrasound is a simple and reliable tool in the evaluation of benign anorectal diseases such as fecal incontinence and anal fistula.

Fecal incontinence

Prevalence

Fecal incontinence can cause significant distress in otherwise functional individuals. Large community-based studies have reported a prevalence of fecal incontinence ranging from 7–15% in women living in the community to 50–70% in nursing home residents. The incidence of fecal incontinence is expected to increase in the aging population. Gross incontinence occurs in 0.7% of the US population and is almost twice as common in women as in men. Obstetrical trauma is one of the most common causes of anal sphincter injury leading to fecal incontinence. Fecal incontinence is present in 20% of postpartum women with an anal sphincter defect. Overt anal sphincter damage due to a third-degree or fourth-degree tear occurs in 0.7% of women undergoing vaginal delivery with posterolateral episiotomy.

Etiology of fecal incontinence

Maintenance of fecal continence requires the following: normal functioning of the anal sphincters and puborectalis muscle, intact anorectal sensation, intact cognitive function, and normal stool consistency. Etiologies of fecal incontinence include (i) weakness of internal or external anal sphincter (e.g. obstetrical trauma from vaginal delivery and episiotomy, prior anorectal surgery, fistula, pudendal neuropathy, diabetes); (ii) weakness of puborectalis muscle (e.g. spinal cord lesion, peripheral neuropathy); (iii) decreased perception of rectal sensation (e.g. diabetes, multiple sclerosis, dementia); (iv) reduced storage capacity (e.g. rectal ischemia, radiation proctitis, inflammatory bowel disease); and (v) overflow state with intact sphincter function (e.g. severe diarrhea, fecal impaction).

Assessment of fecal incontinence

Assessment of fecal incontinence begins with a careful history regarding the nature of incontinence, prior history of anorectal diseases and surgeries, obstetrical history in female patients, neuropathies, and neurologic diseases. Physical examination should include perianal inspection at rest and upon straining as if to defecate, digital rectal examination to check for structural lesion, anal sphincter tone at rest and upon squeezing, and ano-perineal sensation. Patients with internal anal sphincter defects have decreased resting sphincter tone, while patients with external anal sphincter defects have decreased voluntary anal canal squeeze.

Diagnostic tests

Further testing of anal sphincter for structural defect or dysfunction may be pursued when etiology of fecal incontinence is uncertain. Flexible sigmoidoscopy or colonoscopy can be used to exclude mucosal inflammation or mass. Pelvic magnetic resonance imaging (MRI) provides a noninvasive way to investigate the structural integrity of the anorectum. Endoanal ultrasound is further discussed in the following section. Anorectal manometry allows measurement of resting and squeeze anal sphincter pressure. An intrarectal balloon can be used to assess rectal sensation. Decrease of resting or squeeze sphincter pressure with normal sensory testing suggests mechanical sphincter defect. Pudendal nerve terminal latency (PNTL) testing measures the time to induce external anal sphincter contraction after stimulation of pudendal nerve. About 16% of postpartum women would have a conduction delay. The use of electromyography for anal sphincter mapping, usually poorly tolerated by patients, has diminished as endoanal ultrasound becomes available.

Atlas of Endoscopic Ultrasonography, Second Edition. Edited by Frank Gress, Thomas Savides, Brenna Casey, and Everson L. A. Artifon.

Companion website: www.wiley.com/go/gress/atlas

Endoanal ultrasound

Endoanal ultrasound has emerged as a reliable and well-tolerated investigation for defects in internal anal sphincter (IAS) and external anal sphincter (EAS). The accuracy of endoanal ultrasound in detecting anal sphincter defects prior to sphincter repair ranges from 89 to 100% in surgical series. While both endoanal ultrasound and pelvic MRI can be used for evaluation of anal sphincter injury, endoanal ultrasound is often the first choice for anal sphincter imaging due to its wide availability and clearer visualization of IAS. On the other hand, pelvic MRI is more helpful in identifying EAS atrophy and a patulous anal canal, which are suggestive of pathologies beyond anal sphincter injury alone. Endoanal ultrasound can be performed with a rigid radial ultrasound probe or a radial echoendoscope. Figure 16.1 shows a schematic diagram of the anal canal complex. On ultrasound, two rings of tissue can be seen in the normal anal canal (Figures 16.2 and 16.3). The inner hypoechoic ring of tissue corresponds to the IAS, with normal thickness of 1–3 mm. The outer hyperechoic ring of tissue represents the EAS, with normal thickness of 6–10 mm. The IAS increases in thickness and becomes more hyperechoic with age, while the EAS becomes thinner with age. The normal anterior part of EAS seems to be shorter and slopes downward in women,

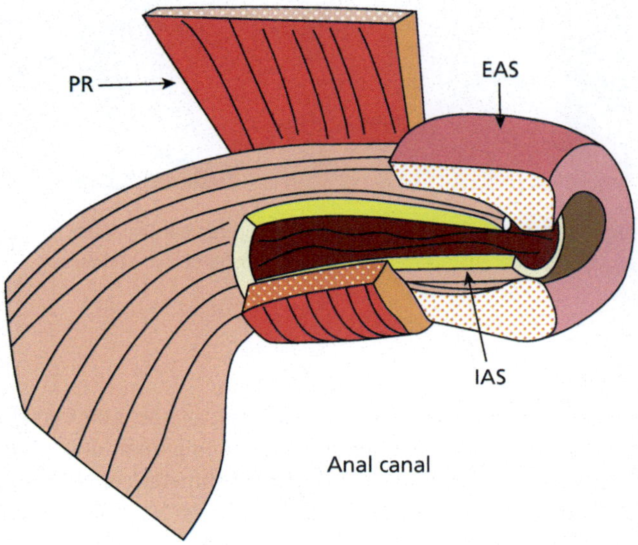

Figure 16.1 Schematic diagram of the anal canal. EAS, external anal sphincter; IAS, internal anal sphincter; PR, puborectalis muscle. Soutrce: courtesy of Ravinder Mittal, MD.

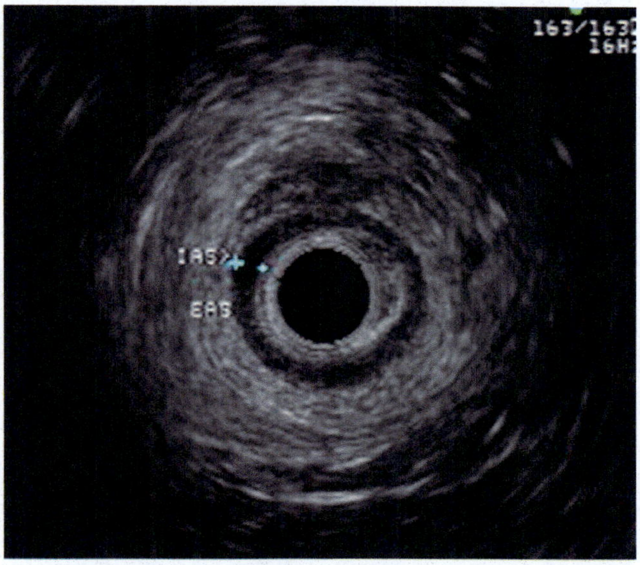

Figure 16.2 Normal anal sphincter complex. The internal anal sphincter (IAS) is black (hypoechoic) and the external anal sphincter (EAS) is white (hyperechoic).

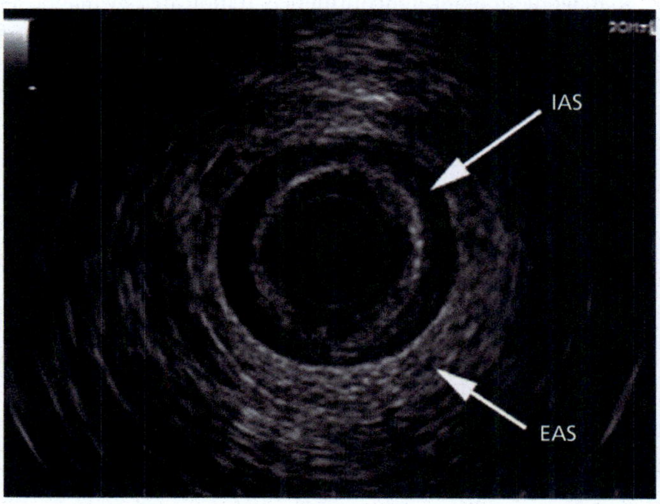

(a)

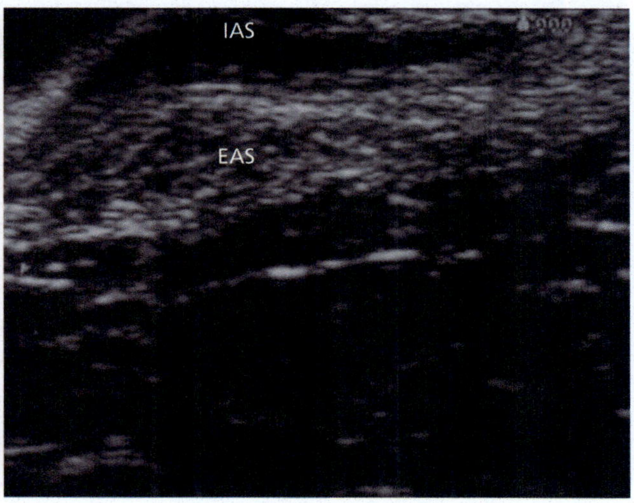

(b)

Figure 16.3 Normal anal sphincter complex. The internal anal sphincter (IAS) is black (hypoechoic) and the external anal sphincter (EAS) is white (hyperechoic): (a) radial array image; (b) linear array image. Source: courtesy of Everson Artifon, MD.

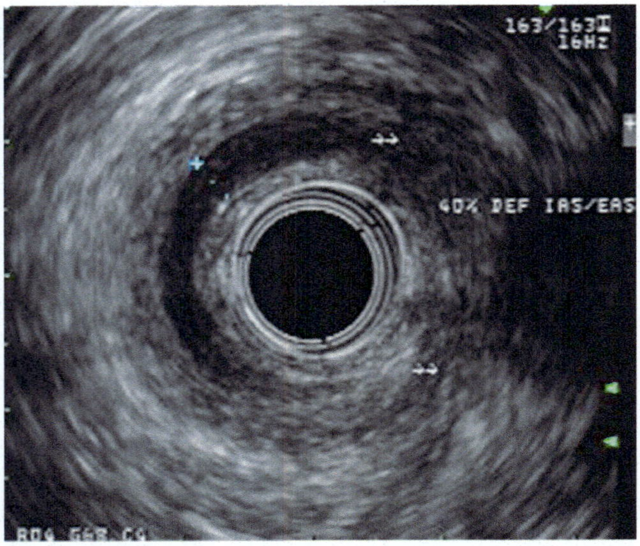

Figure 16.4 Forty percent defect in both the internal hypoechoic anal sphincter (IAS) and the outer hyperechoic external anal sphincter (EAS), likely due to obstetrical trauma.

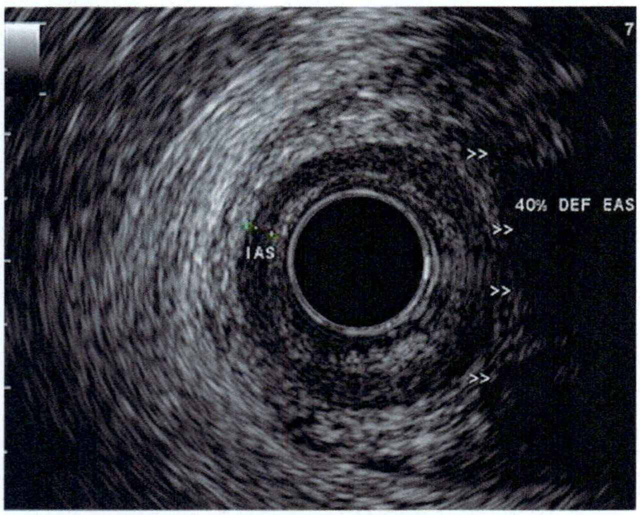

Figure 16.5 Forty percent defect in external anal sphincter (EAS), likely due to obstetrical trauma. Note that the black hypoechoic inner circular muscle layer is circumferentially intact.

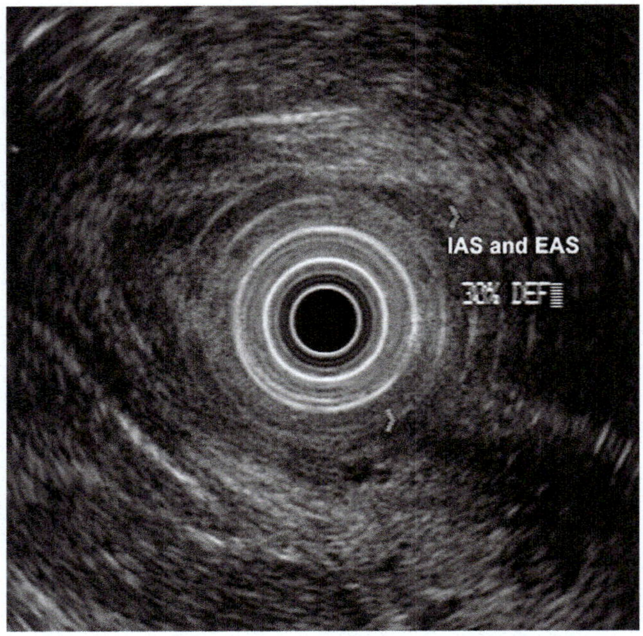

Figure 16.6 Thirty percent defect in both the internal anal sphincter (IAS) and the external anal sphincter (EAS), likely due to obstetrical trauma.

which may sometimes be incorrectly identified as an EAS defect. IAS defects appear as hyperechoic breaks in the normally hypoechoic ring, whereas EAS defects appear as relatively hypoechoic areas in the normally hyperechoic ring (Figures 16.4–16.6). Obstetrical trauma usually involves the anterior aspect of the anal sphincters (Video 16.1).

Transperineal ultrasound

Transperineal three-dimensional (3D) ultrasound offers another approach to evaluate the anal sphincter complex. It is less invasive compared to the endoanal approach and allows visualization of the entire sling of the puborectalis muscle, which is often not possible on endoanal ultrasound (Figure 16.7). The length of the anal sphincter complex and the longitudinal size of sphincter defect can be studied using the 3D images (Figure 16.8).

Treatment

Trial of bulk forming agents, antidiarrheal agents, bowel habit ritualization, and biofeedback is reasonable for initial management of fecal incontinence. If indicated by diagnostic testing or lack of response to conservative management, patients can be referred for surgical management.

Perianal fistula

Perianal fistula can develop secondary to trauma, Crohn's disease, infection, or malignancy. Endoanal ultrasound can be used to study the fistula course and anal sphincter involvement. Fistula tracks are identified as hypoechoic tracts on endoanal ultrasound (Figures 16.9–16.11). Hydrogen peroxide infusion into the fistula generates the formation of small air bubbles, which can enhance visualization of the fistula track by changing it to a hyperechoic structure on ultrasound (Figure 16.12 and Video 16.2). Additional examples are shown in Figures 16.13–16.16.

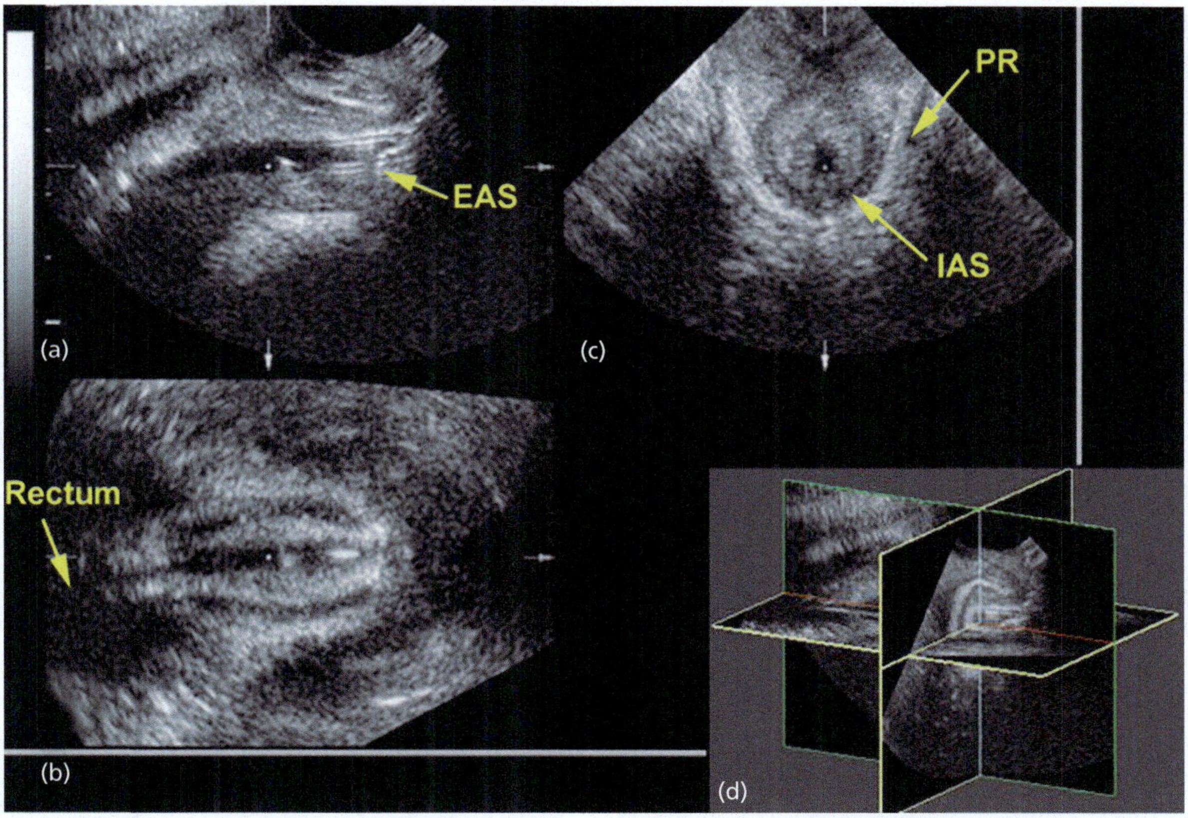

Figure 16.7 Transperineal three-dimensional ultrasound images showing the anal canal in the three orthogonal planes. (a) Sagittal image of the anal sphincter complex. EAS, external anal sphincter. (b) Coronal image of the anal sphincter complex. (c) Transverse image at the proximal anal sphincter showing the internal anal sphincter (IAS) and the puborectalis muscle (PR). Source: courtesy of Ravinder Mittal, MD.

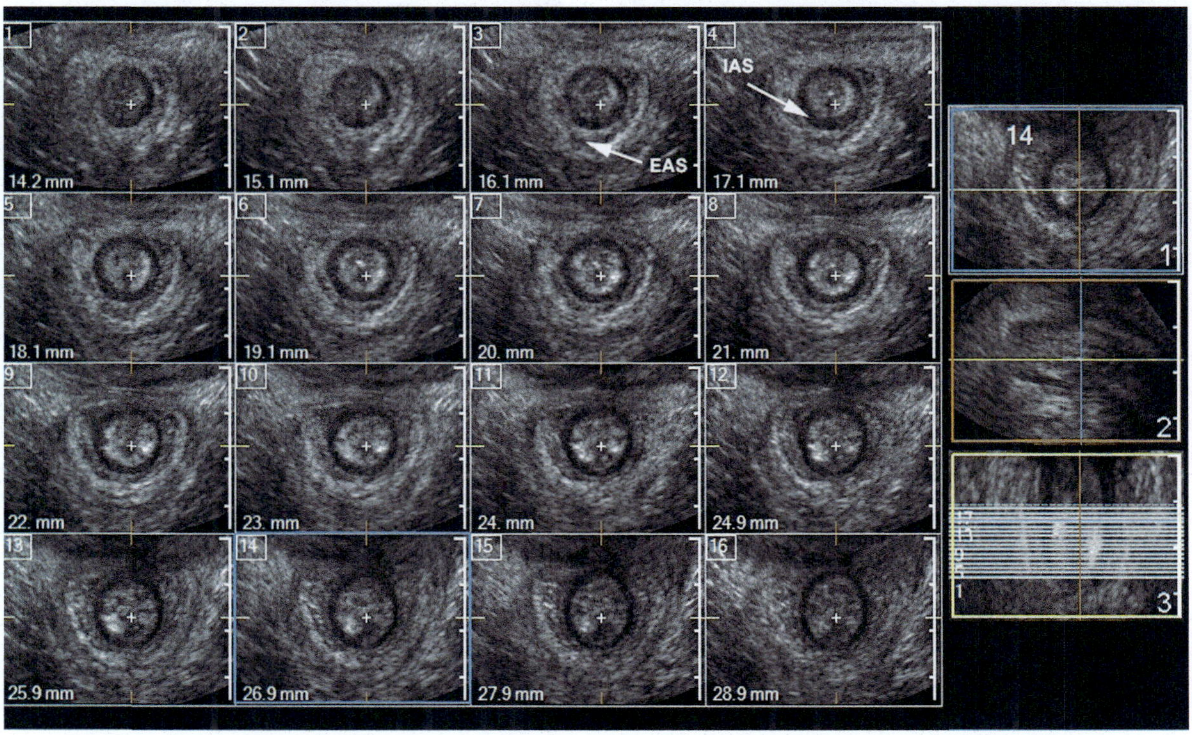

Figure 16.8 Transverse (cross-sectional) 1-mm multislice imaging of the normal anal canal produced by transperineal three-dimensional ultrasound. EAS, external anal sphincter; IAS, internal anal sphincter. Source: courtesy of Ravinder Mittal, MD.

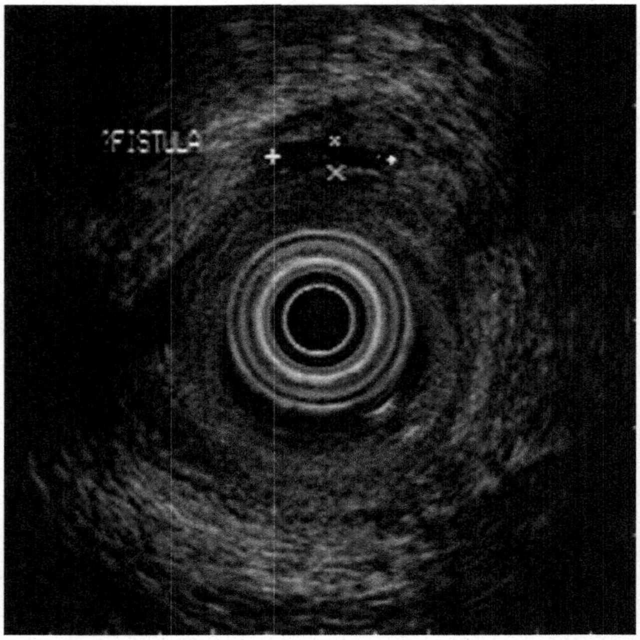

Figure 16.9 Perianal fistula. Note that the anechoic tubular structure is outside of the anal sphincters.

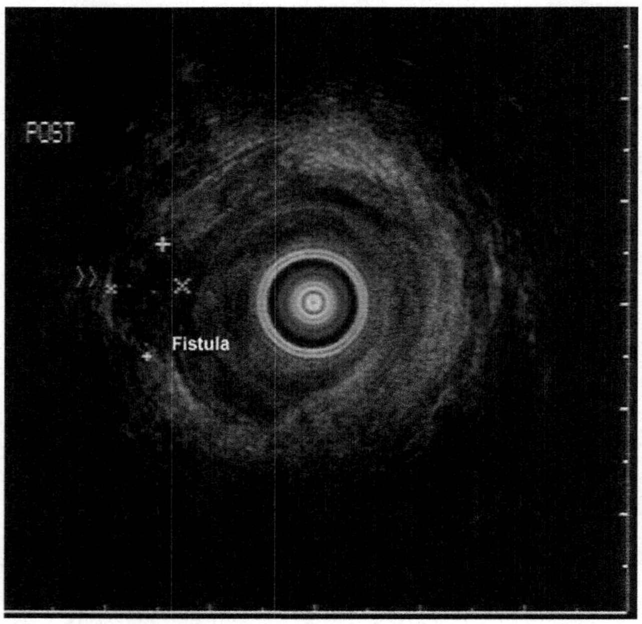

Figure 16.10 Perianal fistula with small perianal abscess measuring 11 × 7 mm.

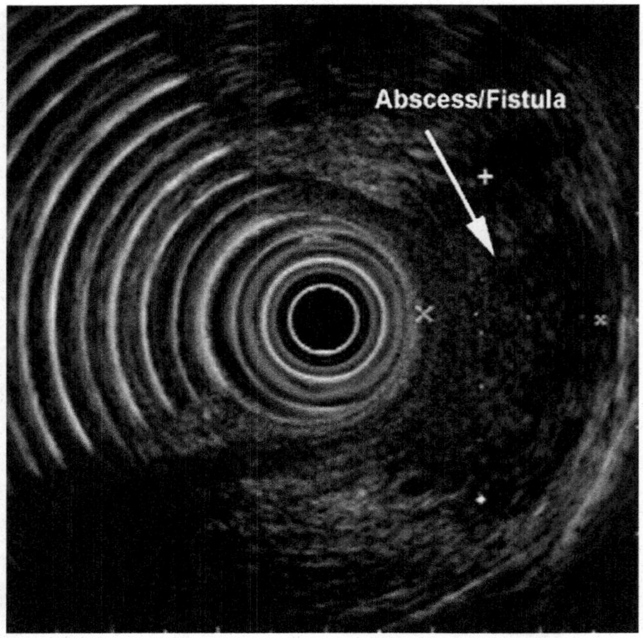

Figure 16.11 Perianal abscess and fistula.

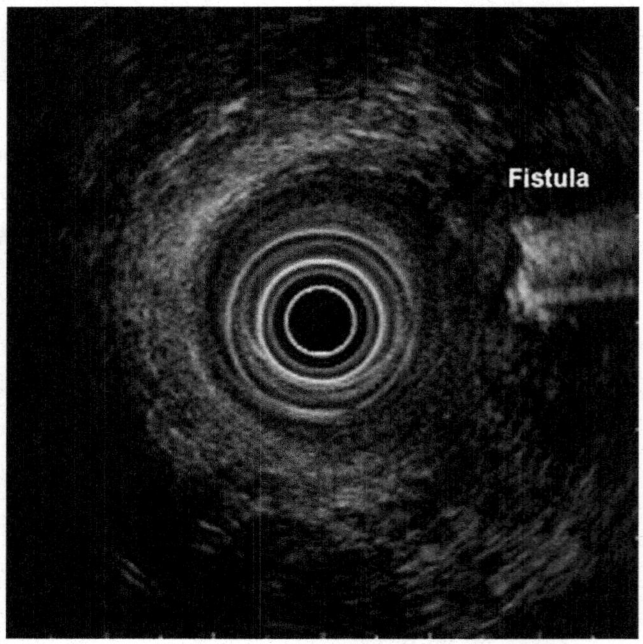

Figure 16.12 Post-hydrogen peroxide injection image of the perianal fistula and abscess shown in Figure 16.11. Note the hyperechoic signal which better delineates the fistula track in the abscess after hydrogen peroxide injection.

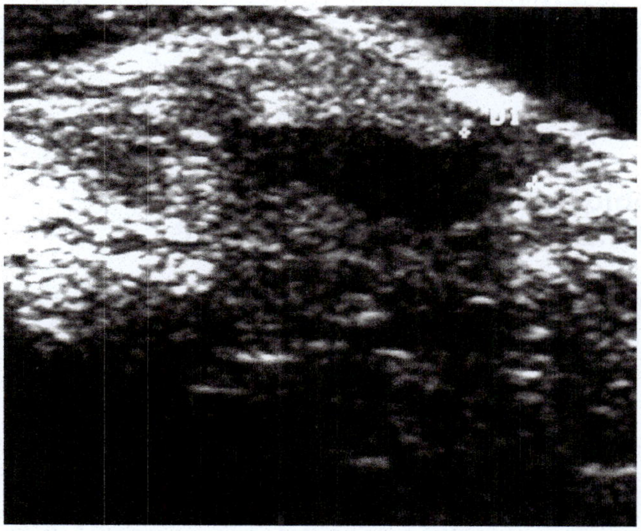

Figure 16.13 Perianal fistula. A hyperechoic path is visible, starting on the skin of the perianal region and coursing through the hyperechoic band which corresponds to the external anal sphincter (outlined with the + markers). Source: courtesy of Everson Artifon, MD.

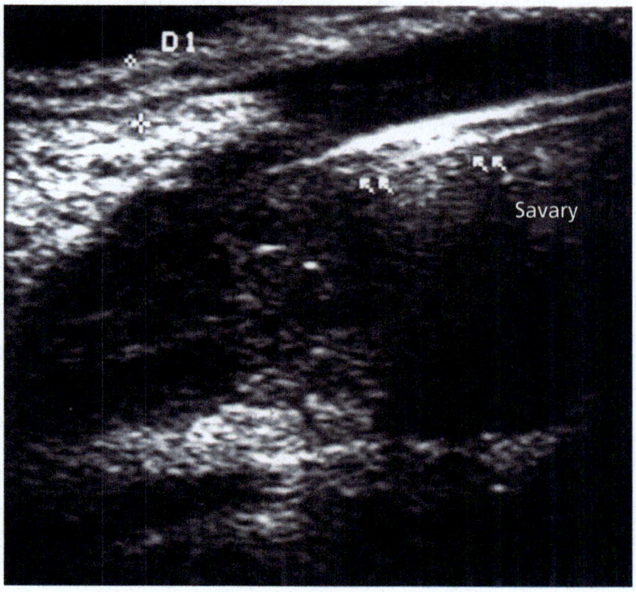

Figure 16.14 The path of a complex perianal fistula is identified by inserting the flexible end of a Savary guidewire through the fistula opening on the skin side. Two hyperechoic lines are seen (Savary wire) that cross the hypoechoic perirectal tissue. Source: courtesy of Everson Artifon, MD.

Chapter video clips

Video 16.1 Endoscopic ultrasound examination of post-obstetrical anal sphincter defect in a patient with fecal incontinence. Source: Aloka.

Video 16.2 Flexible sigmoidoscopy and endoscopic ultrasound examination of perianal fistula and anal sphincter in a patient with Crohn's disease. Source: Olympus.

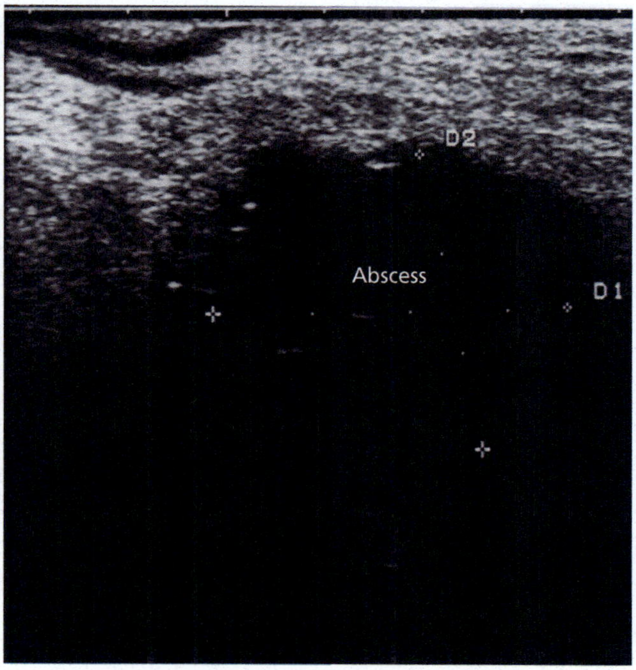

Figure 16.15 Perirectal abscess. A 36-year-old woman with history of Crohn's disease and recurrent perirectal abscesses presented to the hospital with perianal pain and fever. Rectal endoscopic ultrasound was performed under anesthesia, revealing a perirectal abscess (hypoechoic collection) measuring about 36 mm in greatest diameter. Source: courtesy of Everson Artifon, MD.

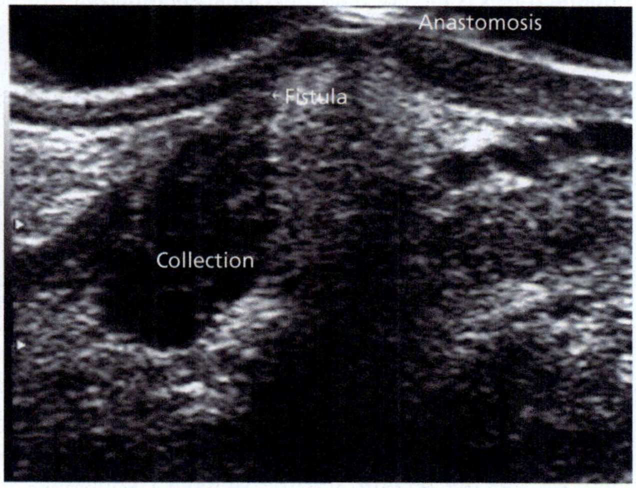

Figure 16.16 Anastomotic abscess. A patient with history of sigmoidectomy for diverticular disease undergoes follow-up colonoscopy. Endoscopic examination reveals the presence of an orifice near the anastomosis, which was draining purulent material. Endoscopic ultrasonography with a linear probe was carried out. In the superior aspect of the image, hyperechoic lines can be noted, corresponding to the staple anastomosis. Inferiorly and to the left of the anastomosis, a heterogeneous, predominantly hypoechoic collection can be seen, representing an abscess that fistulizes to the intestinal lumen. Source: courtesy of Everson Artifon, MD.

17 Endometriosis

José Celso Ardengh[1], Juan Pablo Román Serrano[2], Samuel Galante Romanini[2], Juliana Silveira Lima de Castro[2], and Isabela Trindade Torres[2]

[1] Ribeirão Preto Medical School, University São Paulo, Ribeirão Preto, São Paulo, Brazil; Endoscopy Service Hospital 9 de Julho, Sao Paulo, Brazil

[2] Endoscopy Service Hospital Nove de Julho, Sao Paulo, Brazil

Introduction

Endoscopic ultrasound (EUS) identifies pelvic diseases besides rectal cancer and fecal incontinence. In this context, endometriosis can be identified and classified by changing the therapeutic strategy to be adopted.

Transrectal EUS can identify and stage prostate cancer. Although this indication is not part of the daily clinical practice of medical specialists in the United States, in this chapter we focus on pelvic endometriosis since it can affect the gastrointestinal tract in 3–37% of severe cases.

Definition and location

Endometriosis is the presence of ectopic endometrial stroma outside of the endometrial cavity. Microscopically, it may be associated with macrophages full of hemosiderin; macroscopically, it appears as pigmented (typical) or non-pigmented (atypical) brown, red, or black lesions. It affects approximately 10% of women of childbearing age. It can be deep or extensive and affect adjacent organs such as the rectum and/or sigmoid colon, the bladder, and the ureters. When it invades the ovary, this is known as endometrioma.

This disease is multifocal, and the main locations affected are the pelvic peritoneum (ovarian cavity and uterosacral ligament) and the pelvic organs (ovaries, fallopian tubes, bladder, sigmoid colon, and rectum), although sites of endometriosis can also be found in the liver, lungs, pleura, and other organs. The sites most affected by extragenital endometriosis are the rectum and the sigmoid colon (85% of cases), followed by the cecal appendix and small intestine.

Epidemiology and risk factors

It is estimated that 3–10% of the women in their fertile period have endometriosis. Around 30% can be infertile, and approximately 50% experience chronic pelvic pain. Occurrence in black women is lower than in white women. The diagnosis may be given in the third decade of life. A low body mass index and anxiety levels higher than average are characteristic of the disease. Late diagnosis favors a poor quality of life due to chronic pain, with implications for day-to-day work, and manifests high rates of infertility.

Risk factors include:

- family background, with an affected first-degree relative
- early menarche and late menopause
- nulliparity
- late pregnancy
- short menstrual cycles (<27 days)
- increased menstrual flow and volume
- cervical stenosis and other obstructions to menstrual flow
- white race.

The protective factors include smoking, use of contraceptives, multiparity, and early first pregnancy (<18 years).

Clinical picture

Progressive dysmenorrhea, chronic pelvic pain, dyspareunia, infertility, and intestinal and urinary abnormalities during menstruation are common symptoms. With respect to intestinal abnormality, it is relevant to mention change in intestinal habit (constipation and diarrhea), abdominal distress and/or distension, and cyclical bleeding (hematochezia).

Atlas of Endoscopic Ultrasonography, Second Edition. Edited by Frank Gress, Thomas Savides, Brenna Casey, and Everson L. A. Artifon.

Companion website: www.wiley.com/go/gress/atlas

Diagnosis

The medical history, physical examination, and laboratory tests can diagnose the presence of endometriosis. Confirmation is provided by histopathological analysis through video-laparoscopy, while tests for CA-125 (up to 35 U/ml), carried out between the first and third day of the menstrual cycle, are also helpful in diagnosis. CA-125 sensitivity is higher in stages III and IV endometriosis with extensive disease, adhesions or endometriomas. This test is therefore recommended for monitoring and treatment. The serum amyloid A protein (up to 5 U/ml) is specially requested when intestinal disorder is suspected.

Classification

The American Society for Reproductive Medicine classifies endometriosis according to size, depth, and location in four stages.

- Stage I: minimal disease, with isolated implants and without significant adhesions.
- Stage II: mild, with added superficial implants smaller than 5 cm and dispersed, without significant adhesions.
- Stage III: moderate, with multiple superficial and deep implants and evident peritubal and peritoneal adhesions.
- Stage IV: severe, with multiple superficial and deep implants, including endometriomas and firm and dense adhesions.

Imaging methods

Abdominal and pelvic magnetic resonance imaging (MRI), transrectal ultrasound, EUS, and video-laparoscopy help in the diagnosis because they have high accuracy. Pelvic and transvaginal ultrasound can be normal or reveal ground-glass cysts, but experienced clinicians can determine the involvement of the intestinal wall, including the layers, and good intestinal preparation helps to identify the ectopic spots and determine the intestinal extension of the disease, facilitating the surgical approach. After transvaginal ultrasound, MRI is considered second line for staging of the disease.

EUS

The examination is divided into two steps.

1. Endoscopic evaluation of the mucosa up to the distal sigmoid, the device being advanced in search of stenosis, extrinsic compression, and changes of relief or tension of the mucosa.

2. Echoendoscopic evaluation of the digestive system walls on withdrawal of the echoendoscope. The five or seven echoendoscopic layers are evaluated, depending on the frequency used (5, 7.5, 10, or 12 MHz).

In order to facilitate communication among professionals and summarize the examination findings, the Echo-Logic classification was developed based on the location of the pelvic injury and the degree of penetration into the vaginal wall (Figure 17.1). The degree of penetration into the intestinal wall is represented by the letter T, where T1 represents extraintestinal

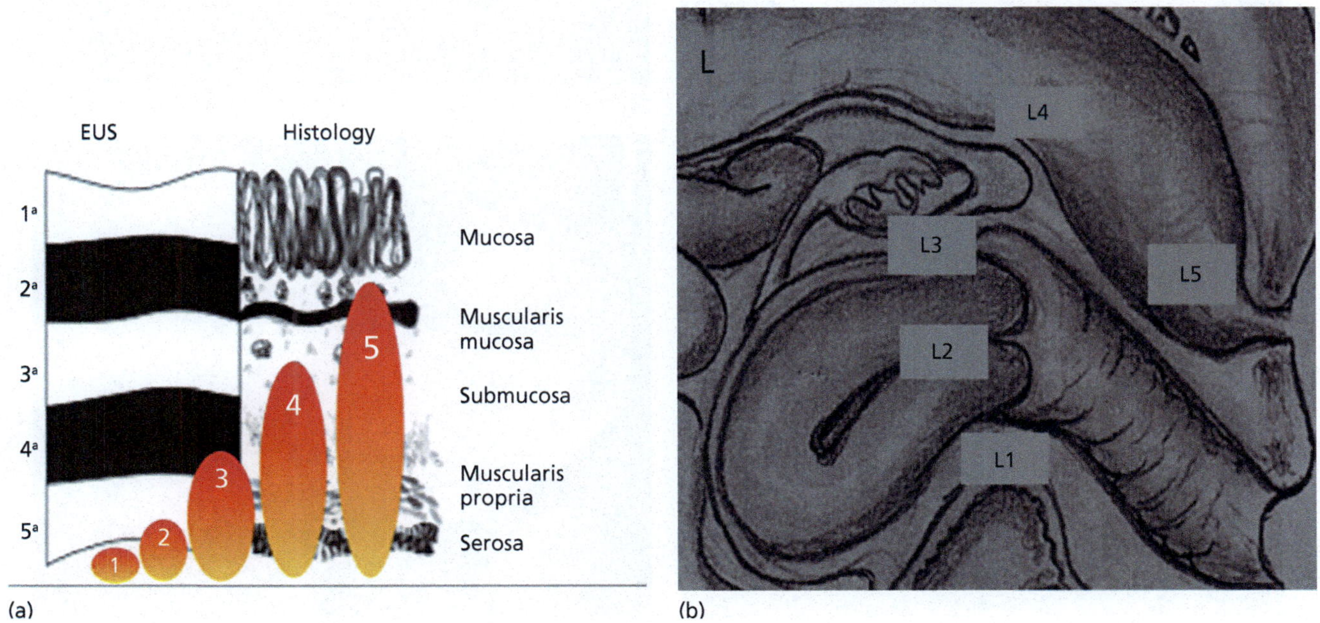

Figure 17.1 (a, b) Classification of intestinal endometriosis according to Rossini and Ribeiro (2002). This classification is based on the dissemination of endometriosis in the intestinal walls as it is observed with EUS (ueT1–ueT5) and also on its location in the pelvis (ueL1–ueL5). u, ultrasound; e, endometriosis classification; L, location; T, tumor.

injury, T2 injury that affects the serosa, T3a injury that affects the longitudinal (external) muscle layer itself, T3b injury that affects the circular (internal) muscle layer itself, T4 injury that affects the submucosa, and T5 injury that affects the muscular wall of the mucosa. Regarding the anatomical location of the pelvis, five sites are represented by the letter L, where L1 represents pre-cervical injury, L2 paracervical (L2R, right; L2L, left), L3 retrouterine, L4 injury in rectovaginal reflection, and L5 injury in the rectovaginal septum. These designations are preceded by the letters EU (ultrasound for endometriosis). For L5 injuries, the distance in millimeters between the injury and the internal anal sphincter is also mentioned.

Endometriosis is defined as infiltration, usually larger than 5 mm, from the muscular layer. These lesions occur as slightly heterogeneous hypoechoic nodules infiltrating the fourth echoendoscopic layer. With higher frequencies (7.5–12 MHz), invasion of all the muscular layer or just the external longitudinal muscular layer can be differentiated. In general, the layer nearest to the serosa is slightly more hyperechogenic than the layer nearest to the intestinal light source due to the higher fibrosis component in this region (Figures 17.2–17.8).

Invasion of the submucosa or mucosa is rare, but is characterized by the interruption of hypoechogenic lines. Other important data for evaluation include location of the lesion, vertical depth, longitudinal extension, circumference of damage of the intestinal loop, submucous infiltration, invasion of adjacent organs, occurrence of pelvic blocking, measurement of the distance from the lesion to the posterior peritoneal reflection, occurrence and quantification of the rectovaginal septum alteration, and appearance of synchronic lesions.

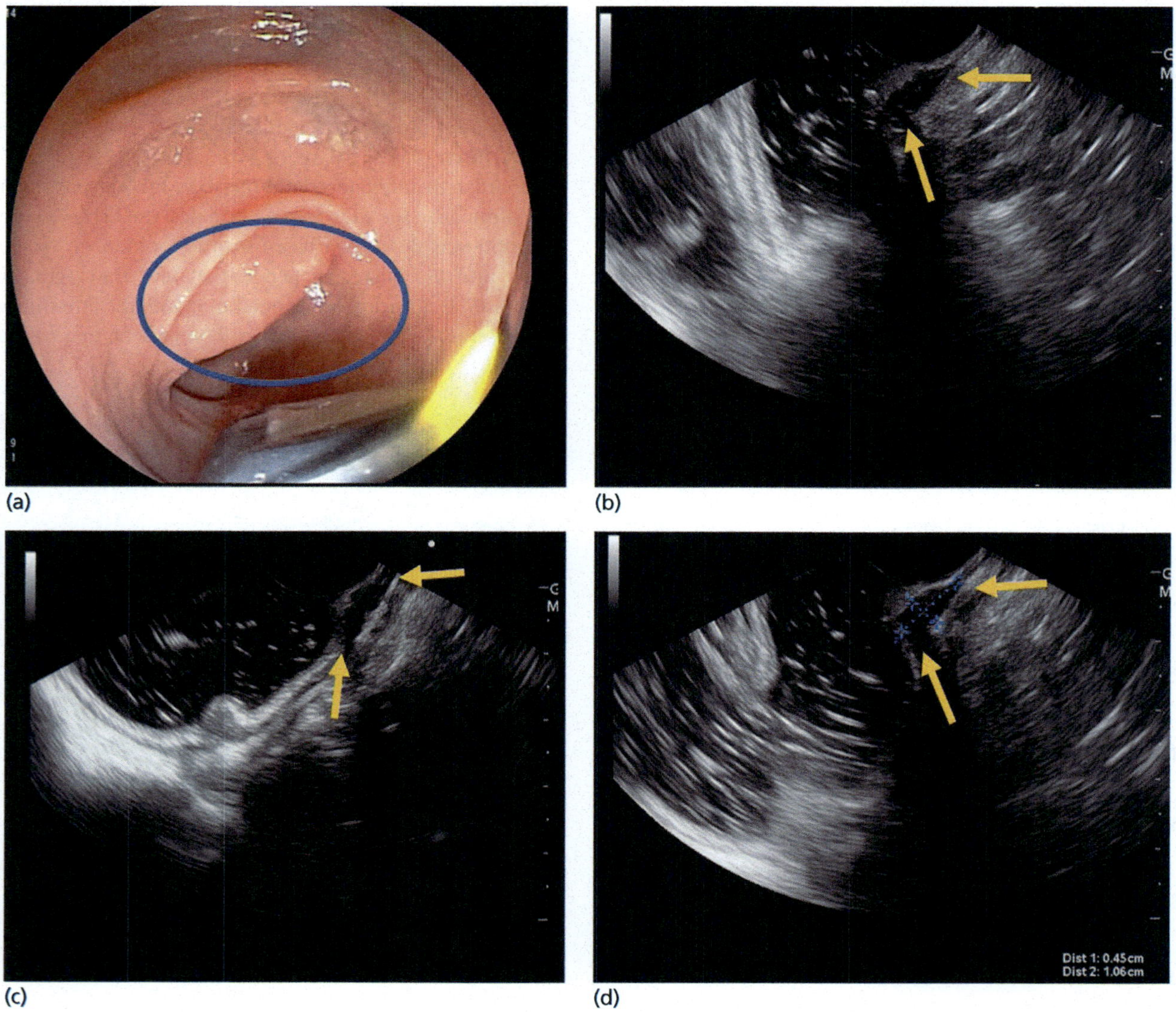

Figure 17.2 Endometriosis sites with alteration of the colonic wall of the rectosigmoid junction, which affects the fourth layer of the appropriate muscle at full depth. (a) Endoscopic view; (b–d) sectoral EUS showing hypoechoic homogeneous area with well-defined borders (arrows).

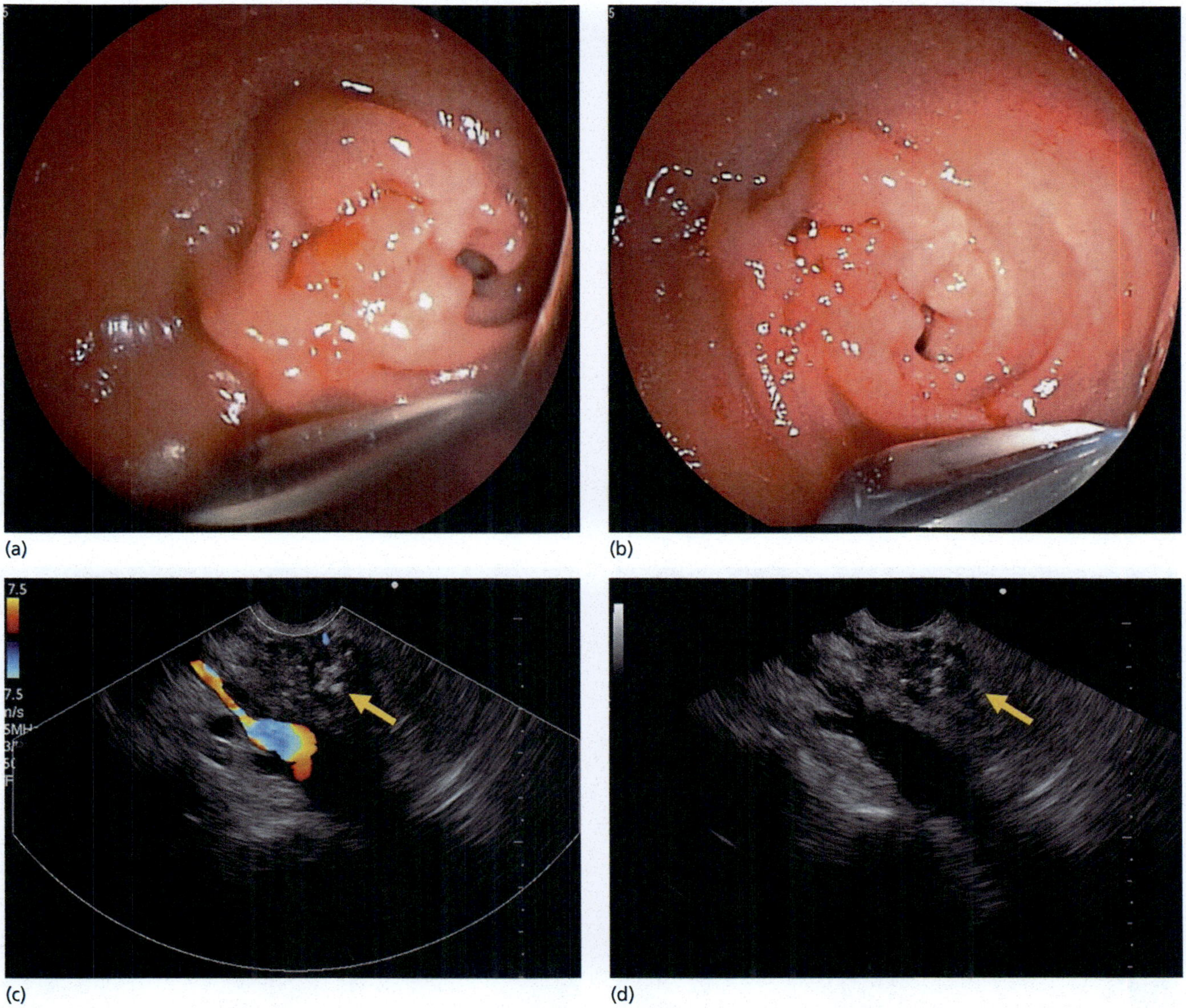

(a) (b) (c) (d)

Figure 17.3 (a, b) Endoscopic view of the area of sigmoid substenosis. (c) Positive Doppler over hypoechoic and heterogeneous site with alteration of all the wall of the sigmoid colon. (d) Hypoechoic heterogeneous ill-defined lesion that has invaded all the layers of the sigmoid colon. Obvious seat of endometriosis with intestinal invasion.

It is important to accurately describe the distance from the lowest identified lesion of the puborectal muscle to the anal sphincter since this information is vital for surgical planning. This is especially true for lesions that affect the rectovaginal septum, which is the hyperechogenic line that starts in the posterior peritoneal reflection and extends to the beginning of the internal anal sphincter.

Other pelvic structures that can be evaluated for endometriotic involvement using EUS are the uterus, ovaries, uterosacral ligaments, and bladder. Ovarian endometriomas have a characteristic "frosted glass" echogenicity (Figure 17.9).

EUS plus fine needle aspiration for the evaluation of endometriosis

Endometriosis is the presence of stroma outside the uterine cavity. The diagnosis of rectosigmoid invasion by colonoscopy is difficult; however, fine-needle aspiration guided by endosonography (EUS-FNA) allows the diagnosis of a subepithelial tumor identified by colonoscopy (Figures 17.10 and 17.11).

EUS-FNA is indicated in patients with nonspecific gastrointestinal symptoms, hematochezia, abdominal pain, and recently initiated constipation, as well as perimenstrual

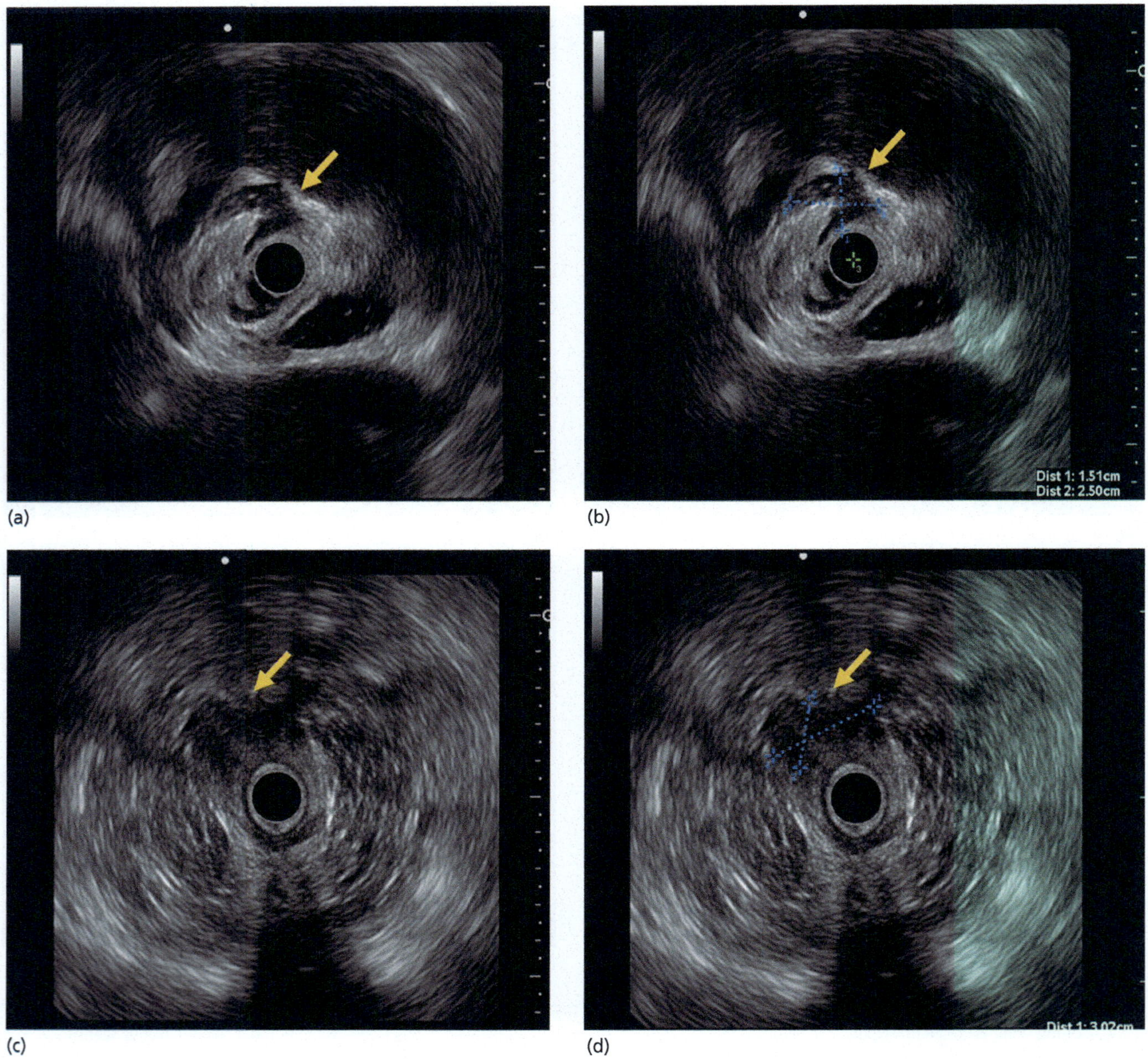

Figure 17.4 Radial scanning with two foci in different locations: (a, b) rectosigmoid junction; (c, d) lower rectum at the rectovaginal septum (yellow arrows).

pelvic pain during menstruation. If a suspicious lesion that invades the fourth layer has been identified on EUS, FNA using a 20G ProCore needle (Cook Medical) is recommended in order to obtain the greatest possible amount of tissue for histopathology.

Cytopathology and histopathology confirm the presence of endometriosis by identifying endometriotic implants with fibrous tissue, blood, foamy macrophages with hemosiderin granules and cysts (Figures 17.12–17.14). EUS-FNA is increasingly used for the diagnosis of endometriosis with rectosigmoid invasion. Sensitivity is only about 40–50%, and therefore video-laparoscopy is still recommended even today as gold standard for the diagnosis of endometriosis of the peritoneal cavity.

Video-laparoscopy

This method is the gold standard for the anatomopathological diagnosis, and can be a very interesting therapeutic tool. It identifies defects, lesions, and white and reddish adhesions (called "candle flame").

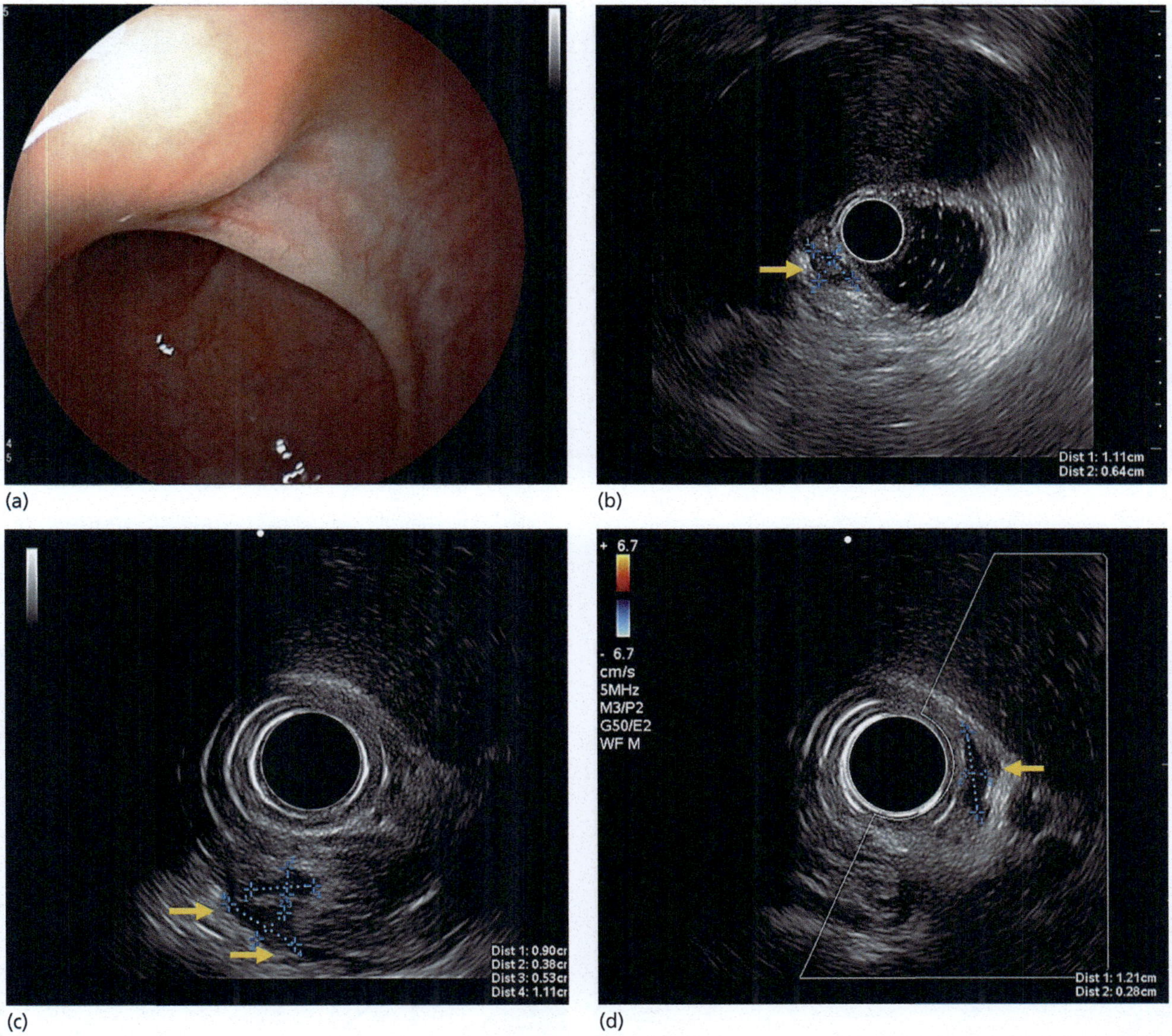

Figure 17.5 (a) Bulging of the upper rectum wall. (b–d) Radial exploration of sites of endometriosis at several positions showing hypoechogenicity and irregularity of borders beyond focal heterogeneity.

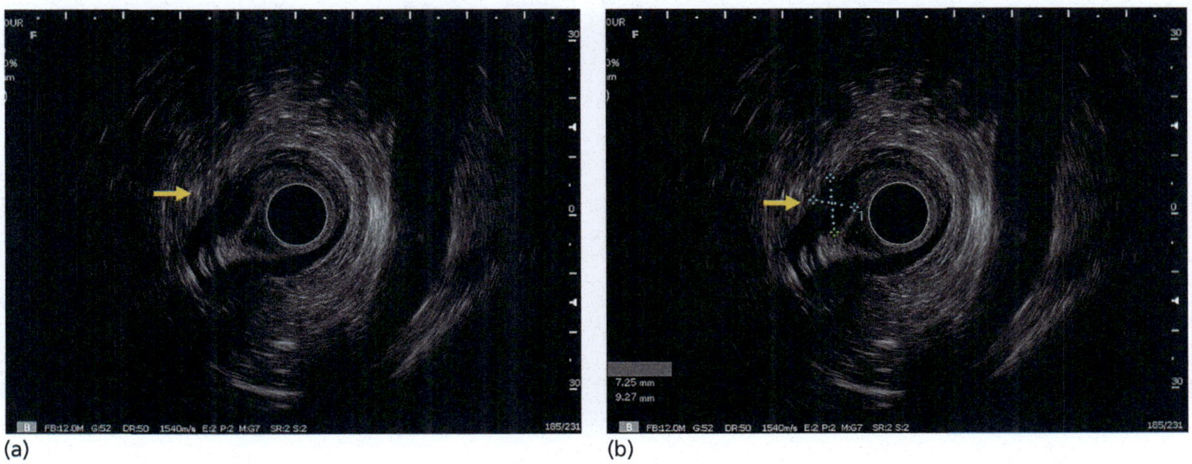

Figure 17.6 (a, b) Radial exploration of sites of hypoechoic, homogeneous, sigmoid endometriosis completely affecting the muscular layer.

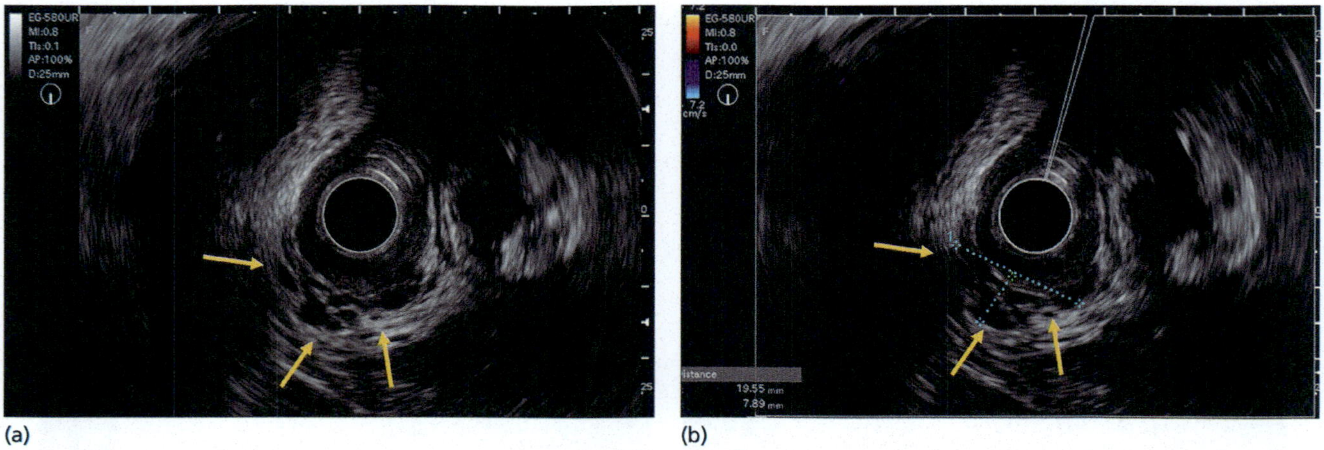

Figure 17.7 (a, b) Radial exploration of a heterogeneous hypoechoic focus with irregular borders that affects the rectovaginal septum (yellow arrows).

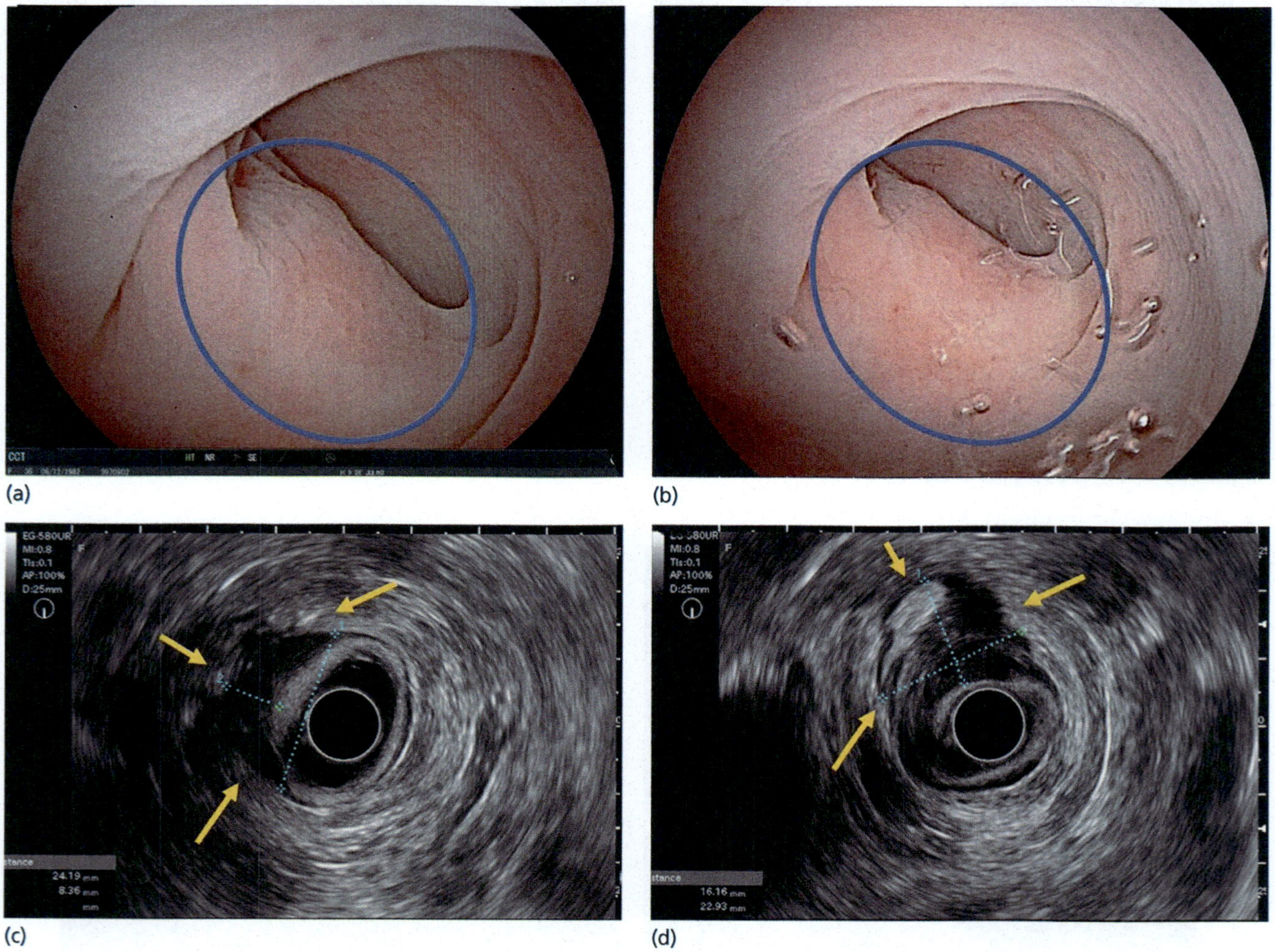

Figure 17.8 (a, b) Endoscopic view of the upper rectum showing bulging of the superficial mucosa. (c, d) Radial scanning of a heterogeneous area with irregular borders (yellow arrows) that surround all the colon wall.

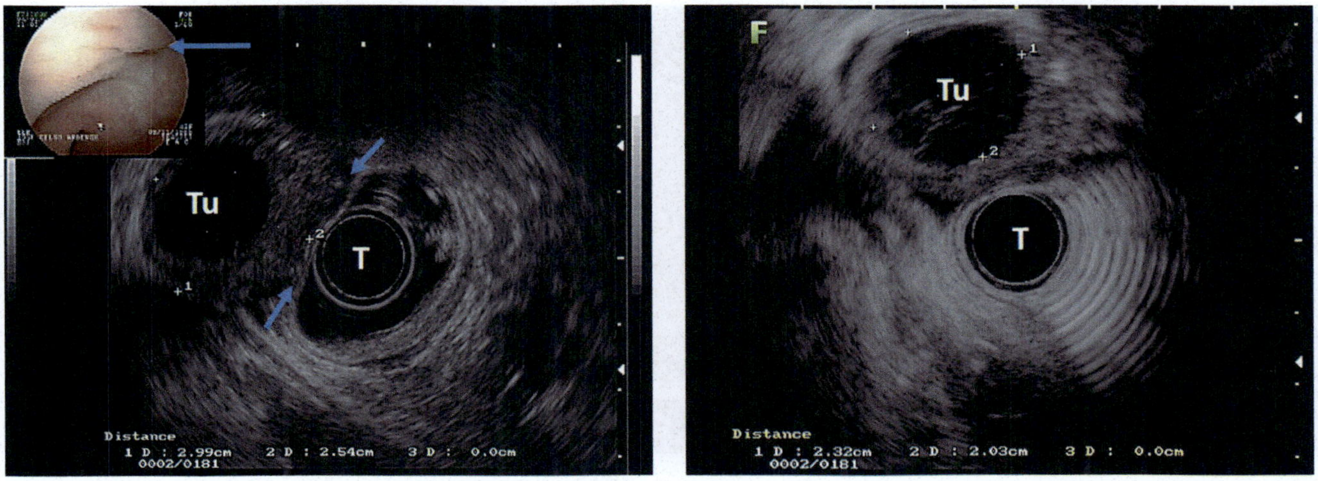

(a) (b)

Figure 17.9 (a, b) Extrinsic sigmoid compression of a left ovary endometrioma with cystic solid composition and thickening of its walls.

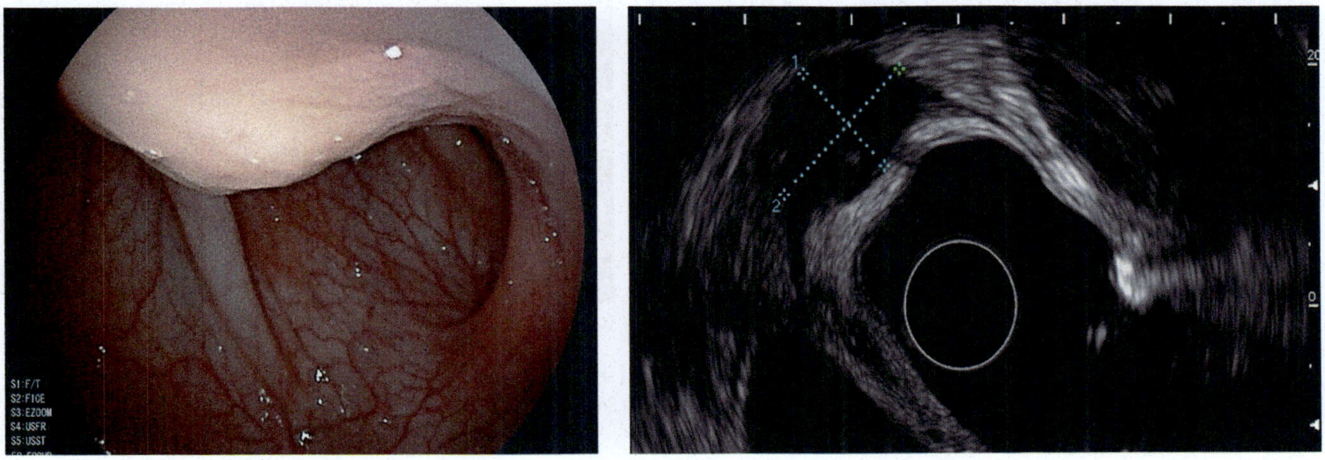

(a) (b)

Figure 17.10 (a) Colonoscopy showing a subepithelial lesion as sigmoid bulging. (b) A hypoechoic lesion affecting the fourth echoendoscopic layer (muscularis propria) indicating deep endometriosis.

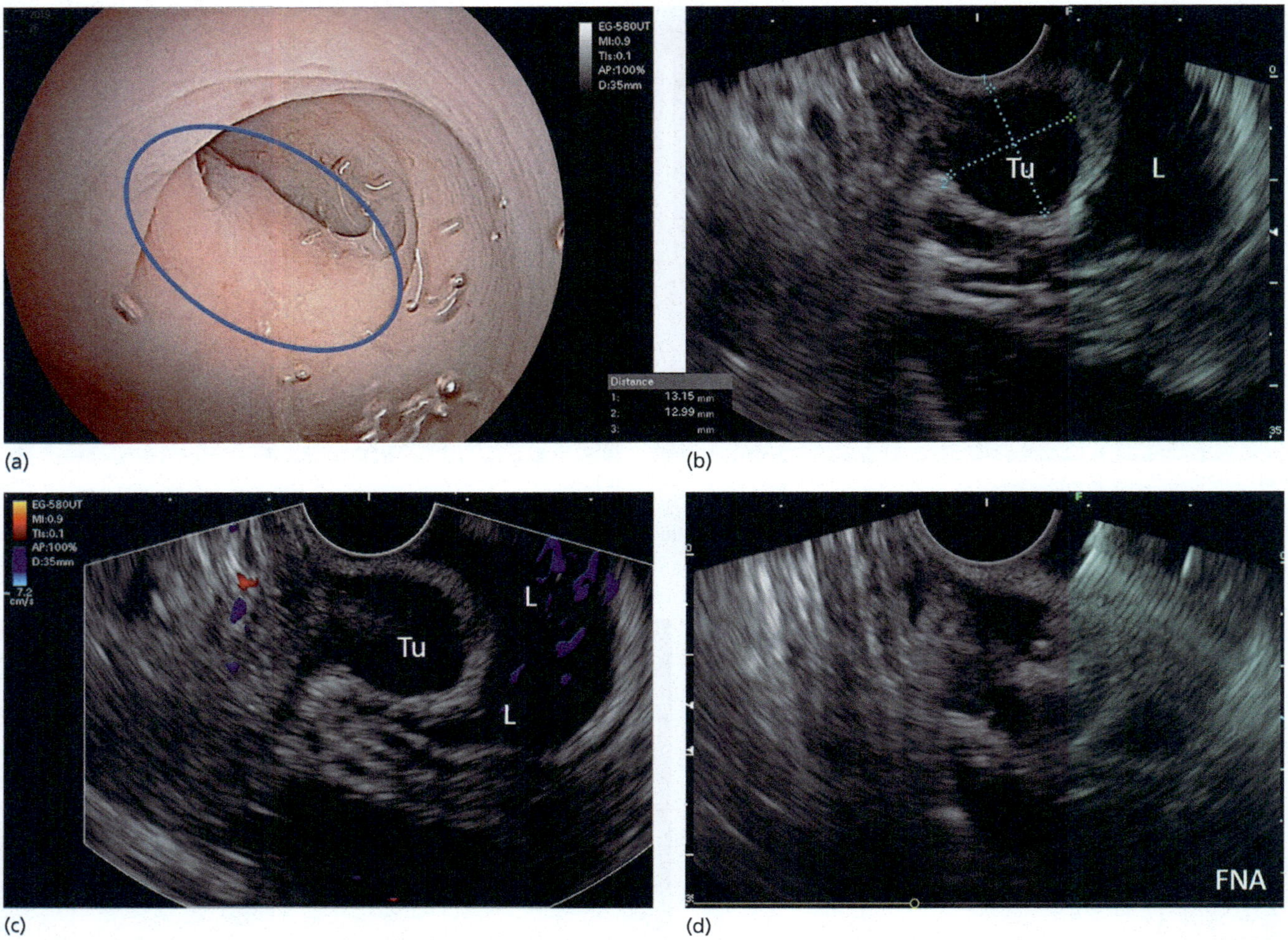

Figure 17.11 (a) Bulging of the rectosigmoid junction. (b, c) Sectoral exploration showing a hypoechoic lesion that has affected all the muscular layers in vertical depth, longitudinal extension, and partial circumference. (d) EUS-FNA with ProCore 20G needle.

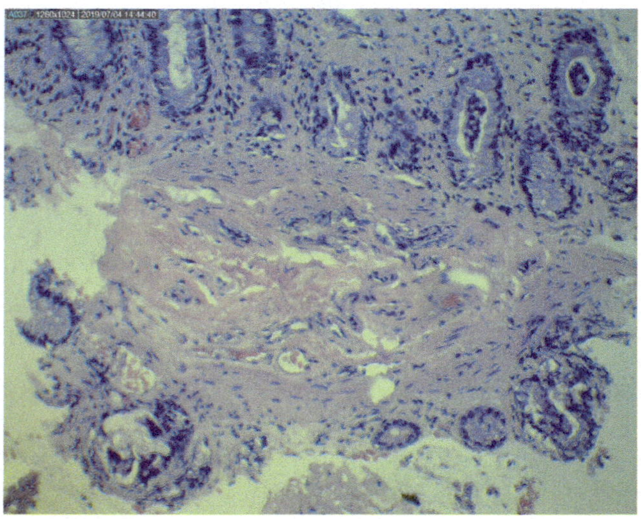

Figure 17.12 Endometrial gland and endometrial stroma and superficial colonic mucosae in tissue sample obtained by ProCore 20G FNA. The histopathological findings confirm the presence of deep endometriosis.

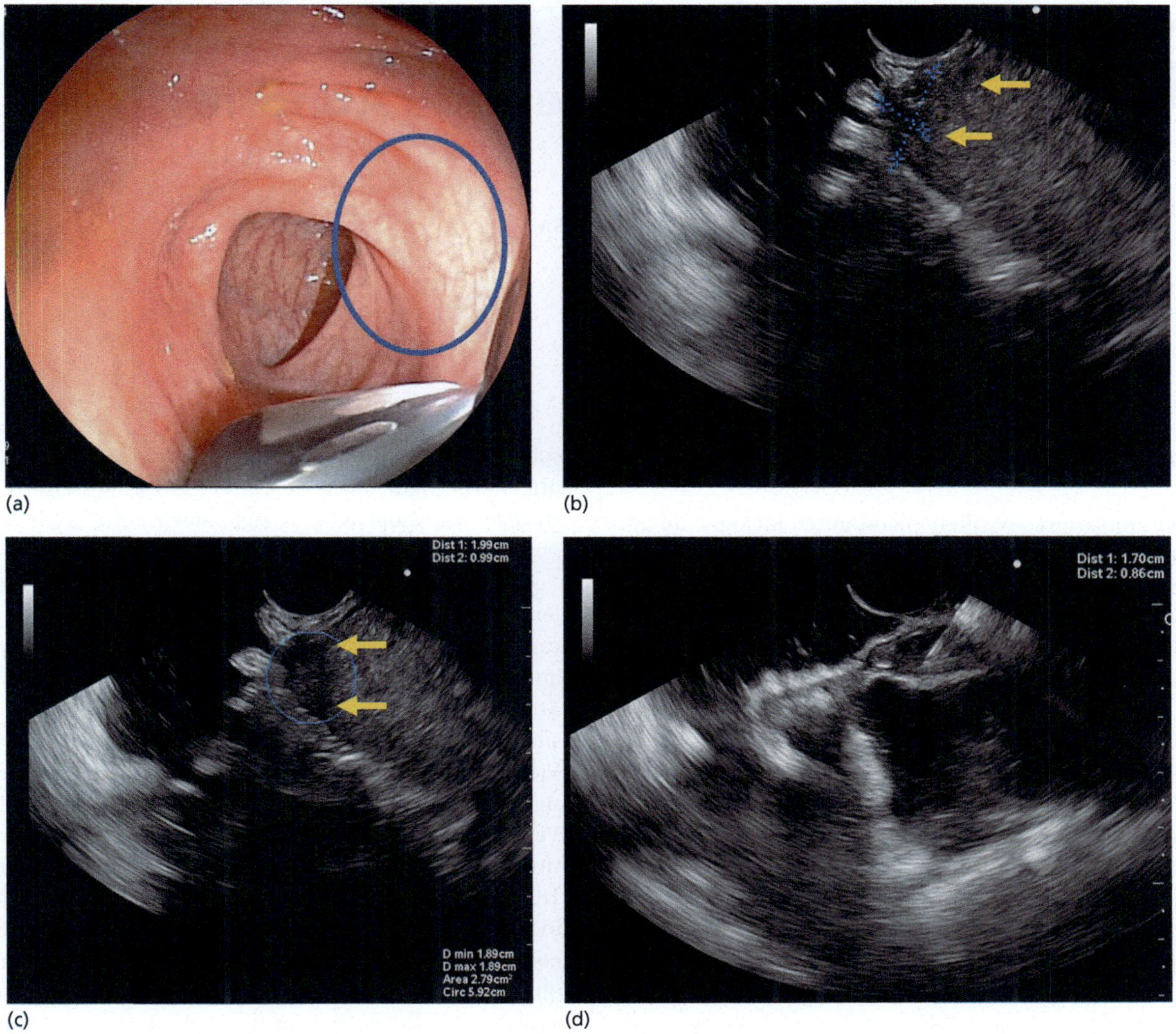

Figure 17.13 Radial scanning EUS of two foci of endometriosis located in two different locations: (a, b) rectosigmoid junction; (c, d) lower rectum at the rectovaginal septum (yellow arrows).

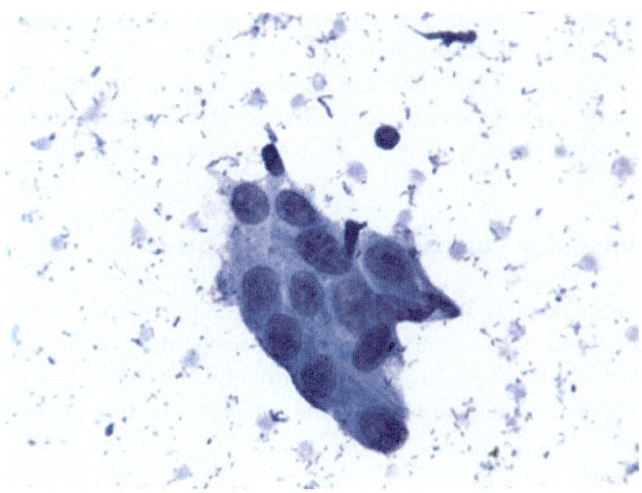

Figure 17.14 Glandular cells aspirated from endometrial lining.

18 Vascular Anomalies and Abnormalities

John C. Deutsch
Essentia Health Care Systems, Duluth, MN, USA

Introduction

Vascular anomalies are often encountered incidentally during an endoscopic ultrasound (EUS) examination. They are frequently ignored as inconsequential (as in the case of atherosclerosis or calcification of the aorta). However, some vascular processes may be responsible for the symptoms which lead to the EUS examination. For example, one may find vascular occlusion of the superior mesenteric artery and celiac artery in a patient with abdominal pain, or splenic vein thrombosis in a patient with gastrointestinal (GI) hemorrhage ultimately due to isolated bleeding gastric varices. Dysphagia can be causes by aortic arch anomalies ("dysphagia lusoria"). Sometimes an unexpected vascular finding can preclude the original reason for the EUS examination as shown in a case discussed in this chapter in which an aortic pseudoaneurysm was identified during an EUS evaluation of early gastric cancer.

This chapter contains images collected during EUS examinations showing a variety of vascular abnormalities that varied from the trivial to important, both symptomatic and asymptomatic. This is not intended to be comprehensive, since there are an unlimited number of conditions which could be described. Rather, this chapter will hopefully help the endosonographer to pay attention to normal and potentially abnormal vascular anatomy, since these features may be pivotal in understanding a patient's condition.

Aortic arch anomalies

Potentially symptomatic aortic arch anomalies are relatively uncommon and occur in a small proportion (1 in 500) of the population. Those which can be easily identified during routine EUS examination include the aberrant right common carotid artery arising directly from the aortic arch. The right subclavian artery arises from the arch distal to the left subclavian artery. The right subclavian artery passes posteriorly to the trachea and esophagus. A right-sided aortic arch can also occasionally be found.

These congenital anomalies can cause swallowing problems (dysphagia lusoria). If the difficulties are severe, one can transect the artery which passes between the esophagus and the vertebrae and reimplant it. After this type of surgery a residual stump can sometimes be identified. Video 18.1 shows an example of an anomalous right subclavian artery. Video 18.2 shows a different patient in whom an anomalous right subclavian artery had been resected and reimplanted. Video 18.3 shows a right-sided aortic arch with a vascular ring formed by an aberrant left subclavian artery, and Video 18.4 shows a different patient with the same features following surgical repair of the vascular ring. As shown in the videos, the aorta is in the right chest (to the left of the vertebrae on the image screen) through its length. At the level of the arch, the left subclavian stump can be seen. An ectatic aorta can sometimes suggest a right-sided aorta (with the aorta in the right chest relative to the vertebrae), but this can usually be sorted out by tracing the aorta for its entire length as in Video 18.5. If the image screen on a radial array instrument is inadvertently flipped, one can also be fooled into thinking structures are on the opposite side of the chest.

There are many different variants (such as double aortic arch) and branching patterns such as the bovine arch. Details concerning these varieties are available on the Internet.

Vascular calcification and plaques

These features are extremely common, although the extent of disease varies. Calcification can be seen in any of the arterial structures (Video 18.6). It is usually without symptoms. The echo signal coming off the calcified structures is very

Atlas of Endoscopic Ultrasonography, Second Edition. Edited by Frank Gress, Thomas Savides, Brenna Casey, and Everson L. A. Artifon.

Companion website: www.wiley.com/go/gress/atlas

bright with acoustic shadowing behind. The shadowing can interfere with visualization of perivascular structures and complicate fine needle aspiration (FNA) of small lesions. The vascular calcifications can sometimes lead to diagnostic confusion (Figure 18.1). Video 18.7 shows the computed tomography (CT) scan of a patient referred to our center for abdominal pain and chronic pancreatitis of unknown cause. Endoscopic ultrasound clearly showed that all calcifications were associated with an artery and that the pancreatic parenchyma was normal. On careful review of the CT scan, this patient appeared to have had a very redundant splenic artery and an accessory splenic artery that was the source of the abnormality seen on CT scan. The abdominal pain appeared to be unrelated to either the pancreas or the calcifications.

However, vascular calcifications can sometimes be the cause of symptoms. The patient shown in Video 18.8 was referred for marked weight loss and abdominal pain suspected to be chronic pancreatitis. Esophagogastroduodenoscopy (EGD) showed what appeared to be an ischemic stomach. Endoscopic ultrasound showed a normal pancreas but obliteration of the celiac and superior mesenteric artery origins by a calcified plaque. This patient underwent urgent revascularization which corrected her pain and helped her weight return towards baseline. Plaques are not always fixed to the vessel wall. Video 18.9 shows that plaques can sometimes be noncalcified and hypermobile, suggesting a risk of embolism.

Aneurysms and pseudoaneurysms

An aneurysm is expansion of a vessel and all layers of the vascular wall. A pseudoaneurysm occurs when there is disruption of the vascular wall. These features can be subtle. Figure 18.2 and Video 18.10 show the area near the aortopulmonary (AP) window in a person undergoing EUS. This appears to be a pathologically enlarged lymph node. Further evaluation demonstrates this to be a pseudoaneurysm. A dramatic example of an apparent aortic pseudoaneurysm is shown in Video 18.11. This was found during evaluation of an early gastric cancer and took precedence over evaluation of the tumor. Figure 18.3 shows an example of an aortic root dissection that was first discovered during EUS for abdominal adenopathy suspected to be due to metastatic colon cancer.

Dilation of smaller arteries is more subtle. Video 18.12 was taken from a patient in whom an outside endoscopist found a subepithelial mass and in which "the biopsies were normal." Endoscopic ultrasound revealed a small splenic artery aneurysm. Video 18.13 shows an asymptomatic celiac artery aneurysm. In addition to degenerative atherosclerotic vascular disease, inflammatory disease such as pancreatitis can cause vascular injury as demonstrated in a patient in whom a splenic artery pseudoaneurysm was found during an exam after a resolved attack of acute pancreatitis. Video 18.14 shows a splenic artery pseudoaneurysm which arose after a bout of gallstone pancreatitis. The vessel was subsequently stented due to risk of hemorrhage.

Venous thrombosis

Thrombosis of the portal vein and its branches are probably the most common site for endosonographers to detect venous thrombosis. It can occur in patient with portal hypertension as shown in Figure 18.4 and Video 18.15 of a patient undergoing EUS who had cirrhosis from autoimmune liver disease. Splenic vein thrombosis can lead to isolated gastric varices. Video 18.16 shows an endoscopy from a patient referred for recurrent GI bleeding suspected to be variceal. The endoscopy shows a normal esophagus and possible gastric varicies which were confirmed during EUS. Careful

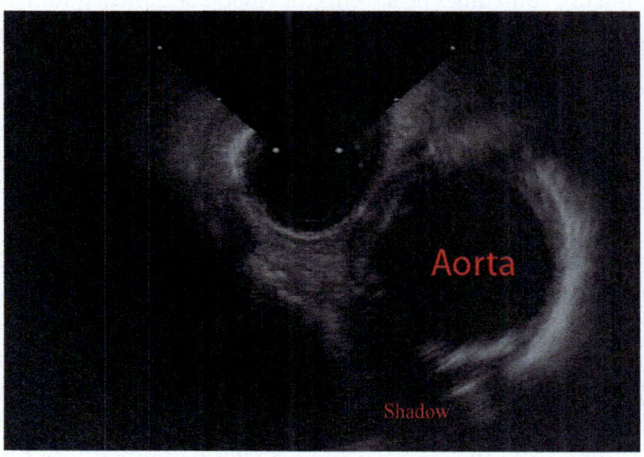

Figure 18.1 A radial array endoscopic ultrasound image of a calcific aortic plaque. The area behind the plaque is shadowed out.

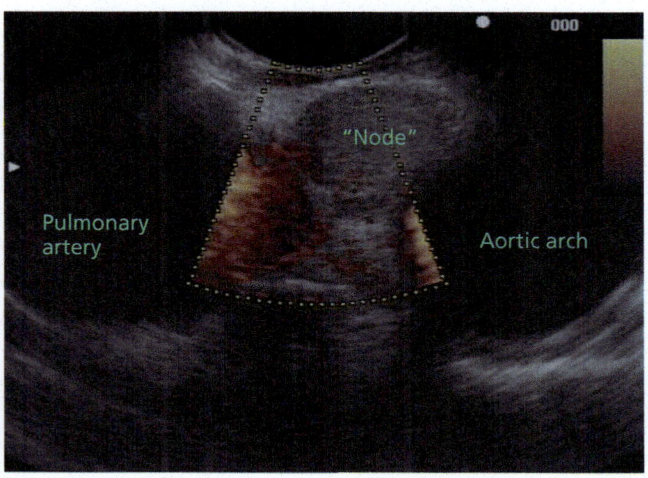

Figure 18.2 A linear array image of the aortopulmonary window with an isoechoic mass that was demonstrated on the video to be a pseudoaneurysm.

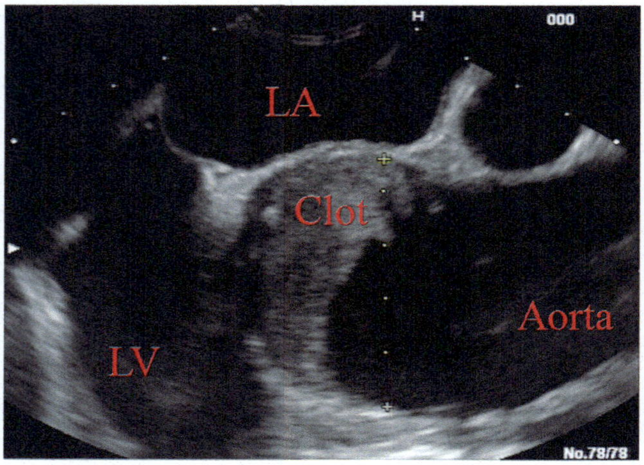

Figure 18.3 A linear array image showing the aortic root with clot due to an unsuspected aortic dissection. LA, left atrium; LV, left ventricle.

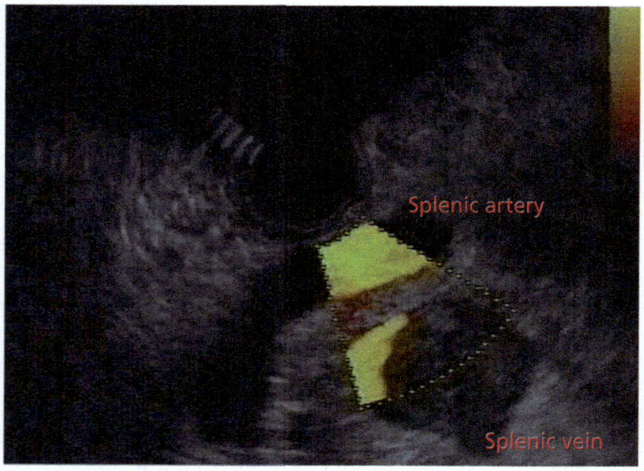

Figure 18.4 Radial array Doppler image of a clot in the splenic vein.

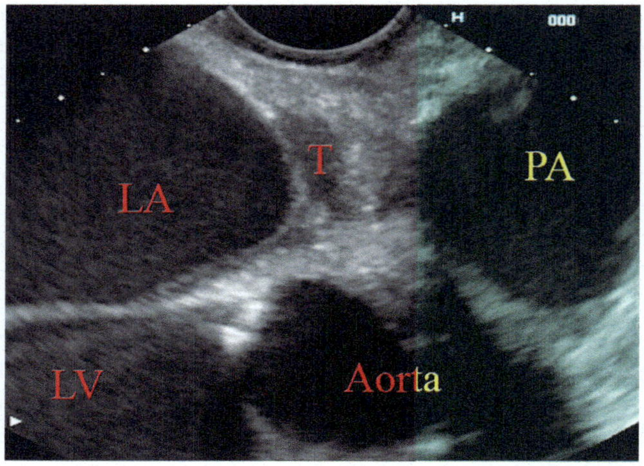

Figure 18.5 A linear array image of a metastasis (T) from breast cancer to the left atrial myocardium. LA, left atrium; LV, left ventricle; PA, pulmonary artery.

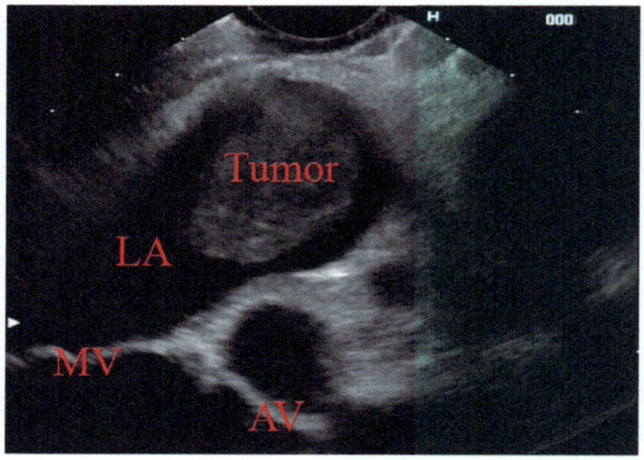

Figure 18.6 A linear array image of a rhabdomyosarcoma infiltrating into the left atrium (LA). The mitral valve (MV) and aortic valve (AV) are shown.

evaluation of the splenic vein revealed venous obstruction from a cystic pancreatic neoplasm near the splenic hilum.

Dieulafoy lesions

Dieulafoy lesions consist of arteries that are ectopically located in the submucosa. These can rupture and cause significant blood loss, but when they are not bleeding they can be very difficult to identify. Endoscopic ultrasound can be used to help identify Dieulafoy lesions as in this case (Video 18.17) in which a pulsatile lesion was seen in the rectal vault.

Neoplasms

Neoplastic tumors can extend into blood vessels and can take on the appearance of thrombus. Although rare, there are neoplastic lesions which can arise in the vascular tree and can sometimes be a source of emboli or obstruction. The most common is probably the atrial myxoma but other lesions include leiomyosarcomas and endothelial tumors. An example of a left atrial myxoma is shown in Video 18.18. Figure 18.5 shows an atrial myocardiac metastasis from breast cancer. Figure 18.6 shows a large rhabdomyosarcoma that has infiltrated into the left atrium.

Miscellaneous aberrancies

Arteries can be abnormally long and tortuous resulting in abnormal EUS imaging. An example is shown in Video 18.19 in which a redundant loop of splenic artery is seen. During EUS, the stomach can actually be pushed into the loop, resulting in images of the splenic artery surrounding the stomach.

Chapter video clips

Video 18.1 Anomalous right subclavian artery off of left-sided aortic arch creating a vascular ring around the esophagus.

Video 18.2 Anomalous right subclavian artery stump created by surgical transection of anomalous right subclavian artery off of left-sided aortic arch.

Video 18.3 Anomalous left subclavian artery off of right-sided aortic arch creating a vascular ring around the esophagus.

Video 18.4 Anomalous left subclavian artery stump created by surgical transection of anomalous left subclavian artery off of right-sided aortic arch.

Video 18.5 Tortuous aorta that is on the right side in the lower chest but crosses midline to the normal left-sided position at the aortic arch.

Video 18.6 Vascular calcification of the brachiocephalic artery and aorta.

Video 18.7 Vascular calcification of anomalous splenic artery that suggested chronic pancreatitis by CT imaging.

Video 18.8 Vascular calcification of celiac and superior mesenteric arteries in setting of gastric ischemia.

Video 18.9 Mobile atheroma.

Video 18.10 Aortic arch pseudoaneurysm that looks like AP window node.

Video 18.11 Aortic pseudoaneurysm.

Video 18.12 Splenic artery bulging into stomach suggesting a subepithelial mass.

Video 18.13 Celiac artery aneurysm.

Video 18.14 Splenic artery pseudoaneurysm.

Video 18.15 Splenic vein thrombosis.

Video 18.16 Splenic vein thrombosis.

Video 18.17 Rectal Dieulafoy lesion.

Video 18.18 Atrial myxoma.

Video 18.19 Tortuous splenic artery creating a loop encircling the stomach.

3 Pancreatico-biliary

19 Duodenal and Ampullary Neoplasia

Brenna Casey[1] and Kumar Krishnan[2]

[1] Massachusetts General Hospital and Harvard Medical School, Boston, MA, USA

[2] Interventional Endoscopy, Harvard Medical School, Massachusetts General Hospital, Boston, MA, USA

German anatomist Abraham Vater (1684–1751) first described a tubular structure which consists of the confluence of the distal common bile duct and main pancreatic duct in the second portion of the duodenum. This convergence is now known as the ampulla of Vater. In about 85% of individuals the pancreatic duct and common bile duct join in the ampulla and form a distal common channel. The normal ampulla starts about 2 mm outside the duodenal wall and penetrates the muscularis propria somewhat more distally, forming an intraduodenal segment 9–25 mm in length.

Tumors of the ampulla of Vater originate from the pancreaticobiliary–duodenal junction, limited by the sphincter of Oddi. Ampullary tumors may present with obstructive jaundice, duodenal obstruction or bleeding, or they may be discovered as an incidental finding at the time of upper gastrointestinal endoscopy or barium radiography for unrelated symptoms. While the presenting symptoms may be very similar to those of pancreatic carcinoma, ampullary malignancies have a much better prognosis. Their evolution appears to follow the adenoma–carcinoma sequence and they are usually discovered at an earlier stage than pancreatic tumors. Ampullary tumors are generally undetectable on transabdominal ultrasound, magnetic resonance imaging (MRI), and computed tomography (CT) due to their small size. Endoscopically they present as polypoid exaggerations of the ampulla. Endoscopic ultrasonography (EUS) provides high-resolution images and permits positioning of the ultrasound transducer in close approximation to the tumor in the duodenum. Endoscopic ultrasonography is specifically useful for T and N staging, which is important in determining the method of resection and ultimately the prognosis of patients with ampullary carcinomas (Figures 19.1 and 19.2).

Endoscopic ultrasound imaging of ampullary neoplasia is achieved by positioning the echoendoscope directly adjacent to the ampulla itself. Acoustic coupling is aided by a synergy created by positioning the water-filled balloon adjacent to the lesion while water is slowly (to avoid formation of bubbles which will obscure the detail of the images) instilled into the lumen of the duodenum (Figure 19.3). Particularly in small tumors, it is essential to avoid overfilling the balloon, as the ampullary lesion may be easily compressed by the balloon resulting in impaired visualization or in some cases overlooking the lesion completely. On the other hand, overfilling of the balloon can compress the tumor and underlying wall layers together, leading to artifact and misinterpretation resulting in overstaging. The patient is usually in the left lateral position, but in some cases a supine position or right lateral decubitus may improve imaging success, especially when the lesions are very small making a stable imaging position challenging. Tumors of the ampulla present as localized wall thickening of the duodenum at the level of the ampulla. The dilated distal common bile duct can be traced into the tumor and neoplastic growth may be seen in the dilated lumen. Smaller tumors are usually echo-homogeneous and echo-poor; inhomogeneous internal echoes occur more frequently with increasing tumor size. An adenoma of the ampulla does not involve the duodenal wall layers whereas a more advanced carcinoma infiltrates the duodenal wall layers or the pancreas. Differentiation of a T1 carcinoma (limited to the ampulla) from an adenoma is not possible by means of EUS.

Tumors of the periampullary regions may be either exophytic polypoid or hypoechoic mass lesions in the area of the ampulla that may be indistinguishable from distal pancreatic carcinomas (Video 19.1). Although biopsies of the polypoid lesions may only show adenomatous tissue, frequently a small focus of malignancy is present. Endoscopic ultrasound is not capable of differentiating a small focus of malignancy within an otherwise benign adenoma. Only in the case of deep infiltrative growth can the endosonographer discern the presence of a malignancy. A recent sphincterotomy and the resulting inflammatory response to the thermal injury

Atlas of Endoscopic Ultrasonography, Second Edition. Edited by Frank Gress, Thomas Savides, Brenna Casey, and Everson L. A. Artifon.

Companion website: www.wiley.com/go/gress/atlas

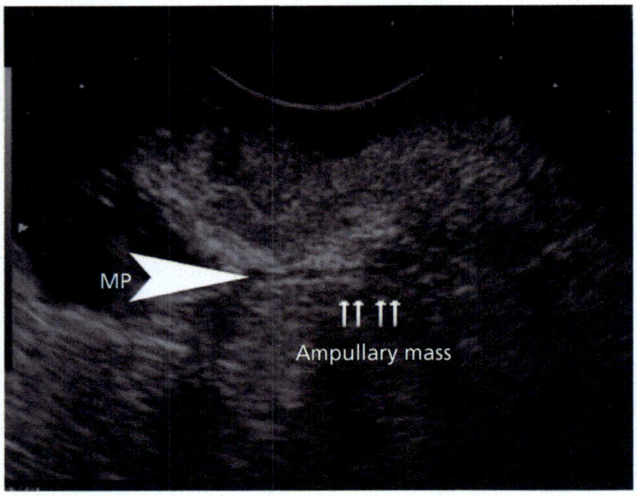

Figure 19.1 The linear array echoendoscope is in the duodenum directly adjacent to the ampulla. There is a large, exophytic, hypoechoic ampullary mass infiltrating the duodenal wall and filling the lumen. The lesion does not penetrate through the muscularis propria (MP, arrowhead).

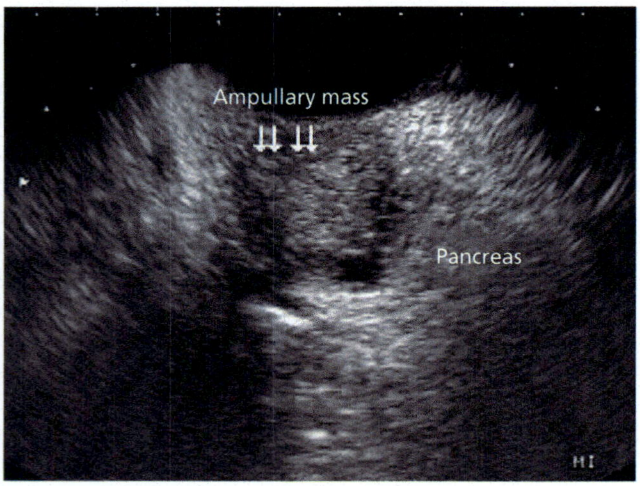

Figure 19.2 A hypoechoic mass is seen here arising from the ampulla. The malignancy is invading through the duodenal wall, surrounding the bile duct and into the pancreas, which makes this lesion a stage T3 ampullary cancer.

may create artifacts which mimic pseudopodia signifying inifiltrative growth. Endoscopic ultrasound cannot replace histology and should be used to stage ampullary lesions of known histological status. For villous adenomas of the ampulla of Vater, extension of the villous tissue into the common bile duct can occasionally be seen.

Staging according to the TNM system is as follows.

TX	Primary tumor cannot be assessed
T0	No evidence of primary tumor
T1	Tumor 1 cm or less (tumor limited to ampulla of Vater for ampullary gangliocytic paraganglioma)
T2	Tumor >1 cm
T3	Tumor invades pancreas or retroperitoneum or into non-peritonealized tissues
T4	Tumor invades visceral peritoneum (serosa) or invades other organs

Metastatic lymph nodes are classified using the same uniformly accepted criteria (size or echo pattern).

Accurate local staging is important in centers where endoscopic ampullectomy is performed. However, in most cases local staging does not alter management, as the lesion is removed during a pancreaticoduodenectomy (Whipple procedure). Endoscopic ultrasound detects small ampullary neoplasms when other imaging modalities reveal biliary or pancreatic ductal dilatation in the absence of a detectable mass. It also permits identification of infiltration through the duodenal muscularis propria and invasion into the pancreatic parenchyma. The accuracy of EUS in assessing the depth of tumor invasion and in detecting local lymph node metastases has been reported to be better than 80% for T stage and 70% for N stage. Overstaging in stage T1 occurs in up to one-third of cases and depends greatly on operator technique. However, infiltration into the pancreas, which is associated with a poorer prognosis, is detected in nearly 90% of cases using EUS. From a surgical standpoint, carcinoma of the ampulla can nearly always be resected unless it infiltrates the peripancreatic vessels, in which case a pancreatic primary infiltrating the ampulla should be considered. Other imaging modalities such at CT, abdominal ultrasound, and MRI, while not useful for T-staging of ampullary carcinoma, are necessary adjuncts for complete N-staging and M-staging prior to surgery and/or initiation of chemotherapy/radiation therapy. Intraductal ultrasound probes are useful for assessing tumor extension into the distal common bile duct in villous or papillary-type lesions prior to consideration for endoscopic resection, particularly in those cases in which the limits of the lesion are not clear on cholangiography. Care must be taken to avoid excessive pressure with the duodenoscope elevator on the intraductal ultrasound (IDUS) probe, as well as attention paid to the acute bend that is formed when the probe leaves the working channel of the duodenoscope and enters the bile duct, which may lead to poor imaging quality as well as probe breakage.

For elderly patients with locally advanced disease who are not good surgical candidates, palliation of obstructive symptoms may be provided by debulking of the lesion, endoscopic sphincterotomy, and biliary stent placement.

Chapter video clip

Video 19.1 An exophytic ampullary mass is seen on endoscopy and biopsies are obtained for histology which reveal an ampullary adenoma.

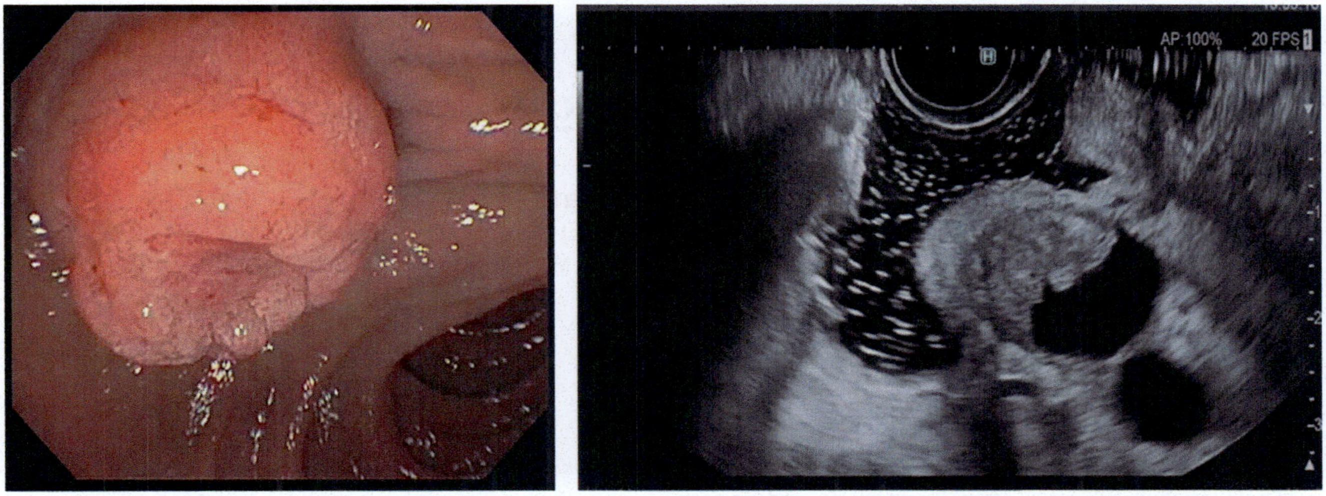

Figure 19.3 An ampullary lesion is noted endoscopically. On EUS, water is instilled into the lumen thus demarcating the lesion well. Further, intraductal extension is noted within the distal common bile duct.

20 Biliary Tract Pathology

Brenna Casey[1] and Kumar Krishnan[2]

[1] Massachusetts General Hospital and Harvard Medical School, Boston, MA, USA

[2] Interventional Endoscopy, Harvard Medical School, Massachusetts General Hospital, Boston, MA, USA

Cancer arising in the extrahepatic bile duct is curable by surgery in fewer than 10% of all cases. Prognosis depends in part on the tumor's anatomic location, which determines resectability. Complete resection is possible in 25–30% of lesions that originate in the distal bile duct, whereas the resection rate is much poorer for more proximal sites. Risk factors for bile duct malignancy include a history of primary sclerosing cholangitis, choledochal cysts, or infections with *Clonorchis sinensis*. Patients may present with jaundice, pain, fever, and pruritus.

Endoscopic ultrasonography (EUS) is an invaluable tool for the evaluation of the biliary tract. The close proximity of the echoendoscope transducer to the extrahepatic biliary tree, the lack of radiation, and the low risk of complications makes it an excellent method for examining the common bile duct. The extrahepatic ductal system can be visualized completely by EUS in 96% of patients. The role of EUS in the evaluation of the biliary tract includes biliary obstruction, suspected choledocholithiasis, indeterminate biliary strictures, idiopathic pancreatitis, unexplained right upper quadrant pain, and mass lesions within and adjacent to the biliary tree (Figures 20.1–20.4). Endoscopic ultrasound plays a key role in T-staging of extrahepatic biliary tumors.

TNM staging is as follows.

Primary tumor (T)

TX	Primary tumor cannot be assessed
T0	No evidence of primary tumor
Tis	Carcinoma in situ
T1	Tumor confined to the bile duct histologically
T2	Tumor invades beyond the wall of the bile duct
T3	Tumor invades the liver, gallbladder, pancreas, and/or unilateral branches of the portal vein (right or left) or hepatic artery (right or left)
T4	Tumor invades any of the following: main portal vein or its branches bilaterally, common hepatic artery, or other adjacent structures such as the colon, stomach, duodenum, or abdominal wall

Regional lymph nodes (N)

NX	Regional lymph nodes cannot be assessed
N0	No regional lymph node metastasis
N1	Regional lymph node metastasis

Distant metastasis (M)

MX	Distant metastasis cannot be assessed
M0	No distant metastasis
M1	Distant metastasis

Differentiating between benign and malignant biliary strictures can be challenging as up to 24% of patients with presumed hilar cholangiocarcinoma are found to have benign disease. Cholangiocarcinoma appears as a round hypoechoic lesion which may arise from a focal point on the bile duct wall or surround the duct wall circumferentially. Endoscopic ultrasound imaging alone is not capable of differentiating inflammatory lesions in the bile duct wall from malignancy and therefore tissue sampling is necessary. Fine needle aspiration cytology may be obtained under EUS guidance using linear array endosonography. In the setting of known malignancy, important staging imaging obtained via EUS should include evaluation of the portal venous system for evidence of tumor invasion.

Intraductal ultrasound (IDUS) is useful in the detection and evaluation of small biliary tumors. Indicators suggestive of malignancy with IDUS include irregular wall thickening, a hypoechoic mass, a papillary projection, and disruption of the normal three-layer wall structure of the bile duct. IDUS is ideally suited for imaging of the proximal biliary tree and facilitates imaging of the right hepatic artery, portal vein, and the hepatic duodenal ligament. It has been shown to improve the accuracy of biliary brushings by directing tissue sampling. Limited depth of imaging with IDUS renders it inappropriate for lymph node staging.

Endoscopic ultrasound has emerged as a sensitive and specific precursor to endoscopic retrograde cholangiopan-

Atlas of Endoscopic Ultrasonography, Second Edition. Edited by Frank Gress, Thomas Savides, Brenna Casey, and Everson L. A. Artifon.

Companion website: www.wiley.com/go/gress/atlas

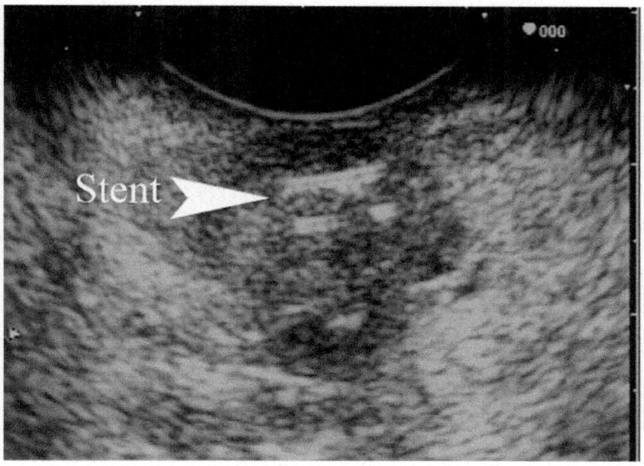

Figure 20.1 In this example of a small bile duct malignancy, a focal hypoechoic mass is seen surrounding the bile duct. A biliary stent is present within the mass.

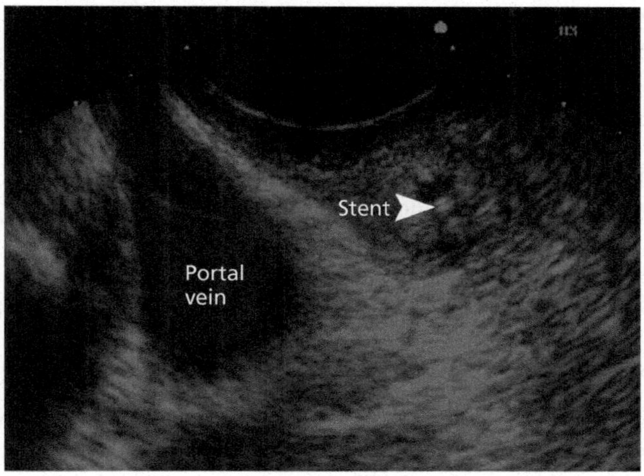

Figure 20.2 The linear array echoendoscope is positioned in the second portion of the duodenum. A hypoechoic mass is seen here within the bile duct surrounding a biliary stent. The portal vein is to the left of the mass and the pancreatic parenchyma can be seen beneath and to the right of the mass.

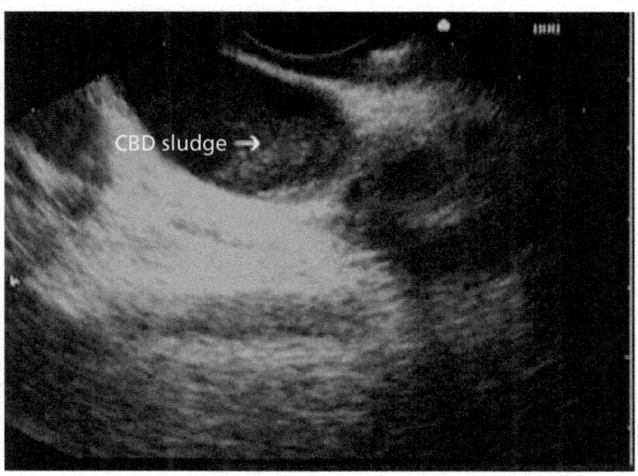

Figure 20.3 This 78-year-old woman has unresectable pancreatic cancer. Endoscopic ultrasound demonstrates a markedly dilated bile duct containing a large amount of biliary sludge. The patient was treated with biliary stent placement.

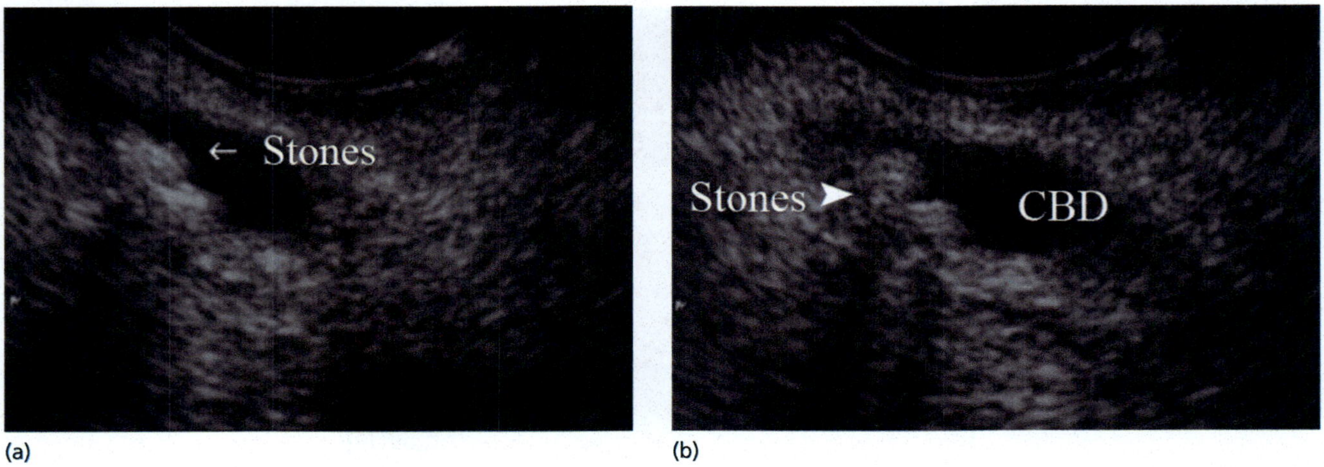

Figure 20.4 This 46-year-old woman presented with elevated liver function tests and right upper quadrant pain. Magnetic resonance cholangiopancreatography (MRCP) revealed a mildly dilated common bile duct with cholelithiasis but no choledocholithiasis. The surgical service has requested clearance of the common bile duct prior to proceeding to cholecystectomy. Endoscopic ultrasound was performed prior to endoscopic retrograde cholangiopancreatography (ERCP) and two common bile duct stones were revealed (a, b). The patient then underwent therapeutic ERCP with successful stone extraction.

creatography (ERCP) for the detection of bile duct stones, and it is more sensitive for the detection of stones of less than 6 mm than magnetic resonance cholangiopancreatography (MRCP). Choledocholithiasis is easily recognized as curvilinear hyperechoic foci with strong acoustic shadowing using either standard or catheter-based EUS. Low-amplitude echoes without acoustic shadowing are considered sludge. While ERCP is more accurate for the detection of choledocholithiasis than EUS by a slim margin, it carries significantly higher risk of complications post procedure and is thus no longer desirable as a diagnostic test. Endoscopic ultrasound is a minimally invasive procedure with a procedural risk identical to that of esophagogastroduodenoscopy (EGD). ERCP should be reserved for planned therapeutics. IDUS is useful during ERCP for detecting small stones and sludge that might otherwise go undetected with ERCP alone.

Chapter video clips

Video 20.1 Cholangiogram revealing a common bile duct stenosis suspicious for malignancy.

Video 20.2 Hyperechoic and shadowing stone in a dilated bile duct.

Video 20.3 Dilated common bile duct secondary to an obstructing mass.

21 Gallbladder Pathology

Sam Yoselevitz and Ann Marie Joyce
Tufts University School of Medicine, Burlington, MA, USA

Introduction

Gallbladder disease is one of the most common gastrointestinal disorders worldwide. It is estimated that there are at least 20.5 million cases of gallbladder disease annually in the United States. Gallbladder pathology encompasses a wide spectrum of disorders including cholelithiasis, cholecystitis, microlithiasis, gallbladder polyps, and carcinoma. Endoscopic ultrasound (EUS) has emerged as a valuable tool in the diagnosis and characterization of gallbladder lesions. EUS is considered to be superior to conventional ultrasound (US) for imaging the gallbladder. With much higher US frequencies, EUS can readily image the structure of the gallbladder and provide high-resolution images of even the smallest of lesions. Clinically, EUS is a useful diagnostic modality for patients who present with suspected gallstone disease despite a normal conventional US. Because EUS can influence clinical management, it is important to understand this technique and to recognize common gallbladder pathology.

Gallbladder stones

Gallstones are the most common biliary pathology. Conventional US is generally considered to be the gold standard for the diagnosis of cholelithiasis, with a sensitivity and specificity of 97% and 95%, respectively. However, multiple studies have demonstrated that EUS is much more sensitive for diagnosing small stones (≤3 mm), particularly in patients who are obese or have other anatomic considerations. In one study of patients with idiopathic pancreatitis by Frossard *et al.*, EUS identified cholelithiasis in 30–40% of cases that that had been missed by conventional US.

On EUS, gallstones appear as hyperechoic foci that cast an acoustic shadow and are found in the dependent portion of the gallbladder (Figures 21.1 and 21.2). Two additional clinically significant gallbladder conditions that are frequently described are sludge (Figure 21.3) and microlithiasis (Figure 21.4). These entities are echogenic in appearance but do not cast an acoustic shadow. Sludge also tends to be more viscous and is not necessarily found in the dependent portion of the gallbladder.

Gallbladder polyps

Gallstones must be distinguished from gallbladder polyps, which can have a similar sonographic appearance. Gallbladder polyps represent a heterogeneous group of lesions in the gallbladder, including premalignant adenomas, cholesterol polyps, inflammatory polyps, and adenomyomas. Other lesions of the gallbladder, such as fibromas, lipomas, and leiomyomas, are extremely rare. Although most gallbladder polyps are benign, some lesions do have the potential for malignant transformation. Current guidelines suggest that gallbladder polyps larger than 10 mm have a higher incidence of malignancy and should be treated with cholecystectomy. However, recent data has shown that up to 29% of polyps between 5 and 10 mm in size can be premalignant. This underlines the importance of EUS in the proper indentification of these lesions.

Gallbladder polyps appear on EUS as single or multiple echogenic foci protruding into the gallbladder lumen without acoustic shadowing. These polyps do not cause destruction of the normal three-layer pattern of the gallbladder wall (Figures 21.5 and 21.6). Although echogenic patterns are highly variable, neoplastic lesions tend to be more heterogeneous in appearance, while benign lesions such as cholesterol polyps have a more homogeneous echo pattern. In a study by Sugiyama et al. in 2000, a total of 194 patients with small gallbladder polyps (<20 mm) underwent both US and EUS. Endoscopic ultrasound correctly predicted the histology

Atlas of Endoscopic Ultrasonography, Second Edition. Edited by Frank Gress, Thomas Savides, Brenna Casey, and Everson L. A. Artifon.

Companion website: www.wiley.com/go/gress/atlas

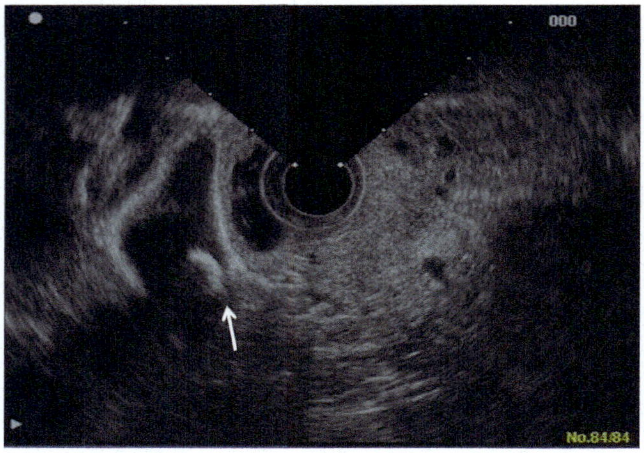

Figure 21.1 Gallbladder stone (arrow) with posterior shadowing.

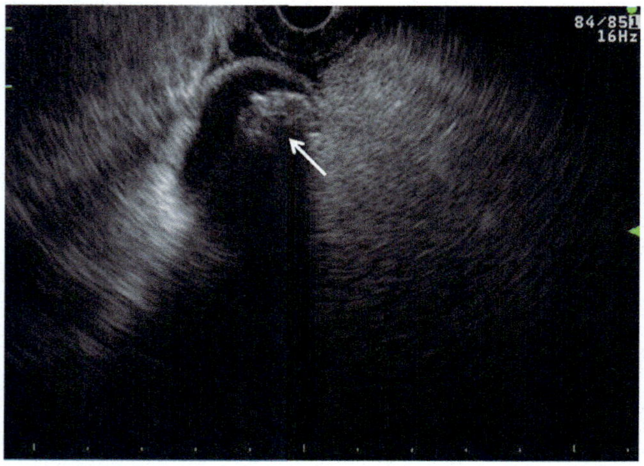

Figure 21.2 Gallbladder stone (arrow) with posterior shadowing.

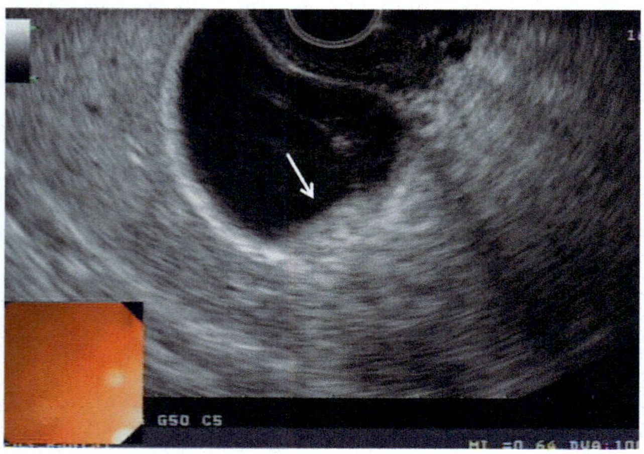

Figure 21.3 Gallbladder sludge (arrow).

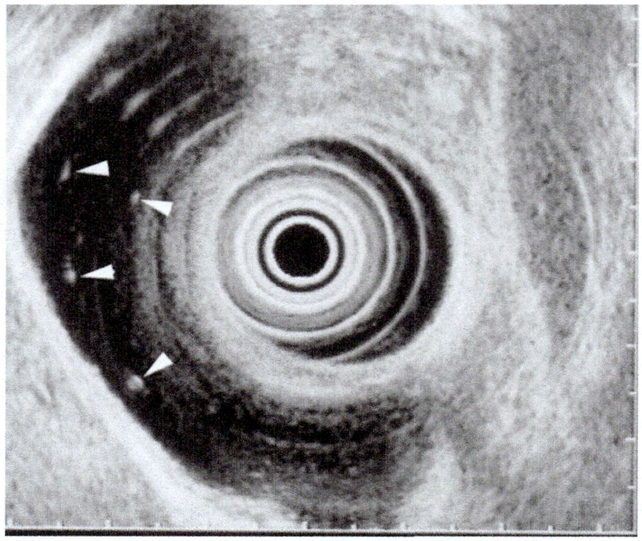

Figure 21.4 Gallbladder microlithiasis (arrows). Source: courtesy of Michael L. Kochman, MD.

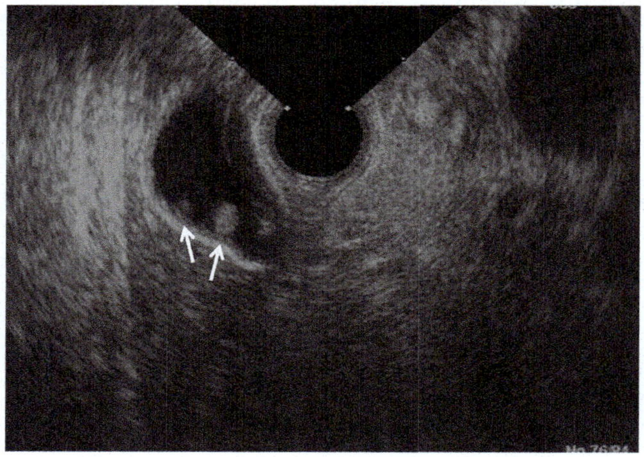

Figure 21.5 Gallbladder polyps (arrows). Notice the lack of shadowing.

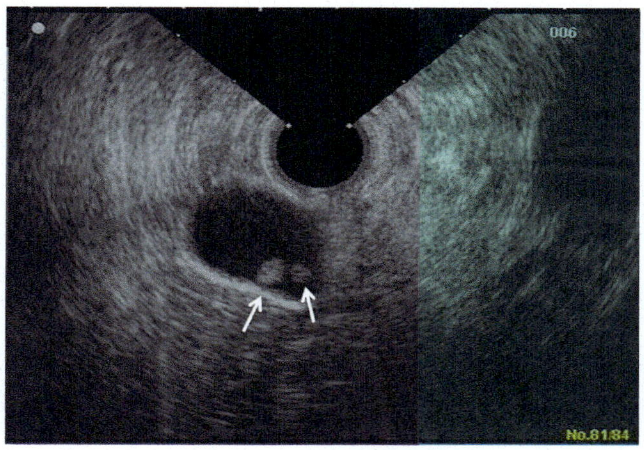

Figure 21.6 Gallbladder polyps (arrows). Notice the lack of shadowing.

in 97% of cases, compared to 76% with conventional US. Studies therefore suggest that EUS should be included as part of the standard work-up for gallbladder polyps.

Gallbladder carcinoma

Malignant lesions of the gallbladder are uncommon, yet unfortunately associated with a very poor prognosis. Gallstones and premalignant gallbladder polyps are the strongest risk factors for the development of gallbladder cancer. Endoscopic ultrasound is useful both in the differential diagnosis of gallbladder lesions as well as in staging tumor extent. In a study by Azuma et al., 89 patients with polyps of less than 20 mm underwent both EUS and conventional US. The sensitivity and specificity for the diagnosis of gallbladder cancer were 92% and 88% respectively with EUS, compared to 54% with US.

Carcinoma of the gallbladder is usually seen on EUS as a hypoechoic mass protruding into the gallbladder lumen or completely filling it. These lesions usually have irregular margins and characteristically destroy the normal three-layer structure of the gallbladder wall (Figure 21.7). Other

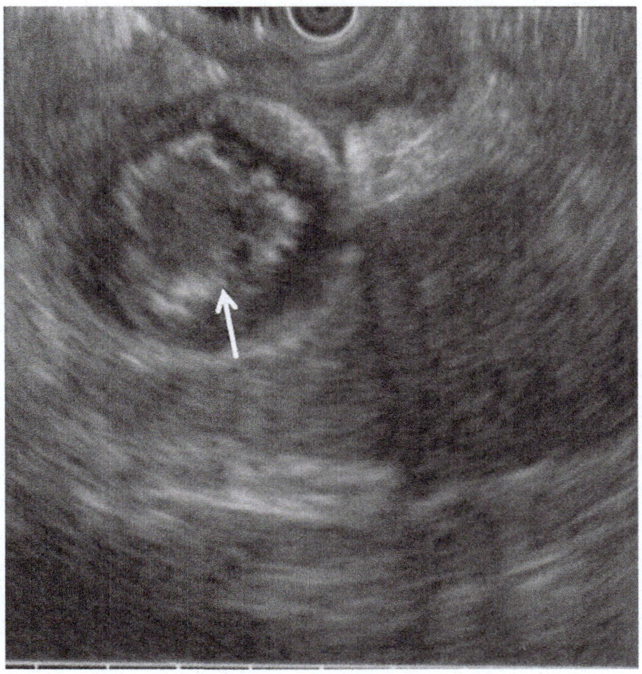

Figure 21.7 Gallbladder carcinoma (arrow).

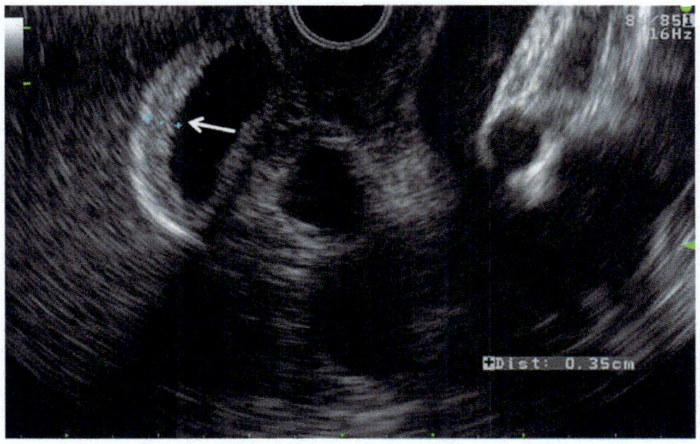

Figure 21.8 Thickened gallbladder wall (arrow).

EUS findings that are suggestive but not diagnostic of gallbladder carcinoma include thickening or calcification of the gallbladder wall, and loss of the normal sonographic interface between the gallbladder and liver. Gallbladder wall thickening, however, may also represent other conditions such as acute or chronic cholecystitis (Figure 21.8).

Endoscopic ultrasound is a useful modality for assessing the depth of invasion of gallbladder carcinoma as well as defining lymph node involvement. Several recent studies have shown that EUS imaging is quite accurate for TMN staging of gallbladder carcinoma, and correlates strongly with postoperative histopathologic findings. In one study by Mitake et al., 39 patients with gallbladder carcinoma were evaluated preoperatively with EUS. Carcinoma considered to be at an early stage with no lymph node involvement was correctly diagnosed in 87.5% of cases. In another study by Sadamoto et al., 41 patients with gallbladder carcinoma evaluated by EUS were analyzed retrospectively. Endoscopic ultrasound was found to be extremely accurate in determining the stage of the tumor, particularly with T1 and T3–4 lesions.

22 Pancreatic Adenocarcinoma

Douglas G. Adler
Peak Gastroenterology Associates, Colorado Springs, CO, USA

Introduction

Adenocarcinoma accounts for 90% of all pancreatic tumors. The highest cure rate is seen in patients with lesions that are localized to the pancreas and do not involve significant local vascular structures. Unfortunately, only 15–20% of patients have potentially resectable disease at the time of diagnosis [1]. Surgery has been and remains the most effective treatment for pancreatic cancer, although 5-year survival rates remain low at 18–33% even in patients who progress to surgery, most commonly following neoadjuvant therapy with chemotherapy, radiation therapy, or a combination thereof [2,3]. Accurate staging of patients with pancreatic adenocarcinoma is critical and allows patients to be appropriately selected to undergo all potential treatments including surgery, chemotherapy, radiation therapy, or palliative care. Endoscopic ultrasound (EUS) is a well-established and minimally invasive technique that has proved invaluable for both accurate locoregional staging of pancreatic adenocarcinoma and as a means of providing tissue from tumors and lymph nodes, thus allowing for a definitive diagnosis.

Tumor identification and diagnosis via fine needle aspiration or fine needle biopsy

The overall staging accuracy of EUS in patients with pancreatic adenocarcinoma is approximately 90–100%. In general, EUS is superior to computed tomography (CT) for the detection of pancreatic cancers. For small pancreatic masses (defined as lesions ≤16 mm), the sensitivity of EUS for tumor detection approaches 100% as compared to 66% using multidetector CT. As determined by EUS, accuracy for resectability is 88–100%. If CT or magnetic resonance imaging (MRI) reveals metastatic disease, then staging is complete (the patient has stage IV disease), and EUS may not be required, at least for diagnostic purposes. In patients with metastatic disease, EUS with fine needle aspiration (FNA) can still be performed if a definitive tissue diagnosis is desired. In patients with metastatic disease, EUS may also be used to perform celiac neurolysis. The sensitivity, specificity, positive predictive value, and negative predictive value of EUS-guided pancreatic FNA for the diagnosis of malignancy in patients with pancreatic cancer has been reported to be 64%, 100%, 100%, and 16%, respectively [4] (Figures 22.1 and 22.2).

Recent work on the EUS evaluation of extravascular migratory metastases has highlighted the fact that tumor cells can migrate along vessels and these can be identified and sampled via EUS. Work in this arena is ongoing [5].

Elastography, the use of sound waves to assess the stiffness of tissue, has been used to guide EUS-FNA or EUS core biopsies to target areas of viable tumor and to minimize sampling of necrotic tissue [6]. Elastography is widely used in Europe, less so in the USA.

It should be noted that EUS-guided fine needle biopsy (EUS-FNB) is now widely performed. This allows core samples to be obtained for histologic evaluation (and not just cytologic evaluation). Tissue can also be used for personalized medicine by oncologists [7,8].

Evaluation of vascular invasion

As mentioned, detection of vascular involvement in patients with pancreatic adenocarcinomas is critical for staging. Unfortunately, the definition of "vascular involvement" invasion has not been uniformly defined in the literature or in clinical practice, and different physicians, institutions, and research studies define this term differently. When evaluating peripancreatic vessels via EUS, tumor can be seen to contact vessels with or without the loss of a clear tissue plane

Atlas of Endoscopic Ultrasonography, Second Edition. Edited by Frank Gress, Thomas Savides, Brenna Casey, and Everson L. A. Artifon.

Companion website: www.wiley.com/go/gress/atlas

(a.k.a. echoplane), be adjacent to vessels, invade blood vessels with tumor visualized in the vascular lumen, thrombose vessels, and/or to encase blood vessels. All of these are considered vascular involvement, but individual surgeons and oncologists may differ about which of these findings may exclude patients for surgery.

If there is vascular involvement/invasion between the tumor and the celiac artery and/or the superior mesenteric artery, the patient has unresectable disease (Figure 22.3). Vascular invasion of the splenic artery or splenic vein are typically not contraindications to surgical intervention. With respect to the portal vein and/or the superior mesenteric vein, vascular invasion into the portal vein, the superior mesenteric vein, or the confluence of these vessels is not a contraindication to surgery, but advanced surgical techniques such as vascular grafting and/or reconstruction may be required for successful pancreaticoduodenectomy (Figures 22.4 and 22.5; Video 22.1).

In patients with pancreatic adenocarcinoma, vascular staging accuracy for EUS has been reported to be 100% versus 81% for CT in one study. Another similar study found EUS to have a sensitivity, specificity, positive predictive value, and negative predictive value for determining superior mesenteric vein and portal venous involvement in patients with pancreatic adenocarcinoma to be 81%, 86%, 87%, and 80%, respectively. This same study also demonstrated that for superior mesenteric artery tumor involvement the sensitivity and specificity, positive predictive value, and negative predictive values have been reported to be 17%, 67%, 17%, and 67%, respectively. These lower numbers reflect that the superior mesenteric artery can be difficult to fully track via EUS once it diverges significantly from the aorta. The limited ability to see the superior mesenteric artery well on EUS is perhaps the greatest limitation of the technique. A meta-analysis found the overall sensitivity of EUS for diagnosing vascular invasion overall to be 73% with a specificity of 90% [9].

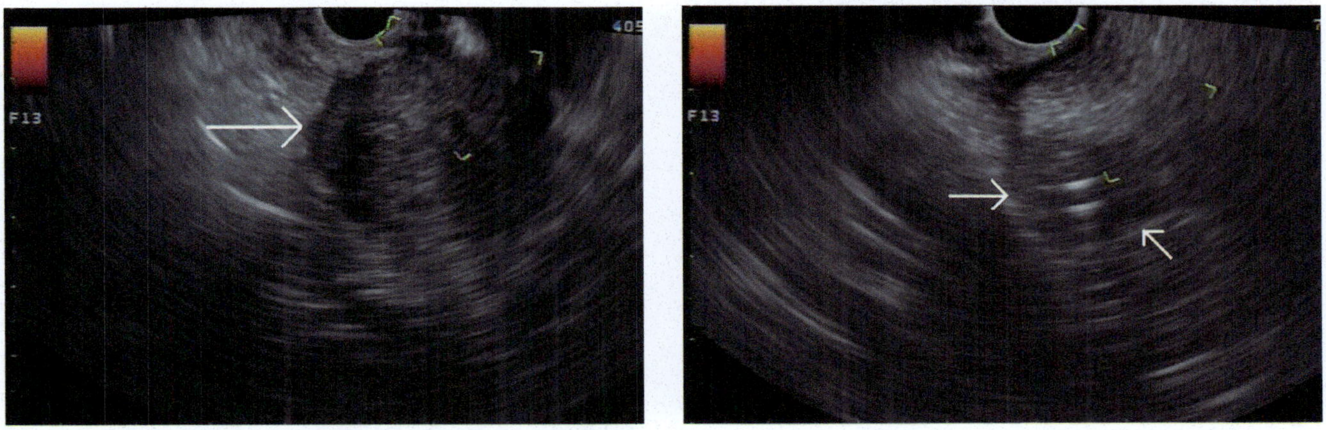

(a) (b)

Figure 22.1 (a) Representative EUS image of a large pancreatic adenocarcinoma (arrow). The tumor is a well-demarcated, hypoechoic mass lesion in the body of the pancreas. (b) Representative EUS image of a small pancreatic adenocarcinoma (arrows). The patient has a 1.5-cm lesion in the head of the pancreas surrounding the common bile duct, which is seen to contain a plastic stent. The walls of the plastic stent appear as bright hyperechogenic lines.

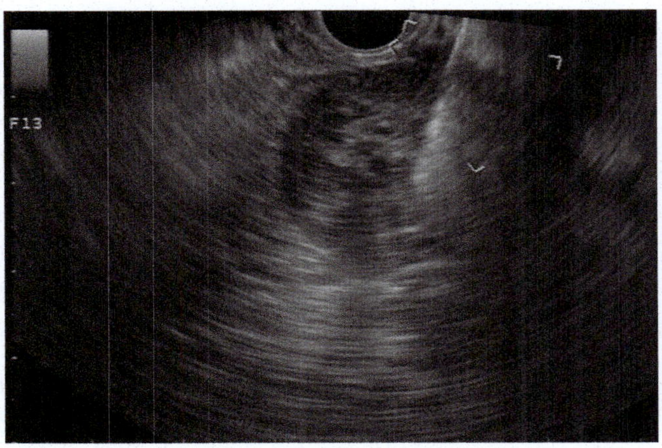

Figure 22.2 EUS-guided FNA of a pancreatic adenocarcinoma with a 22-gauge needle.

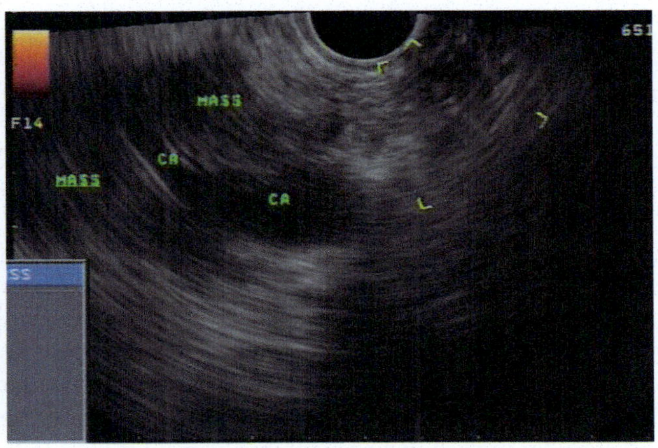

Figure 22.3 EUS image of a pancreatic adenocarcinoma in the body of the pancreas encasing the celiac artery (CA).

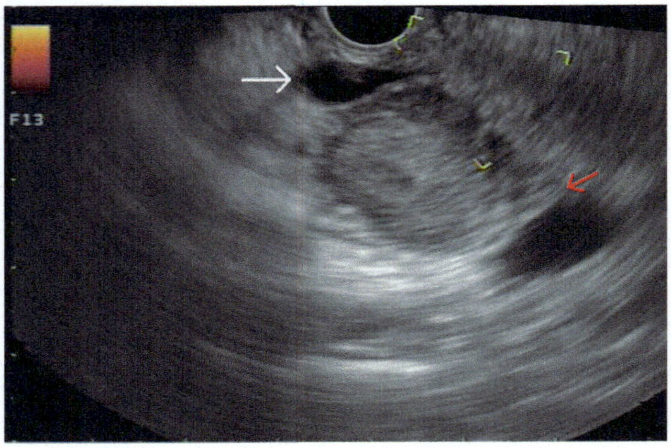

Figure 22.4 A 2-cm pancreatic head mass seen to abut and compress the common bile duct (white arrow, top of image) and to abut the portal vein (bottom of image) with an intact tissue plane between the mass and the vessel (red arrow).

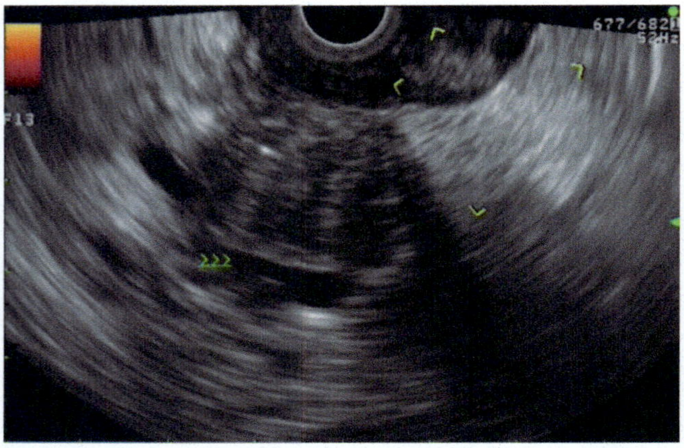

Figure 22.5 Large pancreatic cancer in the head of the pancreas seen to encase the superior mesenteric vein (green arrowheads). Source: Aloka.

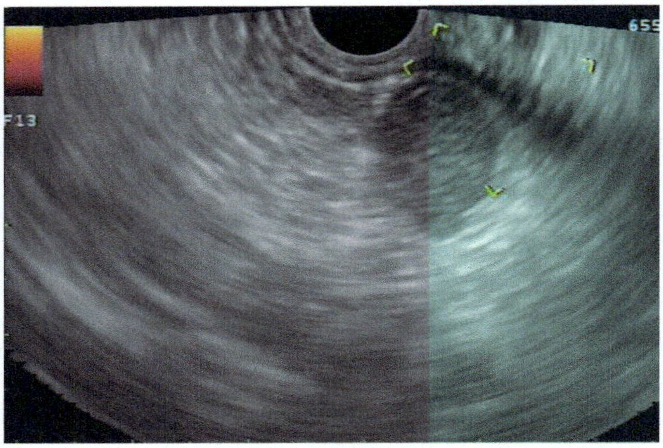

Figure 22.6 A 15-mm peripancreatic lymph node. Node is hypoechoic, round, well demarcated, and greater than 1 cm in size, all of which suggests malignancy.

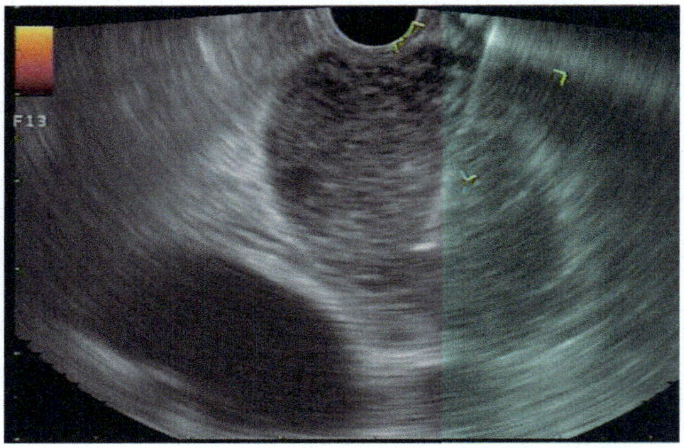

Figure 22.7 EUS-guided FNA of a large, 4-cm peripancreatic node in a patient with pancreatic adenocarcinoma. Cytology revealed malignant cells.

Evaluation of peripancreatic lymphadenopathy

The presence or absence of malignant peripancreatic lymphadenopathy does not play a definitive role in determining if a pancreatic cancer is resectable or unresectable, but the presence of malignant adenopathy can have a powerful effect on overall management. If a cancer appears to be potentially resectable, the identification of malignant lymph nodes may be a justification for neoadjuvant therapy.

When imaged via EUS, malignant lymphadenopathy is suggested by the presence of lymph nodes that are greater than 1 cm in size, hypoechoic, have distinct margins, and are round in shape. Individually, none of these characteristics determine the presence of malignant cells, but when all four of these features are present in the same lymph node, the accuracy for predicting malignant involvement is 80% [10]. Sensitivity, specificity, positive predictive value, and negative predictive value for the detection of celiac axis, portal vein, hepatic artery and superior mesenteric artery lymph nodes via EUS are 44%, 93%, 80%, and 72%, respectively (Figures 22.6 and 22.7).

EUS evaluation of peripancreatic lymphadenopathy is superior to that of CT [11,12]. While not all malignant appearing nodes are sampled, if the appearance of a lymph node is indeterminate for malignant involvement, EUS-guided FNA or FNB of the node in question can be performed for a definitive nodal evaluation. The overall sensitivity, specificity, and accuracy of detection of malignant lymph nodes by EUS are approximately 85%, 100%, and 89%, respectively [13].

Limitations and complications of EUS in patients with pancreatic cancer

Despite its value in patients with pancreatic adenocarcinoma, EUS has some significant limitations. Pancreatic adenocarcinomas may be difficult to detect via EUS (and, of note, CT or MRI) in patients with chronic pancreatitis (due to baseline tissue distortion) or if the tumor is isoechoic with the surrounding pancreatic parenchyma [14,15]. As already mentioned, EUS is relatively insensitive for the detection of superior mesenteric artery involvement. Complete visualization of the entire pancreas can sometimes be difficult, especially in patients with prior bariatric surgery or partial gastrectomy. The pancreatic genu and uncinate process can be challenging to completely image, especially in patients with large body habitus.

Potential complications from EUS with or without FNA can include acute pancreatitis (0–2%), perforation (0.03%), infection/febrile episode (1%), and significant hemorrhage (1.3–4%) [16,17].

The number of EUS practitioners, while steadily increasing, still remains concentrated in large medical centers. One study on EUS training volumes revealed that most three-year gastrointestinal fellows and many fourth-year advanced endoscopy fellows are currently receiving insufficient training in EUS. Further limiting the spread of EUS to the general community, training in EUS is not offered at 14% of US gastrointestinal fellowship programs [18]. In general, the best results are obtained from the most experienced operators.

Conclusion

Pancreatic adenocarcinoma remains a commonly encountered clinical entity. Accurate staging and tissue diagnosis are critical for formulation of optimal management plans. EUS offers high accuracy for staging of pancreatic adenocarcinoma, provides excellent tissue acquisition, and is essentially unrivaled for the detection of small tumors. EUS is also highly effective in evaluating patients for the presence of malignant lymphadenopathy and in assessing vascular involvement.

References

1 Li D, Xie K, Wolff R, Abbruzzese JL.Pancreatic cancer. *Lancet* 2004;363(9414):1049–1057.

2 Pellegrini CA, Heck CF, Raper S, Way LW. An analysis of the reduced morbidity and mortality rates after pancreaticoduodenectomy. *Arch Surg* 1989;124(7):778–781.

3 Lim JE, Chien MW, Earle CC. Prognostic factors following curative resection for pancreatic adenocarcinoma: a population-based, linked database analysis of 396 patients. *Ann Surg* 2003;237(1):74–85.

4 Bhutani MS, Hawes RH, Baron PL, et al. Endoscopic ultrasound guided fine needle aspiration of malignant pancreatic lesions. *Endoscopy* 1997;29(9):854–858.

5 Rustagi T, Gleeson FC, Chari ST, et al. Safety, diagnostic accuracy, and effects of endoscopic ultrasound fine-needle aspiration on detection of extravascular migratory metastases. *Clin Gastroenterol Hepatol* 2019;17(12):2533–2540.e1.

6 Kitano M, Yoshida T, Itonaga M, et al. Impact of endoscopic ultrasonography on diagnosis of pancreatic cancer. *J Gastroenterol* 2019;54(1):19–32.

7 Haseeb A, Taylor LJ, Adler DG. Comparing endoscopic ultrasound-guided core biopsies of solid pancreatic and extrapancreatic lesions: a large single-operator experience with a new fine-needle biopsy needle. *Ann Gastroenterol* 2018;31(6):742–746.

8 Naveed M, Siddiqui AA, Kowalski TE, et al. A multicenter comparative trial of a novel EUS-guided core biopsy needle (SharkCore™) with the 22-gauge needle in patients with solid pancreatic mass lesions. *Endosc Ultrasound* 2018;7(1): 34–40.

9 Puli SR, Singh S, Hagedorn CH, et al. Diagnostic accuracy of EUS for vascular invasion in pancreatic and periampullary cancers: a meta-analysis and systematic review. *Gastrointest Endosc* 2007;65(6):788–797.

10 Bhutani MS, Hawes RH, Hoffman BJ. A comparison of the accuracy of echo features during endoscopic ultrasound (EUS) and EUS-guided fine-needle aspiration for diagnosis of malignant lymph node invasion. *Gastrointest Endosc* 1997;45(6):474–479.

11 Gress FG, Hawes RH, Savides TJ, et al. Role of EUS in the preoperative staging of pancreatic cancer: a large single-center experience. *Gastrointest Endosc* 1999;50:786–791.

12 Chen CH, Tseng LJ, Yang CC, et al. The accuracy of endoscopic ultrasound, endoscopic retrograde cholangiopancreatography, computed tomography, and transabdominal ultrasound in the detection and staging of primary ampullary tumors. *Hepatogastroenterology* 2001;48(42):1750–1753.

13 Williams DB, Sahai AV, Aabakken L, et al. Endoscopic ultrasound guided fine needle aspiration biopsy: a large single centre experience. *Gut* 1999;44(5):720–726.

14 Scaglione M, Pinto A, Romano S, et al. Using multidetector row computed tomography to diagnose and stage pancreatic carcinoma: the problems and the possibilities. *JOP* 2005;6(1):1–5.

15 Bhutani MS, Gress F, Giovannini M, et al. NEST Study (No Endoscopic Detection of Tumor) of missed pancreatic neoplasms by endoscopic ultrasound: an American Endosonography Committee study [abstract]. *Gastrointest Endosc* 1999;49:AB86.

16 Eisen GM, Baron TH, Dominitz JA, et al. Complications of upper GI endoscopy. *Gastrointest Endosc* 2002;55(7):784–793.

17 Adler DG, Jacobson BC, Davila RE, et al. ASGE guideline: complications of EUS. *Gastrointest Endosc* 2005;61(1):8–12. Erratum in *Gastrointest Endosc* 2005;61(3):502.

18 Azad JS, Verma D, Kapadia AS, Adler DG. Can U.S. GI fellowship programs meet American Society for Gastrointestinal Endoscopy recommendations for training in EUS? A survey of U.S. GI fellowship program directors. *Gastrointest Endosc* 2006;64(2):235–241.

Chapter video clip

Video 22.1 EUS video of a large pancreatic head mass abutting the SMV and PV with loss of echoplane between the tumor and the mass. Also note the dilated CBD, which has an indwelling plastic stent. Source: Aloka.

23 Pancreatic Malignancy (Non-adenocarcinoma)

Larissa Fujii-Lau[1], Michael J. Levy[2], and Suresh T. Chari[3]

[1] University of Hawaii, Honolulu, HI, USA

[2] Mayo Clinic, Rochester, MN, USA

[3] MD Anderson Cancer Hospital, Houston, TX, USA

Introduction

Endoscopic ultrasound (EUS) is routinely employed in the evaluation of solid pancreatic masses as it enhances diagnostic accuracy, guides management, and improves patient outcomes. Much has been published regarding the use of EUS for pancreatic adenocarcinoma, which accounts for approximately 95% of all solid pancreatic malignancies. There are fewer EUS data available for endocrine tumors, and even less for lymphoma, solid pseudopapillary tumors, acinar cell carcinoma, and secondary metastatic tumors.

Endocrine pancreatic tumors (Figures 23.1 and 23.2)

Endocrine pancreatic tumors (EPTs) are rare, with an incidence of less than 1 in 100 000. Because of more widespread use and better-quality cross-sectional imaging, EPTs are being incidentally identified more commonly. EUS has been shown to be more sensitive at identifying EPTs than cross-sectional imaging, particularly since a significant proportion of these tumors are less than 20 mm in size.

The majority of EPTs (70–90%) are nonfunctioning, followed by gastrinomas and insulinomas; glucagonomas, somatostatinomas, and VIPomas are less often reported. EUS is often performed to assist with preoperative localization of these tumors to help guide surgical resection, which offers the only chance for cure and is usually recommended due to the malignant potential of EPTs. Endoscopic ultrasound localizes 75–95% of insulinomas; the high EUS detection rate for insulinomas is likely explained by the fact that 99% of insulinomas are contained within the pancreas. Approximately 75–100% of pancreatic gastrinomas are identified by EUS compared with only 0–67% of duodenal gastrinomas.

The EUS appearance of EPTs is similar regardless of the tumor type or functional status, typically appearing as round, well-delineated, homogeneous, mildly hypoechoic lesions, often hypervascular with a surrounding hyperechoic rim. They may also appear isoechoic or hyperechoic, have a hypoechoic border, be cystic, and contain calcifications. The EUS technique for localizing these tumors is identical to that of adenocarcinoma, except that a more deliberate exam may be needed to find these often small lesions. The parapancreatic region should also be carefully examined to search for lymphadenopathy and because the primary tumor may be attached by a pedicle or completely separate from the pancreas, which makes it more difficult to locate than intrapancreatic tumors.

EUS characteristics may also predict the malignant potential, which can be otherwise difficult to discern in the absence of extensive local invasion or distant metastasis. The presence of anechoic regions, an irregular central echogenic area, or pancreatic duct obstruction corresponds with severe hemorrhage, necrosis, or hyaline degeneration, each of which suggests a malignant tumor, although their predictive value is uncertain. If contrast harmonic EUS is performed, a more heterogeneous enhancement has been shown to correlate to more aggressive tumors (defined as G3 tumors or G1/G2 tumors with morphologic and/or histologic findings of metastatic disease).

Endoscopic ultrasound-guided fine needle aspiration (EUS-FNA) or fine needle biopsy (EUS-FNB) helps differentiate benign parapancreatic lymph nodes from primary EPTs, a distinction that can be difficult, especially for insulinomas. Samples obtained by EUS-FNB can also be tested for Ki-67 labeling index which is included in the World Health Organization (WHO) 2017 grading system for EPTs.

There have been case series on EUS-guided fine needle injection (EUS-FNI) of alcohol or radiofrequency ablation for treatment of nonfunctioning EPTs or insulinomas. Localized EUS-guided treatment of these lesions may be considered in patients with small tumors who are not surgical candidates. However, this should only be performed in tertiary referral centers that have a study protocol in place. More studies are

Atlas of Endoscopic Ultrasonography, Second Edition. Edited by Frank Gress, Thomas Savides, Brenna Casey, and Everson L. A. Artifon.

Companion website: www.wiley.com/go/gress/atlas

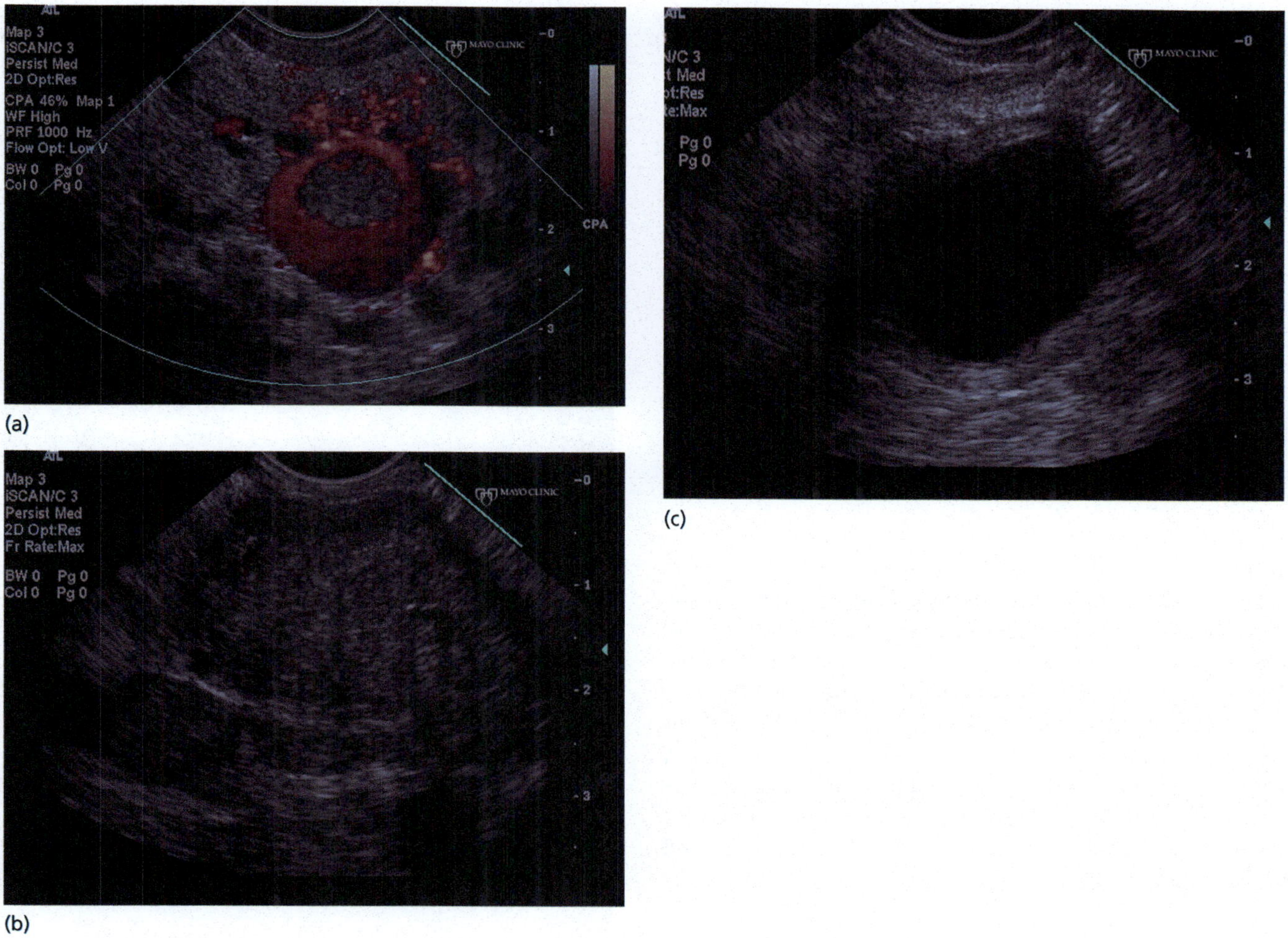

Figure 23.1 Images obtained from a patient with a gastrinoma following helical computed tomography (CT) that revealed a pancreatic cyst that was not felt to represent a gastrinoma. Linear endoscopic ultrasound identified malignant vascular thrombosis as highlighted with the use of power Doppler (a). A large endocrine tumor was identified, which appeared more hypoechoic, irregular, and infiltrating than usual. This mass encompassed most of the pancreatic body and tail (b). The tumor also contained a pancreatic tail cystic component that was seen on CT (c). Source: Mayo Clinic.

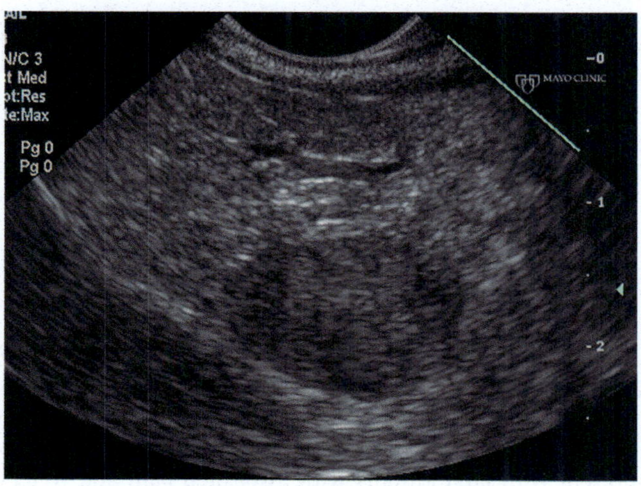

Figure 23.2 Following a negative computed tomography (CT) to search for a presumed insulinoma, linear endoscopic ultrasound identified the insulinoma within the pancreatic body, allowing curative surgical intervention. Source: Mayo Clinic.

required to determine the optimal technique, injectate volume, and follow-up of EUS-guided treatment.

Primary pancreatic lymphoma (Figure 23.3)

Approximately one-third of patients with non-Hodgkin's lymphoma (NHL) develop secondary pancreatic involvement. Primary pancreatic lymphoma is rare and accounts for fewer than 3% of extranodal NHL, and less than 0.5% of all pancreatic malignancies. It is generally treated with chemotherapy and/or radiation therapy, commonly resulting in disease remission and occasionally cure.

Most tumors appear by EUS as a mildly hypoechoic, solid and less often cystic mass that may be single or multiple. It may be difficult to distinguish primary pancreatic masses from commonly accompanying prominent peripancreatic lymphadenopathy. Although the appearance may mimic adenocarcinomas, lymphomas are less hypoechoic, have less

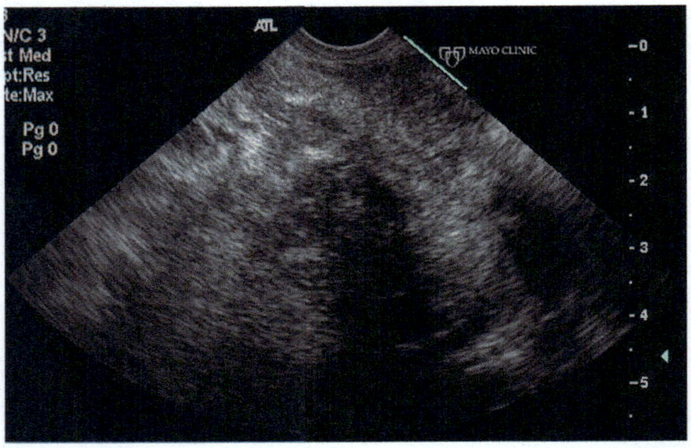

Figure 23.3 Linear endoscopic ultrasound imaging of a patient with a pancreatic lymphoma. Source: Mayo Clinic.

pronounced peritumoral inflammatory changes, and less commonly have vascular invasion and associated pancreatic duct dilatation. Clinical presentation is of little utility as typical "B-type" symptoms, including fever and night sweats, are seldom present. NHL may be diagnosed by EUS-FNA with immunophenotyping by flow cytometry. It is important to have a high suspicion for NHL as several EUS-FNA passes should be placed in a different container specifically for flow cytometry. The diagnostic accuracy may be further improved by obtaining EUS-FNB to further enhance morphologic and architectural assessment.

Solid pseudopapillary tumors (Figure 23.4)

Solid pseudopapillary tumors (SPTs) are rare pancreatic neoplasms that typically develop in young women in the second or third decade of life. They are usually discovered incidentally and typically follow an indolent course. As they can be malignant and develop distant metastases, surgery is the therapy of choice providing curative resection in 95% of patients. Most favor an aggressive resection for malignant disease that includes major venous and even arterial structures and distant metastases. Of note, nodal metastases are unusual and formal lymphadenectomy is not necessary. Continued surveillance of all patients is recommended, and should metastases appear, surgical resection is indicated.

Imaging typically reveals large, well-circumscribed, hypoechoic lesions that may be solid to nearly entirely cystic often containing multiple cystic compartments. EUS-FNA permits diagnosis in most patients; however, the cytology may be confused with endocrine tumors and acinar cell carcinoma. Negative chromogranin and synaptophysin staining exclude an islet cell neoplasm, whereas a negative keratin stain excludes acinar carcinoma. Immunohistochemical analysis of SPTs usually shows strong staining for CD56 and vimentin and β-catenin gene mutations are common.

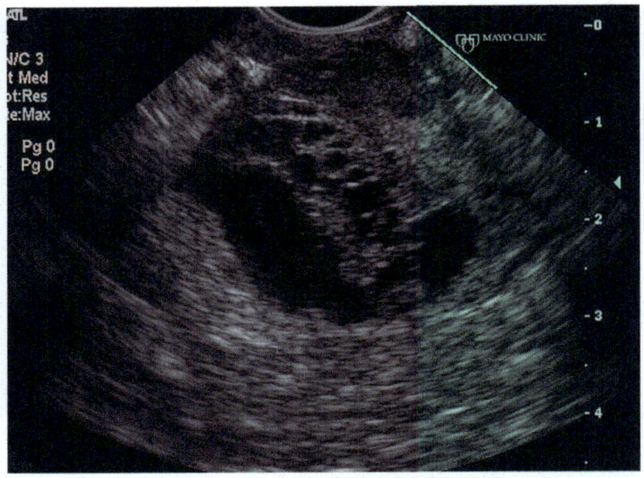

Figure 23.4 Endoscopic ultrasound revealed a large well-circumscribed hypoechoic lesion that contained solid and cystic components with the diagnosis of a solid pseudopapillary tumor established by endoscopic ultrasound-guided fine needle aspiration (EUS-FNA) and later confirmed at surgery. Source: Mayo Clinic.

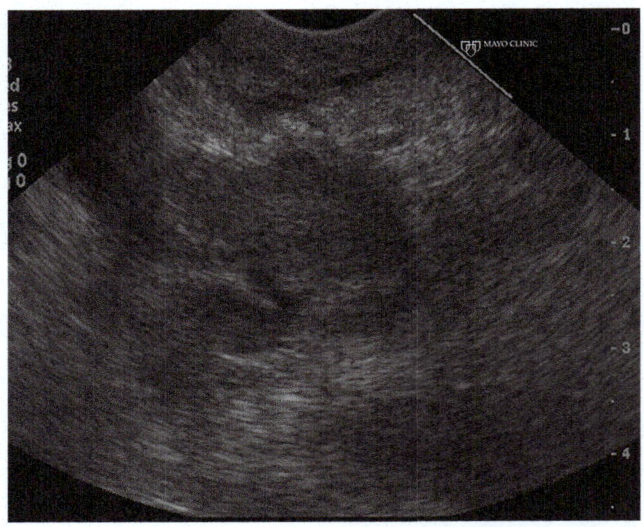

Figure 23.5 A pancreatic head acinar cell tumor is identified by endoscopic ultrasound and confirmed at fine needle aspiration (FNA) leading to pancreaticoduodenectomy. Source: Mayo Clinic.

Acinar cell carcinoma (Figure 23.5)

Although acinar cells comprise over 80% of all pancreatic cells, acinar cell carcinoma (ACC) accounts for less than 1% of all pancreatic neoplasms. They typically develop in males during the sixth or seventh decade of life. Most patients present with large tumors with associated pain and weight loss. Patients may develop lipase hypersecretion syndrome resulting from systemic secretion of pancreatic enzymes and characterized by fever, polyarthritis, subcutaneous fat necrosis, and eosinophilia. There is some debate as to the clinical course of ACC. While some report poor outcomes, most recent studies have found a better prognosis than for pancreatic adenocarcinoma. Despite the typically large size of ACCs, resection margins are usually negative. Surgical resection is the therapy of choice and while nearly all succumb to their disease, the postoperative survival duration is greater (approximately four to five years) than for pancreatic adenocarcinoma. Neoadjuvant therapy may provide effective downstaging and allow resection in a small cohort of patients.

EUS characteristics of ACC are nonspecific. Most are hypoechoic but ACC can also be isoechoic or slightly hyperechoic. There may be cystic components, calcifications, diffuse pancreatic enlargement, or pancreatic duct dilation present. EUS elastography has not been shown to help differentiate ACC from pancreatic adenocarcinoma. However, contrast harmonic EUS has different enhancement properties and ACC more often had a gradual enhancement pattern as compared to the hypoenhancement seen with pancreatic adenocarcinomas.

Immunohistochemical analysis of ACC usually shows strong staining for trypsin, chymotrypsin, and lipase, permitting diagnosis. The most common neoplasm in the differential diagnosis of patients with ACC is well-differentiated EPT. Immunohistochemical stains for the neuroendocrine markers synaptophysin and chromogranin help differentiate these neoplasms. However, mixed acinar–endocrine neoplasms occur and are associated with improved prognosis over pure ACC.

Secondary metastatic tumors (Figure 23.6)

Pancreatic metastases account for approximately 1% of all resected solid pancreatic masses. While over 30 sites of origin have been reported, the most common primary tumors include renal cell carcinoma, lung, breast, colon, melanoma, sarcoma, and ovarian. These tumors are notable for a prolonged delay from initial primary tumor diagnosis until pancreatic metastasis that averages 5–10 years and may occur more than 25 years later. While most metastasize to the pancreatic head, multiple metastases are seen in one-third to half of patients, and diffuse infiltration is also reported. Pancreatic metastases are more often resectable and portend a better prognosis than patients with primary pancreatic adenocarcinoma.

Imaging can vary tremendously for these lesions that may be solid and/or cystic, have variable echodensity, and are often hypervascular. EUS-FNA can usually establish the diagnosis, but EUS-FNB and immunostaining may be necessary for definitive diagnosis. Endoscopic ultrasound further impacts patient care through the detection of multifocal disease undetected by noninvasive imaging. Endosonographers should suspect metastatic tumor in patients with a prior diagnosis of distant neoplasia given the relatively indolent course and improved surgical outcomes with postoperative survival of two to four years.

Summary

Endoscopic ultrasound is routinely used to evaluate pancreatic masses. By offering high-resolution imaging and tissue sampling, EUS can often establish the malignant potential of these masses, enhance staging accuracy, and determine the tumor type to help guide treatment and improve outcomes. Adequate tissue obtained during EUS-FNA or EUS-FNB is required for immunohistologic staining to help differentiate these lesions.

Chapter video clip

Video 23.1 Pancreatic cancer. Source: Mayo Clinic.

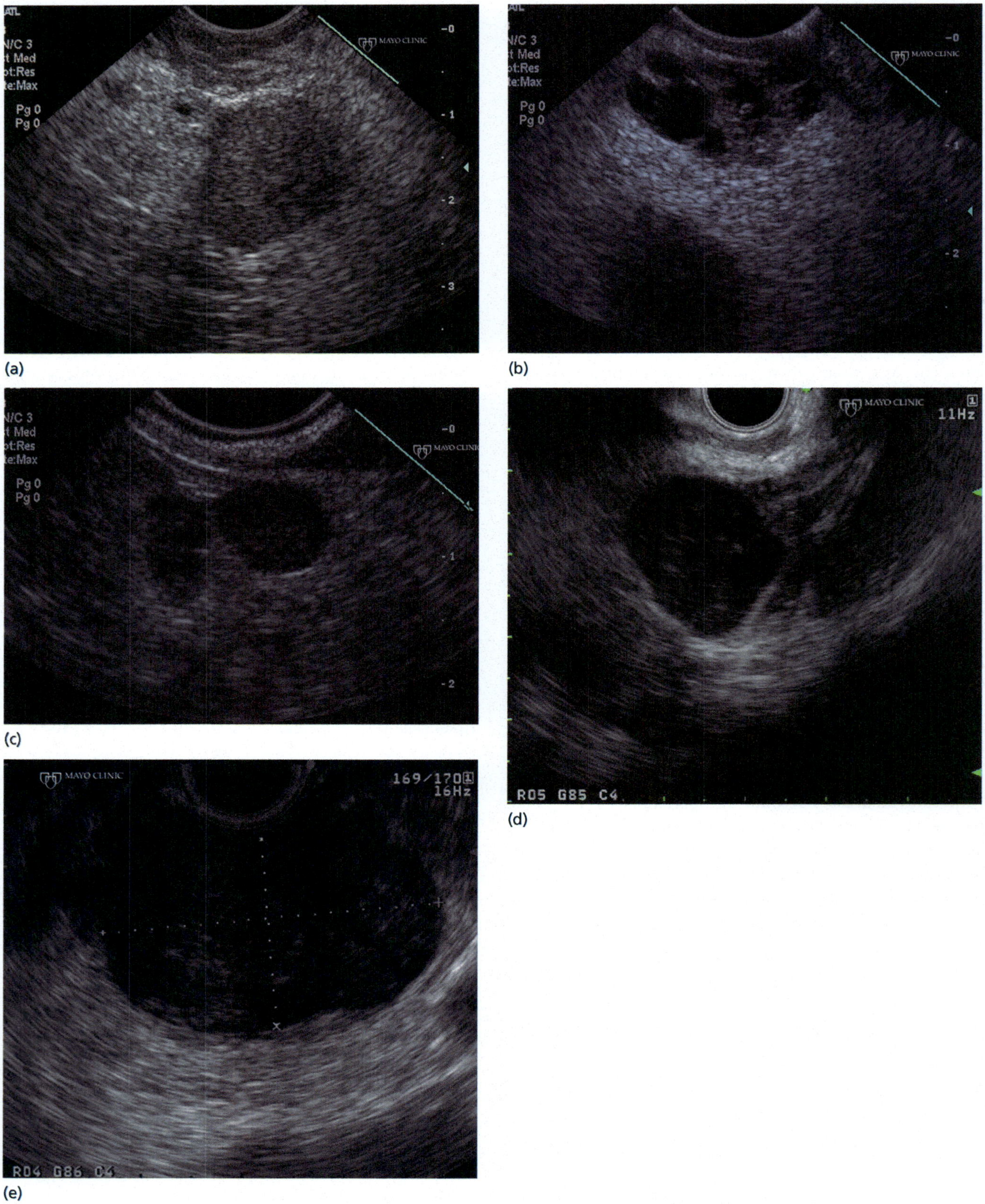

Figure 23.6 The varied appearance of metastatic tumors to the pancreas is demonstrated (a–e). Source: Mayo Clinic.

24 Autoimmune Pancreatitis

Larissa Fujii-Lau[1], Michael J. Levy[2], and Suresh T. Chari[3]

[1] University of Hawaii, Honolulu, HI, USA

[2] Mayo Clinic, Rochester, MN, USA

[3] MD Anderson Cancer Hospital, Houston, TX, USA

Introduction

While the first description of autoimmune pancreatitis (AIP) was by Sarles et al. in 1961, the term "autoimmune pancreatitis" was first introduced by Yoshida et al. in 1995. There are two types of AIP, type 1 being the classic AIP described from Japan. Type 1 AIP is part of a systemic fibro-inflammatory process that afflicts multiple organs including pancreas, bile duct, retroperitoneum, lymph nodes, salivary glands, and kidneys which demonstrate a characteristic IgG_4-rich lymphoplasmacytic infiltrate. Type 2 AIP appears to be a pancreas-specific disorder, sometimes associated with inflammatory bowel disease. Both forms readily respond to steroid therapy. Type 2 can only be definitively diagnosed on histology.

The initial description of AIP highlighted the presence of obstructive jaundice secondary to a pancreatic head mass mimicking pancreatic cancer. As clinical experience evolved there came a greater understanding of the diverse clinical, laboratory, and histologic manifestations of AIP, leading the way to more comprehensive diagnostic criteria such as the Mayo HISORt system that considers the findings of histology, imaging, serology, other organ (non-pancreatic) involvement, and response to steroid therapy. Similarly, international consensus diagnostic criteria (ICDC) for the diagnosis of AIP incorporate five features, including imaging characteristics of the pancreatic parenchyma and duct (obtained with cross-sectional imaging or endoscopic retrograde cholangiopancreatography), serology, other organ involvement, pancreatic histology, and response to steroids. While pancreatic imaging is a key component of the diagnostic systems, notably absent in both criteria is specific mention of the role for endoscopic ultrasound (EUS). This omission of EUS from diagnostic algorithms likely results from the lack of meaningful studies that document the EUS imaging features and a paucity of data pertaining to the utility and safety of EUS-guided fine needle aspiration (EUS-FNA) and EUS-guided fine needle biopsy (EUS-FNB) in this patient cohort. Our aim is to review the spectrum of AIP features identified by EUS and suggest a potential role of EUS-guided tissue sampling.

Endoscopic ultrasound imaging (Video 24.1)

The classic EUS finding in AIP is diffuse (sausage-shaped) pancreatic enlargement with a hypoechoic, coarse, patchy, heterogeneous appearance (Figures 24.1–24.3). When all of these classic features are present, there is a high likelihood of AIP. However, there may be significant overlap between the appearance of AIP and other pancreatic disorders. EUS may reveal isolated or multiple mass lesions that can mimic "unresectable" carcinoma (Figure 24.4). Other less common EUS features include glandular atrophy, calcification, cystic spaces, features of usual chronic pancreatitis, or even a normal gland (Figure 24.5). Unfortunately, there are no pathognomonic EUS findings for AIP. While a few features of AIP are characteristic, none are adequate to allow definitive diagnosis of AIP and their presence in other pancreatic disorders is common. The lack of pathognomonic features and diverse spectrum of EUS findings somewhat limits the utility of EUS imaging alone. This has driven the pursuit of safe and reliable methods for obtaining tissue to enhance diagnostic accuracy.

As the biliary tree is the most common extrapancreatic organ involved in AIP, it should be thoroughly evaluated during EUS when AIP is suspected. Wall thickening of either the bile duct or gallbladder may be appreciated by EUS.

Atlas of Endoscopic Ultrasonography, Second Edition. Edited by Frank Gress, Thomas Savides, Brenna Casey, and Everson L. A. Artifon.

Companion website: www.wiley.com/go/gress/atlas

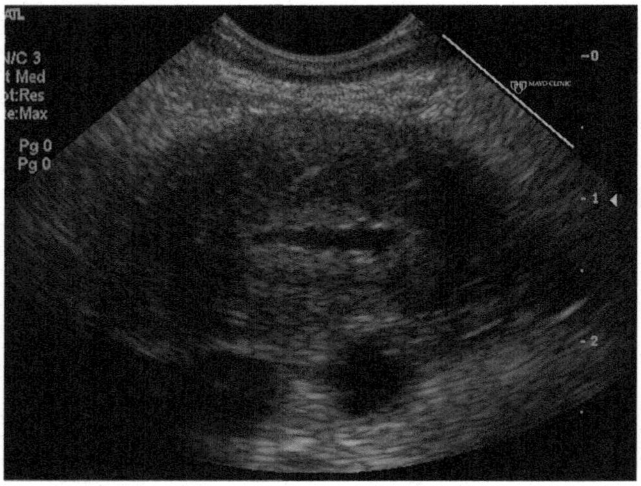

Figure 24.1 Classic endoscopic ultrasound appearance of autoimmune pancreatitis including hypoechoic diffuse (sausage-shaped) pancreatic enlargement with hypoechoic, coarse, patchy, heterogeneous parenchyma.

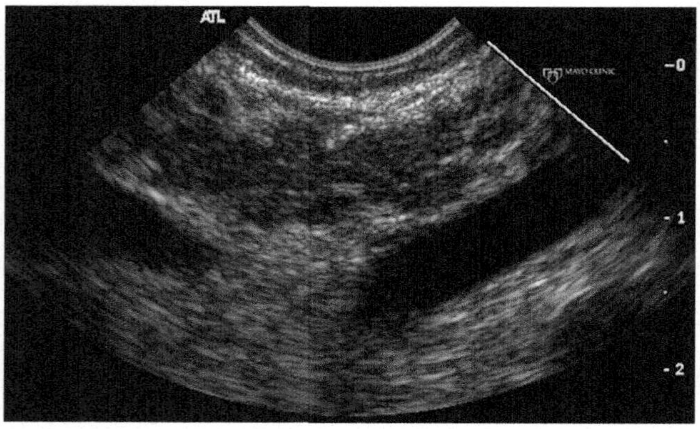

Figure 24.2 Almost classic endoscopic ultrasound appearance of autoimmune pancreatitis with a hypoechoic gland and coarse, patchy, heterogeneous changes without glandular enlargement.

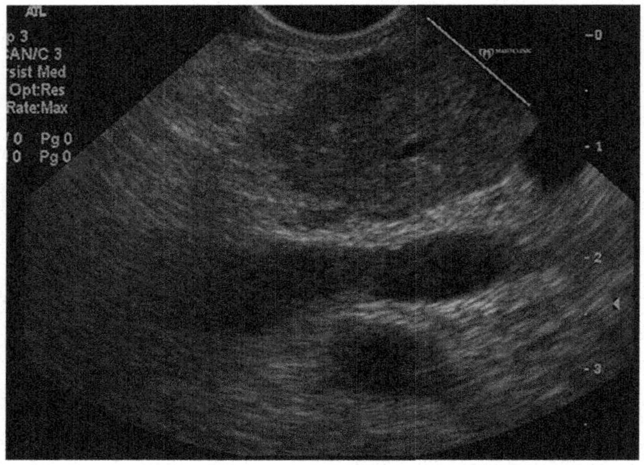

Figure 24.3 Almost classic endoscopic ultrasound appearance of autoimmune pancreatitis with a hypoechoic and enlarged gland without the prominent coarse, patchy, heterogeneous changes.

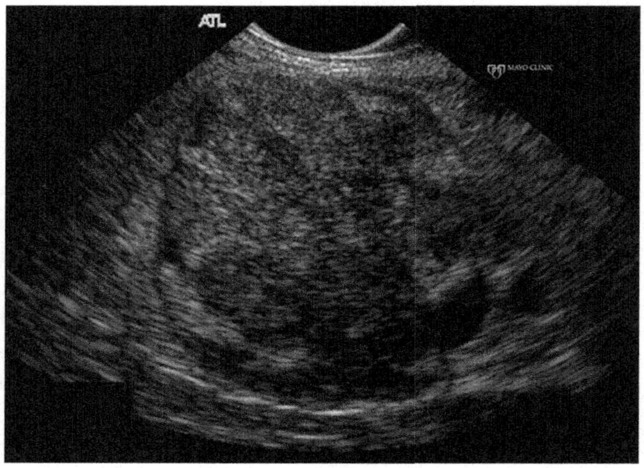

Figure 24.4 Endoscopic ultrasound finding of a mass-like lesion in a patient with autoimmune pancreatitis that may be confused with an "unresectable" pancreatic ductal carcinoma.

Image-enhancing techniques during EUS

Although the use is not widespread, some image-enhancing techniques employed during EUS may be used to help differentiate AIP from pancreatic cancer. In one study on the use of elastography in AIP, five patients with focal AIP were found to have a homogeneous stiff (blue) pattern in the mass and throughout the entire pancreas, which differed from pancreatic cancer or normal pancreas in which the pancreatic parenchyma was predominantly of intermediate stiffness (green).

Using contrast-enhanced EUS, AIP has been shown to be associated with hypervascularity within the mass-like lesion and the surrounding pancreatic parenchyma as compared to pancreatic cancer where the mass is hypovascular in comparison to the surrounding pancreatic tissue

EUS-FNA and EUS-FNB

As the EUS features of AIP overlap with other diseases of the pancreas, tissue sampling has an important role in the evaluation of AIP. Cytologic specimens obtained during EUS-FNA of the pancreas are often inadequate for diagnosing AIP. Typically, a definitive diagnosis requires pancreatic core biopsy obtained at surgery under CT guidance, or by EUS-FNB. Some suggest that the main role of EUS-FNA is to exclude pancreatic adenocarcinoma rather than to diagnose AIP. However, this opinion needs to be viewed with caution

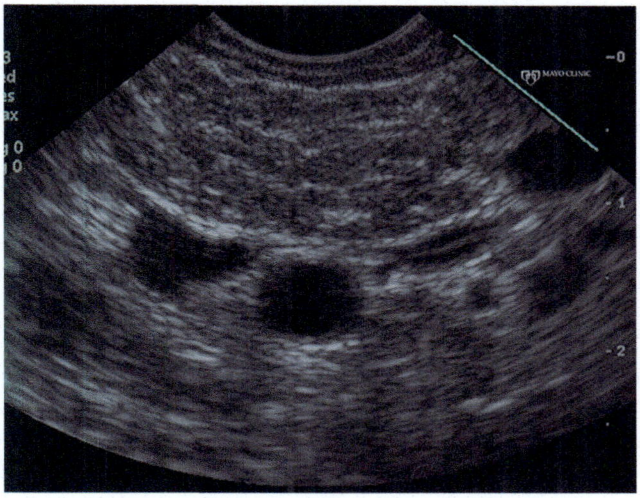

Figure 24.5 Endoscopic ultrasound features of nonspecific chronic pancreatitis in a patient with autoimmune pancreatitis.

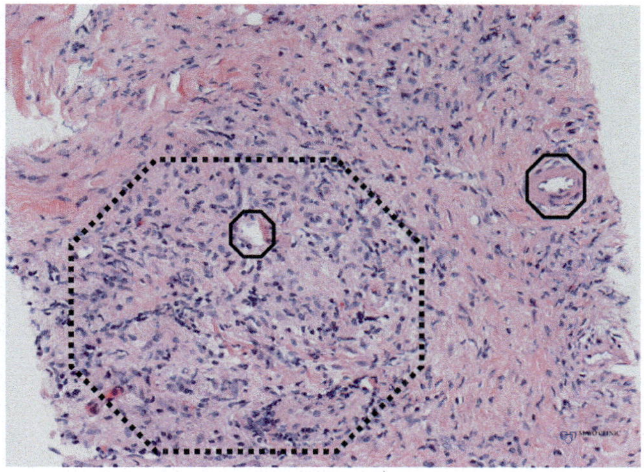

Figure 24.6 Histologic examination of endoscopic ultrasound-guided Tru-cut biopsy (EUS-TCB) specimen reveals an intact artery seen at the right of the image (single solid marker). In addition, an intense infiltration by lymphocytes and histiocytes results in near complete obliteration of the vein (obliterative phlebitis) shown at the left of the image (dashed marker surrounding solid marker). H&E, original magnification ×300.

due to a 10–40% false-negative rate in the diagnosis of cancer using EUS-FNA.

To overcome the inadequate samples obtained at EUS-FNA, larger-caliber cutting biopsy needles have been created in which the goal is to obtain samples with preserved tissue architecture. One of the original needles was the Tru-cut biopsy (TCB) needle. Although no longer available, we have previously demonstrated that EUS-TCB acquires core specimens with preserved tissue architecture permitting histologic diagnosis of AIP similar to the results using other EUS-FNB needles. In updating our initial report, 48 patients (38 male, 10 female; mean age 59.7 years [range 18–87]) with a final diagnosis of AIP have undergone a mean of 2.9 EUS-TCB tests (range 1–7). Autoimmune pancreatitis was histologically diagnosed on EUS-TCB in 35 (73%) patients and the diagnostic sensitivity varied from 33 to 90% among the five endosonographers. Nondiagnostic cases were found to have chronic pancreatitis ($n = 8$), nonspecific histology ($n = 2$), and failed tissue acquisition ($n = 3$). Thirty-seven patients underwent EUS-FNA (mean 3.4 passes, range 1–7 passes) that failed to establish or suggest the diagnosis in any patient. Complications of EUS-TCB included mild transient abdominal pain ($n = 3$) and self-limited intraprocedural bleeding ($n = 1$). No patient required hospitalization or therapeutic intervention. The diagnosis of AIP was strongly suspected prior to EUS in 14 patients as a result of their clinical, laboratory, imaging, and laboratory findings. For 22 patients the diagnosis was considered pre-EUS as part of a broader differential, and in 12 patients the EUS appearance alone led to the initial suspicion of AIP. Serum IgG_4 was more than twice the upper limit of normal in only 23% of patients. No patient with EUS-TCB diagnosis of AIP required surgery. In the patients with false-negative EUS-TCB, the diagnosis was made by HISORt criteria. Over a mean follow-up of 2.6 years no false-negative diagnoses of pancreatic cancer were identified. Our experience demonstrates that large-caliber pancreatic biopsy is safe and provides sufficient material to definitively diagnose AIP, obviating the need for surgical resection.

Recently, more studies have emerged using other EUS-FNB needles in the diagnosis of AIP. However, larger studies and a comparative study of EUS-FNA and EUS-FNB is likely required to understand the role of EUS tissue acquisition in the diagnosis of AIP.

Histologic features

Histologic features of type 1 AIP (lymphoplasmacytic sclerosing pancreatitis, LPSP) include a lymphoplasmacytic infiltrate that surrounds medium- and large-size interlobular pancreatic ducts, and pancreatic venules (obliterative phlebitis) while sparing arterioles, as well as swirling fibrosis centered around pancreatic ducts (storiform fibrosis) (Figure 24.6). Histology accurately distinguishes AIP from other causes of chronic pancreatitis and pancreatic carcinoma. IgG_4 immunostaining of tissue samples identifies IgG_4-positive plasma cells and the presence of moderate (11–30 cells per high-power field [HPF]) or severe (>30 cells/HPF) infiltration is considered diagnostic (Figure 24.7). These findings distinguish AIP from alcohol-induced pancreatitis and the peritumoral inflammation associated with carcinoma. Histologic features of type 2 AIP (idiopathic duct-centric pancreatitis, IDCP) include a lymphoplasmacytic infiltrate with granulocyte epithelial lesions with partial/complete duct obstruction. Tissue immunostaining in IDCP is typically negative, but may reveal mild (1–10 cells/HPF) or moderate (11–20 cells/HPF) IgG_4-positive plasma cell infiltration.

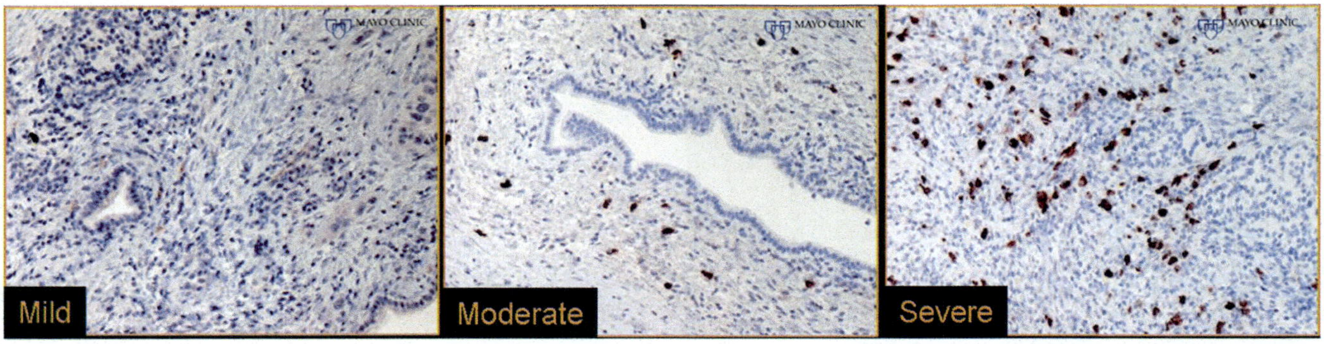

Figure 24.7 IgG_4 immunostaining of the Tru-cut biopsy specimen reveals the findings of mild infiltration (1–10 plasma cells per high-power field [HPF]), moderate infiltration (11–30 cells/HPF) and severe infiltration (>30 cells/HPF).

Summary

The difficulty in diagnosing AIP highlights the need for improved understanding of its EUS imaging features and the development of reliable and safe methods for acquiring core tissue specimens. Until such time, EUS will have a central role in the evaluation of AIP in a minority of centers. We advocate EUS imaging to provide supportive evidence for or against an AIP diagnosis. Because imaging alone cannot firmly establish the diagnosis, FNA is often necessary to exclude underlying malignancy. We recommend EUS-FNB for patients with a compatible clinical presentation in whom there is diagnostic uncertainty and when the findings are likely to alter management. This recommendation assumes the reliable and safe us of EUS-FNB. Further study is necessary to help clarify the diagnostic accuracy and role of EUS imaging and tissue sampling in this patient cohort.

Chapter video clip

Video 24.1 Autoimmune pancreatitis. Source: Mayo Clinic.

25 Pancreatic Cystic Lesions: The Role of EUS

William R. Brugge
Massachusetts General Hospital and Harvard Medical School, Boston, MA, USA

Introduction

The frequent use of cross-sectional radiographic imaging has led to an increase in the identification of cystic lesions of the pancreas. In asymptomatic patients, the cystic lesion most often represents a form of intraductal malignancy. Fluid collections in patients with acute pancreatitis are usually inflammatory in nature. In the management of patients with a cystic lesion, there are usually two predominant questions: "Is the cyst mucinous or non-mucinous?" and "Is the cyst malignant or benign?" Endoscopic ultrasound (EUS) with fine needle aspiration (FNA) can provide critical data to answer these diagnostic questions.

Cystic lesions of the pancreas are often readily apparent by EUS. The lesions appear as anechoic against the "salt and pepper" background of the pancreatic parenchyma. Focal fluid collections can simulate a true cyst of the pancreas, but often there are tell-tale signs of pancreatitis. Occasionally, tumor necrosis can simulate a pancreatic cyst because of the presence of fluid in the mass. Endoscopic ultrasound can provide details of the structural characteristics of the cyst, pancreatic parenchyma, pancreatic duct as well as surrounding structures, but is not sufficient to distinguish malignant from benign lesions (Table 25.1).

Fine needle aspiration of the cyst fluid and analysis of cellular material, amylase level, and tumor markers such as carcinoembryonic antigen (CEA) have been shown to assist in narrowing the differential diagnosis. In studies where surgical correlation is available, EUS with FNA and cytopathology has an accuracy of 55–91%. In particular, a cyst fluid CEA concentration above 192 ng/ml is predictive of a mucinous lesion with 79% accuracy. The presence of a *KRAS* mutation is also indicative of a mucinous lesion.

The diagnostic techniques described are particularly pertinent in those patients who are not surgical candidates or do not have symptoms attributable to the cyst. Endoscopic ultrasound with FNA should be reserved for those cases in which the results would alter clinical management. If a cyst is found in the setting of recurrent acute pancreatitis in a patient who is fit for surgery, resection should be considered and EUS is not indicated.

Pseudocyst

A pancreatic pseudocyst represents an inflammatory fluid collection. There is no epithelial lining within a pseudocyst and surrounding structures form the borders of a pseudocyst. Imaging findings of chronic pancreatitis, including calcifications, increase the likelihood that a cystic lesion is a pseudocyst.

The EUS features of pseudocysts include a thick-walled, unilocular, fluid-filled cavity (Figure 25.1). Aspiration of a pseudocyst reveals thin, brown, amylase-rich fluid. Cytologic examination reveals inflammatory cells and occasionally necrotic debris. The fluid CEA level should be relatively low and without evidence of mucin.

Serous lesions

Serous cystadenoma is the most common type of non-mucinous cyst (Figure 25.2). These lesions typically have a microcystic morphology creating a honeycomb appearance. The microcysts are divided by thin septations that can become fibrotic and form the classic central stellate scar. Macrocystic morphology is seen in a minority of serous cystadenomas. Microscopically, the cyst lining is composed of cuboidal cells with glycogen-rich cytoplasm and dense chromatin.

Atlas of Endoscopic Ultrasonography, Second Edition. Edited by Frank Gress, Thomas Savides, Brenna Casey, and Everson L. A. Artifon.

Companion website: www.wiley.com/go/gress/atlas

Table 25.1 Demographics and characteristics of pancreatic cystic neoplasms.

Cyst type	Most common location	Gender	Solitary or multicentric	Morphology	Malignant potential
Serous cystadenoma	Head	Female	Solitary	Microcystic with honeycombing, minority are macrocystic	Very low
Mucinous cystic neoplasm	Tail	Strongly female	Solitary	Macrocystic, can be septated	High
Intraductal papillary mucinous neoplasm	Multifocal	Equal	Multicentric	Main duct: dilated duct, mixed macrocystic, microcystic Branch duct: cluster of grapes	High
Solid pseudopapillary neoplasm	Body	Strongly female	Solitary	Encapsulated, mixed solid and cystic	Moderate
Cystic endocrine tumor	Tail	Equal	Solitary	Variable	Variable based on type

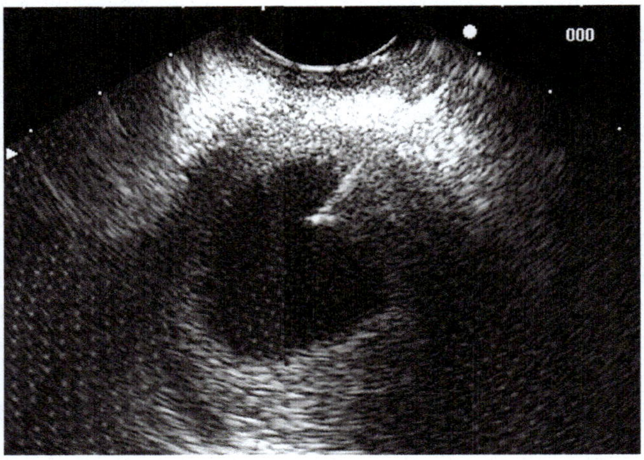

Figure 25.1 Thick-walled cystic lesion undergoing fine needle aspiration (FNA). The lesion was resected and was a pseudocyst.

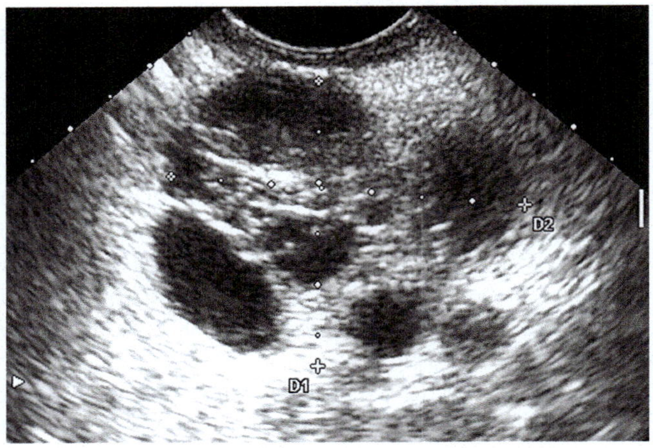

Figure 25.2 Serous cystadenoma. Multicystic lesion in the body of the pancreas with microcystic and macrocystic components and a central scar. The overall size is 2.8 × 3.5 cm.

Mucinous lesions

Mucinous cystic neoplasms (MCNs) are a distinct type of mucinous cyst (Figure 25.3a). They occur almost exclusively in women when they are defined by the presence of ovarian stroma. These tumors are principally located in the tail of the pancreas and mucin may be visible within the cyst cavity (Figure 25.3b). Malignant MCNs may have a mural nodule or mass apparent on EUS (Figure 25.3c). Depending on the degree of cellular atypia, MCNs are classified as adenomas, borderline tumors, or carcinomas. The cysts do not communicate with the pancreatic ductal system and the cyst fluid generally contains mucin and a high concentration of CEA.

Intraductal papillary mucinous neoplasm (IPMN) (Figure 25.4a) generally presents in the seventh decade of life. It can be divided into morphologic subtypes: main-duct IPMN, branch-duct IPMN, and mixed. Main-duct IPMN carries a much greater likelihood of malignancy than branch-duct IPMN. The characteristic imaging features of branch-duct IPMN include multilocular appearance with a cluster-of-grapes configuration, communication with the pancreatic duct, and dilated ductal structures with filling defects representing mucus. In addition, a dilated main pancreatic duct, cyst size greater than 3.0 cm, and mural nodularity are features of IPMN that predict an increased likelihood of malignancy (Figure 25.4b,c).

Other cystic neoplasms

Solid pseudopapillary epithelial neoplasm (SPEN) usually occurs in young women. Although this lesion is rare, recognition is important given its malignant potential and very high cure rate with surgical resection. It is typically large with solid and cystic features. Fine needle aspiration cytopathology may demonstrate branching papillae and myxoid stroma.

Pancreatic cystic endocrine tumors have a male to female ratio of 1 : 1 with a peak incidence in the fifth and sixth decades. Cystic neuroendocrine tumors often have a thick wall

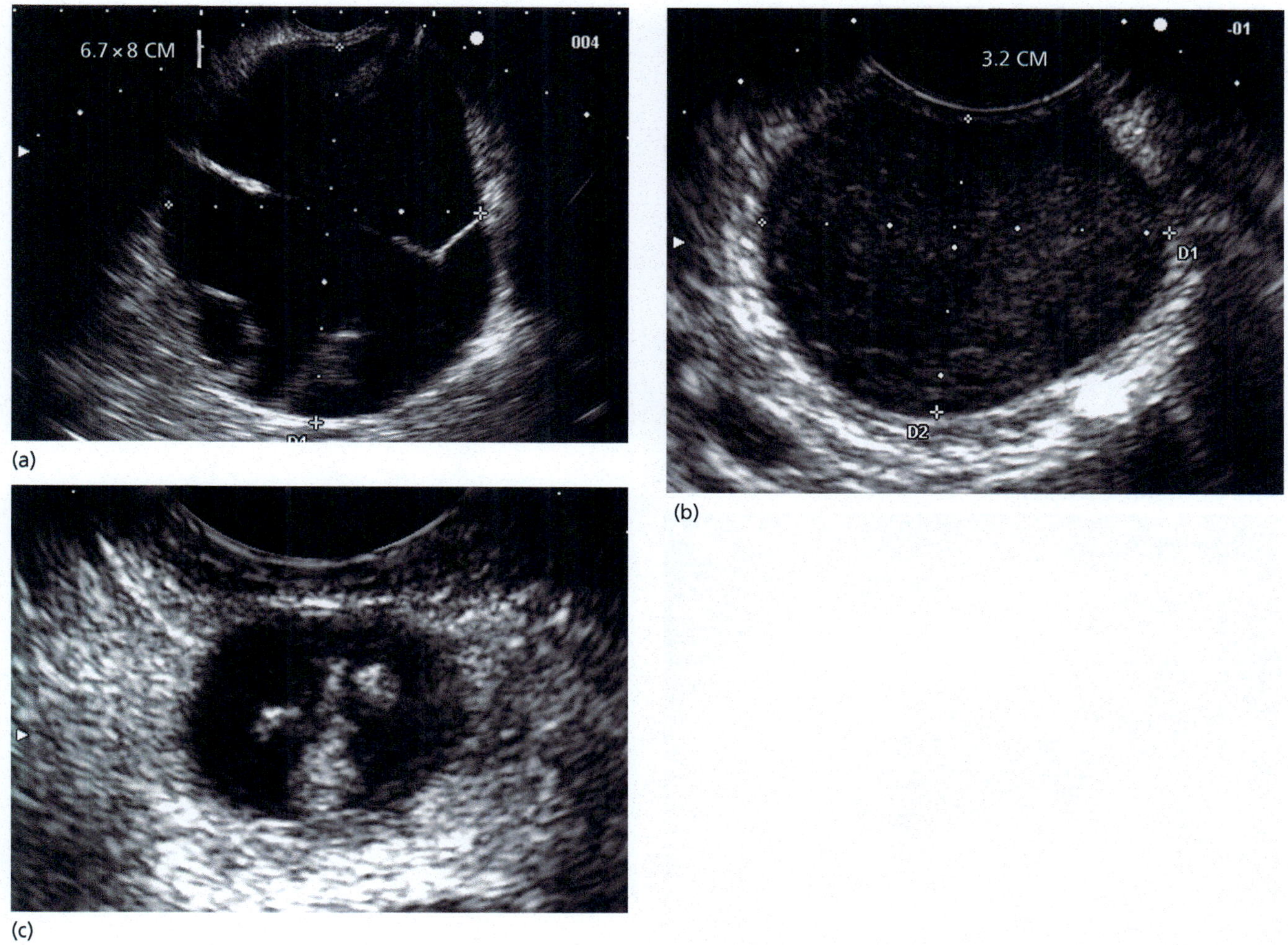

Figure 25.3 (a) Mucinous cystic neoplasm with multiple septations. The lesion was benign when surgically resected. (b) Mucinous cystic neoplasm with mucin visible within the cyst cavity. (c) A 1.5-cm malignant cystic lesion with mucin and debris in the lumen of the cyst.

(Figure 25.5a). Given their high degree of vascularity, EUS with color flow Doppler may demonstrate increased blood flow within these lesions (Figure 25.5b).

Ductal adenocarcinoma can also present with cystic morphology as a result of tumor necrosis. As with solid adenocarcinoma of the pancreas, there is a male predominance, and the typical age of onset is late sixties to early seventies. Endoscopic ultrasound may demonstrate mixed solid–cystic mass with resultant ductal obstruction and possible invasion of adjacent structures.

Chapter video clip

Video 25.1 Pancreatic cystic lesions. Source: Hitachi.

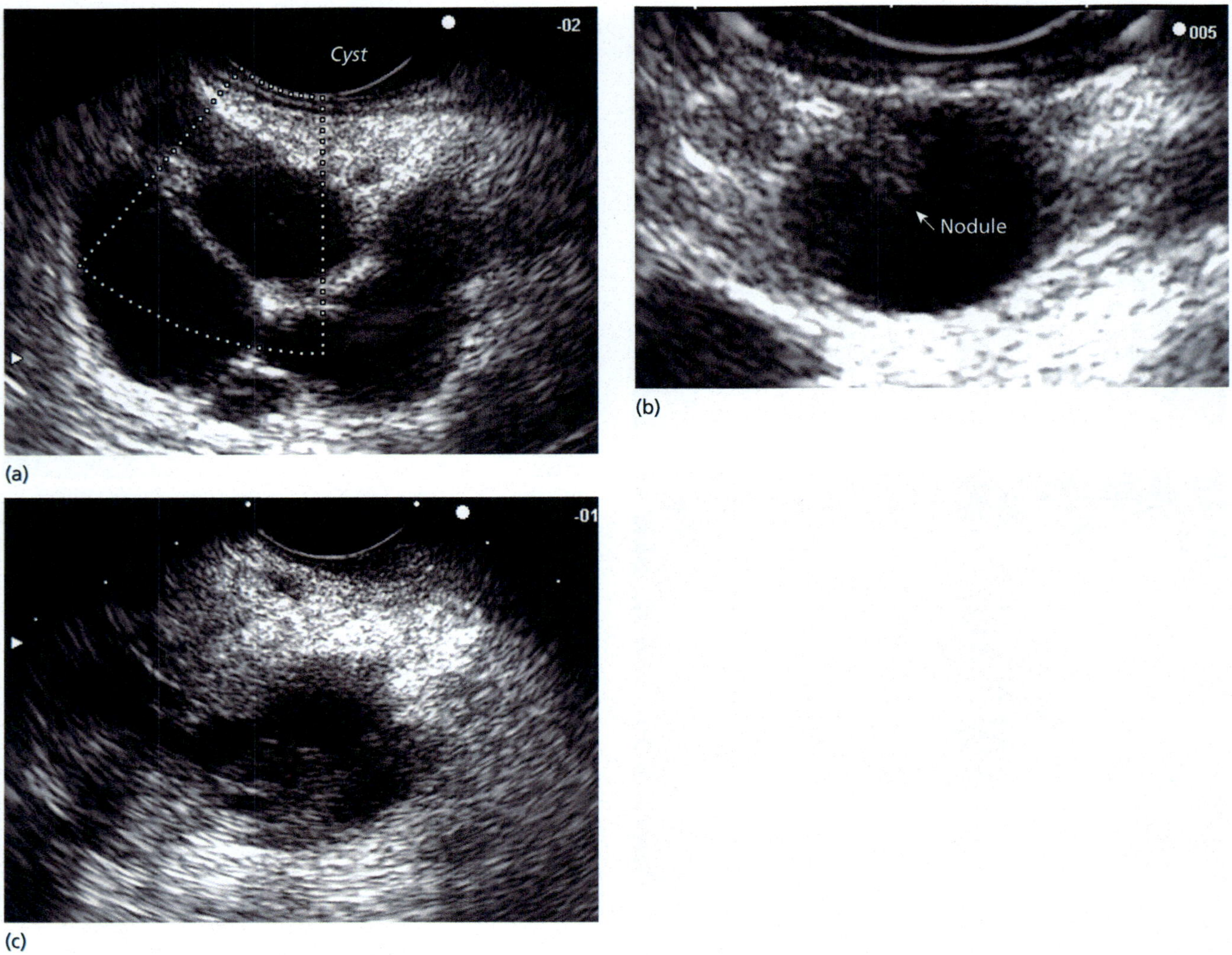

Figure 25.4 (a) Thinly septated intraductal papillary mucinous neoplasm (IPMN) in the head of the pancreas. (b) IPMN with mural nodule suggestive of malignancy. (c) Malignant IPMN with thick wall and large nodule.

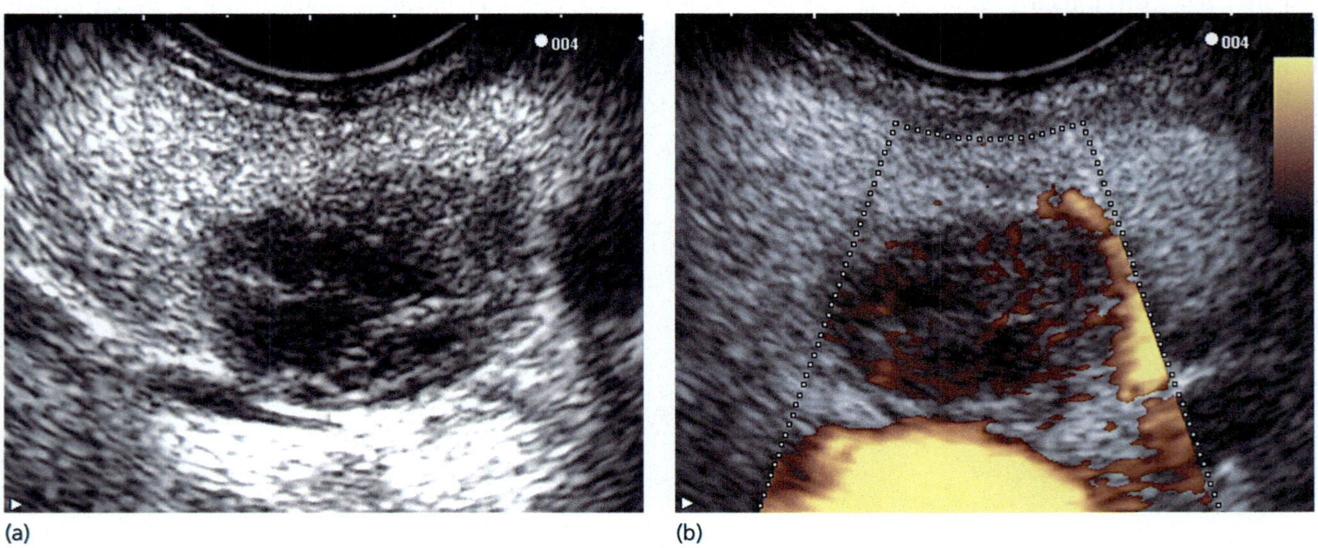

Figure 25.5 (a) Pancreatic cystic endocrine tumor. Note the presence of the thick wall and complex septations. (b) Pancreatic endocrine tumor. Color flow Doppler demonstrates hypervascularity within the solid portions of the mass.

26 Intraductal Papillary Mucinous Neoplasms: The Role of EUS

William R. Brugge
Massachusetts General Hospital and Harvard Medical School, Boston, MA, USA

Introduction

Intraductal papillary mucinous neoplasms (IPMNs) have emerged as the most common mucinous cystic neoplasm and represent a significant clinical entity. Endoscopic ultrasound (EUS) is an important tool for the diagnosis and management of IPMNs.

IPMNs represent a premalignant pancreatic lesion generally characterized by proliferation of the mucinous epithelium with varying degrees of ductal and cystic dilatation. These papillary lesions typically involve the main pancreatic duct with or without side branch involvement. Based on the differential location of the tumor, they can be classified into three types: branch-duct IPMN, main-duct IPMN, and mixed IPMN. IPMNs can further be described according to a continuum of cellular atypia similar to that of colorectal cancer: benign (adenoma/low-grade dysplasia), borderline (moderate dysplasia), and malignant (ranging from carcinoma in situ/high-grade dysplasia to invasive carcinoma).

Several studies have suggested that main-duct IPMNs are associated with higher grade of histology and more rapid growth, compared with branch-duct lesions, which are felt to represent more indolent disease. The exact rate of cell transition from benign to malignant is not clear, although the progression to invasive disease in main-duct IPMN has been estimated to range from five to seven years. There have been estimates of the rate of malignant degeneration ranging from 0.5 to 1.0% per year. Overall, invasive carcinoma arising in association with IPMN has a better prognosis than conventional ductal adenocarcinoma; however, when metastatic, its prognosis is as poor as that of pancreatic adenocarcinoma.

Clinical features

Symptoms for IPMN are vague and often nonspecific, and most patients are asymptomatic, especially those with small (≤3 cm) lesions. When symptomatic, patients usually present with abdominal pain which may represent recurrent pancreatitis. Patients commonly present in the sixth to seventh decade, with the mean age at diagnosis being 65 years.

Obvious main-duct lesions are more likely to present with symptoms masquerading as chronic pancreatitis and other features. Gradual distension of the pancreatic duct due to excess mucin secretion induces recurrent abdominal pain and symptoms of pancreatitis secondary to main-duct IPMN. Because of the presentation and appearance, IPMNs have in fact been misdiagnosed as chronic pancreatitis in the past.

Role of imaging

Multiple modalities can be used to image and stage IPMNs, including computed tomography (CT), magnetic resonance cholangiopancreatography (MRCP), endoscopic ultrasound (EUS), and endoscopic retrograde cholangiopancreatography (ERCP). Using any one of the modalities can provide diagnostic features, evidence of malignancy, and staging information.

Cross-sectional imaging

The resolution of multidetector CT (MDCT) has improved dramatically in the past years. The quality of the digital displays provides excellent imaging of the pancreas and the ductal system. Communication between a cystic branch-duct lesion and the main duct is well visualized on thin-section MDCT. With these improvements, CT provides excellent imaging of IPMN including important features such as septations and nodules (Figure 26.1).

MRCP has also evolved rapidly in the imaging of the pancreas. Breath-hold MRCP is less dependent on patient

Atlas of Endoscopic Ultrasonography, Second Edition. Edited by Frank Gress, Thomas Savides, Brenna Casey, and Everson L. A. Artifon.

Companion website: www.wiley.com/go/gress/atlas

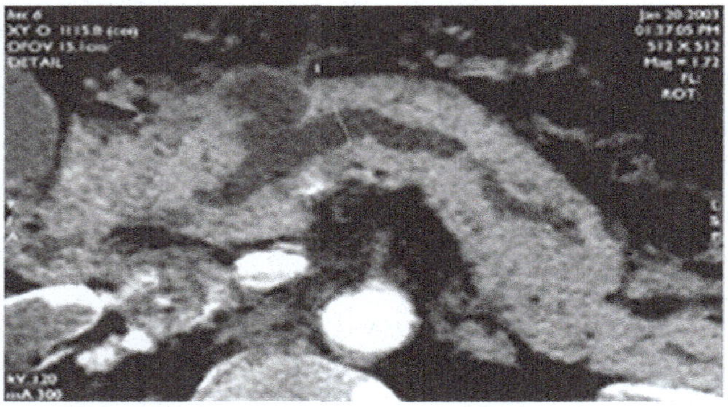

Figure 26.1 Reformatted computed tomography scan demonstrating a side-branch intraductal papillary mucinous neoplasm.

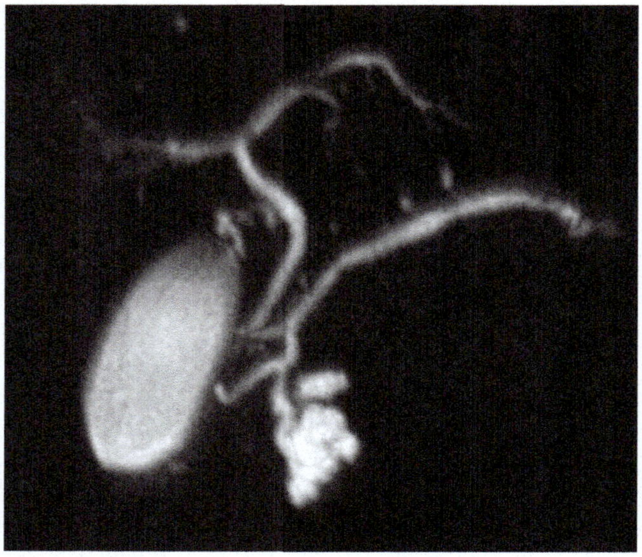

Figure 26.2 Magnetic resonance cholangiopancreatography demonstrating a side-branch intraductal papillary mucinous neoplasm in the head of the pancreas.

cooperation. Studies have shown this technique to be even more effective in detecting connections with the main pancreatic duct than MDCT (Figure 26.2). The use of intravenous secretin improves the quality of MRCP and visualization of the extent of duct involvement. For IPMN evaluation, whether MDCT or MRCP is used, a dedicated pancreatic imaging protocol should be adhered to.

Endoscopic ultrasound evaluation

Endoscopic ultrasound evaluation can be particularly helpful if there is diagnostic uncertainty, although it is not the preferred first-line imaging modality for IPMN. It is also helpful in cases where surgical risk is high, and verification of malignancy is needed before resection, such as in older patients or those with high comorbidities. Endoscopic ultrasound can provide detailed imaging of main-duct IPMN, side-branch disease, and combined duct disease.

The EUS findings of IPMN include cystic lesions, a dilated main pancreatic duct, and/or a parenchymal mass (Figures 26.3–26.5). The diagnosis is usually readily made once multiple cystic lesions have been demonstrated. However, the findings of a viscous fluid during fine needle aspiration (FNA) will confirm the diagnosis. With the diagnosis established, attention should turn towards detection of malignancy. The most obvious targets are a dilated main duct, a nodule arising within a cyst, and a pancreatic mass (Figure 26.6). Of course, signs of metastatic disease such as liver metastases, lymphadenopathy, and ascites are very important findings. Fine needle aspiration of the main pancreatic duct is performed with a 22-gauge needle usually from the gastric body. Pancreatic duct juice is readily aspirated from the main duct. Care should be taken in the

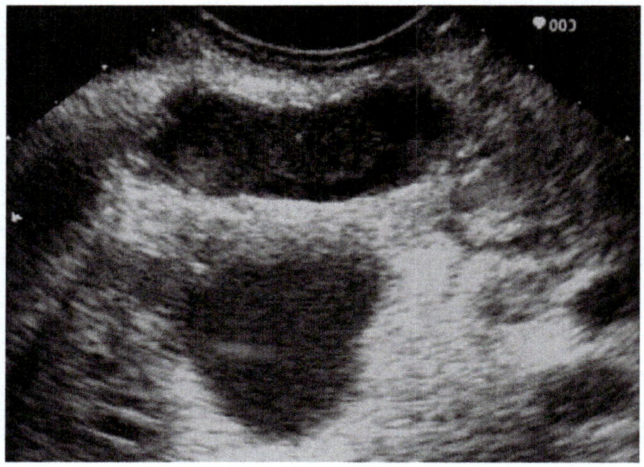

Figure 26.3 Linear endoscopic ultrasound image demonstrating a dilated main pancreatic duct, indicative of a main-duct intraductal papillary mucinous neoplasm.

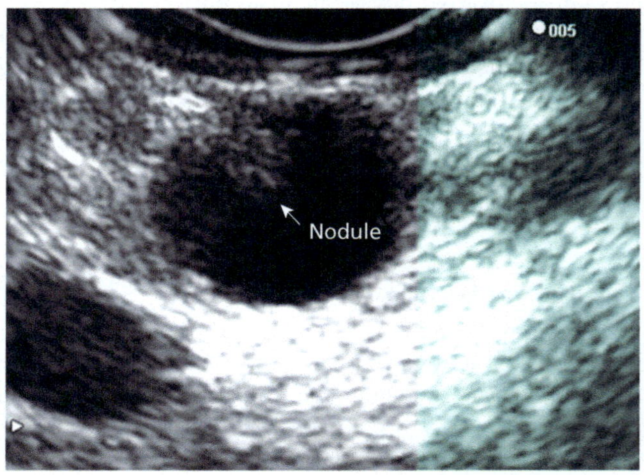

Figure 26.4 Linear endoscopic ultrasound image revealing a small cystic lesion with a mural nodule.

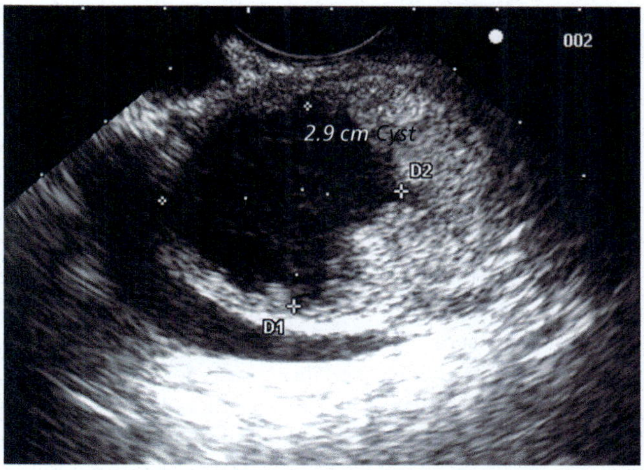

Figure 26.5 Linear endoscopic ultrasound image of a malignant-appearing 2.9-cm cystic lesion, including an adjacent mass.

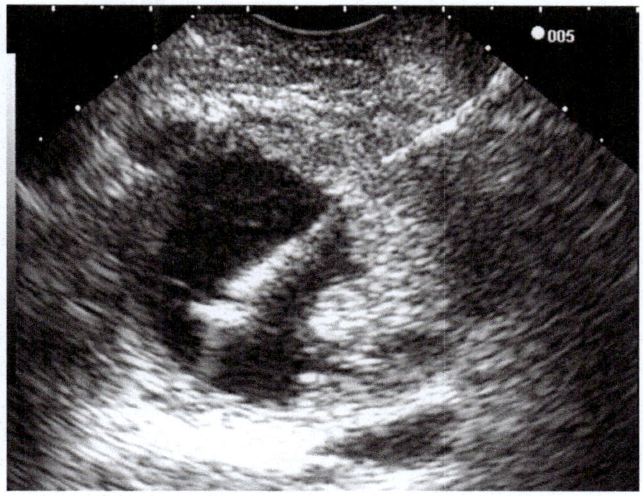

Figure 26.6 Fine needle aspiration of a malignant cystic mass.

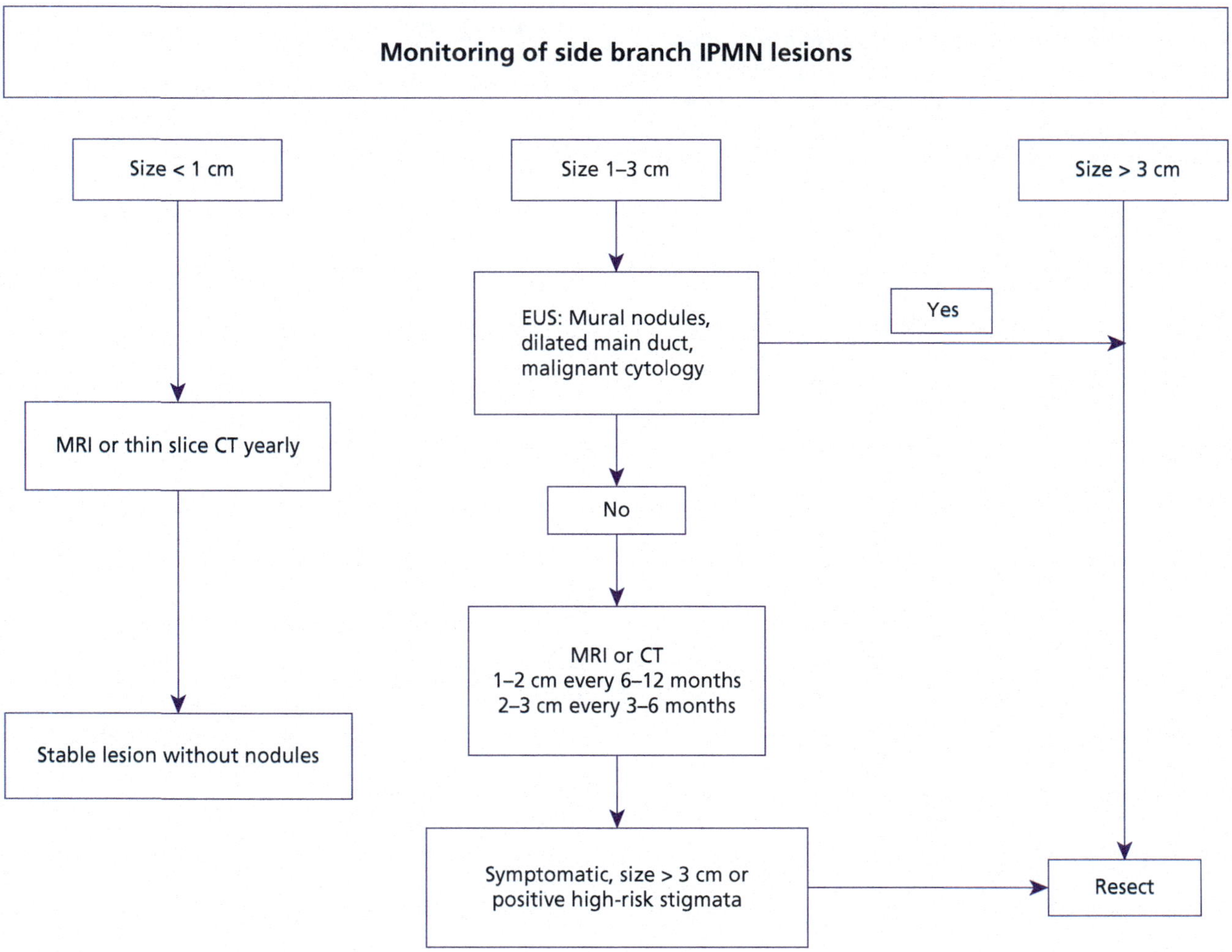

Figure 26.7 International Association of Pancreatology (IAP) algorithm for management of intraductal papillary mucinous neoplasm (IPMN).

aspiration of nodules, because of the risk of bleeding and contaminating the cytologic specimen. The results of FNA should be used to assist in the planning of resection. For example, in the presence of multiple cysts, representative lesions in the head, body, and tail should be used to determine the type of resection.

Cytologic material from aspirated fluid is often inconclusive for IPMN. However, cyst fluid tumor markers, such as carcinoembryonic antigen (CEA) and cancer antigen (CA) 72-4, are important for establishing the mucinous origin of the cyst. *KRAS* is also a very useful marker for a mucinous lesion. The diagnosis of malignancy is usually established with the finding of malignant cytology, aspirated from a cyst, nodule, or mass.

Management of small IPMN (≤3 cm)

Many IPMNs need not be resected and can be followed conservatively due to their low risk for malignancy and slow progression toward invasive cancer. These include IPMNs without symptoms, without main-duct dilatation (>6 mm), without mural nodules, without thick walls/septations, or less than 3 cm in size. Consensus follow-up guidelines have been formulated by the International Association of Pancreatology (IAP): yearly follow-up is recommended for lesions less than 1 cm in size; follow up every 6–12 months is advisable for lesions of 1–2 cm; and follow-up every three to six months is indicated for lesions larger than 2 cm (Figure 26.7).

If symptoms arise, or if any of the above limits regarding size, dilatation, or solid components are surpassed on follow-up, resection is suggested. A greater than 1 cm increase in lesion size over a year is generally considered significant for malignancy. If minimal or no change is observed after two years, then the time frame between follow-up studies can be extended. An algorithm for observing small (≤3 cm) IPMN has been proposed.

When deciding which modality to use, follow-up imaging should be tailored further by considering radiation concerns relative to age. It may be advisable to monitor IPMN patients who are less than 40 years old with MRI and those who are over 40 years old with CT. Steps should still be taken to minimize radiation risk since the cumulative exposure from prolonged and repeated radiological follow-up may be substantial.

Chapter video clips

Video 26.1 How to perform cyst FNA. Source: Hitachi.

Video 26.2 Intraductal papillary mucinous neoplasms. Source: Hitachi.

27 Chronic Pancreatitis

David G. Forcione
Massachusetts General Hospital and Harvard Medical School, Boston, MA, USA

Introduction

Chronic pancreatitis is defined by irreversible morphologic changes of the pancreas often associated with abdominal pain and, in late stages, endocrine and exocrine insufficiency. Data from the United States and Japan have demonstrated that as many as 3% of US male veterans and 17% of Japanese individuals may be affected. In addition to being associated with significant medical morbidity, care of patients with chronic pancreatitis is costly, with estimates of over $2 billion per year in the United States for the over 100 000 outpatients and 50 000 inpatient annual visits.

As with other diseases, early diagnosis offers a better chance of effective treatment outcomes. Since Sivak's original description of the use of endoscopic ultrasound (EUS) to evaluate chronic pancreatitis in 1986, there has been increasing interest and data demonstrating the utility of this imaging modality for early diagnosis. The close proximity of the upper gastrointestinal tract to the pancreas provides endosonographers with an ideal imaging modality of the pancreas. In general, EUS appears safer than endoscopic retrograde cholangiopancreatography (ERCP). Furthermore, there are increasing data that both ductal and parenchymal changes of the pancreas associated with chronic pancreatitis may be seen earlier and more accurately with EUS as compared with conventional cross-sectional imaging modalities. Advances in EUS imaging such as sonoelastography and contrast-enhanced EUS are expected to improve the overall accuracy of the examination. Preliminary data using combined contrast-enhanced EUS and real-time sonoelastography demonstrate these modalities may further improve our ability to discern chronic pancreatitis from pancreatic neoplasia.

Threshold diagnostic criteria and interobserver variability are both common issues that may arise when any imaging modality is the predominant diagnostic tool for a specific disease entity. Chronic pancreatitis is particularly challenging given that the gold standard of diagnosis (i.e. histology) is rarely feasible. Furthermore, EUS is particularly susceptible as an imaging modality to these given the potential subjective nature of the examination. In the past two years, the EUS community has come closer to reducing the potential for this variability through the development of specific EUS-based criteria. The Rosemont Criteria (2009) is a significant step forward towards unifying the role of EUS in diagnosing chronic pancreatitis.

In this chapter, we review the utility of EUS as an imaging modality for chronic pancreatitis.

Clinical overview of chronic pancreatitis

The classification and diagnosis of chronic pancreatitis has evolved since the Marseilles conference of 1963 first established the histopathologic paradigm of fibrosis, inflammation, loss of exocrine parenchyma, ductal dilation, and stones. It soon became clear, however, that conventional radiologic diagnosis, i.e. transabdominal ultrasound (TUS), computed tomography (CT), and magnetic resonance imaging (MRI), was best suited for diagnosing advanced disease and may not have sufficient accuracy for early or mild chronic pancreatitis.

The role of ERCP was incorporated in 1984 by the Cambridge Classification. The Cambridge Classification incorporates features of both the main pancreatic duct and side branch, including dilation and ductal ectasia, to assess the severity of chronic pancreatitis. Although ERCP appeared to be more accurate than conventional cross-sectional imaging at identifying chronic pancreatitis through ductal changes, it continues to be seen as an imaging modality with limited predictive value. As noted with histopathology, autopsy series have demonstrated age-related ductal

Atlas of Endoscopic Ultrasonography, Second Edition. Edited by Frank Gress, Thomas Savides, Brenna Casey, and Everson L. A. Artifon.

Companion website: www.wiley.com/go/gress/atlas

changes of chronic pancreatitis without associated symptoms. Furthermore, as an invasive examination with potential morbidity, the role of ERCP for the diagnosis of early or mild chronic pancreatitis remains to be well established.

Pancreatic function testing (PFT) remains an option for the diagnosis of chronic pancreatitis. Currently, this is performed using standard upper endoscopy and secretin stimulation of the exocrine pancreas. Duodenal aspirates are obtained for bicarbonate and enzymatic (lipase) measurements. Some have incorporated PFT in the diagnostic criteria for chronic pancreatitis. Nonetheless, the role of PFT remains uncertain due to limited availability, patient intolerance, and uncertain validation across larger, more diverse patient populations. Furthermore, patients may have exocrine changes without associated morphologic changes and it is unclear if these patient subsets truly have chronic pancreatitis.

The gold standard for the diagnosis of chronic pancreatitis remains histopathology. Typical morphologic changes include chronic inflammation, fibrosis, and glandular atrophy. These findings may be uniform or patchy in the pancreas. Autopsy series have identified "asymptomatic/normal" individuals with significant atrophy and fibrosis. Furthermore, variation in pathologist interpretation of these findings adds to the potential difficulties in accurate diagnosis using these criteria.

There is increasing evidence that a wide array of insults may be associated with the development of chronic pancreatitis. Whitcomb *et al.* established the TIGAR-O classification in 2001 to incorporate the roles of Toxic (ethanol), Idiopathic, Genetic (*SPINK1*, *PRSS*, and *CFTR*), Autoimmune, Recurrent severe acute pancreatitis, and Obstructive etiologies. All of these entities should be carefully considered in patients being evaluated for chronic pancreatitis. Despite an exhaustive search, the etiology remains idiopathic in up to 20% of patients.

Endoscopic ultrasound imaging of the normal pancreas

In order to best understand the role of EUS in imaging of chronic pancreatitis, it is useful to review some of the fundamentals of normal pancreas imaging with EUS. Data from large series of "normal" TUS and EUS examinations from the 1990s have provided some useful imaging parameters.

Wiersema *et al.* characterized the normal pancreas parenchyma as having uniform echogenicity, typically brighter than the liver. The mean ductal diameters were 2.4 mm in the head (range 0.8–3.6 mm), 1.8 mm in the body (0.9–3.0 mm), and 1.2 mm in the tail (0.5–2.0 mm). Catalano *et al.* made endosonographic observations of the pancreas in 25 "normal" patients. The normal pancreas parenchyma was described to be homogeneous with identification of variable echotexture separating the ventral and dorsal anlage of the pancreas in 68%. The mean ductal diameter in the body was 1.7 mm (range 1–3 mm), and side branches could be appreciated in 32%.

Some studies have also provided some interesting insight into the wide spectrum of findings that may be seen in otherwise healthy individuals. A large TUS series from Japan (130 951 patients) identified that pancreatic duct dilation (>3 mm) may be seen in 0.49% of individuals and tended to be found in older men. In addition, calcifications and cysts were found in 0.05% and 0.22% of patients, respectively.

In summary, these data provide endosonographers with a basic framework for normal parenchymal and ductal imaging and set the basis for establishing some threshold criteria for the diagnosis of chronic pancreatitis.

EUS imaging in chronic pancreatitis: historical perspectives

Since the original description of the role of EUS imaging in chronic pancreatitis by Sivak in 1986, a number of studies have tried to define appropriate criteria for diagnosis. Early classifications incorporated nine criteria for chronic pancreatitis, including five parenchymal and four ductal. These data were almost exclusively derived using radial EUS imaging performed by experts in academic practices. The parenchymal changes included hyperechogenic foci, hyperechogenic strands, lobulation, cysts, and calcifications. Histopathologic correlates of the former three were felt to represent focal fibrosis and glandular atrophy. Ductal changes included a dilated main pancreas duct (>3 mm head, >2 mm body, >1 mm tail), ductal irregularity ("chain of lakes" appearance), hyperechoic ductal margins, and side-branch ectasia (Figures 27.1 and 27.2).

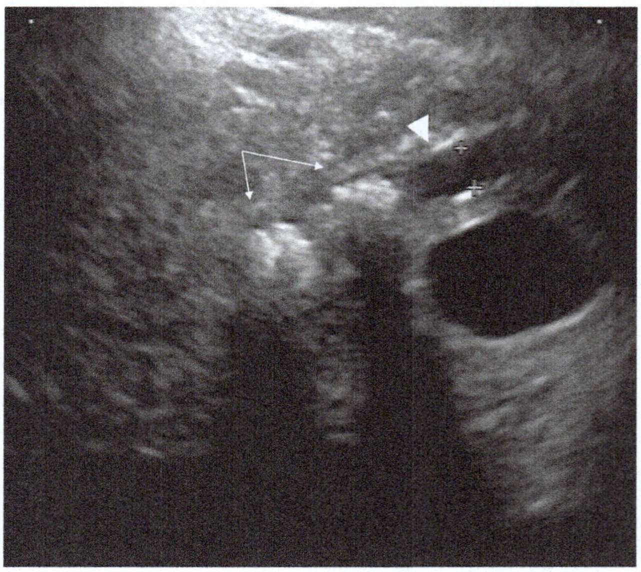

Figure 27.1 Endoscopic ultrasound (linear) showing features of chronic pancreatitis: a dilated pancreatic duct (arrowhead) and two intraductal stones (arrows).

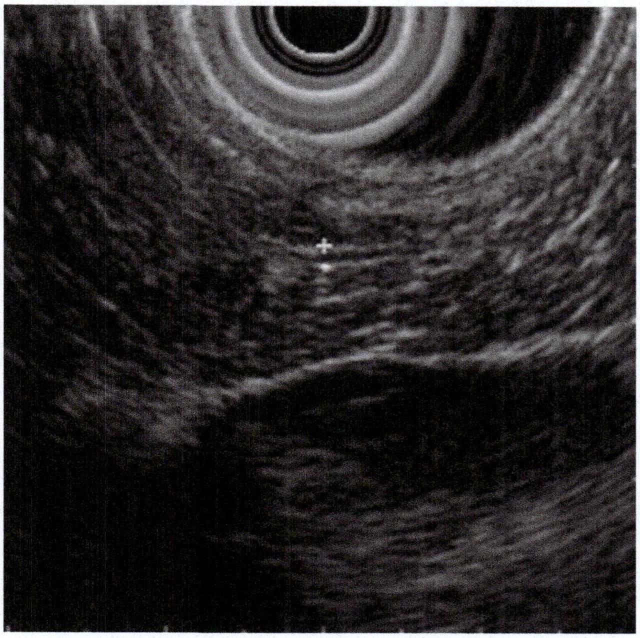

Figure 27.2 Endoscopic ultrasound showing a hyperechoic duct wall (crossmark) in chronic pancreatitis.

Clearly, the number of threshold criteria selected will determine how sensitive and specific the imaging test may be: fewer (<2) threshold criteria are associated with higher sensitivity but lower specificity, and more (<6) are associated with a lower sensitivity and higher specificity. Since these criteria were developed, several studies have been done to define the appropriate threshold criteria. Initial attempts at this defined chronic pancreatitis to be "unlikely" if zero of nine criteria were noted, "likely" if more than five of nine were noted, and "uncertain" if between one and five criteria were noted.

Both comparative and receiver operator curve studies have been done to further define the role of EUS and the number of threshold criteria. Stevens *et al.* compared EUS and ERCP with a threshold of six criteria and found statistical equivalence with ERCP in terms of sensitivity and specificity (68% and 79%, respectively). The authors also considered secretin stimulation pancreatic function testing (SS-PFT). This did not appear to add to the diagnostic accuracy over ERCP and EUS. Furthermore, SS-PFT was felt to be not widely available and potentially inconvenient for patients. Varadarjulu et al. evaluated patients with non-calcific chronic pancreatitis going to surgery and identified more than four EUS criteria as 91% sensitive and 86% specific for the diagnosis. Pungapong et al. identified the combination of EUS and secretin-stimulated magnetic resonance cholangiopancreatography (MRCP) to have a very high sensitivity and specificity at 98% and 100%, respectively. These authors also identified pancreatic juice interleukin-8 levels (after secretin stimulation) to add diagnostic value. Finally, over the last five years, it also has become clear that age and other factors (gender, alcohol use, tobacco, body mass index) may affect the diagnostic threshold and that certain criteria, such as calcifications, may carry greater weight towards a diagnostic end point.

As noted, histopathology remains the diagnostic gold standard for chronic pancreatitis. Unfortunately, this is rarely available outside of surgical or autopsy specimens. Biopsy techniques of the pancreas are limited by the often patchy nature of chronic pancreatitis, safety, availability, and limited tissue acquisition. Linear echoendoscopy provides an opportunity to perform biopsy (fine needle aspiration [FNA] for cytology and core biopsy for histology) of the pancreas using a transgastric or transduodenal technique, and this option has been evaluated for chronic pancreatitis. Hollerbach et al. evaluated EUS-FNA in 27 patients with suspected chronic pancreatitis and found a surprisingly high specificity of 67%. Dewitt et al. evaluated the use of EUS Tru-cut biopsy for core specimen acquisition in 16 patients with chronic pancreatitis. In this study, diagnostic confirmation was achieved in 5.6%. Fourteen of sixteen were either normal or non-diagnostic and one was associated with equipment malfunction. The authors noted a complication frequency of 11%, including acute pancreatitis and pain requiring hospitalization in two patients. The overall kappa value in this study was only 0.25. At this time, the role of EUS-FNA or Tru-cut biopsy remains uncertain and limited by accuracy and technical factors (safety and availability).

EUS imaging in chronic pancreatitis: the Rosemont Criteria

Over the last decade, the true role of EUS for the diagnosis of chronic pancreatitis has been hampered by a number of factors, including interobserver variability, lack of standardization in technique, and nomenclature. There has also been disagreement over the number and appropriate validation of threshold criteria. Furthermore, expense and availability of EUS has limited its impact for routine use in chronic pancreatitis.

In 2007, a group of 37 expert endosonographers from North America and Japan convened in Rosemont, Illinois to review the literature and develop updated diagnostic criteria using EUS for chronic pancreatitis. The group evaluated three areas: parenchymal criteria, ductal criteria, and correlation with histology, and, from these, established an EUS-based diagnostic system. For the first time, attention was also placed on the relative weight of various factors (i.e. major and minor criterion, and rank). Consensus for criteria was established when greater than two-thirds agreement was found. It is important to note that similar to previous classification systems, the criteria were based on radial EUS imaging. This classification system (denoted the "Rosemont Criteria") was formally published in *Gastrointestinal Endoscopy* in 2009.

Table 27.1 The Rosemont Criteria.

Features	Definition	Location	Major criteria	Minor criteria	Rank	Histologic correlate
Parenchymal						
Hyperechoic foci with shadowing	Echogenic structures >2 mm in length and width that shadow	Body, tail	Major A		1	Parenchymal calcifications
Lobularity	Well circumscribed, >5 mm structures with enhancing rim and relatively echo-poor center				2	Unknown
A. With honeycombing	Contiguous >3 lobules	Body, tail	Major B			
B. Without honeycombing	Non-contiguous lobules	Body, tail		Yes		
Hyperechoic foci wthout shadowing	Echogenic structures/foci >2 mm in both length and width without shadowing	Body, tail		Yes	3	Unknown
Cysts	Anechoic round/elliptical structures without septations	Head, body, tail		Yes	4	Pseudocysts
Stranding	Hyperechoic lines >3 mm in length in at least two different directions	Body, tail		Yes	5	Unknown
Ductal						
MPD calculi	With acoustic shadowing	Head, body, tail	Major A		1	Stones
Irregular MPD	Uneven or irregular MPD	Body, tail		Yes	2	Unknown
Dilated side branches	>3 tubular anechoic structures each >1 mm width budding from MPD	Body, tail		Yes	3	Side branch ectasia
MPD dilation	>3.5 mm body, or >1.5 mm tail	Body, tail		Yes	4	MPD dilation
Hyperechoic MPD margin	Echogenic, distinct structure >50% entire MPD	Body, tail		Yes	5	Ductal fibrosis

Source: adapted from Catalano MF, Sahai A, Levy M, et al. EUS-based criteria for the diagnosis of chronic pancreatitis: the Rosemont classification. *Gastrointest Endosc* 2009;69:1251–1261.

The Rosemont Criteria are demonstrated in Table 27.1. Many of the previously described criteria were again found to be important imaging characteristics in diagnosing chronic pancreatitis. Hyperechoic foci with shadowing, cysts, and intraductal calculi were felt to be relevant if found anywhere in the pancreas, whereas all other findings required demonstration in the body and/or tail. After an extensive review of the literature and consensus discussions, the overall kappa for findings in this group of experts was quite good (>0.7). Some of the advantages of the Rosemont Criteria include differential weighting, stricter definitions, and a four-level diagnostic stratification (Table 27.2).

Since the publication of the Rosemont Criteria in 2009, one multicenter comparison study has been reported evaluating standard criteria versus Rosemont Criteria for chronic pancreatitis (Stevens et al.). In this study, 50 video clips (all radial EUS) were evaluated by 14 experts, equally divided into those with extensive experience (>1000 cases) and those with moderate experience (500–999 cases). In this series of clips, 13 had established chronic pancreatitis. The standard criteria threshold was more than four of nine findings. Interestingly, the use of the Rosemont Criteria did not significantly increase interobserver agreement for EUS diagnosis of chronic pancreatitis compared with standard scoring. One

Table 27.2 The Rosemont diagnostic stratification.

Stratum	Criteria
Consistent with chronic pancreatitis	1 major A + >3 minor features 1 major A feature + a major B feature 2 major A features
Suggestive of chronic pancreatitis	1 major A feature + <3 minor features 1 major B feature + >3 minor features >5 minor features
Indeterminate of chronic pancreatitis	3 or 4 minor features, no major features Major B alone or with <3 minor features
Normal	<3 minor features[a], no major features

[a] Except non-shadowing foci, cysts, main pancreas duct dilation, and dilated side branches.

Source: adapted from Catalano MF, Sahai A, Levy M, et al. EUS-based criteria for the diagnosis of chronic pancreatitis: the Rosemont classification. *Gastrointest Endosc* 2009;69:1251–1261.

would therefore conclude that high interobserver agreement is critical for the reliability of any diagnostic test.

The Rosemont Criteria have initiated important steps in the right direction for the EUS diagnosis of chronic pancreatitis – a common nomenclature. Ideally, the system will be further validated in larger patient populations prospectively and against the gold standard of histopathology.

Endoscopic ultrasound imaging in chronic pancreatitis: the future

The utility of EUS as a diagnostic modality for chronic pancreatitis holds great promise. Improvements in imaging quality will continue to evolve. Additional studies are clearly necessary to validate the Rosemont Criteria. Minimally invasive ways of pancreatic tissue acquisition will likely develop and will be an important part of the evaluation of these patients. As with many other complex diseases where tissue acquisition is challenging, multimodal evaluation may be optimal. It is likely that combination evaluation with high-resolution EUS imaging, secretin-stimulated MRCP, and exocrine function testing will provide the most accurate means of morphologic and physiologic assessment.

Chapter video clips

Video 27.1 Chronic pancreatitis.

Video 27.2 Pancreatic duct stones.

28 Liver Pathology

Indraneel Chakrabarty and Ann Marie Joyce
Tufts University School of Medicine and Lahey Clinic Medical Center, Burlington, MA, USA

Introduction

The most common liver pathology seen using endoscopic ultrasonography (EUS) includes cirrhosis, fatty liver, hepatic cysts, and neoplasms. Dilated intrahepatic, extrahepatic, and common bile ducts with or without stones are often seen as well. Endoscopic ultrasonography of the liver can be frustrating as it is often difficult to determine if the liver was viewed in its entirety depending on the patient's body habitus and anatomy. For optimal imaging, the echoendoscope should be set to the lowest possible frequency for maximal hepatic penetration. There are three primary positions for viewing the liver. The duodenal bulb is the best position to evaluate the right lobe of the liver. The balloon over-inflation technique can be used to help lock the scope into the duodenal bulb. From here the scope should be advanced and withdrawn and torqued clockwise and counterclockwise accordingly for maximal views of the right lobe. This should be repeated until the ultrasonographer feels that he or she has viewed the liver to the best of their ability given the patient's size and anatomy. After completion of this exam, the balloon should be deflated and the scope positioned in the antrum. This will give views of both the right and left hepatic lobes. The same technique of torque and advancing the scope forward and backwards should be applied until all views of the liver have been exhausted. The last position is the gastric fundus, which gives optimal views of the left hepatic lobe. It is usually initiated from the gastroesophageal junction using the same techniques as in the latter position until all views are achieved to the ultrasonographer's satisfaction. The endosonographic description of liver pathology is reviewed in this chapter.

Cirrhosis

The two leading causes of cirrhosis in the United States is alcohol abuse followed by hepatitis C. Combined they are the twelfth leading cause of death in the United States as of 2000, accounting for over 25 000 deaths. In addition, approximately 75–85% of acutely infected hepatitis C individuals progress to chronic infection, with up to 20% developing cirrhosis over 20–25 years. Other etiologies include hepatitis B, non-alcoholic steatohepatitis, primary biliary cirrhosis, primary sclerosing cholangitis, autoimmune hepatitis, hereditary hemochromatosis, Wilson's disease, and α_1-antitrypsin deficiency. All patients with cirrhosis are at increased risk of developing hepatocellular carcinoma. In general, cirrhosis is characterized by the replacement of normal hepatic tissue with permanent scar tissue, which leads to disruption of organ function and blocks portal blood flow through hepatic parenchyma leading to the various clinical features of cirrhosis. This scar tissue can often be visualized under EUS as nodular tissue characterized by coarse, diffuse, heterogeneous, echoic parenchyma (Figure 28.1a). The outer wall of the liver often loses its smooth border and can appear irregular or nodular (Figure 28.1b). One of the complications related to cirrhosis is ascites. Ascites can be seen as anechoic areas adjacent to intra-abdominal organs (Figure 28.1c). A sample of the fluid can be obtained through a fine needle aspiration (FNA).

Fatty liver disease

Fatty liver disease (FLD) is an accumulation of large vacuoles of triglyceride or fat within the hepatic parenchyma via the

Atlas of Endoscopic Ultrasonography, Second Edition. Edited by Frank Gress, Thomas Savides, Brenna Casey, and Everson L. A. Artifon.

Companion website: www.wiley.com/go/gress/atlas

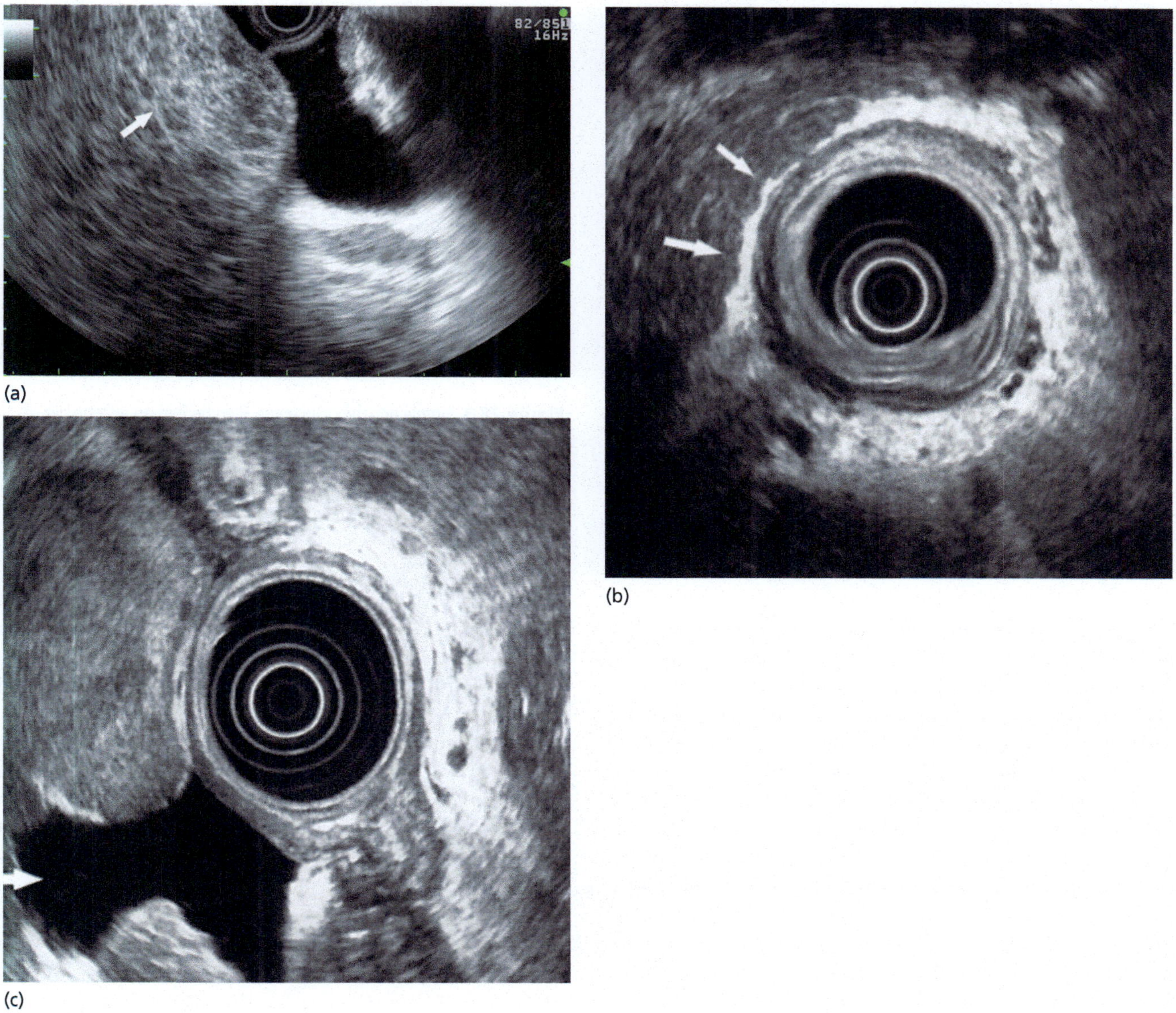

Figure 28.1 (a) Cirrhosis. The cirrhotic liver is characterized by diffuse, coarse, nodular, heterogeneous, echoic parenchyma (arrow). (b) Cirrhosis with nodular surface. The smooth border of the liver is often lost in cirrhotics and can appear irregular or nodular (arrows). (c) Cirrhosis with ascites. Ascites is often seen in cirrhotics as anechoic regions surrounding intra-abdominal organs (arrow).

process of steatosis and is normally reversible. This deposition can often be seen via EUS and is described as hyperechoic or bright parenchyma secondary to fat deposition when compared to normal parenchyma (Figure 28.2). It is usually diffuse but can also be seen in patches as in foci of hyperechoic parenchyma surrounded by normal echoic parenchyma. There are multiple causes for fatty liver, the most common being alcohol abuse (alcoholic fatty liver disease or AFLD) and non-alcoholic fatty liver disease (NAFLD) such as from obesity with or without diabetes. Consequently, FLD is very common in the United States, and it can be difficult to distinguish between AFLD and NAFLD without a proper history. Chronic AFLD is the precursor to developing cirrhosis; however, a small percentage of individuals with NAFLD can also progress to cirrhosis.

Hepatic cysts

Hepatic cysts are fluid-filled spaces found within the hepatic parenchyma. There are three main types of hepatic cysts: hydatid cysts, fibrocystic disease of the liver, and solitary

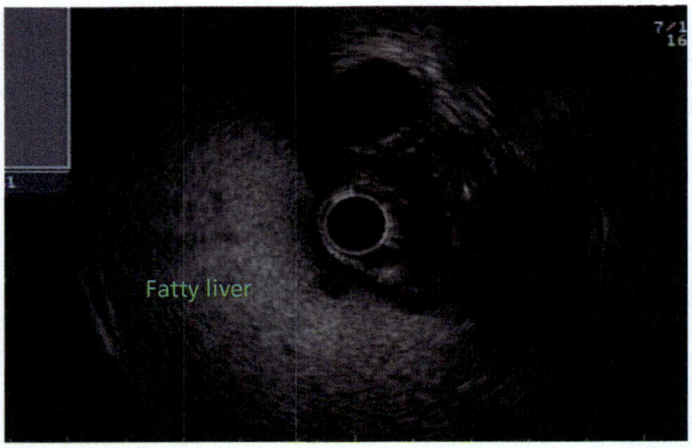

Figure 28.2 Fatty liver is described as diffuse or as foci of hyperechoic or bright parenchyma secondary to fat deposition when compared to normal parenchyma.

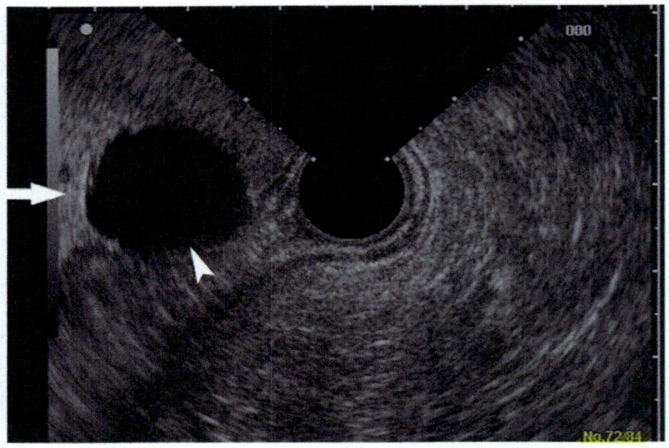

Figure 28.3 Simple hepatic cyst can be seen here as an anechoic fluid-filled structure within the hepatic parenchyma (arrowhead), which demonstrates through transmission beyond the cyst relative to the probe (arrow).

congenital cysts or simple hepatic cysts. Hydatid cysts are caused by various parasitic infections, are often numerous, and often accompanied by right upper quadrant abdominal pain and fever. Fibrocystic disease is a group of rare conditions that result in abnormal remodeling of the ductal plate that give rise to multiple cystic formations within the liver, most commonly seen in polycystic liver disease and often associated with polycystic kidney disease. Simple hepatic cysts are congenital in origin, benign, occur in little over 3% of the population, occur more frequently in women, and are generally less than 5 cm in diameter. They are usually asymptomatic and are often found incidentally. Under endosonography, they are described as anechoic fluid-filled structures within the hepatic parenchyma and normally demonstrate through transmission beyond the cyst relative to the probe. Through transmission is increased enhancement beyond a fluid-filled structure because the intensity of the transmitted ultrasound undergoes less attenuation as it propagates through the cyst and as the reflected signal returns to the transducer. Observing through transmission is helpful in diagnosing whether an anechoic structure is a cyst (Figure 28.3). Doppler endosonography may be necessary to exclude a vessel.

Neoplasms

Malignancy involving the liver is either due to primary liver cancer or secondary to metastatic liver disease. The most common form of primary liver cancer in adults is hepatocellular carcinoma and is the fifth most common cancer in men, eighth in women, and ranks fourth in annual cancer mortality rates. Cholangiocarcinoma is rarer accounting for only 7% of liver tumors in the United States. Even rarer is fibrolamellar hepatocellular carcinoma, accounting for only 0.85% of all primary liver cancers. However, metastatic liver disease is more common than primary liver cancer and is mostly associated with pancreatic, colon, breast, lung, and other cancers that originate from the gastrointestinal tract. The endosonographic findings of metastatic liver disease are similar to those of hepatocellular carcinoma. They are often described as a lesion within the hepatic parenchyma with an outer hypoechoic border and a heterogeneous echogenic center (Figure 28.4a,b). This hypoechoic border is normally referred to as acoustic shadowing, which occurs secondary to refraction from the interface between normal tissue and neoplasm. Hepatic metastases are generally echo-poor and without a distinct border (Figure 28.4a). In addition, hypoechoic to anechoic regions within a tumor could also represent necrosis. Suspicious lesions in the liver can be aspirated using EUS (Figure 28.4b) for diagnostic purposes.

Cavernous hemangiomas are the most common benign tumors of the liver and are thought to be a congenital malformation or a hamartoma that increases in size as the liver grows from birth. Cavernous hemangiomas can be difficult to diagnosis with ultrasonography as the appearance is quite variable and nonspecific by ultrasound. They can appear as irregular echogenic to hypoechoic lesions surrounded by normal hepatic parenchyma (Figure 28.4c). A computed tomography (CT) scan confirmed this lesion as a hemangioma.

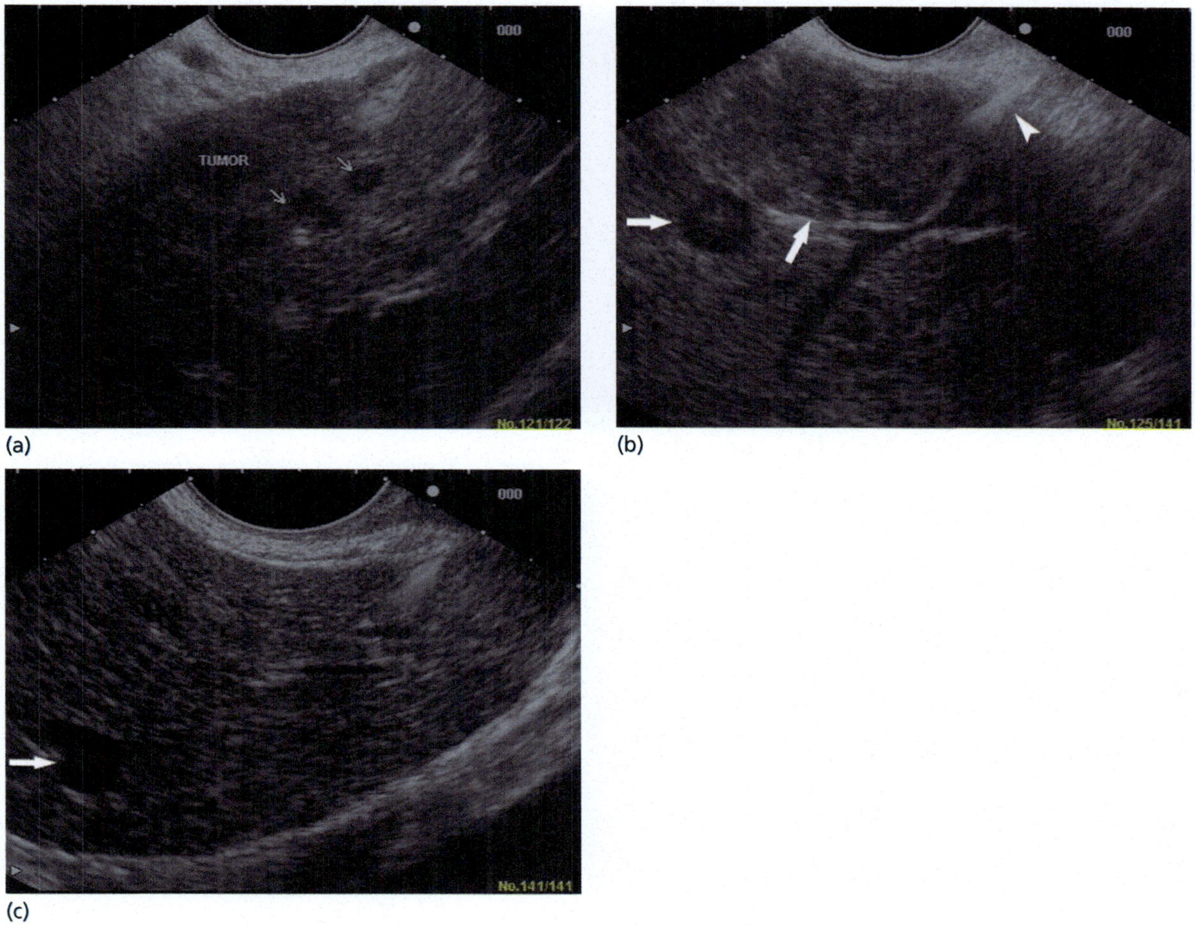

Figure 28.4 (a, b) Metastatic liver disease. Lesions found within the hepatic parenchyma with an outer hypoechoic border and a heterogeneous echogenic center demonstrating acoustic shadowing (arrows). An FNA needle can be seen in (b) (arrowhead). (c) Cavernous hemangioma. An irregular hypoechoic lesion seen within the hepatic parenchyma (arrow). Note the lack of through transmission. A CT scan confirmed this lesion as a hemangioma.

Dilated intrahepatic ducts

Dilated intrahepatic ducts can also be seen on endosonography. There are numerous causes for dilated intrahepatic ducts, ranging from a distal obstruction secondary to stones or from strictures secondary to anastomotic stricture post liver transplant, primary sclerosing cholangitis, to cancers such as cholangiocarcinoma. Smaller intrahepatic ducts eventually give rise to the main left and right hilar intrahepatic ducts, which are normally 1.0–1.5 mm in diameter. These eventually become the left and right hilar external hepatic ducts, which eventually merge to form the common hepatic duct that flows into the common bile duct. Extrahepatic ducts are discussed in more detail in Chapter 2. Thus, dilated hilar intrahepatic ducts larger than 1.5 mm (Figure 28.5) may be concerning for a pathological process in the right clinical setting and should be worked up.

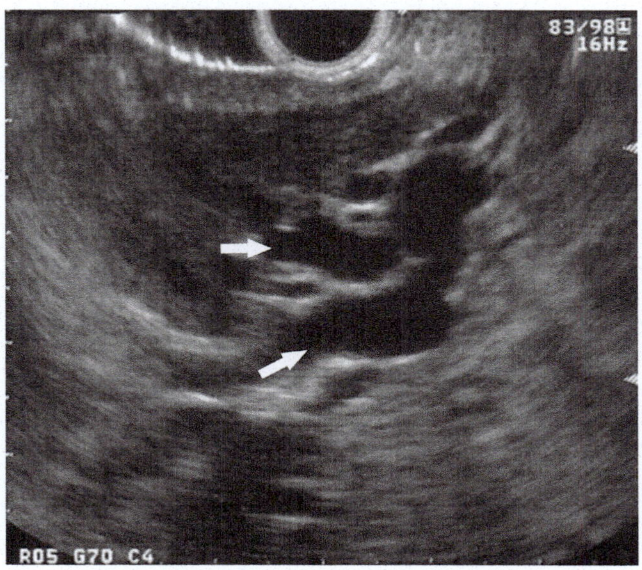

Figure 28.5 Dilated intrahepatic ducts (arrows) are visualized here and are more than 1.5 mm in diameter.

4 How to Section

29 How to Interpret EUS-FNA Cytology

Cynthia Behling
Pacific Rim Pathology Group, Sharp Memorial Hospital, San Diego, CA, USA

Introduction

Endoscopic ultrasound (EUS) is an ideal method for obtaining tissue from submucosal lesions in the gastrointestinal tract or from organs near the gastrointestinal tract. A pathologic interpretation of the tissue biopsy in addition to the EUS characteristics helps to accurately determine the nature of the lesion. The pathologist represents an important member of the patient care team, since microscopic evaluation is key in determining the nature of the sampled lesion. This chapter illustrates some common lesions as well as technical issues. The chapter is divided into three sections which relate pathology and EUS: the technical quality of the material; the quality of interpretation; and the integration of pathologic and clinical information. The goal of the pathologist is to contribute to a successful EUS service by providing accurate and precise diagnostic information.

Although EUS-guided sampling is a relatively newer way of obtaining tissue, the means of preparing the cells or tissue, obtained from endoscopic ultrasound-guided fine needle aspiration (EUS-FNA), referred to in general as a "biopsy," are well-developed and standardized procedures in most cytology/anatomic pathology laboratories. In this chapter, the term "biopsy" refers to any tissue sample obtained via EUS guidance. A "biopsy" could be an FNA, representing cells obtained through a small needle and dispersed onto slides, or a core, representing an intact piece of tissue. The advantages and disadvantages of each type of biopsy are discussed later.

Technical quality of EUS biopsy material

There are a number of techniques and strategies which can optimize the technical quality of EUS biopsy material.

Personnel

Before developing an EUS service, it is important to involve a pathologist or cytotechnologist in planning for specimen handling. Selection of biopsy type and other procedures depends on the personnel and laboratory resources available. Use of a liquid-based cytologic preparation such as ThinPrep™ or SurePath™, direct smears, core biopsy, or some combination of these methods depends on the lesion, pathologist and endoscopist preference, staffing, location of the endoscopy suite in relation to the laboratory, and the relative sensitivity, specificity, and diagnostic accuracy of the various technical choices.

Personnel issues are key in planning for the actual EUS service. For example, at some institutions, the laboratory is physically close to the endoscopy suite and a laboratory technologist travels to the site to prepare aspirate smears, while in other practices the gastrointestinal endoscopy staff are trained to make slides. If laboratory personnel will help prepare specimens, the scheduling of procedures should be done in consideration of the laboratory schedule and any ancillary tests such as flow cytometry, which might require special processing.

Biopsy type: aspirate or core

There are two ways of obtaining biopsy material from a lesion. One is to cut out a small piece of the lesion with a cutting needle and the other to aspirate individual cells and small fragments of tissue. Core biopsies provide tissue architecture, that is, the relationship of the lesional cells and their surrounding stroma are maintained. In core biopsies, vascular and duct structures usually remain intact (Figure 29.1a). In an aspirate sample, the cells are dispersed and evaluated primarily for their individual characteristics, although some microarchitecture remains (Figure 29.1b).

Hematoxylin and eosin (H&E)-stained 3–5-µm sections are cut from tissue obtained with a core biopsy, and are typically

Atlas of Endoscopic Ultrasonography, Second Edition. Edited by Frank Gress, Thomas Savides, Brenna Casey, and Everson L. A. Artifon.

Companion website: www.wiley.com/go/gress/atlas

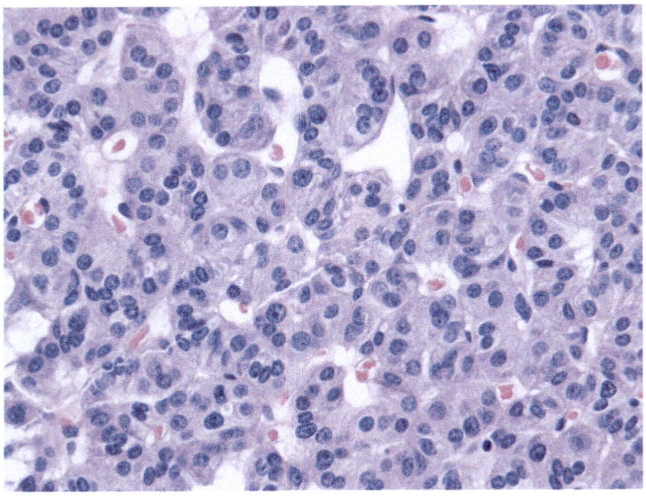

(ai)

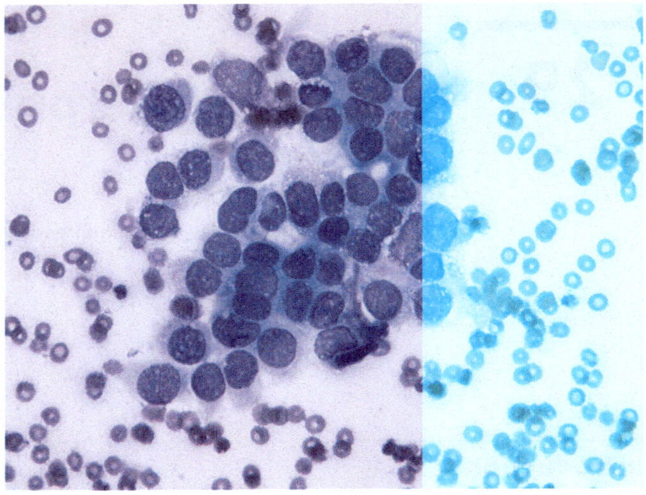

(bi)

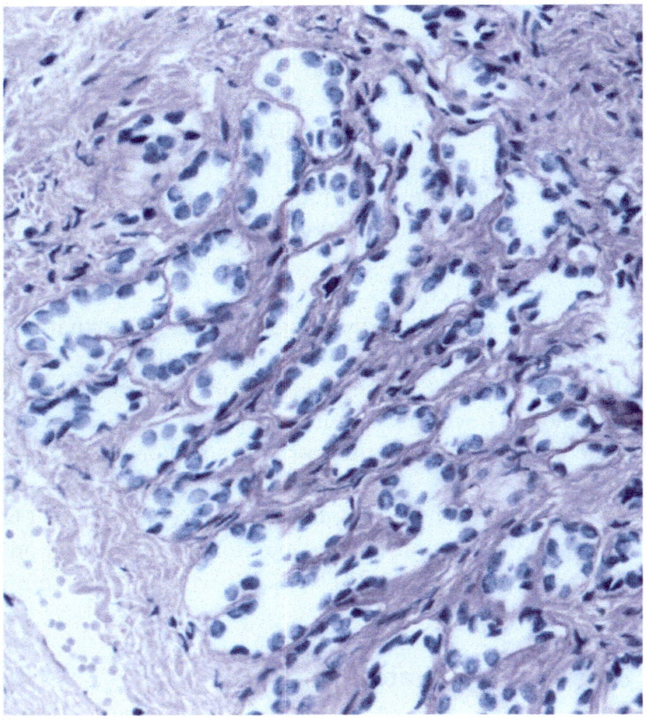

(aii)

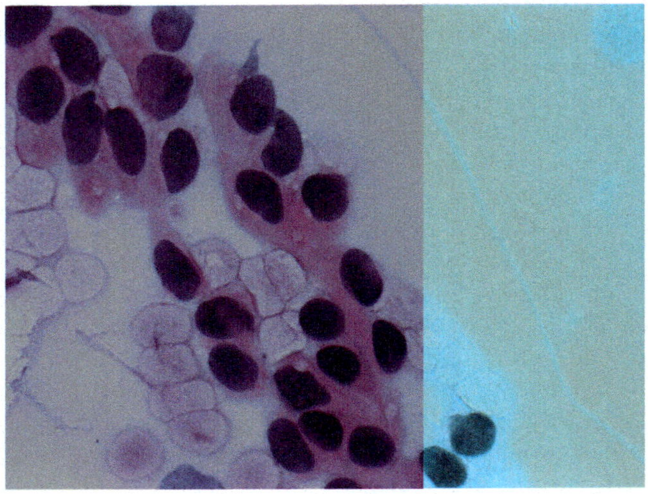

(bii)

Figure 29.1 (a) Core biopsies demonstrate intact tissue architecture and structures such as ducts, vessels, and stromal relationships. (ai) Pancreatic neuroendocrine tumor showing fine vascular structures and rosette formation. (aii) Diastase digested PAS stain of a serous cystadenoma of the pancreas showing small cysts in a fibrous stroma. (b) The dispersed preparation of cells from a fine needle aspirate allow evaluation of individual nuclear and cytoplasmic features as well as microarchitecture. (bi) Pancreatic neuroendocrine tumor cells have finely dispersed chromatin, small nucleoli, and little cytoplasm. (bii) Fine needle aspirates from serous tumors usually contain few cells with oval nuclei arranged in small glandular structures.

fixed in formalin, processed, and embedded in a paraffin block. The procedure is essentially identical to the way in which mucosal biopsies from the gastrointestinal tract are processed. These are the familiar blue and pink, hematoxylin and eosin slides with which all pathologists and gastroenterologists are familiar. For FNA, biopsies are dropped onto a glass slide and then dispersed as a monolayer by drawing a second slide over the fluid drop.

An aspirate biopsy is usually obtained with a "fine" needle, which is 22 gauge or smaller. In this type of biopsy, the material flows or is actively aspirated into the needle and then dispersed onto a slide or placed directly into a preservative or fixative for processing. Smears are prepared in a manner similar to that used in making blood smears. A small drop of the aspirate is placed on one end of the slides and then carefully pulled along the slide to make a dispersed layer of individual

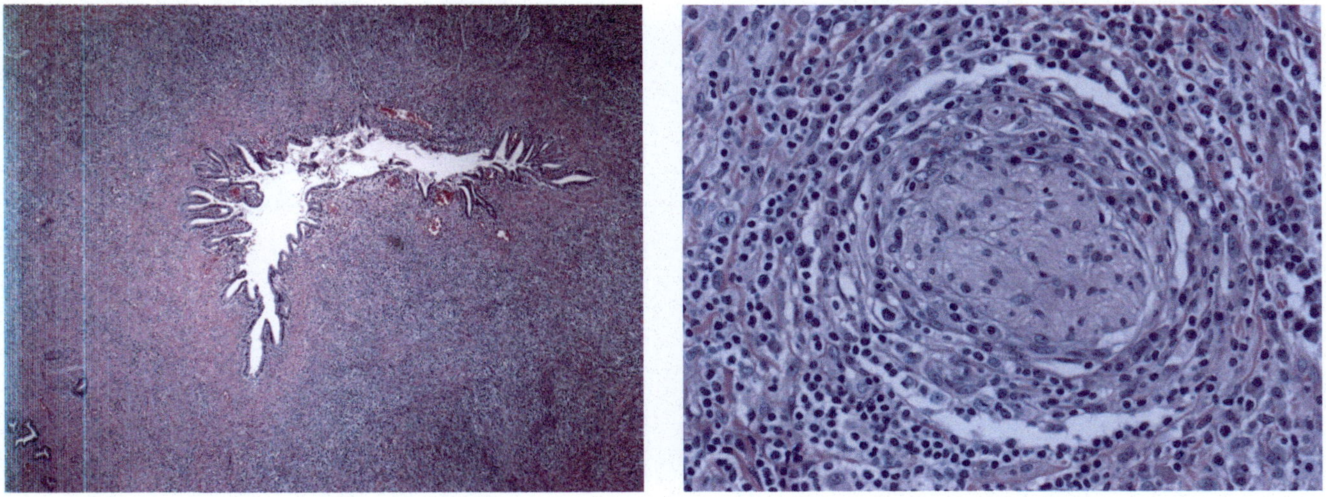

(a) (b)

Figure 29.2 Diagnostic features of autoimmune pancreatitis rely on the demonstration of duct centric inflammation (a), and a dense plasmacytic infiltrate, often surrounding nerves (b).

and small groups of cells. The features of the cells appear somewhat different in smears than in tissue sections and also depend on the type of smear preparation and staining. In many pathology laboratories, aspirate smears are prepared as both air-dried and alcohol-fixed smears.

Different criteria are used in interpreting tissue sections and cytology smears. In the tissue sections evaluable features include formation of structures such as glands, invasion of stroma or nerves, inflammatory changes in duct structures, and many others (Figure 29.2). Preservation of the architecture allows observation of features such as the shape of glands, quality of the surrounding stroma, and the presence of vasculitis. Aspirate smears rely on visualization of nuclear and chromatinic detail, nuclear membrane contour, and cytoplasmic quality (Figure 29.3), emphasizing features of individual cells.

Endoscopic ultrasound-guided sampling lends itself to either aspiration or acquisition of a tissue core (with few exceptions). In some procedures both types of biopsy are obtained, in order to capitalize on the advantages of both preparations. However, for some diseases such as autoimmune pancreatitis or lymphoma, diagnostic criteria may be dependent on features of intact tissue.

Core biopsy tissue remaining in the paraffin block after the initial sections are taken can be used for special stains. Special stains are not limited to tissue biopsies; however, since a portion of the aspirated material from each needle pass can be aliquoted into cell culture media such as RPMI or into a preservative and the sample centrifuged and the pellet processed, embedded, and sectioned. This cell block made from aspirated material can be similarly used for ancillary studies (Figure 29.4).

While examination of tissue sections is the core practice of pathologists, not all pathologists practice cytopathology and, in general, more pathologists are comfortable interpreting tissue sections. For this reason and others, some believe that a tissue core is a better choice. The issue of core versus aspirate can be debated, although the two methods are complementary. Various strategies of "dual sampling" or sequential sampling, that is, using FNA when the core is macroscopically inadequate, have been examined. For some situations, such as autoimmune pancreatitis, a core biopsy may provide better diagnostic material. The tissue architecture of a core biopsy may be useful for traditional diagnostic criteria for lymphomas, and can help distinguish invasive and in situ malignancies or very well differentiated malignancies such as some pancreatic carcinomas. In addition, core biopsy may require fewer needle passes for diagnostic material. Endoscopic ultrasound-guided core biopsies are a recent technical development and have not been studied as completely as EUS-FNA, so the true diagnostic accuracy remains to be determined.

A potential advantage of core biopsy is that tissue remains in the paraffin block and is available for special stains or other studies as needed. Core biopsy may lead to a more confident benign diagnosis when used in combination with FNA for mediastinal lesions but may be less sensitive in pancreas.

Potential disadvantages to core biopsy include more tissue damage. Deployment of a Tru-cut or other needle for core biopsy may also depend on the characteristics and location of the lesion as well as clinical and imaging differential diagnosis.

Cell block

Preparation of a cell block from aspirate material can preserve material for special studies in a manner similar to a core biopsy. A cell block is made by placing the aspirate in a

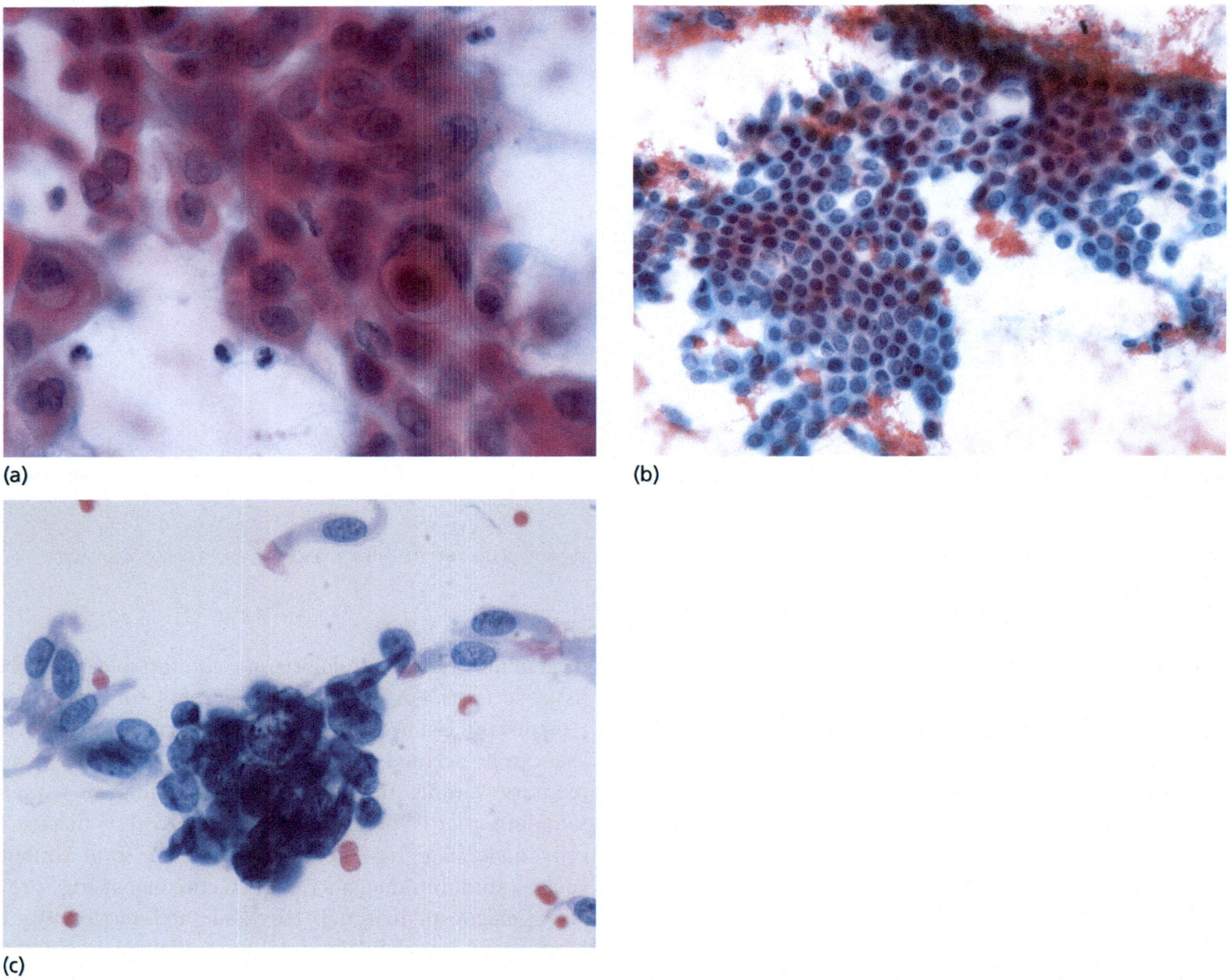

Figure 29.3 Aspirate smears demonstrate fine cellular detail such as squamous differentiation (a), uniform sheets of epithelium with goblet cells from the duodenum (b), or nuclear molding in a small cell carcinoma (c).

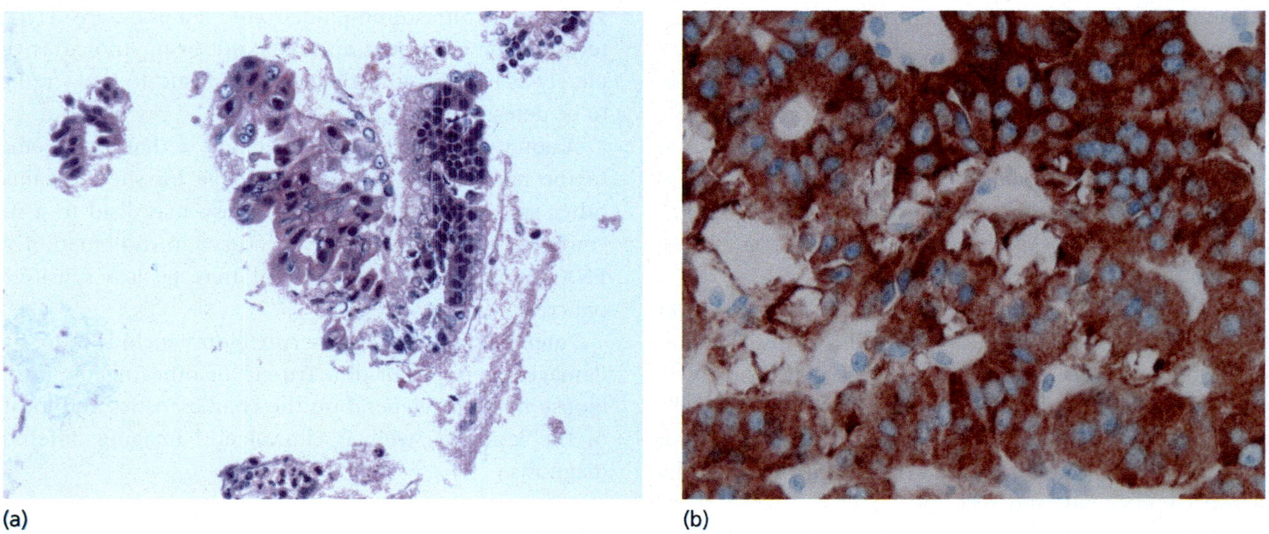

Figure 29.4 Cell blocks, prepared from fine needle aspirate material and placed in liquid-based cytology media or RPMI, can be used for both pathologic interpretation and special stains. (a) Atypical tufting, hyperplastic epithelium (*left*) adjacent to benign ductal epithelium (*right*). (b) Neuroendocrine staining of an islet cell tumor.

preservative media such as RPMI, centrifuging the media to create a cell pellet, and then fixing the cells in formalin and processing the pellet as a tissue biopsy.

A cell block has some but not all the attributes of a biopsy. While the sections may seem more familiar to pathologists, formalin fixation and paraffin embedding is not optimal for preserving cytologic detail and cell block is not usually a "stand-alone" preparation. Cell blocks are however useful as a repository of lesional tissue on which special stains can be performed.

Technical aspects of the needle can influence the quality of the biopsy. Smaller needle sizes (such as 25 gauge) yield adequate numbers of cells. Larger biopsies (22 gauge) may increase the number of cells but at the expense of tissue trauma and bleeding. In general, minimal heparinization of the needle before passes reduces clotting of the material (Figure 29.5).

At some institutions a cell block is made from leftover material rinsed from the needle and may not contain cells from the lesion. One way to ensure that the cell block contains useful material is to aliquot drops of material to the cell block media at the same time the slides are made. This procedure is discussed below.

A new method is that of brush cytology performed through the FNA needle. In a preliminary study, this method showed promise for cystic pancreatic lesions because it yielded more cellular specimens, but will require more testing and validation.

Ideal aspirate smears are thin, well dispersed, and do not have large clotted material or clumps. Also ideal is the preparation of both air-dried and alcohol-fixed slides, since the former lend themselves to quick modified Romanowsky stains such as Diff-Quik™ for immediate cytologic evaluation, the exaggeration of any nuclear pleomorphism, and help identify intracellular or extracellular mucin, while the latter (alcohol-fixed) allow evaluation of nuclear detail, chromatin quality, and keratinization of cells (Figure 29.6).

Needle size

Needle size for core biopsy is limited by compatibility with the endoscope. Needle size for aspirate is also limited by availability, but the choice of needle size can influence the cytology preparation. Needles as small as 25 gauge have been shown to produce adequate numbers of cells for diagnosis. Furthermore, small needle sizes theoretically produce less tissue injury and less bleeding, decreasing the risk that diagnostic cells will be obscured by blood.

Smaller needle size may also be beneficial in patients with coagulopathy to reduce the risk of bleeding in organs where air or fluid leak may occur or in organs where tissue trauma could increase complications. Larger-gauge needles can be

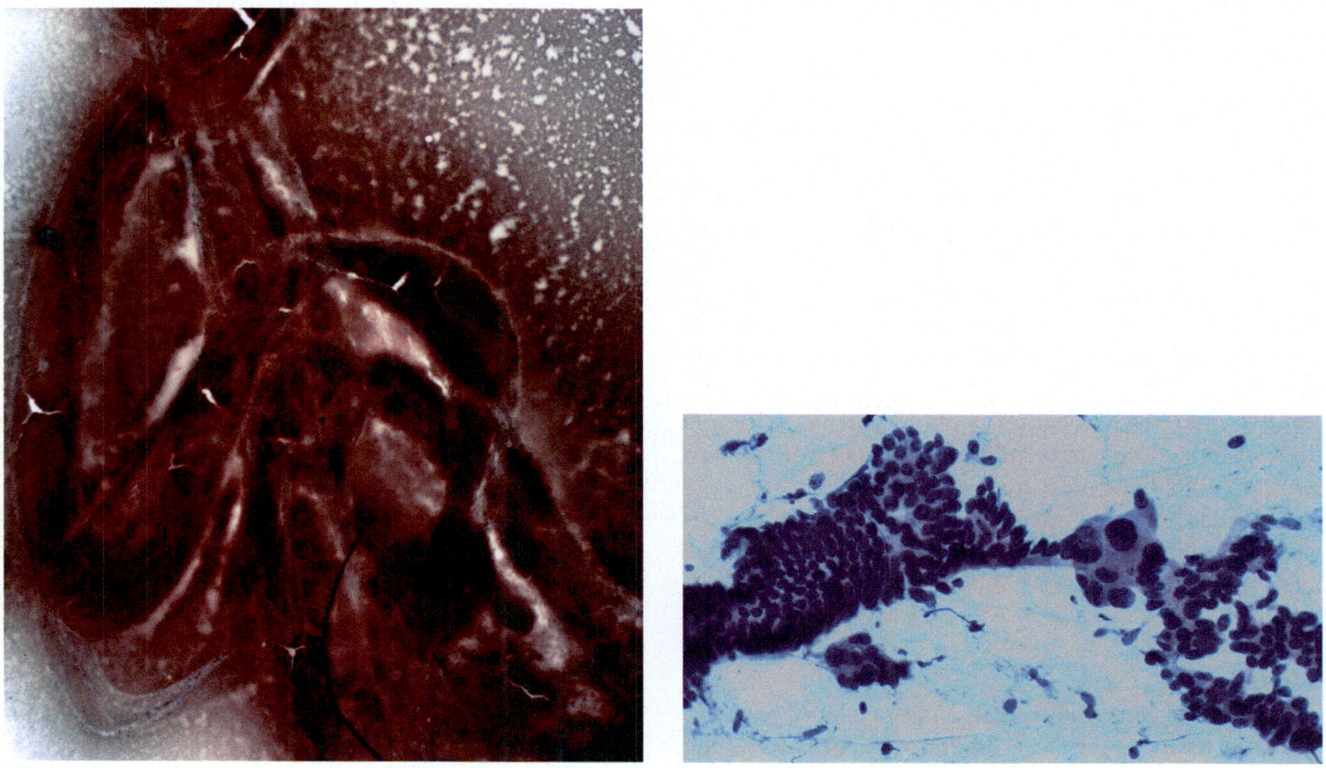

(a) (b)

Figure 29.5 Clotted blood within the needle obscures lesional tissue (a). Optimally heparinized aspirates allow lesional cells to distribute themselves on the slide as an easily visualized monolayer (b).

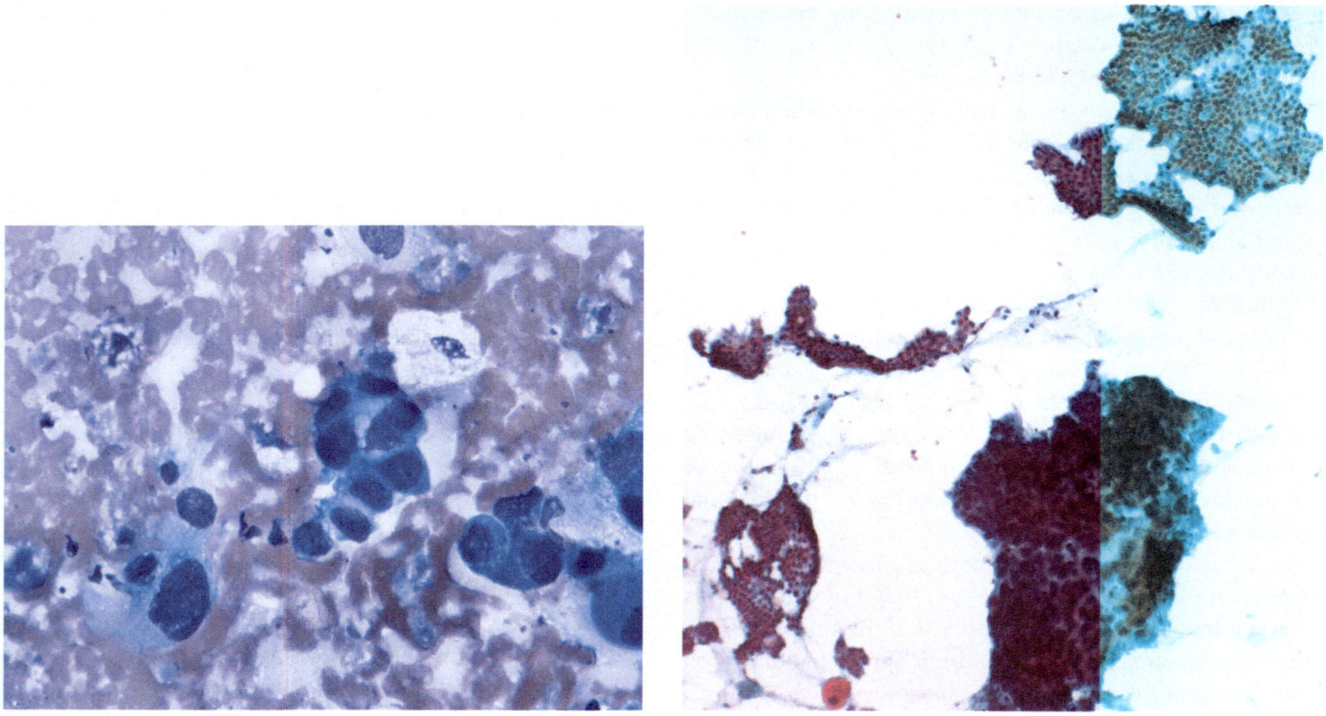

(a) (b)

Figure 29.6 Air-dried slides stained with a modified Romanowsky stain demonstrate cellular pleomorphism as in this pancreatic adenocarcinoma (a). Squamous differentiation, also from a pancreatic tumor, is highlighted by the bright orange staining of keratin by a Papanicolaou (Pap) stain (b).

used where a larger volume of cells is needed such as a work-up for lymphoma.

Needle preparation

Heparin may be used in aspirate procedures to decrease clot formation in the needle lumen. Typically, the stylet is completely removed from the needle and then the needle flushed with heparin. Air is then flushed through the needle to expel the excess heparin. The stylet is then replaced and the needle is ready for use. Use of heparin may have particular application to EUS aspirates in which the needle is extremely long. Clotting can interfere with the preparation of aspirate smears and lead to artifacts such as the clumping of cells. However, too much heparin can also distort the cells, and thus flushing excess heparin from the needle with air is a necessary step in the procedure.

If clots do form, the material trapped inside can be salvaged by gentle microdissection or by scraping the clotted material from the slide and placing it in media for the cell block.

Suction

Application of suction during fine needle biopsy serves to hold the tissue against the cutting edge of the needle. This may increase the number of cells that are sampled for some lesions. Before withdrawing the needle, however, suction should be released to prevent the air-drying of cells when air rushes into the needle as it is removed, and also to prevent the theoretical risk of contamination of the needle tract. However, not all studies document an increased diagnostic yield when suction is used, and, for vascular organs, use of suction may increase blood contamination of the specimen. In addition to increasing the blood in a specimen, suction can induce cytologic artifact. However, this is rarely a problem in practice and, in general, fewer insufficient specimens are obtained when suction is used.

Slide preparation and staining

Technical aspects of slide preparation can influence specimen quality and ultimately adequacy. The manner in which material is expressed onto the slide helps ensure optimal slide preparations. A trained technical assistant (nurse, laboratory technician, or other person) holds the tip of the catheter needle over the end of a labeled glass slide while the needle is advanced approximately 1 cm from the catheter by another assistant (often the endoscopy technician). The stylet is slowly advanced into the needle. This causes a very controlled passage of single drops of material out of the tip. Alternate drops of the material are placed on a slide and into RPMI-1640 medium. The optimal distribution of the material for both cell block and smears is ensured by this technique but it requires a very controlled expulsion of the material from the needle to avoid large "globs" of material on the slides. If there is too much material on a slide, the diagnostic cells could be obscured or, worse, drip off the slide. After several slides are prepared the remaining material is placed into media for cell block. After all the slides are prepared the remaining material is rinsed from the needle with a few milliliters of saline and then air to expel any remaining material into the RPMI. RPMI-1640 is a cell culture medium that is used as a transport medium to preserve the cells until they are made into a cell block or sent for flow cytometry or other special study.

Usually between two and six slides are prepared from each pass, depending on the amount of material obtained. More than six slides usually add little to the diagnostic yield and make the cytotechnologist and pathologist unhappy, since screening and then reviewing many slides containing only one or two cells of interest is quite time-consuming and inefficient.

After the material is placed onto the slides, the drops of aspirated material are quickly spread downward onto the slides using another clean glass slide. This method is identical to that used to prepare a blood smear and requires practice. Too much pressure destroys the cells, while too little causes the cells to remain clumped or be obscured by blood or mucus. Ideally, half of the slides are air-dried and the remainder immediately immersed in 95% ethyl alcohol for later Papanicolaou (Pap) staining. The air-dried slides can be stained with a Diff-Quik stain for immediate cytologic evaluation by the pathologist, if available. Immediate cytologic evaluation is discussed below. When the procedure is finished, the alcohol-fixed slides and RPMI-cell suspension are transported to the laboratory for standard Pap staining and cell block preparation respectively. To prepare a cell block, thrombin is added to the material in RPMI and the mixture centrifuged into a pellet. The pellet is resuspended and then the resulting clot removed, wrapped in lens paper, placed in a tissue cassette, fixed in formalin, and routinely processed for paraffin embedding and H&E or immunostaining. If indicated, material for flow cytometric immunophenotyping or other studies is removed from the RPMI before adding the thrombin.

Although preparing both air-dried and alcohol-fixed slides may seem like extra work, the two preparations are complementary and are used to demonstrate different cytologic features of lesions. Air-dried smears are stained using a modified Romanowsky stain, such as Diff-Quik. As the cells dry, they spread over the glass and there is an exaggeration of pleomorphism if present. Air-dried smears also highlight intracytoplasmic material, and extracellular substances such as mucin. Air-dried, Diff-Quik-stained smears are also ideal for evaluating lymphoid lesions.

Alcohol fixation preserves nuclear features. Alcohol-fixed slides can be stained with H&E or Pap stains. The Pap stain highlights nuclear detail, chromatin quality and, if present, keratinization of squamous cells.

Liquid-based preparations

Liquid-based cytology is becoming a standard means of preparing many cytology samples, and has been especially successful in gynecologic practice. Its use for other samples, including those derived from EUS-FNA, is increasing. In this method, the sample is placed into a proprietary fixative and slides prepared by an automated process. The automated sampling and slide preparation is designed to minimize technical problems associated with manual preparation of smears. Two methods are US Food and Drug Administration (FDA) approved. The first is produced by Cytyc Co., Marlborough, MA (ThinPrep™) and the second by TriPath Inc., Burlington, NC (SurePath™). The advantages of a liquid-based preparation are the very consistent and high-quality preservation of the cells and improved screening, since the cells are dispersed in a monolayer and are confined to a smaller area of the slide than conventional smears. Another advantage is the decreased technical effort involved in slide preparation. Smears do not have to be made at the time of aspiration, rather the material from the aspirate can be entirely placed into the fixative and transported to the laboratory. This method is especially appealing if the laboratory or the pathologist is located at a distance from the endoscopy suite.

However, liquid-based cytology is more expensive due to the use of proprietary media for fixation, and the method causes some alterations in cytologic detail that need to be considered in interpretation. For example, the procedure decreases the mucin in a specimen. Although for some specimens this is a desirable effect, mucin can be a helpful background feature in the interpretation of mucinous pancreatic neoplasms. The liquid-based preparation techniques may also cause disaggregation of cells and cause loss of microarchitecture. Finally, because the fixative is alcohol based, there may be some degradation of antigens, making immunohistochemistry less reliable.

Interpretation of the cells which are obtained by EUS-FNA or core biopsy procedures is made by a pathologist. Some cytology specimens are first screened by a cytotechnologist and then reviewed by a pathologist. A persistent and known pitfall of interpretation of the aspiration specimens is the frequent presence of contaminating cells from the tubular gastrointestinal tract. An easy distinction is not always possible but awareness of the issues should help in interpretation.

Quality of the interpretation

Pathologists are becoming more familiar with EUS-obtained material; however, most have limited experience with these specimens. Fortunately, there are a number of courses pertaining to EUS-FNA which can serve to educate pathologist or endoscopist about pathology issues.

Just as the endoscopist's ability to perform EUS-FNA rises on a steep learning curve, so does the pathologist's ability to interpret the material obtained via EUS biopsy. Endoscopic ultrasound-guided biopsies provide access to material organs and tissues which were previously uncommonly sampled, and therefore the pathologist may have little experience in interpreting these specimens. There are some peculiarities of samples obtained via EUS, such as "noise" or contaminating cells from the digestive system which need to be distinguished from lesional cells.

Characteristic features of all the possible lesions in the organs amenable to sampling by EUS-guided biopsy is beyond the scope of this chapter, but a few of the distinctive or commonly sampled lesions are illustrated (Figure 29.7). Review of cytologic diagnosis of mediastinal lymph nodes obtained from EUS-FNA shows good reproducibility between pathologists. Performance is better for pathologists with more experience.

At centers with experience, false-negative and false-positive diagnoses are rare. In general, a false-negative result occurs when the lesion is not sampled, while false-positive results are due to the pathologist's interpretive error or contamination of the extraluminal aspirate with luminal tumor. Adherence to criteria for diagnosis of malignancy and basic cytologic principles can minimize the possibility of false-positive diagnoses, although in published studies false-positive diagnoses are minimal.

Integration of pathologic and clinical information

Rapid cytologic evaluation

In an ideal situation, a rapid cytologic evaluation is performed during the procedure to assess the adequacy of each pass and to determine if other studies are needed. During immediate cytologic evaluation, a pathologist microscopically examines the air-dried Diff-Quik stained slides prepared at the site. If the material is adequate for diagnosis, then the procedure is stopped. If there is necrosis or no material, then the endoscopist can redirect the needle to another part of the lesion. The goal of rapid evaluation is to optimize the procedure by reducing the number of unsatisfactory or atypical diagnoses as well as reduce the overall number of passes. Rapid evaluation may provide a preliminary diagnosis and reduces the number of false-negative procedures due to inadequate sampling.

The literature supports a role for rapid evaluation in optimizing EUS-FNA; however, the practice is variable among institutions. Although rapid evaluation improves diagnostic yield, some pathologists are reluctant to provide rapid evaluation due to inadequate reimbursement for the increased amount of pathologist time. On an institutional level, however, there may be significant cost savings by reducing the number of repeat procedures due to inadequate specimens. Ways to minimize cost include calling the pathologist after several passes have been prepared instead of having them present for the whole procedure, using a cytotechnologist to assess adequacy instead of a pathologist, having the slides transported to the pathologist in real time, or making a gross assessment of the slides without microscopic evaluation.

The ability to redirect the needle during an EUS procedure is one of the chief advantages of FNA with rapid evaluation over a single needle core. The real-time image of EUS-FNA allows the needle to be placed directly in the tissue of interest. For some tumors, it may be useful to target the edge of the lesion in order to avoid a necrotic center, while for other lesions the center may have a better yield of tumor cells. For example, an aspirate at the edge of a pancreatic cancer may yield only chronic pancreatitis. While precise direction of the needle is not always necessary, a thoughtful approach coupled with rapid interpretation may increase yield in difficult lesions.

Role of the laboratory in EUS

It is important for the pathologist to understand that, in many instances, the EUS procedure is intended to be a diagnostic test rather than a screening test.

Education of the pathologist and laboratory about the direct role they play in the EUS procedure and the patient care algorithm will help ensure the success of the EUS biopsy service. The indications for the procedure and pertinent clinical and imaging details for each patient should be discussed. It is important to know if the procedure is performed for screening, diagnosis, or to obtain material for culture or flow cytometry of genetic testing.

Archiving of slides and reports, and the creation of a database containing pathology and EUS information should be considered as part of a quality assurance and competency program. Records of clinical information, EUS features of a lesion, diagnosis, and other data can allow assessment of individual practitioner competency (endosonographer and pathologist), diagnostic accuracy of the service, and the utility of various techniques such as immediate cytologic evaluation.

Pathologists and their staff should understand the limitations of EUS biopsy, know the technical aspects of their part of the process, and be well trained. Laboratory services in the United States are regulated at state and national levels by the Clinical Laboratory Improvement Amendments of 1988 (CLIA'88), the Laboratory Accreditation Program of the College of American Pathologists (CAP), and others. A high-quality laboratory provides the best possible service to the patient. Specific details of practice guidelines and other standards are available from the College of American Pathologists and the American Society of Cytopathology.

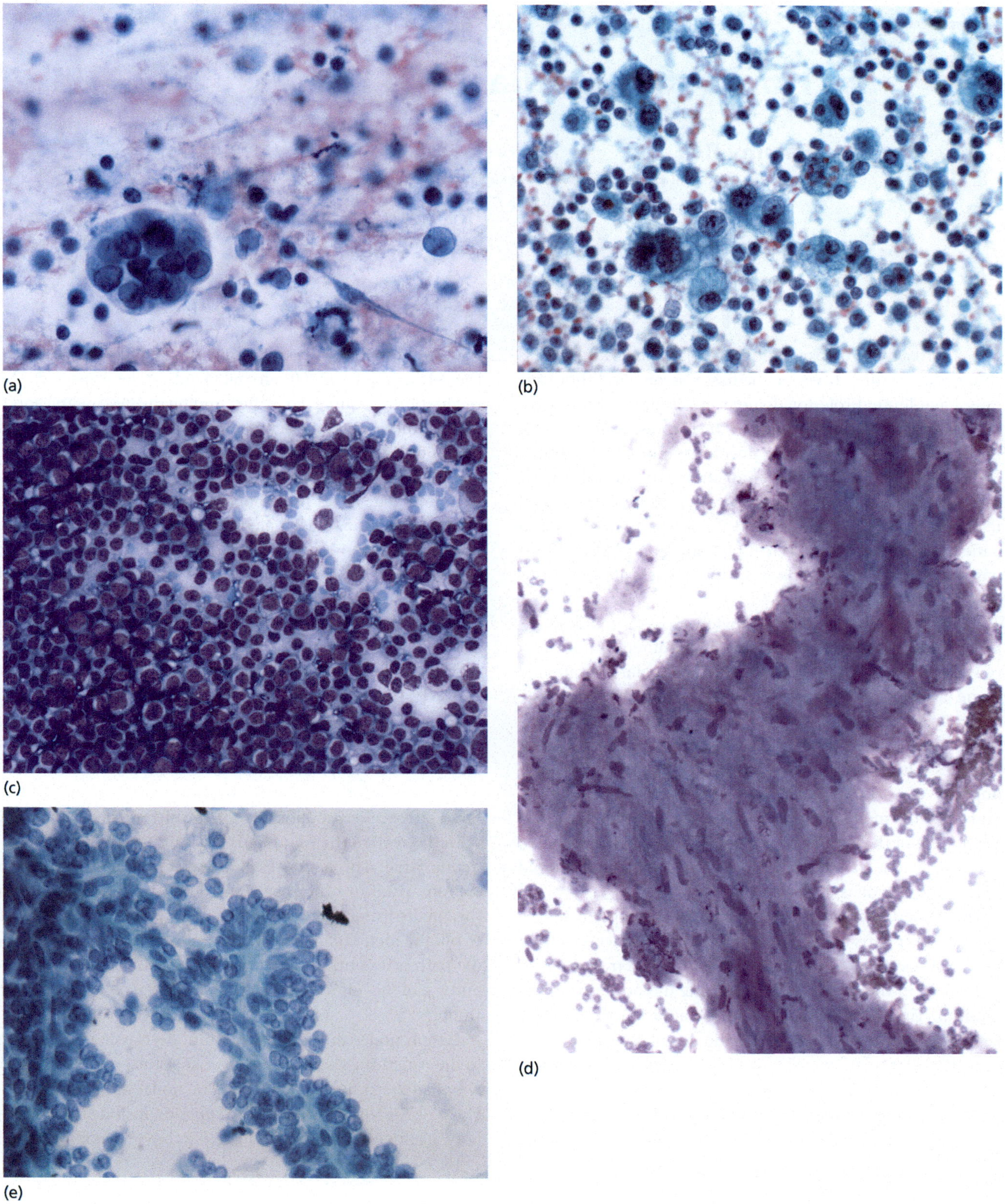

Figure 29.7 Distinctive or commonly encountered in endoscopic ultrasound-guided fine needle aspiration (EUS-FNA) biopsies include (a) metastatic adenocarcinoma in mediastinal lymph nodes; (b) metastatic renal cell carcinoma; (c) lymphoma; (d) gastrointestinal stromal tumors; (e) pancreatic solid pseudopapillary tumor.

30 How to do Mediastinal FNA

Sammy Ho
Montefiore Medical Center/AECOM, Bronx, NY, USA

The approach to biopsy lesions in the mediastinum has changed over time. Invasive mediastinoscopy and thoracotomy have limited role for tissue acquisition, particularly in the posterior mediastinum, due to the increased use of endoscopic ultrasound-guided fine needle aspiration (EUS-FNA). Most recent literature has demonstrated its overall safety, reliability, and accuracy. There is convincing evidence that EUS-FNA is an accurate method for mediastinal staging in patients with non-small cell lung cancer (NSCLC), which has become the main indication for transesophageal EUS-FNA (Table 30.1).

Attempts should be made to review cross-sectional imaging prior to EUS-FNA, often using a computed tomography (CT) scan of the thorax, to help formulate a plan for targeted tissue acquisition as well as characterizing any anatomic aberrancies.

Due to the duration of the time spent with echoendoscope in the esophagus during mediastinal FNA, proper sedation is imperative as is vigilance for periprocedural aspiration. Sudden movements have to be avoided to prevent injuries. Suctioning of the stomach for secretions and minimal use of air and water instillation within the esophagus should reduce the risk of aspiration.

The same linear-array echoendoscope equipment that is used in other parts of the gastrointestinal (GI) tract is utilized for the assessment of mediastinal lesions. The transducer is positioned in the esophagus to examine the posterior mediastinum. Tip of the echoendoscope is adjusted to view the ventral aspect toward 12 o'clock, the dorsal aspect toward 6 o'clock, the cranial toward 9 o'clock, and the caudal toward 3 o'clock position on the screen.

Evaluation of the mediastinum using the linear-array echoendoscope should follow a standardized approach. Beginning with the tip of the echoendoscope in the proximal stomach, the celiac nodes and left adrenal gland can be inspected. The mediastinum is surveyed by first finding the descending aorta. Slow withdrawal of the echoendoscope in 3–4 cm increments and 360-degree rotations can encompass the entire posterior mediastinum. When the transducer is positioned on the posterior and left side of the esophagus, it is possible to examine the thoracic aorta, the left pleura, and the left lung. When the transducer is positioned on the right side of the esophagus, one can visualize the azygos vein as far as its arch, situated between 24 and 25 cm from the incisors. By having the transducer pointing toward the anterior side of the esophagus in the middle part of the posterior mediastinum, the cardiac region can be examined, including the left atrium, the left ventricle, the pulmonary artery, and the aortic root.

Most of the mediastinal lesions are in close proximity to the esophageal wall. Hence, positioning of the echoendoscope to enable visualization and sampling is relatively easier than in other areas of the GI tract. It is important to have an excellent apposition of the tip of the instrument with the wall of the esophagus to avoid "recoil" of the echoendoscope. The actual EUS-FNA technique is similar to the one used in other areas in the GI tract. Generally, in the medistinum, one to three needle passes are sufficient to obtain adequate material. Presence of vessels in the needle path is a contraindication to EUS-FNA, and this possibility can be effectively excluded using color or power Doppler.

Lymph nodes in the mediastinum are classified according to the American Thoracic Society mediastinal staging map for lymphadenopathy (Figure 30.1). The nodal stations amendable to EUS-FNA, from inferior to superior, include the pulmonary ligament (stations 9R and 9L), lower paraesophageal

Atlas of Endoscopic Ultrasonography, Second Edition. Edited by Frank Gress, Thomas Savides, Brenna Casey, and Everson L. A. Artifon.

Companion website: www.wiley.com/go/gress/atlas

Table 30.1 TNM staging system for lung cancer (7th edition).

Primary tumor (T)			
T1	Tumor ≤3 cm diameter, surrounded by lung or visceral pleura, without invasion more proximal than lobar bronchus		
T1a	Tumor ≤2 cm in diameter		
T1b	Tumor >2 cm but ≤3 cm in diameter		
T2	Tumor >3 cm but ≤7 cm, or tumor with any of the following features: Involves main bronchus, ≥2 cm distal to carina Invades visceral pleura Associated with atelectasis or obstructive pneumonitis that extends to the hilar region but does not involve the entire lung		
T2a	Tumor >3 cm but ≤5 cm		
T2b	Tumor >5 cm but ≤7 cm		
T3	Tumor >7 cm or any of the following: Directly invades any of the following: chest wall, diaphragm, phrenic nerve, mediastinal pleura, parietal pericardium, main bronchus <2 cm from carina (without involvement of carina) Atelectasis or obstructive pneumonitis of the entire lung Separate tumor nodules in the same lobe		
T4	Tumor of any size that invades the mediastinum, heart, great vessels, trachea, recurrent laryngeal nerve, esophagus, vertebral body, carina, or with separate tumor nodules in a different ipsilateral lobe		
Regional lymph nodes (N)			
N0	No regional lymph node metastases		
N1	Metastasis in ipsilateral peribronchial and/or ipsilateral hilar lymph nodes and intrapulmonary nodes, including involvement by direct extension		
N2	Metastasis in ipsilateral mediastinal and/or subcarinal lymph node(s)		
N3	Metastasis in contralateral mediastinal, contralateral hilar, ipsilateral or contralateral scalene, or supraclavicular lymph node(s)		
Distant metastasis (M)			
M0	No distant metastasis		
M1	Distant metastasis		
M1a	Separate tumor nodule(s) in a contralateral lobe; tumor with pleural nodules or malignant pleural or pericardial effusion		
M1b	Distant metastasis		
Stage groupings			
Stage IA	T1a–T1b	N0	M0
Stage IB	T2a	N0	M0
Stage IIA	T1a, T1b, T2a	N1	M0
	T2b	N0	M0
Stage IIB	T2b	N1	M0
	T3	N0	M0
Stage IIIA	T1a, T1b, T2a, T2b	N2	M0
	T3	N1,N2	M0
	T4	N0,N1	M0
Stage IIIB	T4	N2	M0
	Any T	N3	M0
Stage IV	Any T	Any N	M1a or M1b

Source: adapted from Goldstraw P, Crowley J, Chansky K, et al. The IASLC Lung Cancer Staging Project: proposals for the revision of the TNM stage groups in the forthcoming (seventh) edition of the TNM classification of malignant tumours. *J Thorac Oncol* 2007;2:706.

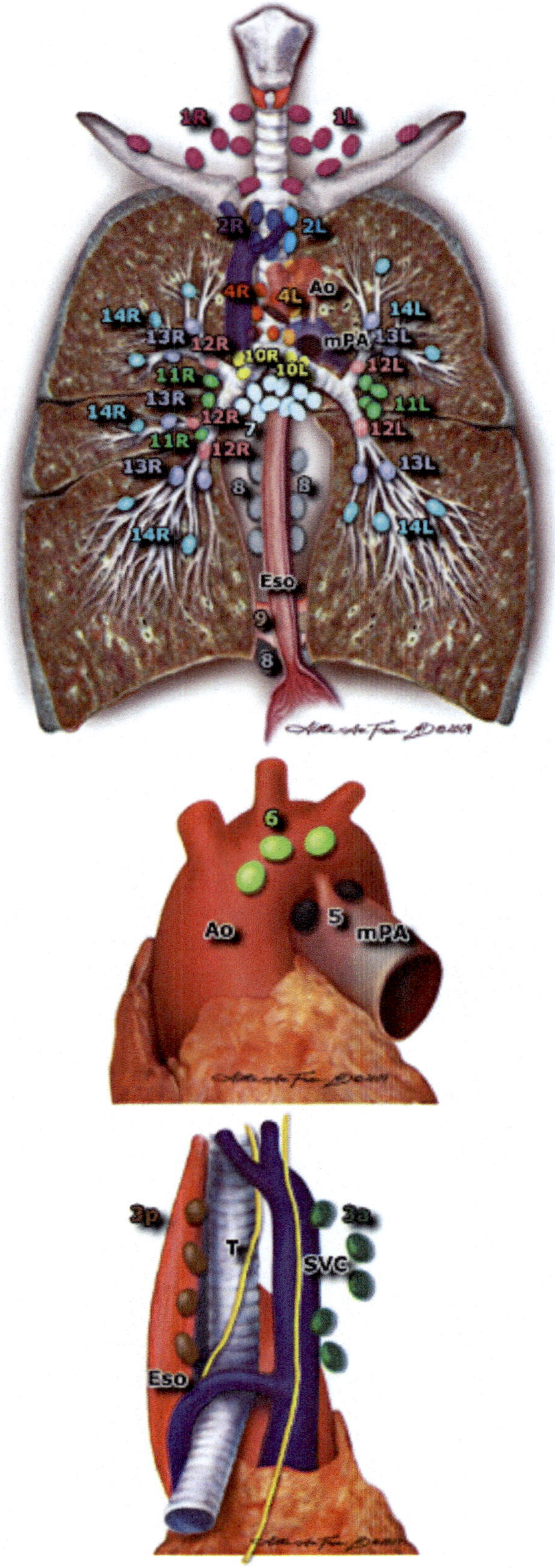

Supraclavicular zone

1 Low cervical, supraclavicular, and sternal notch nodes

Superior mediastinal nodes

Upper zone

2R Upper paratracheal (right)
2L Upperparatracheal (left)
3a Prevascular
3p Retrotracheal
4R Lower paratracheal (right)
4L Lower paratracheal (left)

Aortic nodes

AP zone

5 Subaortic
6 Para-aortic (ascending aorta or phrenic)

Inferior mediastinal nodes

Subcarinal zone

7 Sub carinal

Lower zone

8 Paraesophageal (below carina)
9 Pulmonary ligament

N1 nodes

Hilar/interlobar zone

10 Hilar
11 Interlobar

Peripheral zone

12 Lobar
13 Segmental
14 Subsegmental

Figure 30.1 The International Association for the Study of Lung Cancer (IASLC) lymph node map, including the proposed grouping of lymph node stations into "zones" for the purposes of prognostic analyses. Source: Rusch VW, Asamura H, Watanabe H, et al. The IASLC Lung Cancer Staging Project: a proposal for a new international lymph node map in the forthcoming seventh edition of the TNM classification for lung cancer. *J Thorac Oncol* 2009;4(5):568–577. © 2009, Elsevier.

(stations 8R and 8L), subcarinal (station 7), AP window (station 5), and para-aortal (station 6) nodes. When more than one lymph node group is present, the clinically most important location that is also accessible is selected. If two lesions in anatomically different areas are to be sampled, it is advisable to use two different needles, to avoid cross-contamination and possible misinterpretation of results.

Chapter video clips

Video 30.1 EUS-FNA of a small subcarinal node. Source: Hitachi.

Video 30.2 EUS-FNA of a subcarinal node in conjunction with elastography. Source: Hitachi.

31 How to do Pancreatic Mass FNA

Yunseok Namn and Jonathan M. Buscaglia
Stony Brook University Hospital, Renaissance School of Medicine at Stony Brook University, Stony Brook, NY, USA

Introduction

Gastrointestinal specialists are frequently consulted for the diagnosis and management of solid lesions within the pancreas. These masses are often malignant and include pancreatic ductal adenocarcinoma, neuroendocrine tumors, lymphoma, and metastatic disease presenting as a solid pancreatic lesion (e.g. renal cell carcinoma). Benign lesions include focal chronic pancreatitis and autoimmune pancreatitis (AIP). Endoscopic ultrasound (EUS) is the most sensitive imaging modality of the pancreas and remains pivotal for the evaluation of these solid masses. It allows for safe, minimally invasive characterization of pancreatic pathology with the ability for tissue acquisition in the form of ultrasound-guided fine needle aspiration (FNA). The overall adverse event rate of EUS-FNA is low, ranging between 1 and 2%. The risk of bleeding, which is usually self-limited and without need for transfusions, is considered the most common complication. Pancreatitis is a rare complication and may occur more commonly after FNA of a cystic rather than a solid lesion.

The chief advantage of EUS-guided FNA is the ability to target small intrapancreatic masses and low-grade malignancies that are often not accessible by computed tomography (CT) guidance. The decreased risk of malignant peritoneal contamination with EUS compared to CT-guided FNA of pancreatic lesions is an added potential advantage.

EUS-FNA has an extremely low false-positive rate with a positive predictive value of nearly 99%. Based on a large meta-analysis, EUS-FNA demonstrated an overall sensitivity of 85–91% and specificity of 94–98%. Various studies have shown a negative predictive value of 75%, with the majority of false-negative cases resulting from sampling error.

To optimize the diagnostic yield of EUS-FNA of pancreatic lesions, preprocedural considerations should include reviewing the patient's history, physical exam findings, and pertinent blood work. It is especially important to review all relevant cross-sectional imaging such as a CT scan or magnetic resonance imaging (MRI). This provides the endosonographer with specific clues that may facilitate a more thorough and complete examination, such as the exact location of a lesion or its relationship with major vascular structures. Furthermore, knowledge of additional pathologic features such as hepatic metastases or abdominal ascites may be important if FNA results are non-diagnostic, and they can frequently influence intraprocedural decision-making. Figures 31.1–31.7 demonstrate typical examples of the sonographic appearance of masses in the pancreas during EUS evaluation.

The technique

We often begin our examination with a radial echoendoscope and image the pancreas from the uncinate process to the tail of gland. This allows for a more thorough examination of the pancreas given the 270–360 degree imaging capability. It also facilitates a more complete evaluation of the pancreatic neck and tail, as well as the mediastinum. After the location of the mass is identified, we then introduce the curved linear array echoendoscope. Depending on the lesion location, FNA is performed transgastrically for lesions of the pancreatic genu, body, and tail. Transduodenal FNA is generally performed for lesions in the uncinate process and head of the pancreas. Transduodenal FNA is often more technically difficult due to the torque on the echoendoscope and the use of extreme upward tip deflection necessary for masses involving the uncinate process.

Once the lesion is positioned favorably in a 5 o'clock to 7 o'clock position below the EUS probe, FNA is performed with the appropriate needle under constant EUS guidance. Multiple needles are available for FNA and include a 19-gauge (G), 22-G, and 25-G needle. The choice of needle is based on the type of lesion targeted. For solid mass lesions, a

Atlas of Endoscopic Ultrasonography, Second Edition. Edited by Frank Gress, Thomas Savides, Brenna Casey, and Everson L. A. Artifon.

Companion website: www.wiley.com/go/gress/atlas

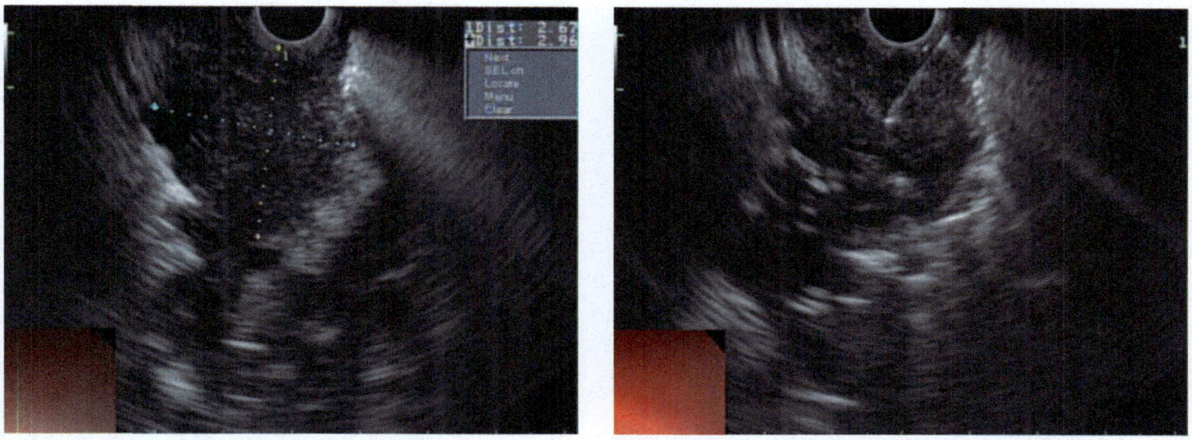

(a) (b)

Figure 31.1 (a) Hypoechoic, irregular, 3-cm adenocarcinoma in the head of pancreas. (b) Mass positioned in the 6 o'clock to 7 o'clock position during fine needle aspiration.

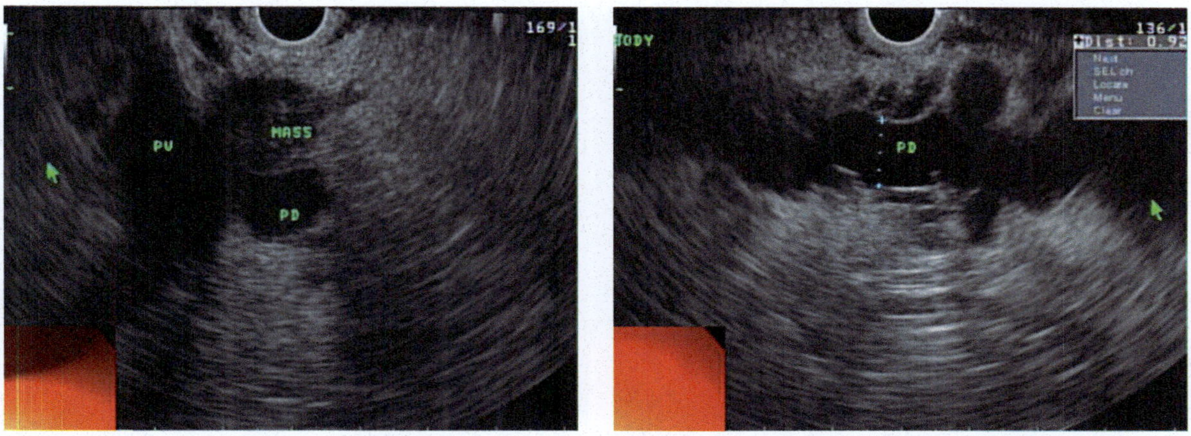

(a) (b)

Figure 31.2 (a) Small adenocarcinoma in the head of pancreas adjacent to the portal vein (PV) and a dilated pancreatic duct (PD). (b) Downstream dilation of the PD in the body of the pancreas.

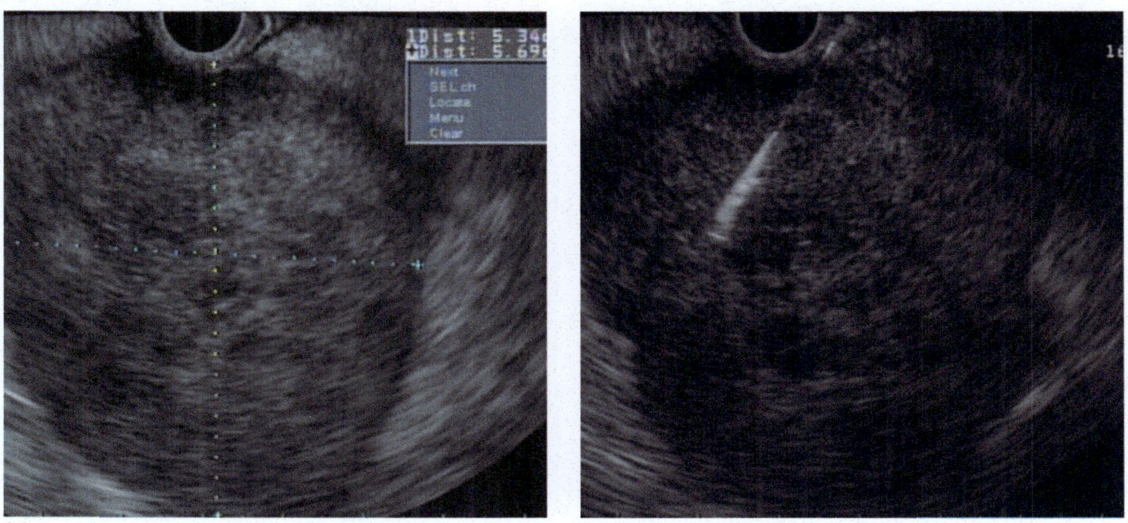

(a) (b)

Figure 31.3 (a) Large 5-cm adenocarcinoma in the tail of pancreas. (b) Mass positioned at the 6 o'clock position during fine needle aspiration with a 25-gauge needle.

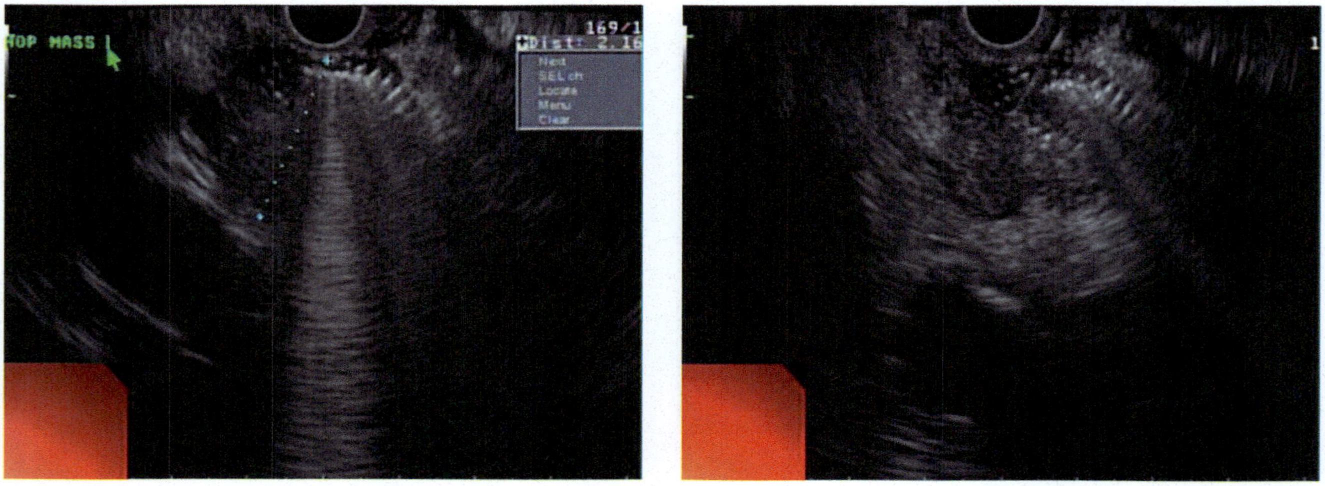
(a) (b)

Figure 31.4 (a) A 2-cm mass in the head of pancreas with acoustic interference from a metal stent within the common bile duct. (b) Fine needle aspiration through the metal stent to sample tissue from the inferior portion of the mass.

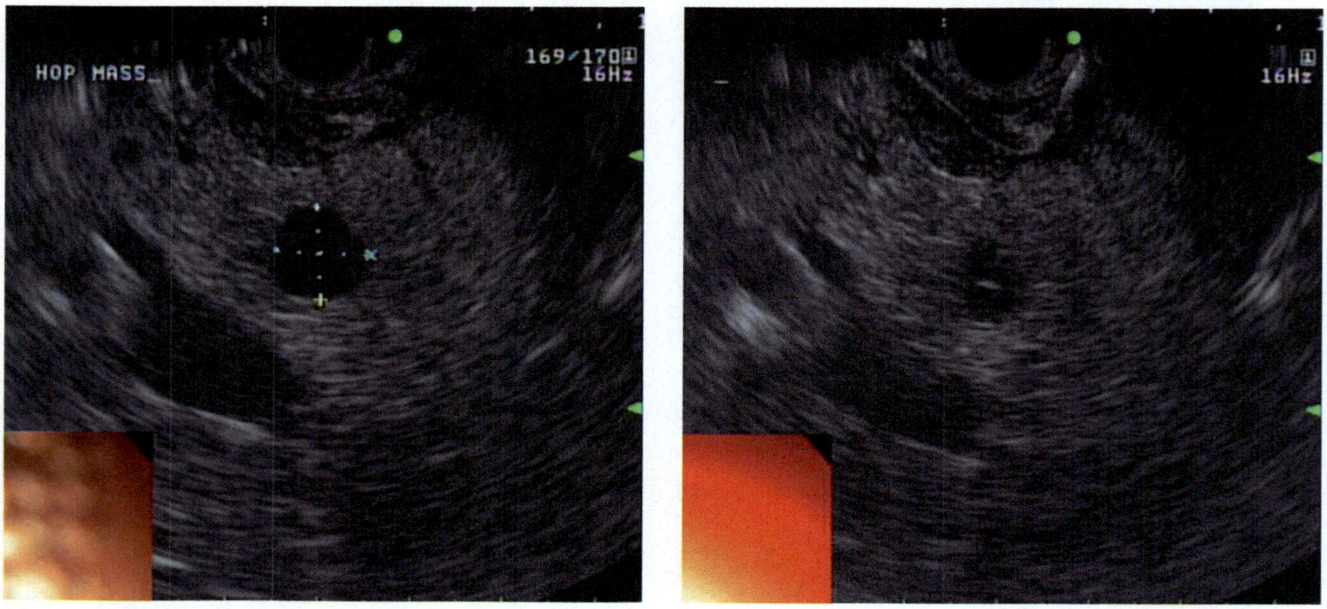

(a) (b)

Figure 31.5 (a) Small 1-cm hypoechoic neuroendocrine tumor in the head of pancreas. (b) Fine needle aspiration needle tip visible in the center of the mass.

19-G needle is generally discouraged due to the potential risk for bleeding, as well as the lack of data demonstrating a diagnostic advantage with larger-caliber FNA needles. In general, we prefer to use the 25-G needle because of its flexibility and thus ease of use in difficult positions with excessive torque on the echoendoscope to access the pancreatic head and uncinate region from the first or second portion of the duodenum.

In straighter positions, such as within the stomach, we often use a 22-G needle. Prior to FNA, the tip of the EUS probe is positioned in a fashion to minimize the distance between the lesion and the probe itself. This allows for greater precision when advancing the needle through the gastrointestinal tract and into the pancreas. Color Doppler is often used to exclude any intervening vessels just before FNA.

When the FNA needle is in place inside the echoendoscope channel and appropriately fastened at the end of the scope, the stylet is pulled back approximately 1 cm to create a sharpened needle tip. Both dials controlling tip deflection on the echoendoscope are locked to ensure scope stability.

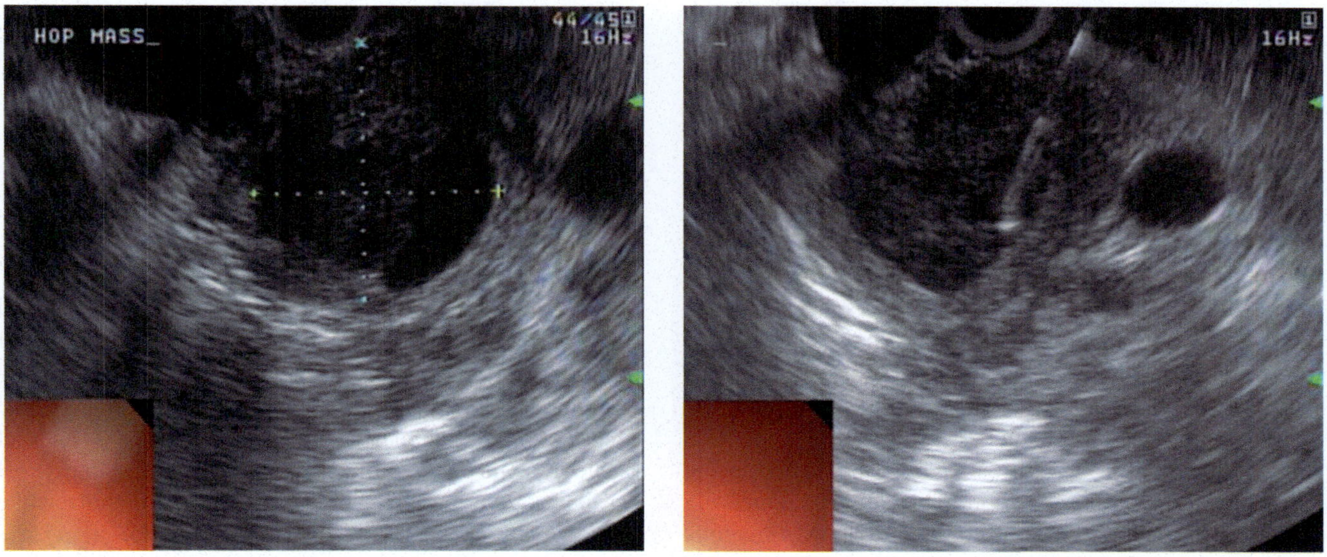

(a) (b)

Figure 31.6 (a) Cystic neoplasm with malignant degeneration in the head of pancreas. (b) Fine needle aspiration targeting the solid components of the mass for higher diagnostic yield.

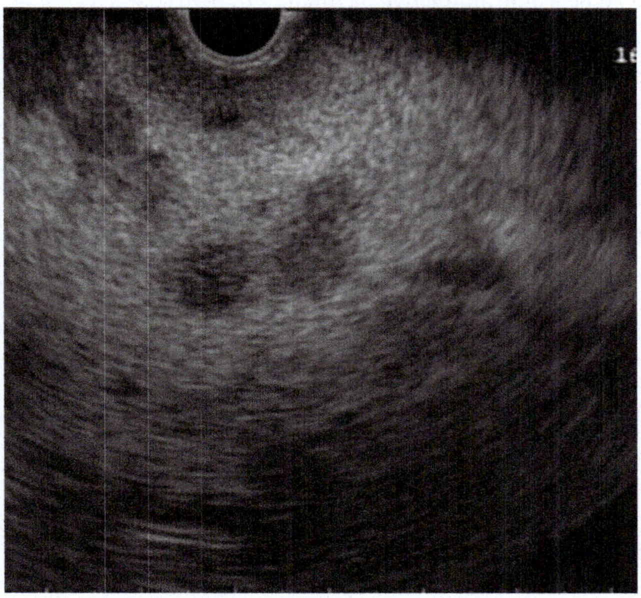

Figure 31.7 Hepatic metastases visualized during EUS examination for a pancreas mass.

Transgastric FNA can be challenging due to the thick gastric wall. To prevent tenting of the needle against the lumen, the gastric wall can first be suctioned to increase the angle at which the needle passes, followed by a quick spearing motion of the needle with sufficient force to penetrate the wall. This assures accurate entrance of the needle tip into the lesion. Once the FNA needle tip lies sufficiently within the center of the lesion, the stylet is pushed forward to purge any gastrointestinal contaminant obtained at the time of wall puncture. The stylet is then completely removed, and a 10- or 20-ml syringe may be fastened to the operator end of the needle in order to apply suction to the needle's lumen. This technique is often referred to as "dry suction" FNA. It is important to know that other techniques exist, such as the "wet suction" in which the needle lumen and syringe are filled with water before applying suction, as well as the "slow pull" technique in which no syringe is used and the stylet is simply pulled from the needle lumen as the operator is making several passes with the needle tip in the center of the lesion. The needle is then passed back and forth swiftly (multiple rapid thrusts) within the mass along separate linear planes while keeping the needle tip visible at all times to break up tissue for better cytologic yield. We recommend this "fanning" technique using the elevator and subtle tip deflections of the large echoendoscope dials to sample different areas as opposed advancing the needle back and forth through the same portion of the mass (Video 31.1).

In large solid masses, the center of the lesion is often soft and necrotic; therefore, the peripheral firm portions of the mass should be aspirated to maximize the cytologic yield. Prior to removal of the needle, suction should be turned off to prevent intestinal contamination. The needle is then removed completely from the echoendoscope channel, and an air-filled syringe is used to flush the aspirated material onto glass slides. If clot is present within the needle, the stylet is inserted to push the material forward. A thin smear is then made and immediately rinsed with an alcohol fixative. For in-room staining, a separate thin smear may be made and then air-dried. Next, a Diff-Quik™ stain is usually performed which allows for immediate evaluation by either the endosonographer or the cytotechnician.

The number of passes with the FNA needle depends on the presence of rapid on-site evaluation of cytology (ROSE), which is a valuable tool for optimizing diagnostic yield. The immediate evaluation of sample quality by the pathologist helps determine if the acquired sample was satisfactory for cytologic study and theoretically reduces the number of punctures. Some studies have shown that ROSE can improve the overall diagnostic yield of FNA by up to 10–15%. If ROSE is present, additional passes with the needle depend on the adequacy of the specimen delivered to and assessed by the cytotechnician. When ROSE is not available, we generally perform three separate passes with the needle, and then await a future and final cytopathologic interpretation. If para-tumor or celiac axis lymph nodes are noted, FNA with a separate needle can be performed in a similar fashion. This may be especially important in making an accurate diagnosis for a necrotic mass lesion in which adequate tissue acquisition is often difficult.

As an adjunctive diagnostic tool, contrast-enhanced EUS can be used to assess the vascularization and perfusion patterns of pancreatic masses. Pancreatic adenocarcinoma has a distinct hypovascular appearance while other pancreatic processes, such as neuroendocrine tumors and chronic/autoimmune pancreatitis, have either a hypervascular or isovascular appearance. EUS elastography is another technique that can help distinguish pancreatic cancer from other inflammatory masses based on tumor elasticity.

Box 31.1 Tips for EUS-FNA of solid pancreatic masses

- Review clinical data prior to endoscopy
- Choose appropriate needle size
- Sample lesion with quick "thrusts" in multiple linear planes
- Aim for margins of necrotic masses
- Arrange for on-site cytopathology if possible

Final considerations

Fine needle aspiration is an important tool in the diagnosis and management of pancreatic masses. Studies have shown the overall accuracy of EUS-FNA ranges between 71 and 94% in this setting. It is important to review all pertinent clinical data (especially cross-sectional imaging) prior to performing endoscopy to optimize the diagnostic yield. The choice of the needle may depend on the location and size of the lesion. Once the lesion is targeted and placed in optimal position, FNA is performed under total EUS guidance while visualizing the needle tip at all times. Factors that may increase the diagnostic yield of FNA include sampling the lesion in multiple planes through the "fanning" technique, targeting the firmer peripheral margins of the necrotic mass, and arranging for rapid on-site evaluation of cytology (Box 31.1). Contrast-enhanced EUS and EUS elastography can be useful adjunctive techniques to help characterize, differentiate, and stage focal pancreatic masses.

Chapter video clip

Video 31.1 EUS-FNA of a pancreatic mass. Source: Stony Brook University.

32 How to do Pancreatic Cyst FNA

Ahmad Najdat Bazarbashi and Linda S. Lee

Division of Gastroenterology, Hepatology and Endoscopy, Brigham and Women's Hospital, Harvard Medical School, Boston, MA, USA

Introduction

Pancreatic cysts remain a challenge to diagnose and manage. Evaluation should focus on whether the cyst is malignant and, if not, the risk of malignant transformation. While magnetic resonance imaging (MRI) should be performed on all patients with pancreatic cysts if possible, endoscopic ultrasound (EUS) is an important complementary diagnostic tool for indeterminate cysts and cysts with concerning features. The value of EUS lies not only with its imaging of the cyst size, border, content, and surrounding structures, but also in its ability to aspirate cyst fluid and tissue via fine needle aspiration (FNA) or fine needle biopsy (FNB) for analyses. Because tissue diagnosis via FNA of pancreatic cysts is often limited by the paucicellular specimens, other diagnostic tests and tools have been explored including cyst fluid analysis and, more recently, FNB. EUS-FNB may safely increase diagnostic yield and requires further study. What tests to send for cyst fluid analysis continue to evolve and may include amylase, carcinoembryonic antigen, glucose, molecular analysis, cytology and/or histology.

Prior to EUS, the patient should undergo a thorough history and focused physical examination including history of pancreatitis, family history of pancreatic cancer, and smoking and alcohol intake as these may influence the differential diagnosis of the pancreatic cyst. Anticoagulation should be held after discussion with the prescribing clinician. Radiology images should be carefully reviewed to understand the patient's anatomy and location of the pancreatic cyst(s), and to anticipate any potential difficulties in finding and sampling the lesion. When consenting patients, the endosonographer should detail the nature of the procedure, risks, benefits and alternatives. Risks to highlight include bleeding, infection, abdominal pain, pancreatitis, and perforation. Realistic expectations should be set for the patient, indicating that cyst fluid analysis and FNA/FNB are imperfect and do not always provide definitive diagnosis of the cyst. Antibiotic prophylaxis has been recommended by the American Society for Gastrointestinal Endoscopy for EUS-FNA of pancreatic cystic lesions (typically a fluoroquinolone administered peri-procedure and for three days afterwards).

Technique (Video 32.1)

Esophagogastroduodenoscopy (EGD) is often performed prior to EUS to ensure there are no anatomical abnormalities that may interfere with passing the echoendoscope or with visualizing the pancreas and surrounding structures, for example an unknown surgery. Linear echoendoscope is preferred over radial echoendoscope since it allows for FNA or FNB. EUS examination should proceed methodically to avoid missing visualizing certain areas. One may begin by identifying important anatomical structures such as the liver (Figure 32.1) and aorta/celiac trunk (Figure 32.2). The pancreas can be found by gently pushing the echoendoscope forward in the stomach after identifying the celiac trunk and following the SMA to the pancreas or by rotating 180 degrees from the thickest portion of the left lobe of the liver. The genu, body, and tail are examined from the transgastric station (echoendoscope positioned towards the posterior wall of stomach; Figure 32.3), while the uncinate process and head of the pancreas are usually visualized transduodenally (echoendoscope in the duodenal bulb for the head and second portion of the duodenum for the complete head and uncinate process; Figure 32.4).

Once the cyst is identified, it should be evaluated for size, shape, echogenicity, contents (mucin, septations, nodule, solid mass), thickness of wall, and communication with main pancreatic duct (Figure 32.5). Mucus appears hypoechoic relative to the adjacent tissue with a well-defined hyperechoic rim while nodules are isoechoic/hyperechoic

Atlas of Endoscopic Ultrasonography, Second Edition. Edited by Frank Gress, Thomas Savides, Brenna Casey, and Everson L. A. Artifon.

Companion website: www.wiley.com/go/gress/atlas

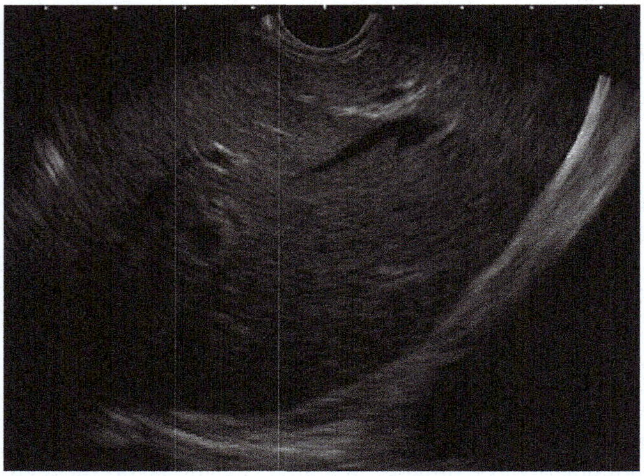

Figure 32.1 EUS of left lobe of liver.

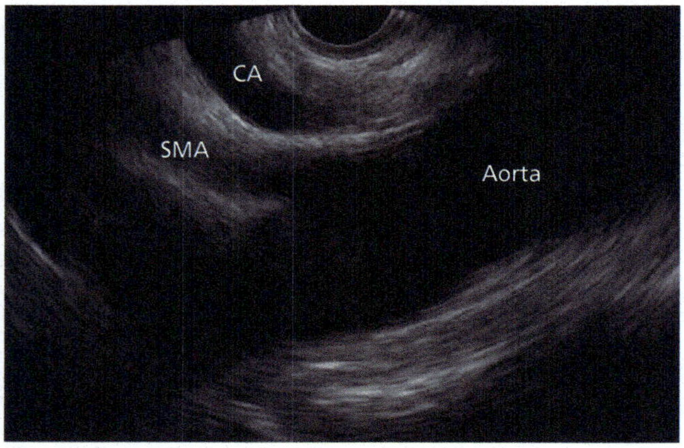

Figure 32.2 EUS of aorta, celiac artery (CA), and superior mesenteric artery (SMA).

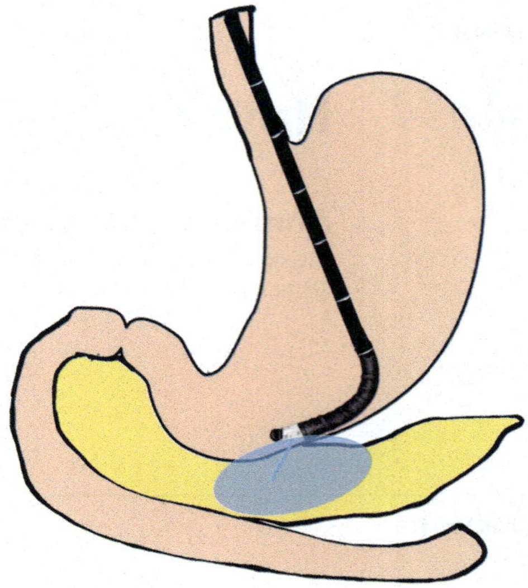

Figure 32.3 Transgastric EUS examination of pancreas (genu, body, tail).

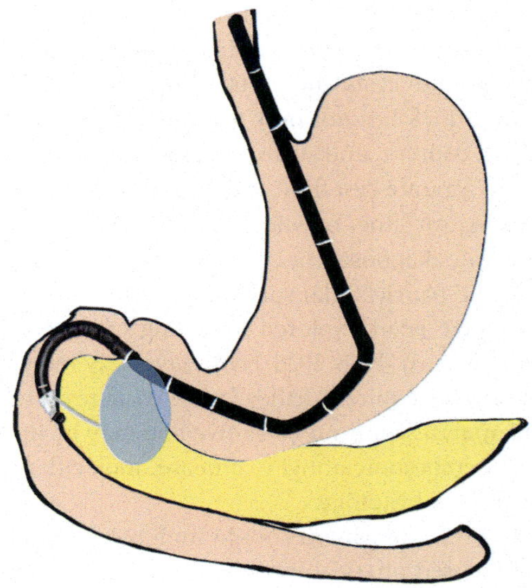

Figure 32.4 Transduodenal EUS examination of pancreas (head and uncinate process).

without a smooth border or hyperechoic rim. In preparation for biopsy, the cyst should ideally be located near the 6 o'clock position as close to the tip of the echoendoscope as possible using the large dial (Figure 32.6), and Doppler imaging used to ensure no vessels lie in the path of the needle (Figure 32.7).

For FNA/FNB, 22G needles are usually used although thinner 25G needles may be considered for transduodenal punctures, especially into the uncinate process. This is because transduodenal punctures are often more difficult than the transgastric approach due to the angulated, long position of the echoendoscope in the duodenum. However, suctioning viscous fluid may be challenging through smaller-caliber needles while 19G needles facilitate faster and easier aspiration of large and mucinous cysts. After removing the biopsy cap and advancing the needle device down the accessory channel of the echoendoscope, it is attached to the Luer lock at the accessory channel port. Both large and small dials on the echoendoscope should be locked to ensure slight movements or deviations are minimized during needle advancement. The position of the sheath may be adjusted using the bottom adjustable slider on the needle (Figure 32.8), which allows use of the various needles with the different brands of echoendoscopes. Once the sheath is visible, the sheath adjusting knob should be locked. The stylet should be pulled back slightly to expose the needle tip with certain FNB needles. How far to advance the needle can be estimated by measuring the distance from the tip of the echoendoscope into the cyst, and the adjustable needle knob (Figure 32.8) should be locked in place accordingly to prevent the needle from traversing too far. The needle is then slowly advanced out of the sheath; however, if difficulty is encountered, do not force the needle out as this may

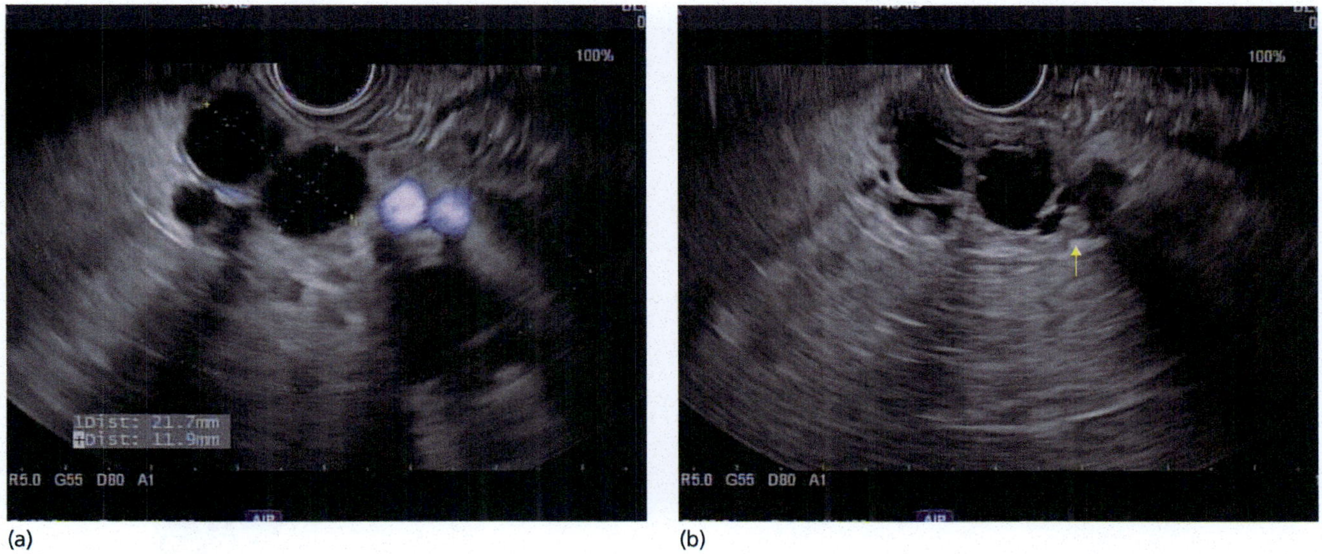

Figure 32.5 (a) EUS of anechoic septated lobular cyst in tail of pancreas. (b) EUS of anechoic septated lobular pancreatic cyst with nodule (yellow arrow) proven malignant on surgical resection. Source: Frank G. Gress.

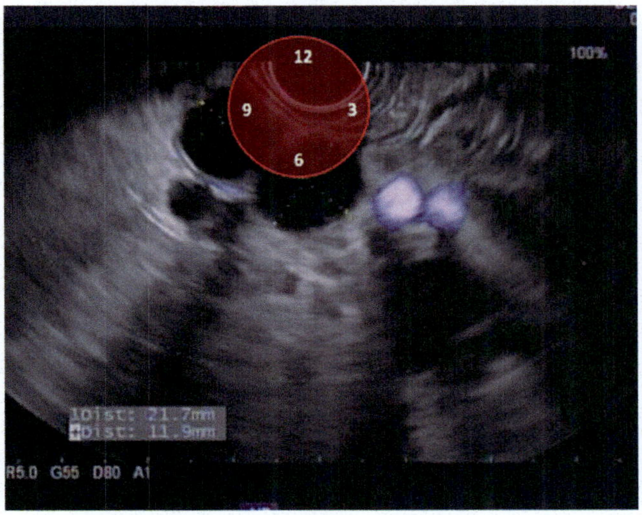

Figure 32.6 Position lesion at 6 o'clock for FNA/FNB. Source: Frank G. Gress.

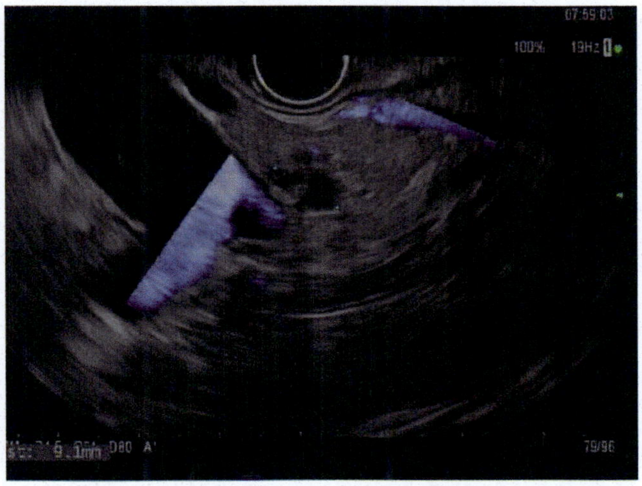

Figure 32.7 EUS with Doppler showing blood vessels (purple) in path of needle. Source: Frank G. Gress.

damage the echoendoscope. Adjust the position of the echoendoscope and unlock the dials to help the needle to exit easily. Once the needle is visible, slowly advance it to the gastric/duodenal wall, adjust the angle of entry as needed using the elevator, recheck Doppler to ensure no vessels are in the path of the needle, and thrust it rapidly and firmly into the cyst (Figure 32.9). The stylet may be pushed in completely to expel any gastric or duodenal wall tissue that may have been captured, after which it is completely removed and a 10- or 20-ml syringe attached to the needle handle for suctioning cyst fluid. To prepare the syringe, air is completely expelled, the stopcock closed, and then the plunger pulled back and turned to lock into position to create a vacuum (Figure 32.10). Ideally the cyst is aspirated completely with one pass. Observe the cyst fluid accumulating in the syringe, and if frank blood is filling it, aspiration should stop. FNA/FNB of the collapsed cyst wall may be performed with short to-and-fro movements. If nodules or solid components were noted, these should be sampled in a similar fashion to solid pancreatic masses.

Once aspiration is complete, suction should be turned off with or without removing the syringe before the needle is withdrawn from the lesion to avoid contamination of the collected specimen. The fully withdrawn needle is locked in

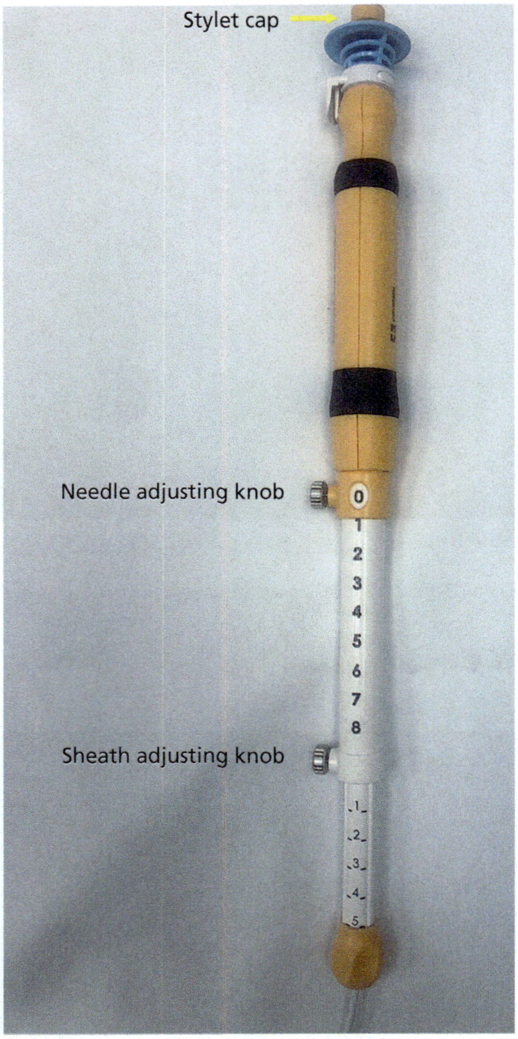

Figure 32.8 EUS needle handle. Source: Frank G. Gress.

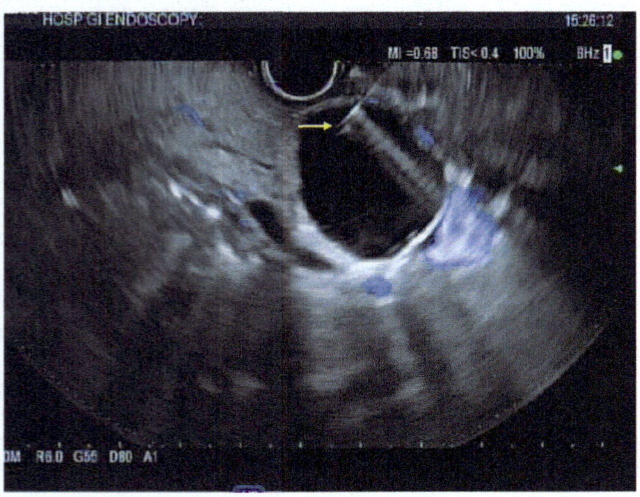

Figure 32.9 FNA needle within pancreatic cyst (yellow arrow indicates tip of needle). Source: Frank G. Gress.

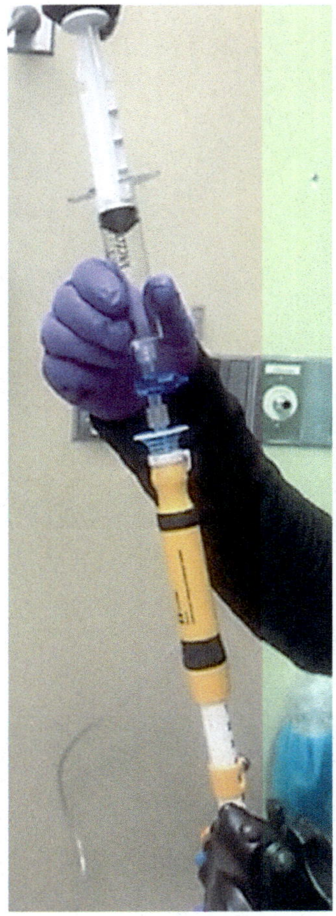

Figure 32.10 Vacuum syringe. Source: Frank G. Gress.

position and then the needle removed from the echoendoscope. The fluid should be grossly examined for its color which may range from bloody to brown, serosanguinous, white, or serous (Figure 32.11). String sign should be assessed, if possible, by placing a drop of fluid between the index finger and thumb, pressing both together and then slowly pulling them apart to look for development of string-like material, which is consistent with a mucinous cyst (Figure 32.12). Alternatively, one may observe for string sign in fluid being expressed from the tip of the EUS needle. The cyst fluid should be placed into a container for cyst fluid analyses. Tissue within the needle may be sent for cytology (FNA) or histology (FNB).

Summary

EUS is an important diagnostic tool for evaluating pancreatic cystic lesions that are indeterminate or have concerning features on radiology imaging. Careful review of imaging is important. Regarding the technique of sampling pancreatic cysts, FNB needles may safely provide higher diagnostic yield than FNA needles and require further study. While smaller-gauge needles are easier to use in a transduodenal

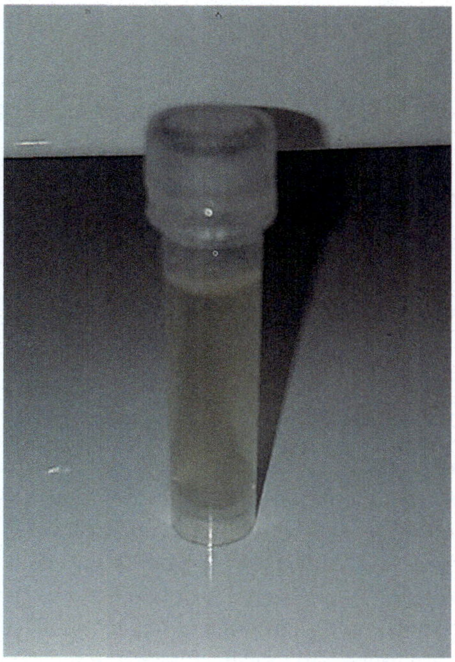

Figure 32.11 Serous fluid aspirated from large pancreatic cyst. Source: Frank G. Gress.

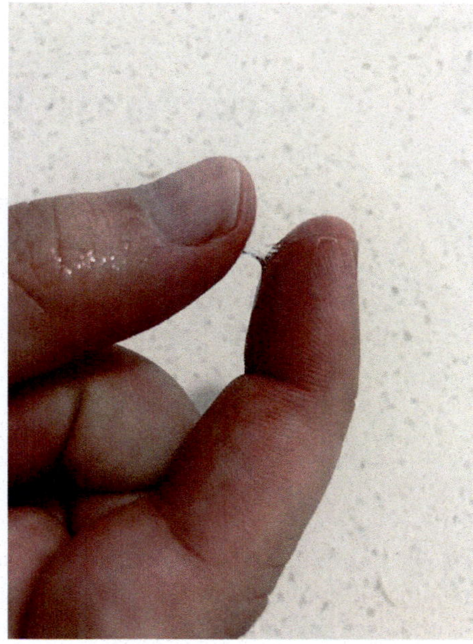

Figure 32.12 String sign consistent with mucinous cyst. Source: Frank G. Gress.

approach, suctioning viscous fluid through them may be more challenging than with a larger-gauge needle. Ideally one pass is used to aspirate the cyst completely, and the collapsed cyst wall may be sampled. Cyst fluid should be assessed for string sign, if possible, and sent for the desired testing. Nodules and solid masses must be sampled as well. Antibiotics should be administered periprocedurally.

Chapter video clip

Video 32.1 Technique of pancreatic cyst EUS-FNA.

33 How to do Pancreatic Pseudocyst Drainage

Shyam Varadarajulu[1] and Vinay Dhir[2]

[1] University of Alabama at Birmingham Medical Center, Birmingham, AL, USA
[2] Institute of Advanced Endoscopy, Mumbai, India

Introduction

Pseudocysts (PCs) are fluid-filled cavities surrounded by a non-epithelial wall composed of inflammatory material. Drainage is required for large PCs that are persistent and symptomatic. Historically, PCs that produce a luminal compression on the stomach or duodenal wall are treated endoscopically by transmural drainage and those not causing a luminal compression by surgery or percutaneous techniques. Accumulating evidence over the past decade suggests that endoscopic ultrasound (EUS) is a safe and effective modality for drainage of PCs, irrespective of the presence or absence of a luminal compression. Unlike conventional transmural drainage, which is a relatively "blind" technique, EUS guidance enables the puncture of a PC under real-time imaging thereby minimizing the potential for complications such as bleeding and perforation. Also, unlike percutaneous techniques, the procedure does not predispose to fistula formation or restrict patient mobility. Compared to surgery, EUS-guided drainage is less invasive, less costly, and is associated with shorter length of hospital stay.

Patient selection

The majority of the PCs larger than 4 cm in size and located adjacent to the gastric or duodenal wall are suitable for EUS-guided drainage. Pseudocysts located in the tail region of the pancreas do not cause a luminal compression and may require puncture from unusual locations such as the distal esophagus. Although hitherto considered a relative contraindication, multiple large PCs can be accessed individually and drained successfully under EUS guidance when located close to the gastrointestinal (GI) lumen. Cysts smaller than 4 cm in size are not suitable for stent placement. If treatment is required in such cases, complete cyst aspiration under EUS guidance can be undertaken in one session. Alternatively, if the PC communicates with the main pancreatic duct, transpapillary stenting may be appropriate. Multiseptated cysts in general do not respond well to endotherapy as the non-evacuated portions of the cyst tend to persist and suboptimal drainage predisposes to infection. Also, the presence of large amounts of necrotic debris warrants endoscopic necrosectomy or surgery. Transluminal stenting per se is inadequate therapy for necrotic fluid collections.

Requisite instruments and accessories

A curvilinear array echoendoscope with a channel diameter of 3.7 mm or more is needed for stent depolyments. A 19-gauge endoscopic ultrasound-guided fine needle aspiration (EUS-FNA) needle is required for passing a 0.035-inch guidewire into the PC. Pseudocyst puncture can also be performed with a needle knife catheter, or with a one-step needle wire device (available in Europe), or a cystotome. Over-the-wire balloon catheters are required for dilation of the transmural tract and double pigtail plastic stents for facilitating drainage of cyst contents. Nasocystic catheters may be required for continuous irrigation of the abscess cavity or necrotic contents. It is important to perform the procedures in a room equipped with fluoroscopy to monitor guidewire exchange and stent deployment.

More recently, fully covered lumen-apposing metal stents (LAMS) have become available for performing single-step drainage procedures. These stents are incorporated in both a cautery and non-cautery-enhanced delivery platform and are available in diameters that range from 8 to 20 mm. The wide lumen of the stent facilitates quick drainage of cyst contents and the bilateral flanges at both ends minimize the risk of stent migration.

Atlas of Endoscopic Ultrasonography, Second Edition. Edited by Frank Gress, Thomas Savides, Brenna Casey, and Everson L. A. Artifon.

Companion website: www.wiley.com/go/gress/atlas

Assessment of the pseudocyst by EUS prior to drainage

A careful evaluation of the PC should be undertaken prior to puncture. The size, location, and number (single or multiple) of PCs should be determined. Most PCs are unilocular with predominantly clear contents and well-defined walls (Figure 33.1). Multilocular cysts and those with mucinous contents or thick nodular walls need to be aspirated to rule out a neoplastic process (Figure 33.2). Also, a thorough survey of the pancreatic gland must be undertaken prior to drainage as a proximal tumor can cause a reactive PC. Some PCs located in the distal body or tail of the pancreas may cause splenic vein thrombosis and collaterals may be present between the cyst and gastric wall (Figure 33.3). In such cases, a puncture site should be chosen after excluding the presence of intervening vasculature (Figure 33.4). It is important that the PC is located within 1–2 cm of the GI lumen to avoid perforation or stent migration.

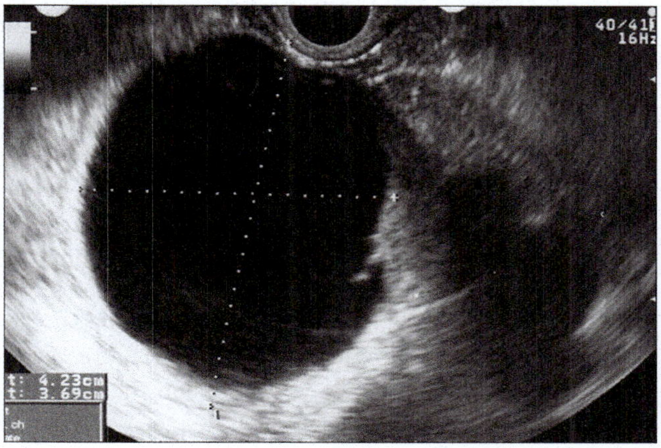

Figure 33.1 A large unilocular pseudocyst with clear contents as visualized under EUS guidance.

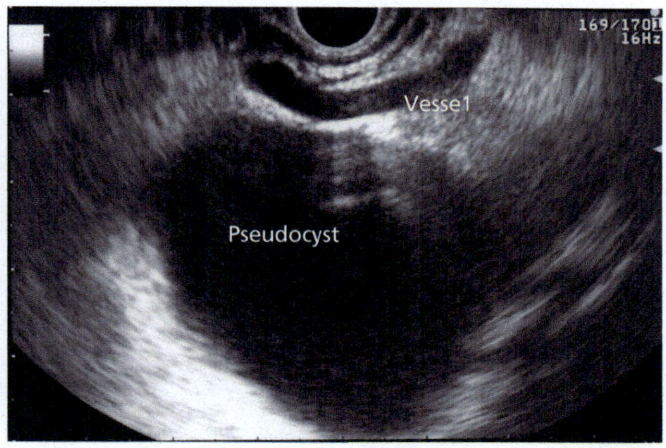

Figure 33.3 Presence of intervening vasculature between the EUS transducer and the pseudocyts.

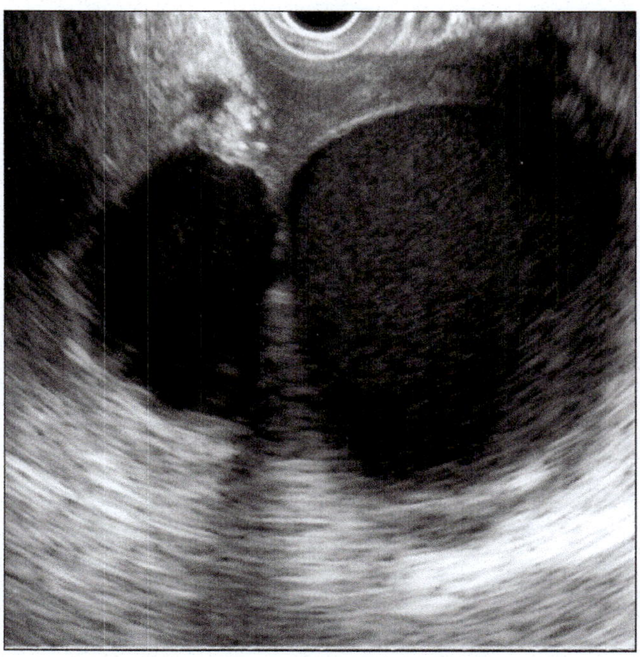

Figure 33.2 Two pseudocysts are seen at EUS: the promixal lesion on FNA analysis was a mucinous neoplasm and the distal lesion a reactive pseudocyst.

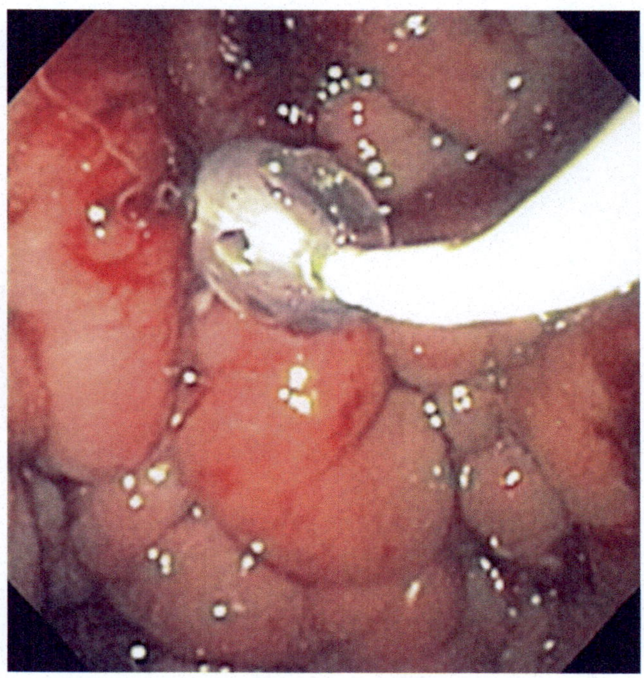

Figure 33.4 Endoscopic ultrasound guidance enables access to the pseudocyst by providing an appropriate window in a patient with gastric varices.

Technique for placement of plastic endoprosthesis

Pseudocyst puncture

Antibiotic prophylaxis is recommended prior to puncture of any cystic lesions. Pseudocyst puncture can be done with a 19-gauge needle (Video 33.1) without the need for cautery (Figure 33.5). Alternatively, cautery-assisted cyst puncture can be performed with help of a needle knife catheter or the Giovannini one-step needle wire device. Puncture should preferably be done at a site where the echoendoscope is relatively straight. An angulated echoendoscope may cause resistance to passage of accessories and stents. As angulation is sometimes unavoidable when accessing a PC from the fundus of the stomach, we prefer not to use electrocautery in such situations as it may result in tangential catheter passage and perforation. The use of fluoroscopy aids in maintaining a straight position of the tip of the echoendoscope (Figure 33.6).

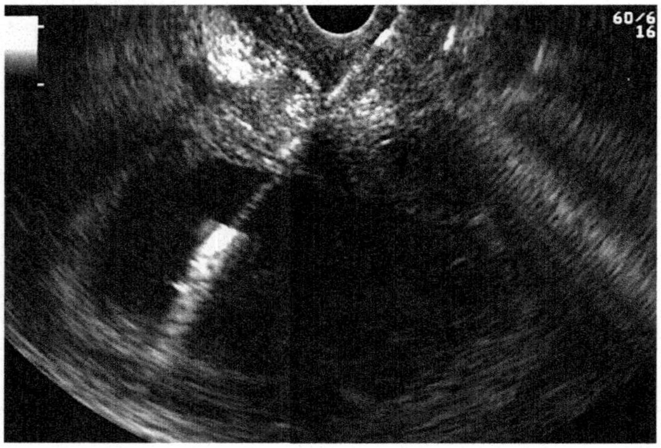

Figure 33.5 Pseudocyst accessed with a 19-gauge FNA needle.

Transmural tract dilation

Once the needle is seen in the PC, fluid should be aspirated for analysis (Gram stain, culture, chemistry, or tumor marker studies). A 0.035-inch guidewire is then coiled within the PC (Figure 33.7). The tract can then be dilated sequentially using a 5-French (Fr) endoscopic retrograde cholangiopancreatography (ERCP) catheter (Figure 33.8), Soehendra biliary dilator, 5.5-Fr inner catheter of the Giovannini one-step system, or the inner catheter of the cystotome. It is important to keep the guidewire taut as otherwise there may be resistance to passage of dilators. Subsequent dilation is then undertaken using an 8–15 mm over-the-wire balloon dilator (Figure 33.9). Large-diameter balloons can be used when the cyst contents are turbid to facilitate better drainage. When using large-diameter balloons it is important to ascertain that there is proper effacement between the PC and the GI lumen so as to avoid perforation.

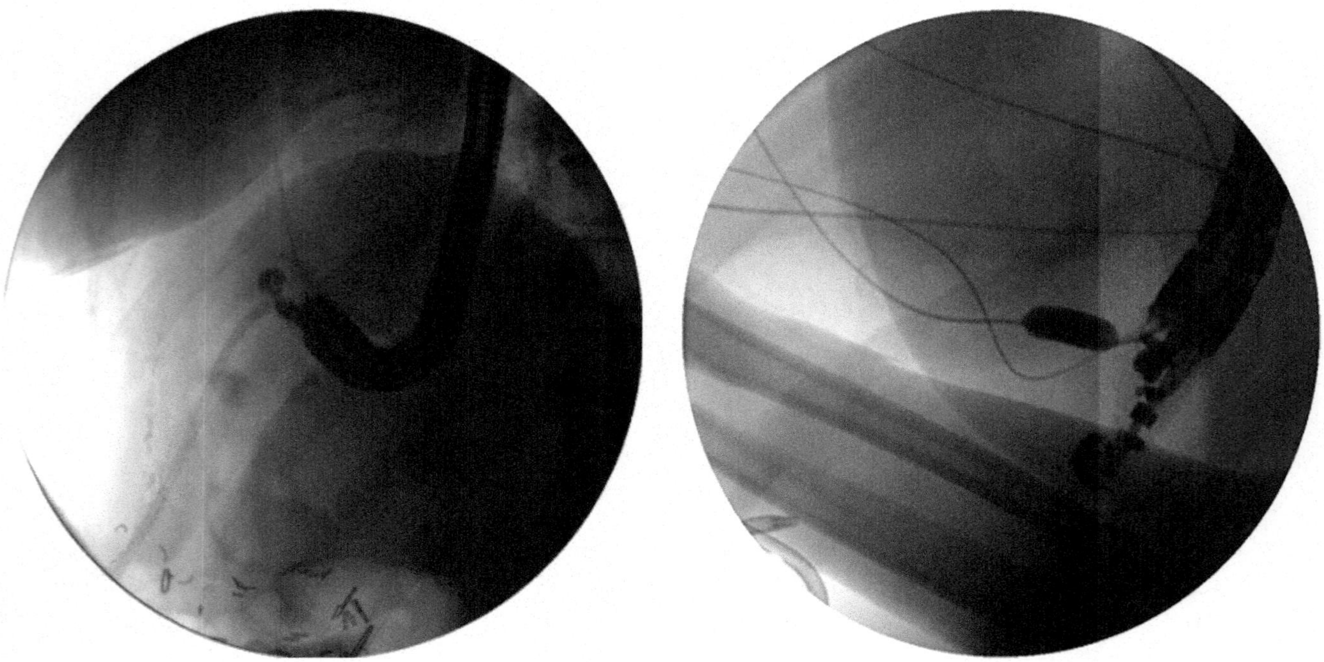

(a) (b)

Figure 33.6 (a) Acute angulation encountered when the echoendoscope is located in the gastric fundus. (b) The tip of the echoendoscope is subsequently straightened with aid of fluoroscopy to facilitate passage of accessories.

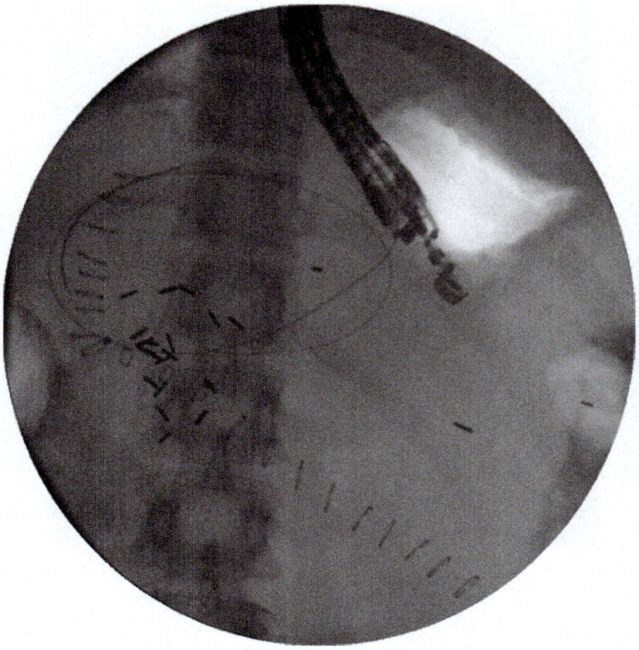

Figure 33.7 A 0.035-inch guidewire is coiled within the pseudocyst under fluoroscopic guidance.

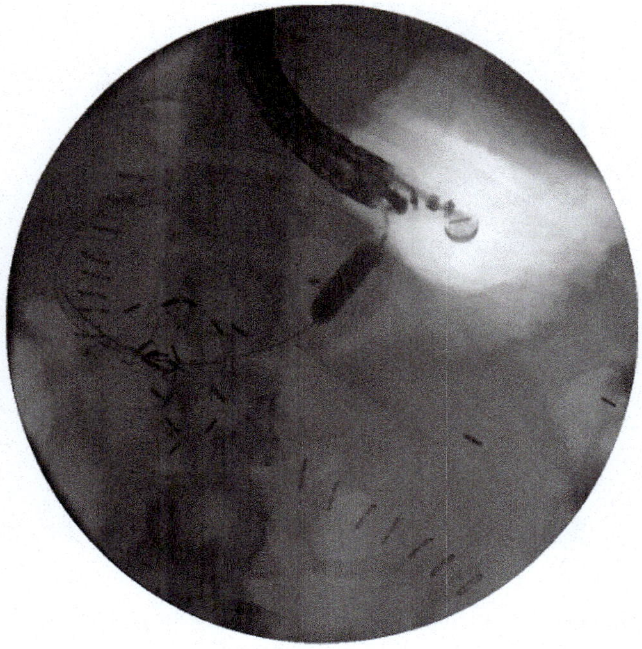

Figure 33.9 The transmural tract is subsequently dilated using an 8 mm over-the-wire biliary balloon dilator.

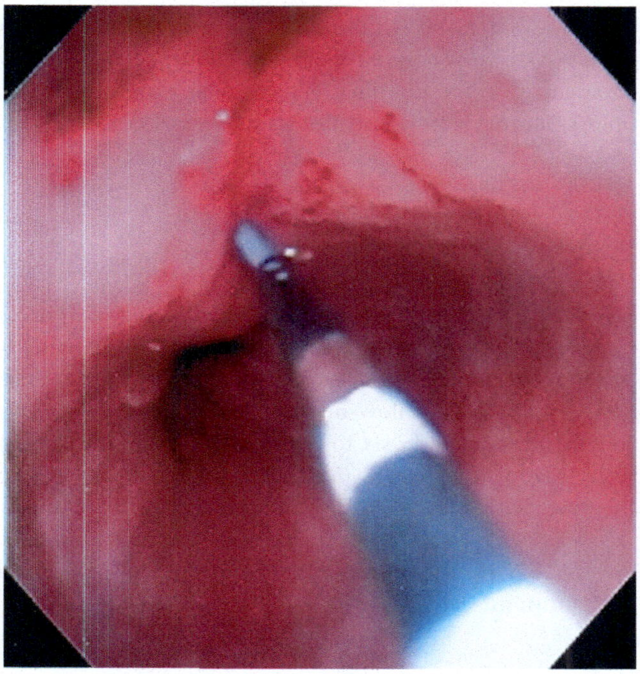

Figure 33.8 The transmural tract is dilated using a 5-Fr endoscopic retrograde cholangiopancreatography (ERCP) cannula.

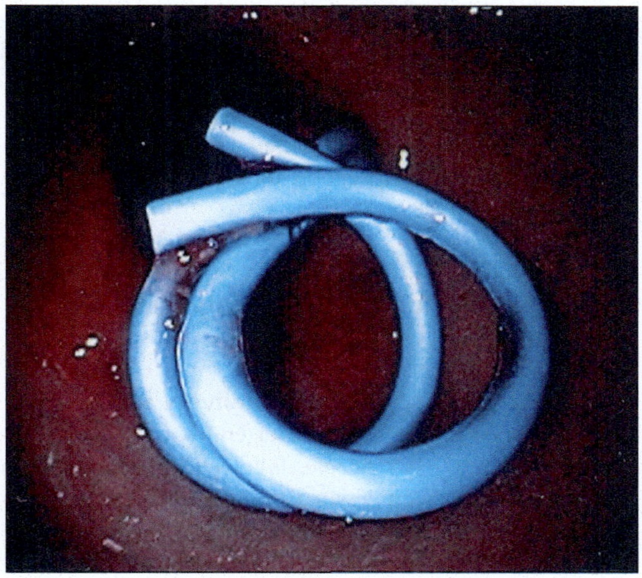

Figure 33.10 Multiple 7-Fr transmural stents are deployed (fluoroscopy view) to facilitate drainage of pseudocyst contents.

Stent deployment

Depending on the fluid consistency, a 7 or 10-Fr double pigtail stent is deployed after transmural tract dilation (Figure 33.10). It is preferable to place more than one stent in large cysts. Multiple wires can be placed at one time if 7-Fr stents are being deployed. Multiple wires should not be placed when 10-Fr stents are deployed due to the small diameter of the echoendoscope channel. In such cases, it is better to cannulate again for subsequent deployment of individual 10-Fr stents. During stent deployment, it is vital to keep the tip of the echoendoscope straight to avoid resistance. Sometimes, the thick viscous fluid from the PC can

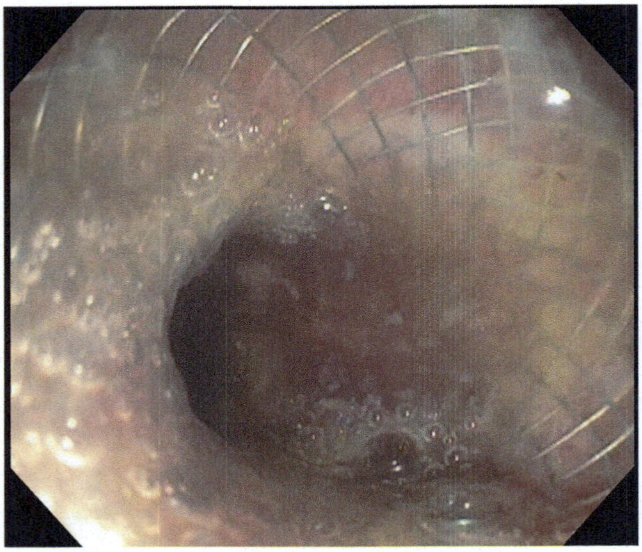
(a)

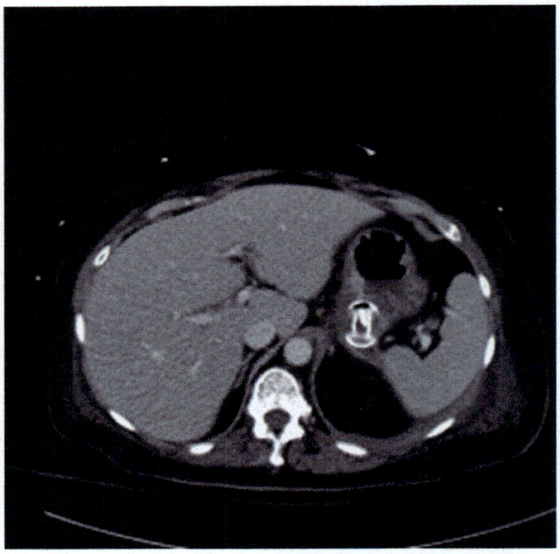
(b)

Figure 33.11 (a) Endoscopic view of the proximal flange of the LAMS in the stomach lumen with drainage of cyst contents. (b) CT of the abdomen demonstrating the LAMS placed for drainage of pseudocyst.

clog the biopsy channel and create friction during stent passage. This can be minimized by spraying PAM® (a cooking lubricant) through the biopsy channel prior to stent passage. Pseudocysts with large amounts of debris may require placement of a nasocystic drainage catheter (in addition to stents) to facilitate continuous irrigation and evacuation of cyst contents over a few days.

Technique for lumen-apposing metal stent placement

Non-electrocautery-enhanced delivery system

The pseudocyst is punctured under endosonographic guidance using a 19G FNA needle, followed by insertion of a 0.025- or 0.035-inch guidewire through the needle, which is looped inside the cavity. The transmural tract is then sequentially dilated using first an ERCP cannula, needle knife catheter or a cystotome, followed by a 4–6 mm dilating balloon. Excessive dilation must be avoided in order to prevent stent migration. LAMS on a delivery system is then inserted over the guidewire into the pseudocyst cavity. The distal flange is first deployed under endosonographic guidance, followed by deployment of the proximal flange under either endosonographic or endoscopic view.

Electrocautery-enhanced delivery system

The pseudocyst is directly punctured (without the need for a guidewire) using the electrocautery-enhanced tip of the stent delivery system under endosonographic guidance. The delivery system is then advanced into the PC and the distal flange is deployed first under endosonographic guidance, followed by deployment of the proximal flange under endosonographic or endoscopic view (Figure 33.11 and Video 33.2).

Post-procedure follow-up

After the procedure, the patient is observed for signs of infection, bleeding, or pancreatitis. The majority of patients can resume oral intake the same day. Antibiotics are continued for 48 hours. A follow-up computed tomography (CT) is usually undertaken in six to eight weeks (for plastic stents) or in three to four weeks (for LAMS) to assess response to therapy. However, following the procedure, if a patient develops persistent pain, unremitting fever, chills or leukocytosis, a CT scan should be obtained to rule out procedural complications.

Chapter video clips

Video 33.1 Technique of EUS-guided pseudocyst drainage. Source: The University of Alabama.

Video 33.2 Technique of EUS-guided LAMS placement for drainage of pancreatic fluid collection.

34 How to do EUS-guided Pancreatic Cyst Chemoablation

Matthew T. Moyer[1] and John M. DeWitt[2]

[1] Division of Gastroenterology and Hepatology, Penn State Hershey Medical Center, Hershey, PA, USA
[2] Division of Gastroenterology and Hepatology, Indiana University Medical Center, Indianapolis, IN, USA

Background

Few areas in medicine are as controversial as the diagnosis and management of mucinous-type pancreatic cysts. Guidelines on the subject are often discordant and based on expert opinion, with the 2017 Fukuoka and 2018 American College of Gastroenterology (ACG) guidelines the most recent and generally the most widely accepted [1,2]. Endoscopic ultrasound (EUS)-guided pancreatic cyst chemoablation is a promising, rapidly evolving, and minimally invasive approach for the treatment of mucinous-type pancreatic cysts. Here, we present a clinical and technical review of EUS-guided ablationE with our recommendations on the indications, contraindications, and appropriate patient selection, and a technical review of the performance of the procedure as well as follow-up.

A lethal malignancy, pancreatic cancer carries a dismal five-year survival rate of 8% and has the lowest survival rate of any major cancer. It is projected to surpass colorectal cancer as the second-leading cause of cancer-related death by 2030 unless breakthroughs in prevention and therapy occur, as we have seen in colorectal cancer [3–5]. The etiology of approximately 80% of pancreatic cancer is ductal adenocarcinoma; however, at least 20% of pancreatic cancer stems from the progressive degeneration of mucinous-type pancreatic cysts [6]. Occurring in over 2% of US adults overall, the prevalence of pancreatic cysts has grown dramatically over the last 20 years due to an aging population and advances in imaging techniques, leading to a public health dilemma. The majority of pancreatic cysts are neoplastic and include mucinous cystic neoplasm (MCN) and intraductal papillary mucinous neoplasm (IPMN) which carry significant potential for malignant transformation [4]. The overall risk of progression to malignancy for a mucinous cyst ranges from 1 to over 50% and is generally linked to its number of high-risk features, per consensus criteria [1,2]. Identification of a mucinous pancreatic cyst requires the patient and clinician to choose between indefinite radiographic surveillance by computed tomography (CT) or magnetic resonance imaging (MRI) or surgical resection, both of which have considerable limitations. Radiographic surveillance is nontherapeutic and carries significant financial and psychological burdens, while surgical resection poses a substantial risk for serious adverse events (20–40%) and mortality (1–5%). In fact, a recent randomized controlled trial showed the mortality of Whipple surgery to be as high as 10%, even in high-volume centers [7–10]. Moreover; subtotal pancreatectomy still requires postoperative and long-term surveillance for IPMNs. This clinical dilemma presents a pressing need to develop a minimally invasive but effective and efficient approach for this patient population in desperate need of improved treatment options. In this respect, EUS-guided pancreatic cyst chemoablation has emerged as an innovative and promising minimally invasive approach for the treatment of pancreatic cysts [11–13].

EUS-guided pancreatic cyst ablation was first described using cyst lavage with dehydrated alcohol; however, cyst ablation using alcohol lavage alone was hampered by low efficacy and an adverse event rate of 2–24%, generally felt to be due to the inflammatory and toxic effects of the alcohol on pancreatic parenchyma and/or neighboring vessels. Consequently, the use of alcohol lavage alone for cyst ablation has largely been abandoned. The more contemporary approach of cyst ablation involves cyst aspiration followed by three to five minutes of alcohol lavage, followed by near-complete aspiration and then instillation of paclitaxel 6 mg/ml, which is often partially diluted due its high viscosity. Complete ablation rates using this two-step technique are reported at 50–79% and this significant increase in efficacy over alcohol alone has resulted in this combination therapy becoming the most widely reported approach for pancreatic cyst ablation over the last 10 years, offering complete

Atlas of Endoscopic Ultrasonography, Second Edition. Edited by Frank Gress, Thomas Savides, Brenna Casey, and Everson L. A. Artifon.

Companion website: www.wiley.com/go/gress/atlas

ablation rates similar to that seen in other ablative strategies in gastroenterology. However, despite its increased efficacy, a significant limitation of alcohol lavage and paclitaxel injection continues to be serious adverse events of pancreatitis, peritonitis and venous thromboembolism, occurring in up to 10% of patients, again likely due to the potent inflammatory and toxic effects of alcohol on the adjacent pancreatic parenchyma and neighboring vessels. A summary of all studies using a prospective design and employing alcohol or alcohol followed by chemoablation is shown in Table 34.1.

In 2017, the randomized, prospective, double-blind CHARM trial was published, demonstrating the clinical value of a completely alcohol-free chemoablation approach. In this study, 39 patients were randomized to initial alcohol or saline lavage, with both arms then treated with a chemoablation cocktail tailored specifically for pancreatic neoplasia (38 mg gemcitabine mixed with 6 mg/mL of paclitaxel). At one year, 61% of patients in the alcohol arm achieved complete ablation, compared with 67% in the alcohol-free arm, showing that alcohol is not required for effective pancreatic cyst ablation when a chemotherapy cocktail specifically designed for pancreatic neoplasia is used. More importantly, the rate of adverse events was significantly lower in the alcohol-free arm ($P = 0.01$) with minor adverse events of abdominal pain (22%) and serious adverse events of pancreatitis (6%) both limited to the alcohol arm, collectively showing that the removal of alcohol from pancreatic cyst ablation reduces adverse events to rates similar to those of EUS-FNA [21]. The results of this randomized clinical trial indicate that an alcohol-free EUS-guided ablation approach is an improved therapeutic option for the treatment of mucinous-type pancreatic cysts and has led to a larger, randomized, prospective, multicenter, National Institutes of Health-funded trial which incorporates several technical improvements with results expected in the next five years [22].

There have been concerns raised regarding the long-term durability of pancreatic cyst ablation since the tumor is ablated and not surgically resected [23]. However, in a recent comprehensive evaluation of long-term efficacy, Choi et al. [24] reported the results of 164 patients who underwent EUS-guided ablation with ethanol followed by paclitaxel. In this study, 72% of patients achieved complete cyst ablation, and over a six-year follow-up period 98% of these remained in complete remission. The authors concluded that this treatment approach is an effective and durable alternative to surgery in appropriately selected patients.

Pretreatment evaluation

It is our recommendation that patients considered for EUS-guided cyst ablation should undergo a full evaluation in a clinic setting where their clinical, radiographic and endoscopic status can be reviewed in discussion with the clinician. Important issues to discuss are the natural history of these tumors, the rationale, risks and benefits of an ablation strategy, areas of uncertainty, and conventional options of surveillance and/or surgical resection as appropriate. A detailed informed consent is mandatory, and it is the recommendation of a soon-to-be published international white paper that these procedures be performed by an interventional endoscopist with formal training in EUS from a credentialed program who is familiar with interventional EUS procedures. Additionally, it is our recommendation that these procedures be performed in a high-volume referral center in a multidisciplinary environment, with appropriate follow-up and a formal quality assurance process.

Patient selection

In order to be effective, EUS-guided pancreatic cyst ablation should not be performed on lesions with certain high-risk features or a high likelihood of malignancy that may impede effective treatment. Conversely, therapy should be avoided in small low-risk pancreatic cysts with little chance of malignant progression and more appropriate for radiographic surveillance as per guidelines. Ablative strategies should be focused on cystic tumors that are technically amendable to ablation and do not show overt signs of malignancy.

Only cysts with a significant likelihood of progression to malignancy can be reasonably considered candidates for ablation. For that reason, the first step in the evaluation is to use clinical, radiographic, cytologic, and chemical analysis from EUS-FNA to diagnose and risk stratify a mucinous type cyst [25]. High-quality data indicate that the overall risk of developing malignancy in a pancreatic cyst measuring 1.5 cm or smaller (without other worrisome features) is less than 1% [26]. Additionally, performing effective EUS-guided cyst ablation in lesions smaller than 1.5 cm is technically difficult, and as the FNA needle itself has a volume of 0.8 ml this prohibits meaningful exchange of chemotherapeutic agent. A minimum size of 2 cm had been previously proposed for surgical resection in patients who are good surgical candidates due to an increased cumulative risk of malignant progression in cystic lesions starting at this size over a patient's lifetime [27]. Consequently, it is our recommendation that mucinous pancreatic cysts ranging in size from 2 to 6 cm meet appropriate size criteria and are the typical range reported in most trials to date [11–13].

The overall structure of a cyst is also an important consideration because multiseptated mucinous cysts (ex. "cluster of grapes" type IPMN) present a technical challenge to ablation since treatment must reach each discrete loculated chamber within a cyst in order to ensure complete ablation. Thus, most trials to date have favored treatment of unilocular or oligolocular cyst morphology and have avoided ablation

Table 34.1 Summary of EUS-guided ablation trials (only studies with a prospective design are included).

	Author, year	Study type	Protocol (no. of patients)	Complete (CR) or partial resolution (PR)	Clinically significant adverse events[a]
EtOH lavage only	Gan et al. (2005) [14]	Prospective (pilot)	5–80% EtOH (25)	35% CR 7% PR	0%
	Dewitt et al. (2009) [15]	Prospective (RCT)	80% EtOH (25) Saline (17)	33% CR 0% CR	24% (4% pancreatitis, 20% abdominal pain) 12% (abdominal pain)
	Gomez et al. (2016) [16]	Prospective (pilot)	80% EtOH (23)	9% CR 44% PR	8% (4% pancreatitis, 4% abdominal pain)
EtOH lavage + paclitaxel infusion	Oh et al. (2008) [17]	Prospective	88–99% EtOH + paclitaxel (14)	79% CR 14% PR	21% (7% pancreatitis, 14% abdominal pain)
	Oh et al. (2009) [18]	Prospective	99% EtOH + paclitaxel (10)	60% CR 20% PR	10% (abdominal pain)
	Oh et al. (2011) [19]	Prospective	99% EtOH + paclitaxel (47)	62% CR 13% PR	4% (2% pancreatitis, 2% abdominal pain)
	DeWitt et al. (2014) [20]	Prospective	100% EtOH + paclitaxel (22)	50% CR 25% PR	23% (10% pancreatitis, 13% abdominal pain)
EtOH lavage + paclitaxel/gemcitabine infusion vs. saline lavage + paclitaxel/gemcitabine infusion	Moyer et al. (2017) [21]	Prospective (RCT)	80% EtOH + paclitaxel/gemcitabine (18) Saline + paclitaxel/gemcitabine (21)	61% CR 67% CR	28% (6% pancreatitis, 22% abdominal pain) 0%[b]

[a] Clinically significant adverse events are presented as an aggregate of the two most common (pancreatitis and abdominal pain). Based on the reported results, it cannot be determined if adverse events overlapped (e.g. a patient who developed pancreatitis also reported abdominal pain). Rare types of adverse events were single events and include peripancreatic fluid collection [19], splenic vein obliteration [19], development of an inflammatory gastric wall cyst [20], and peritonitis [20].

[b] Note the significant drop in adverse events when alcohol-free EUS-guided cyst ablation was used, indicating a significant increase in safety when an alcohol-free protocol is used.

EtOH, ethyl alcohol; RCT, randomized controlled trial.

in lesions with more than four or five discrete loculations [11–13]. When reviewing previous trials and the experience at our centers, our general recommendations for indications and contraindications for pancreatic cyst ablation can be summarized as follows and used to guide therapy.

Indications

Patients with previously identified pancreatic cysts ranging from 2 to 6 cm in diameter which are consistent with mucinous-type cysts as per guidelines [25] including indeterminate-type cysts.

Contraindications

- Pregnancy.
- Less than a three to five year life expectancy (does not merit treatment of a precancerous lesion).
- Inability to safely undergo a 30–60 minute procedure with monitored anesthesia.
- Signs of malignancy or cytology suspicious for malignancy.
- Benign cysts with little or no malignant potential (pseudocyst, serous cystadenoma, lymphangioma, or duplication cyst) as determined by clinical, radiographic, cytologic, and chemical analysis.

Relative contraindications

Cysts with the following high-risk features.

- Main pancreatic duct dilation greater than 5 mm.
- Epithelial-type mural nodules.
- Pathologically thick walls or septations.
- Cytology showing high-grade dysplasia.
- Signs of common bile duct or pancreatic duct obstruction, solid mass component within or associated with a cyst, pathologic lymphadenopathy associated with the cyst, pancreatic duct stricture associated with tail atrophy.
- Septated cysts with more than four to five discrete individual compartments.
- Irreversible coagulopathy, neutropenia, or thrombocytopenia with platelets below 30×10^9/l.

Technical aspects of the procedure

Patient preparation for pancreatic cyst ablation is similar to that for standard EUS-FNA. A discussion with the anesthesiologist is important to ensure that the patient will be relatively still during the actual ablation process and if excessive movement (such as coughing or retching) is felt to be likely, general anesthesia with paralysis should be considered. The ablative agents, including a lavage agent (if used), as well as the chemotherapy infusion (i.e. paclitaxel or paclitaxel plus gemcitabine) should be prepared prior to the procedure and laid out with the infusion device for ease of access during the procedure. The delivery, handling, and disposal of chemotherapy ablation agents should be standardized as per your institution's policies. After a full endosonographic evaluation, the FNA needle is introduced into the center of the cyst, carefully aspirating nearly the entire cyst contents. It is our practice to use a 22-gauge FNA needle for most cysts measuring 2–3 cm in diameter, and a 19-gauge needle for cysts over 3 cm or previously known to have a highly viscous fluid. If alcohol lavage is used, the near-complete cyst aspiration will be followed by alternately filling and aspirating the cyst with alcohol for three to five minutes, using an amount equal to the mucinous fluid originally aspirated. A rim of fluid should be kept around the needle tip at all times to avoid damaging the cyst wall and possibly injecting alcohol into the surrounding parenchyma. After the lavage agent is aspirated out (leaving a small amount of alcohol around the needle tip), the chemoablation agent is infused, replacing no more agent than is required to refill the cyst to its original volume and dimensions [11].

Based on the results of the randomized prospective CHARM trial, it is our practice to use a completely alcohol-free approach, which is simpler, faster, and safer than ablations that include alcohol lavage. In this approach, the lavage step of the procedure is eliminated and instead, after initial cyst aspiration, a mixture of gemcitabine (38 mg/mL) and paclitaxel (6 mg/mL) is infused into the cyst, using an amount equal to the volume of mucin originally aspirated and refilling the cyst to its original dimensions (Figure 34.1). Paclitaxel is highly viscous, and the infusion of the chemotherapy agent in a timely fashion through a 22- or 19-gauge FNA needle requires moderately high pressure, so an infusion apparatus such as a syringe strapped to a high-pressure gun or infusion device is often used [21] (Figure 34.2). Antibiotics are recommended as per ASGE guidelines on pancreatic cyst management, and it has been our approach to observe these patients for one hour postoperatively.

Postoperative care and follow-up

DiMaio et al. [28] demonstrated that serial cyst ablations (similar to the concepts for treating dysplastic Barrett's esophagus) are more effective than a single ablation session for pancreatic cystic tumors. Therefore, it is the approach at our institutions to schedule two to three alcohol-free gemcitabine–paclitaxel chemoablation infusions at three-month intervals where residual cyst at the second and third endoscopies measuring over 15 mm in diameter are retreated. This is followed by clinic evaluation and follow-up cross-sectional imaging 12 months after the last ablation with either enhanced MRI (preferred) or CT scan to measure treatment response and assess for complications (Figures 34.3 and 34.4). The definition of treatment response has been standardized over multiple studies and is based on cyst volume ($^4/_3\pi r^3$, where r is cyst radius) and is defined as complete

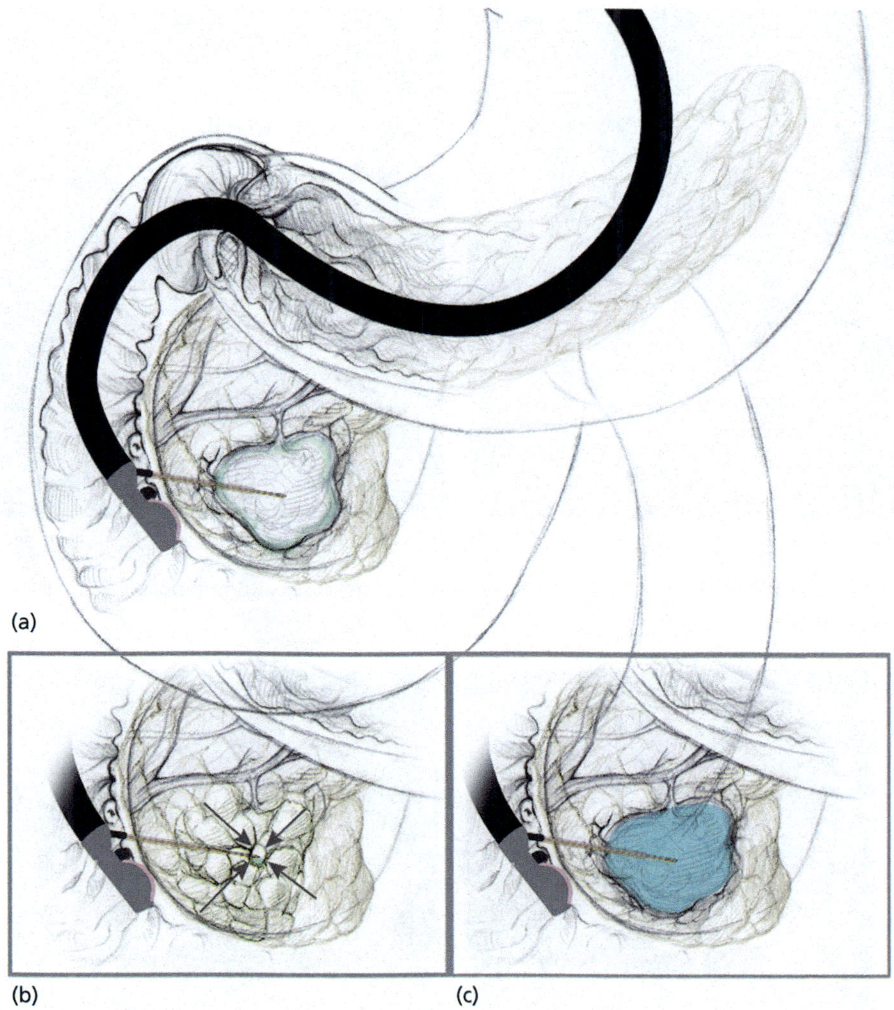

Figure 34.1 The alcohol free EUS-guided cyst ablation process. The FNA needle is introduced into the center of the cystic lesion (a). This is followed by near-complete aspiration of the mucinous fluid from all compartments, leaving a small amount of fluid around the needle tip to assure that the walls of the cyst are not injured (b). The cyst is then immediately refilled with the chemoablation agent, infusing the same volume as was originally aspirated, refilling the cyst to its original dimensions and volume (c). This alcohol-free approach is simpler, faster, and safer than protocols which use alcohol lavage as part of the ablation process.

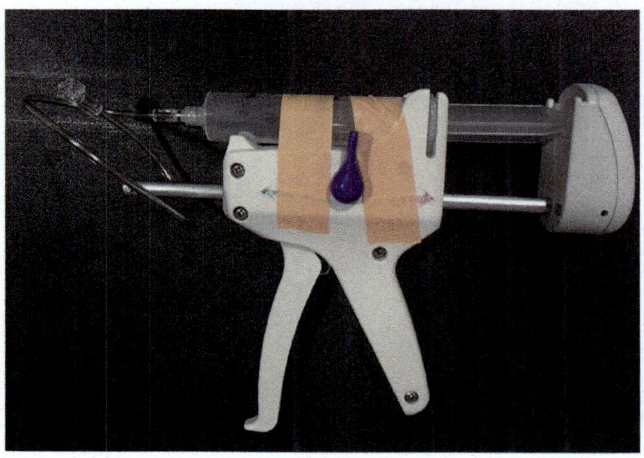

Figure 34.2 A high-pressure gun, syringe, and short connector tubing assembly which can be used to quickly infuse viscous ablation agents into a cyst after the mucinous fluid is aspirated.

(≥95% reduction of cyst volume), partial (94–75% reduction), or non-response (<75% reduction) at one-year follow-up [15–21]. It is our practice that patients then return for follow-up imaging one year later and subsequently re-enter a surveillance program using the post-treatment measurements and cyst characteristics to govern surveillance frequency [1,2].

It is important to acknowledge that even if a treated cyst achieves the definition of complete ablation, the patient's risk of developing pancreatic adenocarcinoma has likely been significantly reduced but not completely eliminated. Histologic assessment of residual cyst epithelium is not possible without surgical resection and there are no high-quality studies to date proving that cyst ablation prolongs life expectancy. Two large retrospective multicenter Japanese studies demonstrate that in patients under long-term surveillance for IPMN (some of which had been treated

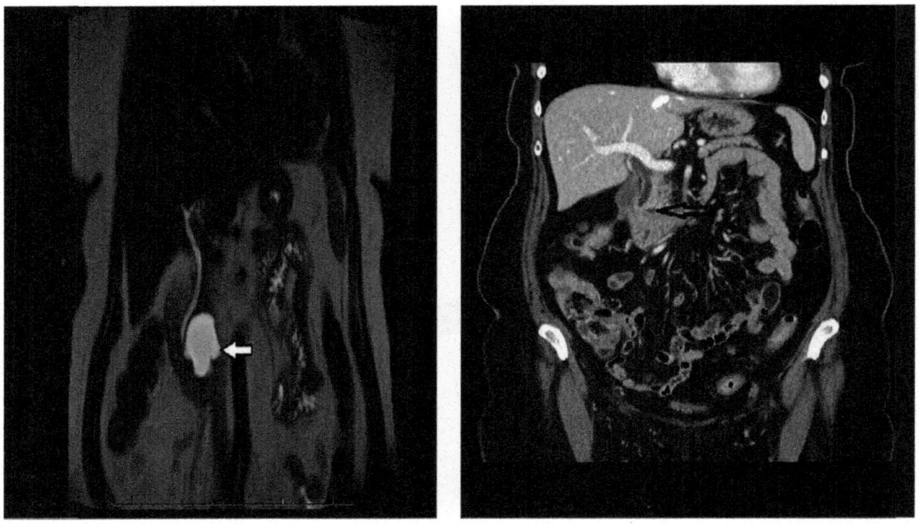

(a) (b)

Figure 34.3 (a) Magnetic resonance image showing a 76-year-old female with a 4.2-cm mucinous-type (premalignant) pancreatic cyst (white arrow) before EUS-guided chemoablation. (b) CT image showing a 4-mm residual defect at one year (black arrow).

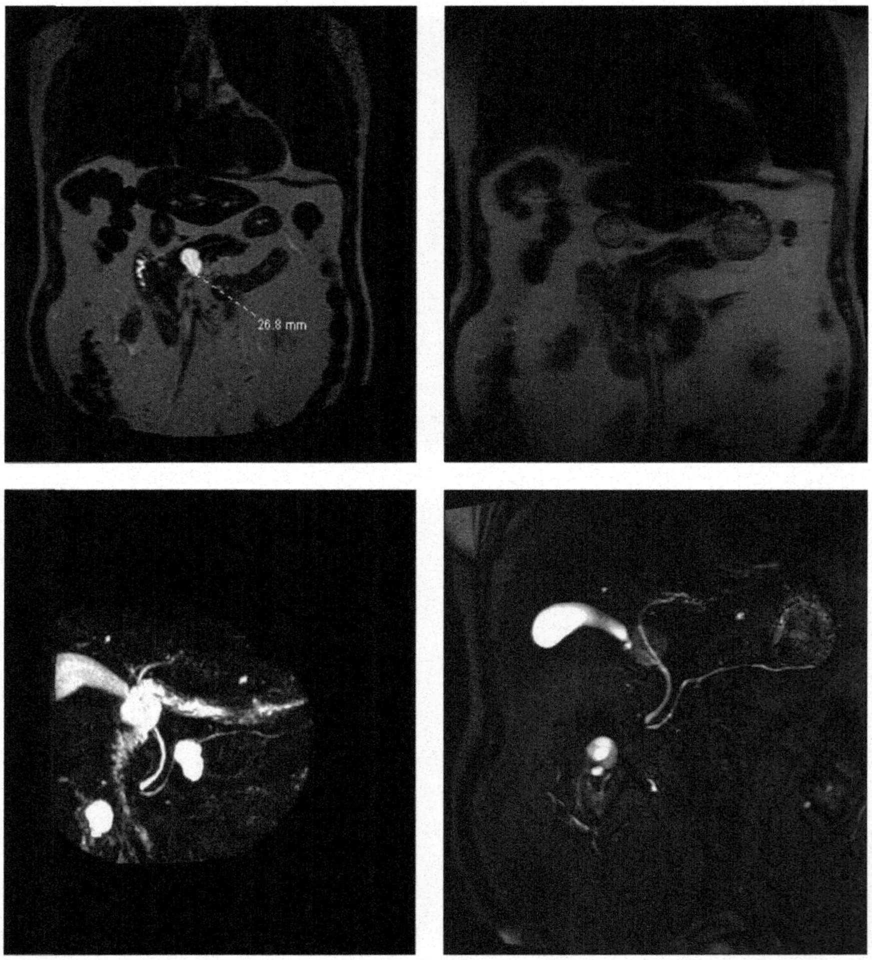

(a) (b)

Figure 34.4 (a) MRI (*top*) and magnetic resonance cholangiopancreatography (MRCP) (*bottom*) of an 83-year-old male with a 2.7-cm intraductal mucinous pancreatic neoplasm prior to EUS-guided chemoablation. (b) Follow-up MRI (*top*) and MRCP (*bottom*) reveals no evidence of residual cyst at six-month follow-up evaluation.

surgically), there remains a 2–4% risk of developing a metachronous pancreatic malignancy in the remaining pancreas [29,30]. Additionally, recent evidence shows an ongoing and progressive risk of malignant transformation of IPMNs during long-term surveillance [26]. Consequently, even patients who achieve a complete ablation should remain in surveillance as long as further therapy would be appropriate; furthermore, whether a surgical, ablative or surveillance strategy is employed, the current understanding is that long-term surveillance will be required until patient age and/or comorbidities make further surveillance unwarranted.

Conclusions

EUS-guided pancreatic cyst ablation is a promising, rapidly evolving, and minimally invasive technique for the treatment of premalignant pancreatic cystic neoplasms, which currently have therapeutic options limited to either indefinite surveillance or major pancreatic surgery. Careful patient selection is paramount, as is careful attention to the technical aspects of the procedure, postprocedure care, clinical follow-up, and quality assurance. Recent clinical evidence indicates the durable treatment response of cyst ablation when a complete response is achieved and a significantly improved safety profile with an alcohol-free ablation protocol. This emerging technique significantly expands treatment options for appropriately selected patients; however, as is typical in most novel and innovative procedures, areas of uncertainty and controversy exist. Additional studies are needed to further develop the technique and to determine which patients are most appropriately offered this emerging treatment option based on efficacy, safety, patient satisfaction, and cost.

Chapter video clip

Video 34.1 How to perform EUS pancreatic cyst ablation.

References

1. Tanaka M, Castillo CF, Kamisawa T, et al. Revisions of international consensus Fukuoka guidelines for the management of IPMN of the pancreas. *Pancreatology* 2017;17(5):738–753.
2. Elta GH, Enestvedt BK, Sauer BG, Marie Lennon A. ACG clinical guideline: diagnosis and management of pancreatic cysts. *Am J Gastroenterol* 2018;113:464–479.
3. Rahib L, Smith BD, Aizenberg R, et al. Projecting cancer incidence and deaths to 2030: the unexpected burden of thyroid, liver, and pancreas cancers in the United States. *Cancer Res* 2014;74:2913–2921.
4. Ryan DP, Hong TS, Bardeesy N. Pancreatic adenocarcinoma. *N Engl J Med* 2014;371:1039–1049.
5. American Cancer Society. *Cancer facts and figures 2018*. Atlanta, GA: American Cancer Society, 2018.
6. Fernandez-Del Castillo C, Tanaka M. Management of pancreatic cysts: the evidence is not here yet. *Gastroenterology* 2015;148:685–687.
7. Clancy TE. Surgery for pancreatic cancer. *Hematol Oncol Clin North Am* 2015;29:701–716.
8. McPhee JT, Hill JS, Whalen GF, et al. Perioperative mortality for pancreatectomy: a national perspective. *Ann Surg* 2007;246: 246–253.
9. Amini N, Spolverato G, Kim Y, Pawlik TM. Trends in hospital volume and failure to rescue for pancreatic surgery. *J Gastrointest Surg* 2015;19:1581–1592.
10. van Hilst J, de Rooij T, Bosscha K, et al. Laparoscopic versus open pancreatoduodenectomy for pancreatic or periampullary tumours (LEOPARD-2): a multicenter, patient-blinded, randomized controlled phase 2/3 trial. *Lancet Gastroenterol Hepatol* 2019;4(3):199–207.
11. Oh HC, Brugge WR. EUS-guided pancreatic cyst ablation: a critical review (with video). *Gastrointest Endosc* 2013;77:526–533.
12. Cho MK, Choi JH, Seo DW. Endoscopic ultrasound-guided ablation therapy for pancreatic cysts. *Endosc Ultrasound* 2015;4:293–298.
13. Moyer MT, Maranki JL, DeWitt JM. EUS-guided pancreatic cyst ablation: a clinical and technical review. *Curr Gastroenterol Rep* 2019;21:19.
14. Gan SI, Thompson CC, Lauwers GY, et al. Ethanol lavage of pancreatic cystic lesions: initial pilot study. *Gastrointest Endosc* 2005;61:746–752.
15. DeWitt J, McGreevy K, Schmidt CM, Brugge WR. EUS-guided ethanol versus saline solution lavage for pancreatic cysts: a randomized, double-blind study. *Gastrointest Endosc* 2009; 70 :710–723.
16. Gomez V, Takahashi N, Levy MJ, et al. EUS-guided ethanol lavage does not reliably ablate pancreatic cystic neoplasms (with video). *Gastrointest Endosc* 2016;83:914–920.
17. Oh HC, Seo DW, Lee TY, et al. New treatment for cystic tumors of the pancreas: EUS-guided ethanol lavage with paclitaxel injection. *Gastrointest Endosc* 2008;67(4):636–642.
18. Oh HC, Seo DW, Kim SC, et al. Septated cystic tumors of the pancreas: is it possible to treat them by endoscopic ultrasonography-guided intervention? *Scand J Gastroenterol* 2009;44(2):242–247.
19. Oh HC, SeoDW, Song TJ, et al. Endoscopic ultrasonography guided ethanol lavage with paclitaxel injection treats patients with pancreatic cysts. *Gastroenterology* 2011;140(1):172–179.
20. DeWitt JM, Al-Haddad M, Sherman S, et al. Alterations in cyst fluid genetics following endoscopic ultrasound-guided pancreatic cyst ablation with ethanol and paclitaxel. *Endoscopy* 2014;46(6):457–464.
21. Moyer MT, Sharzehi S, Mathew A, et al. The safety and efficacy of an alcohol-free pancreatic cyst ablation protocol. *Gastroenterology* 2017;153:1295–1303.
22. Moyer MT, DeWitt JM, Gordon S, et al. Chemotherapy for the ablation and resolution of mucinous cysts: CHARM II: a randomized, prospective, multi-center trial. https://clinicaltrials.gov/ct2/show/NCT03085004.
23. Castillo CF. EUS treatment of pancreatic cysts: let's keep the alcohol (and the chemotherapy) locked in the cupboard. *Gastroenterology* 2011;140:2144–2151.

24. Choi JH, Seo DW, Song TJ, et al. Long term outcomes after endoscopic ultrasound-guided ablation of pancreatic cysts. *Endoscopy* 2017;49:866–873.

25. ASGE Standards of Practice Committee. The role of endoscopy in the diagnosis and treatment of cystic pancreatic neoplasms. *Gastrointest Endosc* 2016;84:1–9.

26. Pergolini I, Sahora K, Ferrone CR, et al. Long-term risk of pancreatic malignancy in patients with branch duct intraductal papillary mucinous neoplasm in a referral center. *Gastroenterology* 2017;153:1284–1294.

27. Weinberg BM, Spiegel BM, Tomlinson JS, et al. Asymptomatic pancreatic cystic neoplasms: maximizing survival and quality of life using Markov-based clinical nomograms. *Gastroenterology* 2010;135:531–540.

28. DiMaio CJ, DeWitt JM, Brugge WR. Ablation of pancreatic cystic lesions: the use of multiple endoscopic ultrasound-guided ethanol lavage sessions. *Pancreas* 2011;40(5):664–668.

29. Maguchi H, Tanno S, Mizuno N, et al. Natural history of branch duct intraductal papillary mucinous neoplasms of the pancreas: a multicenter study in Japan. *Pancreas* 2011;40:364–370.

30. Tanno S, Nakano Y, Koizumi K, et al. Pancreatic ductal adenocarcinomas in long-term follow-up patients with branch duct intraductal papillary mucinous neoplasms. *Pancreas* 2010;39:36–40.

35 How to do Celiac Plexus Block

Sam M. Serouya[1] and Adam J. Goodman[2]
[1] NYU Langone Grossman School of Medicine, New York, NY, USA
[2] NYU Langone Health, New York, NY, USA

Introduction

Pain that develops as a result of pancreatic cancer (Figure 35.1) or chronic pancreatitis (Figure 35.2) is often difficult to manage. Up to 90% of patients with advanced pancreatic cancer report pain that significantly impacts their quality of life. Various methods have been used to treat these patients including narcotic analgesia, antidepressants, pancreatic enzymes, octreotide, denervation procedures, and palliative or decompression/drainage procedures. Opioid analgesics can sometimes effectively treat pain, but are often inadequate and can be associated with numerous side effects including constipation, delirium, nausea, and the potential for addiction. Non-pharmacologic methods of pain control, such as celiac plexus block or neurolysis, may improve quality of life and minimize drug-related side effects.

The celiac plexus lies anterior to the aorta at the level of the celiac artery (Figure 35.3). Most of the sensory nerves returning from the pancreas and other intra-abdominal viscera pass through the celiac ganglion and splanchnic nerves and interruption of these fibers may lessen pain in pancreatic malignancies and chronic pancreatitis. Celiac plexus block (CPB) is a temporizing treatment where a steroid and long-acting local anesthetic are injected into the celiac plexus to control pain associated with chronic pancreatitis. Celiac plexus neurolysis (CPN) is used in patients with pancreatic cancer and refers to the injection of alcohol or phenol, a more permanent agent, into the celiac plexus in an attempt to ablate the nerve fibers that transmit pain.

The history of CPN dates back to 1914 when Kappis and colleagues described an intraoperative procedure. Many decades later, in 1996, the first endoscopic ultrasound (EUS)-guided CPB/CPN was described by both Faigel and colleagues, and Wiersema and colleagues. Then, in 1999, Gress and colleagues described the first case of EUS-guided CPB for chronic pancreatitis.

The efficacy of CPN for the treatment of cancer pain has been demonstrated in a number of studies, with pain control in 70–90% of patients up to three months after the procedure. CPB may have a role in the treatment of pain related to chronic pancreatitis. One study consisting of 18 patients with chronic pancreatitis noted a reduction in pain in 50% (5/10) of patients undergoing EUS-guided CPB compared with 25% (2/8) of patients undergoing computed tomography (CT)-guided blocks. The benefit persisted for up to 24 weeks in 30% of responders. Other studies have demonstrated significant improvement in overall pain scores in approximately 55% of patients at up to eight weeks of follow-up; however, only 10% of patients noted a persistent benefit beyond 24 weeks. These studies have also demonstrated that response to the first EUS-CPB is associated with response to subsequent blocks, thus suggesting repeat procedures will be of benefit to the patient.

Technique (Video 35.1)

Patients with inoperable pancreatic cancer and pain requiring narcotic analgesics are potential candidates for CPN. Selection of patients with pain related to chronic pancreatitis for CPB is less clear; however, patients wishing to avoid narcotics or those with pain refractory to high doses of narcotics may be appropriate candidates. Patients should be selected carefully, with contraindications including platelets less than 50×10^9/l, coagulopathy, disulfiram use, and prior bowel obstruction secondary to CPB/CPN.

Prior to the procedure the patient is hydrated with intravenous saline (500–1000 ml), in order to prevent postprocedural hypotension. The patient is then placed in the left lateral decubitus position and sedation is administered. The linear array echoendoscope is advanced to just below the gastroesophageal junction where a sagittal view of the aorta

Atlas of Endoscopic Ultrasonography, Second Edition. Edited by Frank Gress, Thomas Savides, Brenna Casey, and Everson L. A. Artifon.

Companion website: www.wiley.com/go/gress/atlas

is obtained through the posterior gastric wall. The aorta is traced to the celiac trunk, the first large vessel emerging off the aorta, and the second branch is usually easily identified as the superior mesenteric artery (Figure 35.4). Identifying both the celiac and superior mesenteric arteries helps to confirm correct location. Color flow Doppler should be used to exclude any intervening vessels.

The stylet is removed from a fine needle aspiration (FNA) needle and the entire system is flushed with normal saline to remove any air as this can interfere with imaging. Using real-time imaging, the FNA needle is inserted immediately lateral and anterior to the aorta at the level of the celiac trunk via a transgastric approach (Figure 35.5). A small amount (2 ml) of 0.9% saline is injected to clear the needle. An assistant then aspirates a 10-ml syringe filled with 0.9% saline for approximately 10 seconds. This is to confirm that the needle is not within any of the regional blood vessels.

Injections into the celiac axis can be performed in two ways: one in which the injection is performed with the entire amount of medication infused at a single site at the base of the celiac artery take-off, and one in which injections are performed by rotating to each side of the celiac trunk. For CPB, 20 ml of preservative-free bupivacaine (0.25%) followed by 80 mg of triamcinolone is injected, followed by 3–5 ml of saline. For CPN, 20 ml of bupivacaine (0.25%) followed by 20 ml of dehydrated alcohol is injected at the base

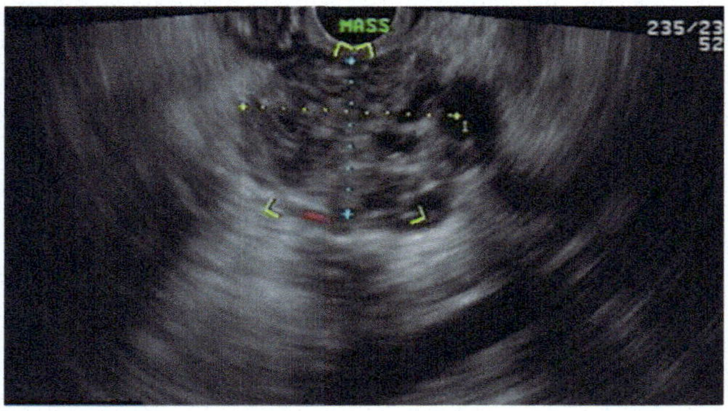

Figure 35.1 Hypoechoic pancreatic mass as seen by EUS.

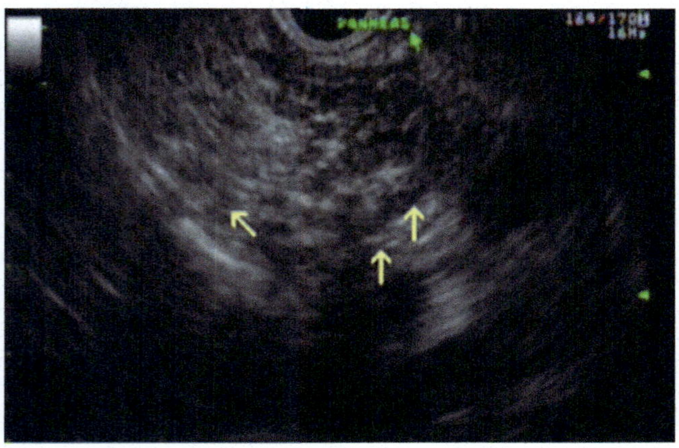

Figure 35.2 Endoscopic ultrasound demonstration of lobularity, one of the major criteria to help diagnose chronic pancreatitis by EUS.

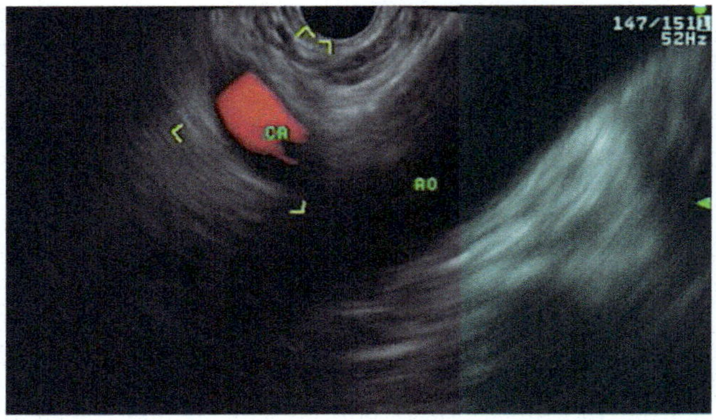

Figure 35.3 Celiac axis (CA) as seen by EUS. AO, aorta.

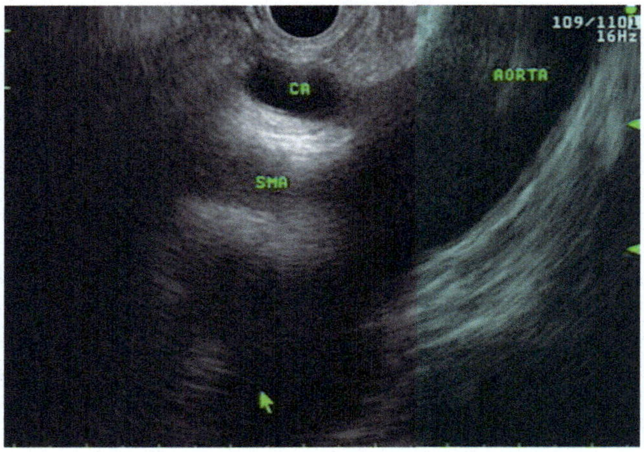

Figure 35.4 Celiac axis confirmed by the aorta, celiac artery (CA) and superior mesenteric artery (SMA).

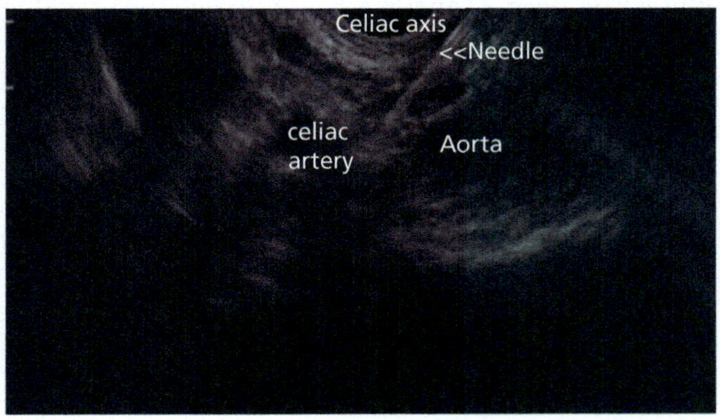

Figure 35.5 Insertion of the EUS-guided fine needle aspiration needle into the area of the celiac axis.

of the celiac artery. After alcohol injection, the needle is flushed with 3 ml of saline prior to withdrawal.

Alternatively, two separate injections are performed by rotating to each side of the celiac trunk. With this technique, 10 ml of bupivacaine (0.25%) and 10 ml of dehydrated alcohol in CPN and 10 ml of bupivacaine (0.25%) followed by 40 mg (1 ml) of triamcinolone in CPB are injected on each side of the celiac trunk. The aspiration test is repeated before each injection. It is believed that the two techniques have similar results.

The examination usually takes 30 minutes and is performed on an outpatient basis. Recovery time is usually two hours. Before discharge, orthostatic blood pressure changes should be checked, and patients should be counseled regarding potential complications.

Complications

Endoscopic ultrasound-guided CPB and CPN are generally effective, safe, and well-tolerated procedures. The three most common complications are transient hypotension (20–40%) due to dilation of the splanchnic vasculature, transient diarrhea (4–38%) due to blockade of the sympathetic innervation of the abdominal viscera and unopposed parasympathetic activity, and transient increase in pain (9%). These symptoms are usually limited to two days post procedure. Less common complications include unilateral paresis or paraplegia, pneumothorax, loss of sphincter function, retroperitoneal bleeding, renal puncture, and prolonged gastroparesis. In addition, cephalic spread of the neurolytic agent may result in involvement of the cardiac nerves and plexus. Infectious complications are uncommon but potentially serious. In a series of 90 patients, only one patient developed an infectious complication (a peripancreatic abscess), which resolved with a two-week course of antibiotics.

Chapter video clip

Video 35.1 How to do celiac plexus block.

36 How to Place Fiducials for Radiation Therapy

Antonio R. Cheesman, Satish Nagula, and Christopher J. DiMaio
Icahn School of Medicine at Mount Sinai, New York, NY, USA

Introduction

Traditional radiation therapy (RT), involving the delivery of high doses of toxic radiation to a target field, is wrought with the unfortunate consequence of acute and chronic injury to healthy tissue adjacent to the tumor. The development of real-time image-guided radiation therapy (IGRT) systems allows for the safe delivery of focal high-dose RT to target lesions while minimizing the amount of collateral damage to normal tissue. These techniques, such as stereotactic radiosurgery and intensity-modulated RT, allow for the precise delivery of RT by being able to verify the target location and track its movement during the respiratory cycle. IGRT is dependent on reference points by which the target lesion can be identified and tracked. Fiducials are inert radiographic markers which are implanted into the target lesion for this purpose. Given the ability of endoscopic ultrasound (EUS) to allow for close proximity to structures in the mediastinum, abdomen, and pelvis that may not otherwise be accessible by percutaneous approaches, the use of EUS-guided fiducial placement into both luminal and extraluminal targets has become an accepted technique.

Equipment

Fiducials and needles

Several types of fiducial markers and delivery systems exist. Traditional fiducials are cylindrical gold seeds measuring 3–5 mm in length by 0.75–1.2 mm in diameter, and are deployed using a 19-gauge fine needle aspiration (FNA) needle.

Newer fiducial designs aim to reduce fiducial migration. Coiled fiducials (Visicoil; IBA Dosimetry, Memphis, TN) are flexible gold coil markers measuring 5–30 mm in length by 0.35–1.1 mm in diameter, and are deployed using a needle-carrier delivery device that fits a 22-gauge FNA needle. (Figure 36.1 and Video 36.1) Notched fiducials (Gold anchor; Naslund Medical Inc., Chicago, IL) are 10–20 mm in length by 0.28–0.4 mm in diameter, and can be deployed using a 22- to 25-gauge FNA needle. These have notches every 2 mm and can take a linear or circular configuration by withdrawing the needle versus pushing the fiducial forward during deployment. Band fiducials (X-seed and X-mark; ONC Solutions Inc., Acton, MA) are 5 mm or 10–30 mm long by 0.85 or 1.15 mm in diameter and consist of separate gold bands overlying a central axle, permitting tissue ingrowth. These fiducials are deployed using 17- or 18-gauge needles and thus may have limited applications for EUS-guided implantation given the lack of availability of these FNA needle sizes.

Multi-fiducial delivery systems also exist. These include a two 5-mm long by 0.43–0.75-mm diameter fiducial system deployed using a 19- or 22-gauge needle (Beacon™ FNF Pre-loaded Needle; Medtronic, Minneapolis MN) and a four 5-mm long by 0.43-mm diameter fiducial system delivered using a 22-gauge needle (EchoTip® Ultra Fiducial Needle; Cook Medical, Bloomington, IN).

Finally, novel radiopaque hydrogel markers (TraceIT Tissue Marker; Augmenix Inc., Bedford, MA) have been designed to fade after three months, and consist of iodinated polyethylene glycol hydrogel particles which can be delivered using a 25-gauge FNA needle.

The available literature suggests traditional fiducials maintain better visibility, newer devices appear to offer limited benefit in migration rates, while wider-diameter fiducials requiring 19-gauge needles are associated with limited endoscope angulation resulting in suboptimal target visualization and increased technical failure rates.

Atlas of Endoscopic Ultrasonography, Second Edition. Edited by Frank Gress, Thomas Savides, Brenna Casey, and Everson L. A. Artifon.

Companion website: www.wiley.com/go/gress/atlas

Techniques

Fiducial loading and deployment

Fiducials not preloaded on a delivery system can be loaded into EUS needles and deployed using various techniques. The *back-loading, dry deployment* method requires withdrawal of the stylet 2–3 cm from the needle tip, back-loading the fiducial into the needle lumen and sealing the needle tip using bone wax; deployment is performed by advancing the stylet. Otherwise, the *back-loading, hydraulic deployment* technique requires complete removal of the stylet, filling the needle channel with sterile water, back-loading the fiducial into the needle lumen and sealing the needle tip using bone wax; deployment is achieved by injecting 1–2 ml of sterile water through the needle channel. Finally, the *back-loading, wet-fill* method is performed by retracting the stylet while the needle is submerged in sterile water, and back-loading the fiducial into the needle lumen without the need to seal the needle tip owing to surface tension; deployment is performed by pushing the stylet.

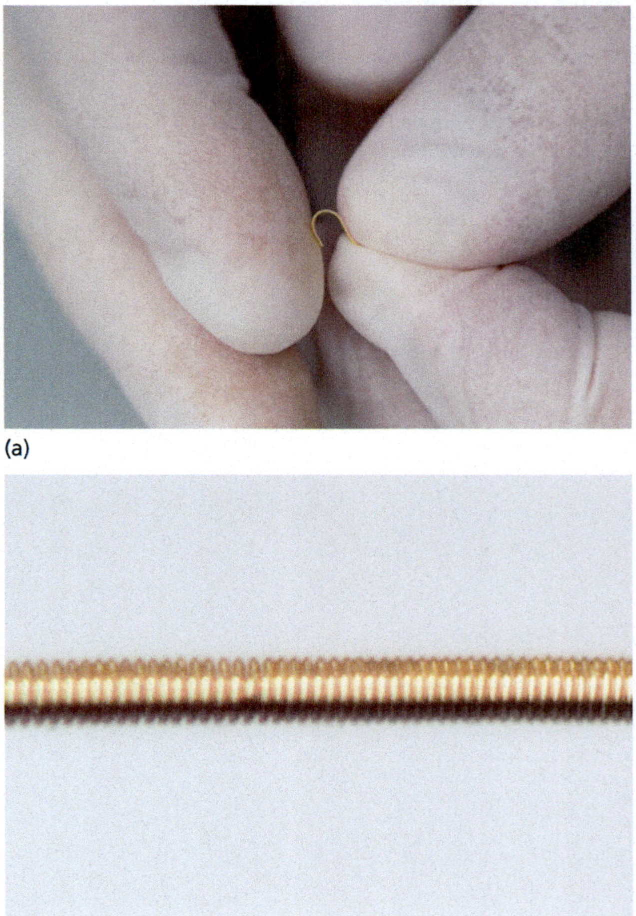

(a)

(b)

Figure 36.1 Gold coil fiducial marker is (a) flexible and (b) has a coiled design.

Contrary to the latter techniques, where placement of each fiducial involves needle withdrawal, the *push-stylet technique* or *front-loading approach* allows for insertion of multiple fiducials without needle withdrawal. This is performed by inserting the needle into the target lesion without a preloaded fiducial, fully withdrawing the stylet, front-loading the fiducials through the needle handle and advancing them by reinserting the stylet.

Finally, coiled fiducials (Figure 36.2 and Videos 36.1 and 36.2), multi-fiducial delivery systems, and radiopaque hydrogel markers have carrier delivery devices that facilitate loading and deployment.

EUS-guided fiducial placement (Video 36.3)

EUS-guided fiducial placement is performed with standard linear echoendoscopes. Doppler is typically used to identify and avoid vessels in the path of the needle. Once a safe window has been identified, the needle is inserted into the target lesion under EUS guidance (Figure 36.3).

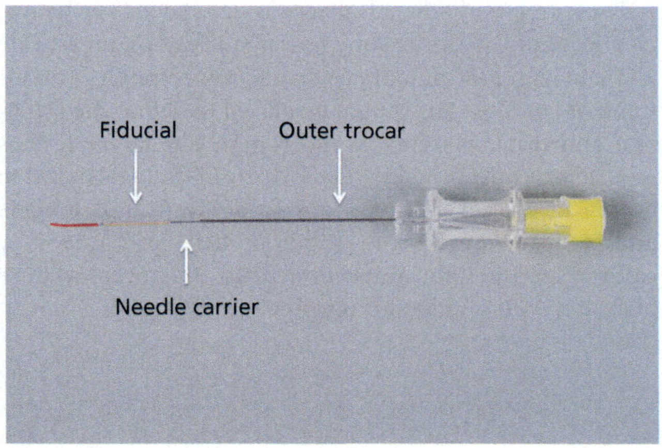

Figure 36.2 Gold coil fiducial preloaded on needle-carrier delivery device.

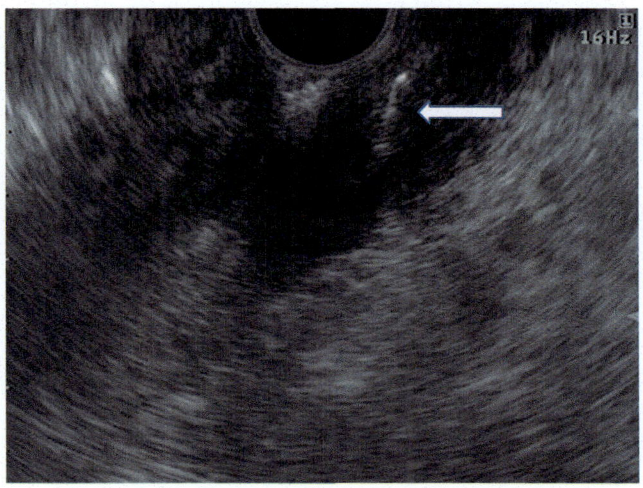

Figure 36.3 Endoscopic ultrasound image (linear array) of fiducial within an adenocarcinoma of the gastroesophageal junction.

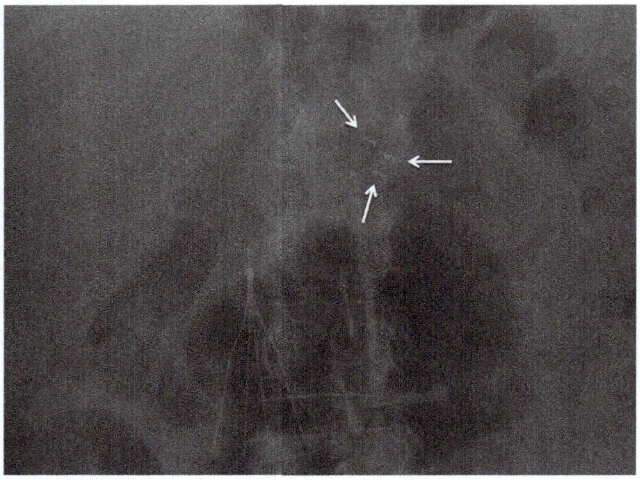

Figure 36.4 Abdominal radiograph (anteroposterior view) demonstrating three fiducials (arrows) located in an adenocarcinoma of the pancreatic head.

The number of fiducials placed is dependent on the size and location of the lesion. For small lesions measuring 1–3 cm (e.g. gastroesophageal junction tumors), a minimum of two fiducials should be placed to define the proximal and distal margins of the tumor. For larger lesions (e.g. pancreatic tumors), three to four fiducials should be placed in varying locations to define tumor borders and planes (Figure 36.4). Different IGRT protocols may call for specific fiducial locations, and thus preprocedure planning with a radiation oncologist is critical.

Periprocedural care

The use of either a sterile or clean non-sterile technique is acceptable when handling the fiducial markers, EUS needle, and bone wax. Antibiotic prophylaxis is typically administered intraprocedurally to all patients, although the benefit of this practice is unknown.

Standard postprocedure monitoring of patients should be performed. Complications related to EUS-guided fiducial placement are rare, but site-specific pain and infectious and inflammatory complications have been reported.

Fiducial migration into adjacent soft tissue and vascular structures, or even loss into the luminal space, can occur. Treatment-planning computed tomographic imaging is typically obtained five to seven days after endoscopic placement to confirm fiducial position and relationship to the target lesion.

Chapter video clips

Video 36.1 EUS-guided insertion of a gold coil fiducial: device design.

Video 36.2 EUS-guided insertion of a gold coil fiducial: loading the fiducial.

Video 36.3 EUS-guided insertion of a gold coil fiducial: case examples.

37 How to Inject Chemotherapeutic Agents

V. Raman Muthusamy and Kenneth J. Chang
University of California, Irvine, Orange, CA, USA

Endoscopic ultrasound (EUS)-guided fine needle injection (FNI) has been used to directly administer chemotherapeutic agents within pancreatic and esophageal tumors. Agents used to date include an allogeneic mixed lymphocyte culture and antitumor viral therapy using viral vectors encoding tumor necrosis factor (TNF)-α or granulocyte-macrophage colony-stimulating factor (GM-CSF). These agents can directly or synergistically assist in achieving tumor lysis. We describe here our specific technique for performing such procedures in pancreatic tumors using TNFerade™ (GenVec Inc., Gaithersburg, MD), a replication-deficient adenovector encoding human TNF-α and regulated by a radiation inducible promoter Egr-1, although the technique is similar for other antitumor agents.

Prior to each TNFerade injection, which requires five weekly injections in conjunction with chemoradiation therapy, attire approved by the institutional biosafety committee should be worn by all personnel involved in the procedure, given that a viral vector is being utilized. Typical gear includes material that achieves complete head covering, safety goggles, specially fitted masks to form a complete oral/facial shield, a gown, and gloves. The TNFerade solution is prepared by the pharmacy and is provided to the gastrointestinal laboratory immediately prior to the procedure. We typically use a 22-gauge fine needle aspiration (FNA) needle (EchoTip™, Cook Medical, Bloomington, IN) to administer the antitumor agent. Prior to inserting the FNA needle into the biopsy channel of the echoendoscope, we remove the stylet within the needle. For TNFerade, in which 2.0 ml is actually injected into the tumor, a total of 2.6 ml is usually provided in a 3.0-ml syringe by the pharmacy so that the entire needle channel can be primed prior to intratumoral injection. This is accomplished by attaching the 3.0-ml syringe to the FNA needle via the Luer lock on the handle. The needle is then primed by injecting the therapeutic agent into the needle until the entire dead space of the needle (usually 0.2–0.4 ml) contains fluid and fluid is witnessed exiting the needle tip. Fluid injection is then continued until exactly 2 ml remains in the syringe, at which point the needle is ready for use. Once the needle enters the tumor, the remainder of the fluid in the syringe is injected so that exactly 2 ml is delivered intratumorally.

We use a standard linear array echoendoscope (GFUC-140P, Olympus America, Center Valley, PA), operating at 5 MHz frequency to achieve maximal imaging depth, to perform all EUS-guided FNI procedures. Prior to FNI of the tumor, we routinely assess the lesion at its maximal cross-section and measure its size, circumference and area, and estimate tumor volume (Figure 37.1). This is important initially to set a baseline tumor size and during subsequent weekly injections to assess tumor response or progression. We also perform a careful standard EUS exam to assess for the presence or development of metastatic disease. A detailed review of previous images/videos is critical to ensure comparable regions are measured during subsequent exams in order to measure tumor response. We have noted that as therapy progresses, the echotexture within the tumor may become brighter, possibly indicating the development of fibrosis within the treated lesion. We believe this finding corresponds to a region of the tumor that has achieved a good response to therapy. Areas that are anechoic often indicate a region of tumor necrosis. In contrast, we believe that portions of the lesion that are hypoechoic represent residual areas of viable tumor.

Our technique of EUS-guided FNI involves identifying the most hypoechoic area(s) of the lesion to inject. Once the target has been identified, we place the 22-gauge needle into the biopsy channel of the echoendoscope and Luer-lock it in place. We then line up the needle-tip to the targeted (hypoechoic) area of the lesion. Having an assistant hold the echoendoscope to stabilize its position at this juncture is often helpful. We then slowly advance the

Atlas of Endoscopic Ultrasonography, Second Edition. Edited by Frank Gress, Thomas Savides, Brenna Casey, and Everson L. A. Artifon.

Companion website: www.wiley.com/go/gress/atlas

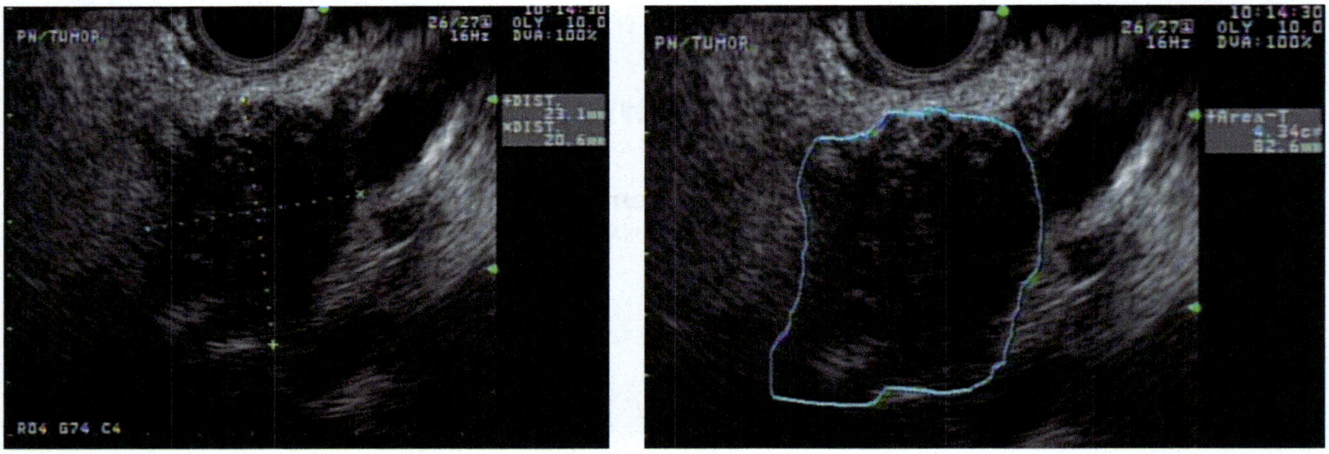

(a) (b)

Figure 37.1 Initial assessment of tumor size by endoscopic ultrasound (EUS) imaging. (a) Measurement of the tumor in maximal cross-section on EUS imaging prior to injection therapy. (b) This image highlights the ability of EUS to measure tumor area and circumference and, using this data, even estimate volume. Source: Chang KJ, Lee JG, Holcombe RF, et al. Endoscopic ultrasound delivery of an antitumor agent to treat a case of pancreatic cancer. *Nature Clin Pract Gastroenterol Hepatol* 2008;5:107–111.

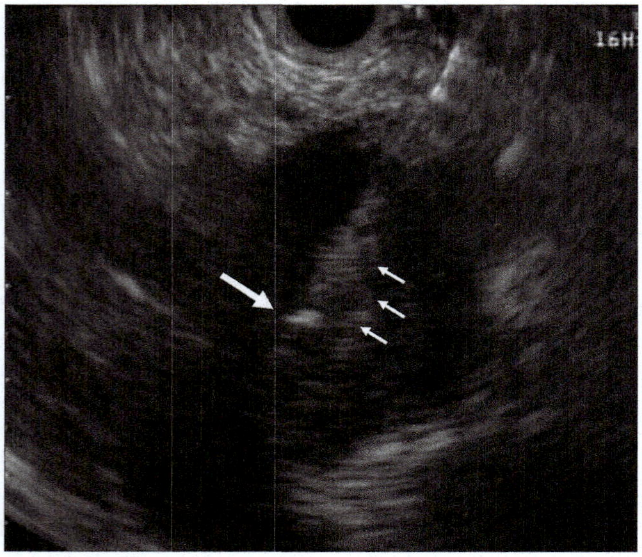

Figure 37.2 Endoscopic ultrasound (EUS)-guided fine needle injection (FNI) of a pancreatic lesion using a 22-gauge needle. The needle tip (large arrow) and the blush resulting from the injection of the chemotherapeutic agent around the needle (small arrows) can be seen. Source: Chang KJ, Lee JG, Holcombe RF, et al. Endoscopic ultrasound delivery of an antitumor agent to treat a case of pancreatic cancer. *Nature Clin Pract Gastroenterol Hepatol* 2008;5:107–111.

needle deep into the lesion using standard EUS-guided FNA technique. Upon reaching the deepest portion of the lesion, we slowly withdraw the needle and slowly inject the therapeutic agent into the well created by the FNA needle. A gradual, methodical withdrawal and injection is recommended to keep the entire injected solution within the tumor. We avoid injecting into anechoic (necrotic) regions and only inject on withdrawal (Figure 37.2). The needle can be realigned and redirected into other hypoechoic areas of the tumor in a fan-like fashion (Video 37.1). This is done by changing the angle of the elevator when the needle has reached the superficial portion of the tumor (that closest to the gastrointestinal lumen on imaging) and re-advancing the needle into a new portion of the tumor. Again, withdrawal is done slowly and injection is performed during needle withdrawal only. This process can be repeated until the entire 2 ml in the syringe has been injected, at which time the needle is removed from the lesion and withdrawn from the echoendoscope and the procedure is complete. A typical intratumoral injection lasts only two to three minutes in duration.

Antibiotics are administered orally three hours before the procedure and at 12 and 24 hours after the procedure. We typically administer a 500-mg dose of oral ciprofloxacin at these time points. The patient is recovered in a standard fashion in the endoscopy unit and then discharged to receive chemoradiation therapy. We believe that careful attention to chemotherapeutic injection technique is essential to achieving maximal results with these agents. An example of a vigorous response to such therapy is illustrated in Figures 37.3–37.5, which show a dramatic weekly reduction in size of a pancreatic tumor (Figure 37.3), with no residual tumor present in the gross resected specimen (Figure 37.4) or on histology (Figure 37.5).

Chapter video clip

Video 37.1 EUS-guided FNI of TNFerade into a pancreatic adenocarcinoma.

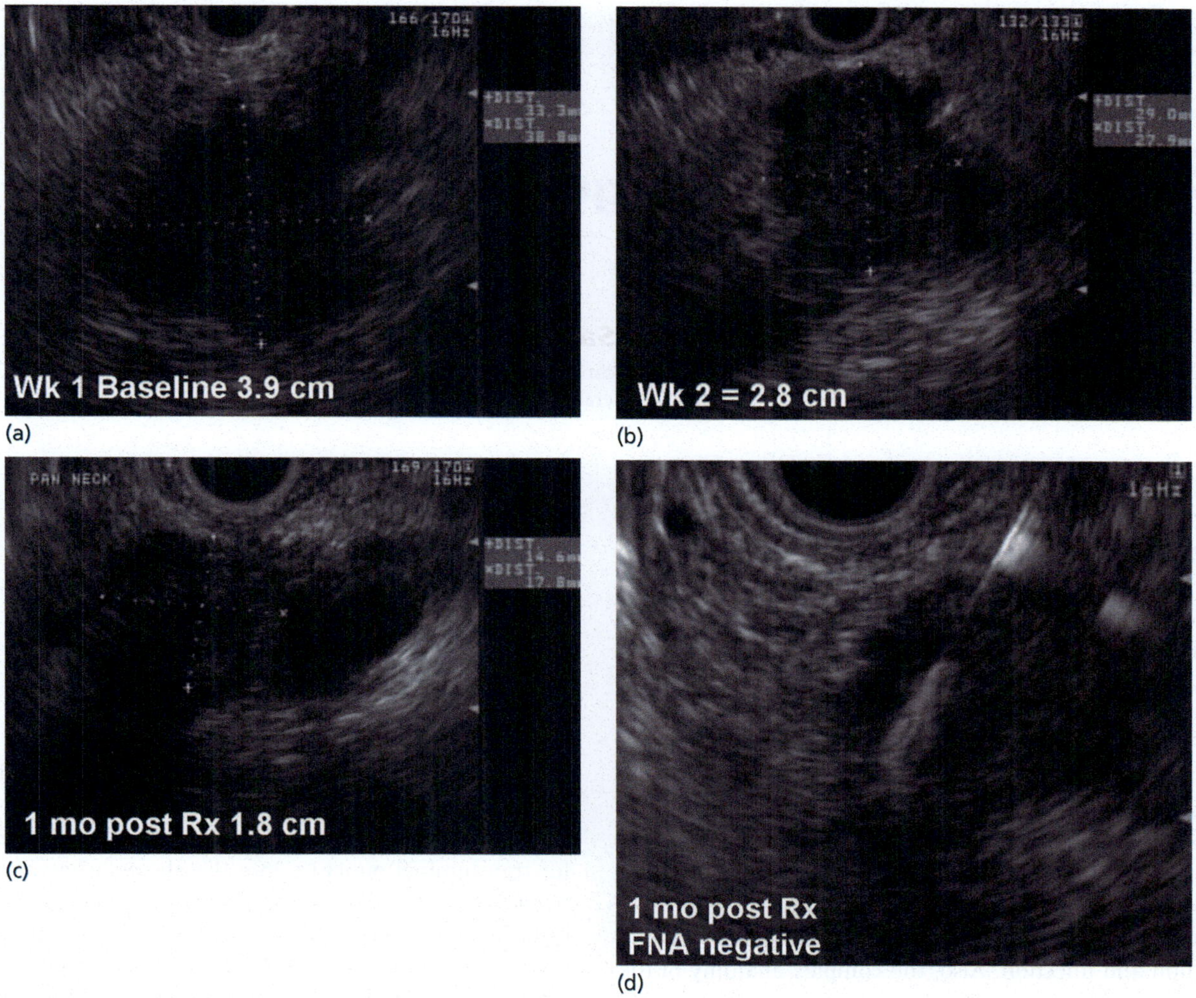

Figure 37.3 Tumor assessment during weekly injections of chemotherapeutic agents. These images show the assessment of tumor response at baseline: (a) week 1; (b) week 2; and (c) one month after completion of therapy (five weekly injections). (d) Fine needle aspiration being performed of the residual lesion one month after therapy. Source: Chang KJ, Lee JG, Holcombe RF, et al. Endoscopic ultrasound delivery of an antitumor agent to treat a case of pancreatic cancer. *Nature Clin Pract Gastroenterol Hepatol* 2008;5:107–111.

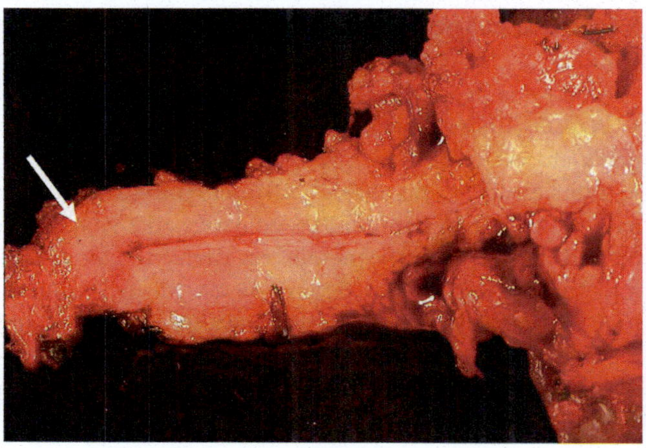

Figure 37.4 Gross specimen of the resected pancreas in Figure 37.3 revealing no residual tumor remaining. The area of the treated tumor can be seen (arrow). Source: Chang KJ, Lee JG, Holcombe RF, et al. Endoscopic ultrasound delivery of an antitumor agent to treat a case of pancreatic cancer. *Nature Clin Pract Gastroenterol Hepatol* 2008;5:107–111.

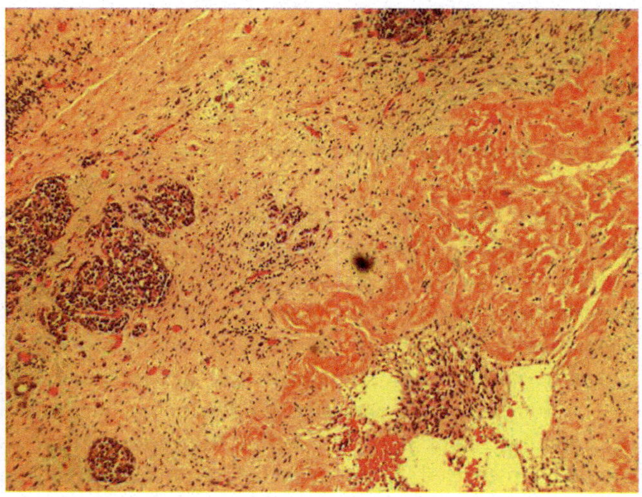

Figure 37.5 Histology from the specimen in Figure 37.4 demonstrating a complete pathologic response. Source: Chang KJ, Lee JG, Holcombe RF, et al. Endoscopic ultrasound delivery of an antitumor agent to treat a case of pancreatic cancer. *Nature Clin Pract Gastroenterol Hepatol* 2008;5:107–111.

38 How to do EUS-guided Pelvic Abscess Drainage

Shyam Varadarajulu[1] and Sandeep Lakhtakia[2]
[1] University of Alabama at Birmingham School of Medicine, Birmingham, AL, USA
[2] Asian Institute of Gastroenterology, Hyderabad, India

Introduction

Development of pelvic abscess is a well-recognized complication in patients undergoing low anterior resection for rectal cancer or following medical conditions such as inflammatory bowel disease. Traditionally, these abscesses are drained surgically or image guided (ultrasound or computed tomography [CT]) via the percutaneous, transrectal, or transvaginal routes. Although effective, surgical drainage is associated with a prolonged hospital stay, particularly when performed to manage a postoperative complication. The percutaneous drainage technique is less invasive than surgery but limits patient mobility and predisposes to fistula formation and infection. Also, the complex anatomy of the pelvis with surrounding bones, vascular structures, and other organs makes percutaneous access to the abscess cavity a technical challenge. By virtue of its ability to image and access extraluminal lesions, endoscopic ultrasound (EUS) has emerged as a minimally invasive therapeutic alternative for drainage of pelvic abscesses.

Patient preparation

A CT of the pelvis must be obtained to get a clear understanding of the abscess location prior to performing pelvic abscess drainage (Figure 38.1). Patients should be administered prophylactic antibiotics prior to the intervention and continued on oral antibiotics for two to three days. Bowel preparation with polyethylene glycol solution or enema is mandatory to minimize the chance of contamination and for adequate visualization. The procedure is best performed under fluoroscopy to visualize guidewire exchange and placement of stent or drain within the abscess. Patients should be instructed to void urine before the procedure as a distended bladder may impair visualization of small abscesses during EUS.

Devices and accessories

A therapeutic linear array echoendoscope with a working channel of 3 mm or more should be used to facilitate deployment of transluminal stents or drainage catheter. A 19-gauge EUS-guided fine needle aspiration (FNA) needle is required for transluminal puncture into the abscess cavity, followed by passage of a 0.035-inch guidewire allowing it to coil inside the abscess cavity. A standard 4.5/5.0 French (Fr) endoscopic retrograde cholangiopancreatography (ERCP) cannula or a needle knife catheter is then railroaded over the guidewire into the abscess cavity. An over-the-wire balloon dilator (8–15 mm) is needed for subsequent dilation of the transmural tract. A double pigtail plastic stent (7 or 10 Fr) or drainage catheter is required to facilitate evacuation of the abscess cavity.

Procedural technique

The following steps are undertaken in sequence (Video 38.1).

- A rectal EUS examination is first undertaken to locate the pelvic abscess.
- After ensuring the absence of intervening vasculature using color Doppler, under EUS guidance a 19-gauge needle is used to puncture the abscess cavity to gain access into the fluid collection (Figure 38.2). Normal saline is used to flush the abscess cavity using a 20-ml syringe and reaspirated to clean out the cavity of as much pus as possible. A sample of the aspirate should be sent for Gram stain and culture.

Atlas of Endoscopic Ultrasonography, Second Edition. Edited by Frank Gress, Thomas Savides, Brenna Casey, and Everson L. A. Artifon.

Companion website: www.wiley.com/go/gress/atlas

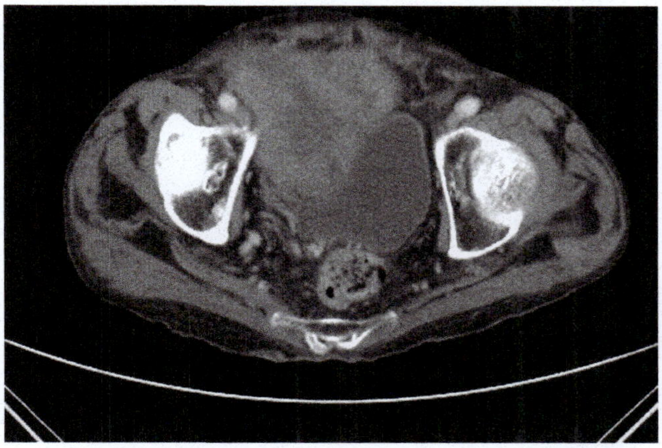

Figure 38.1 Computed tomography (CT) scan of the pelvis revealing an 8 × 7 cm abscess cavity.

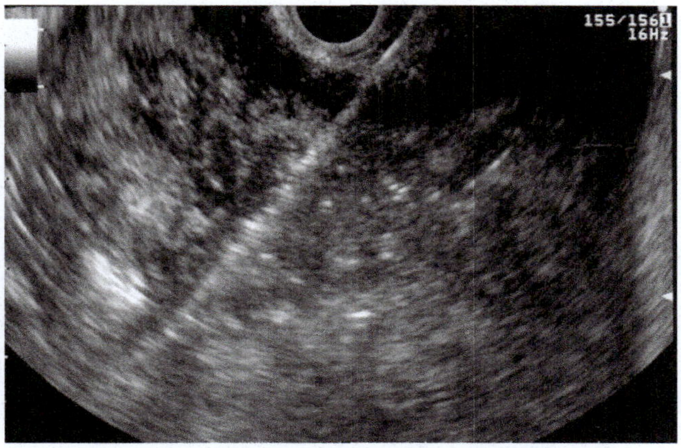

Figure 38.2 Passage of a 19-gauge fine needle aspiration (FNA) needle into the pelvic abscess under EUS guidance.

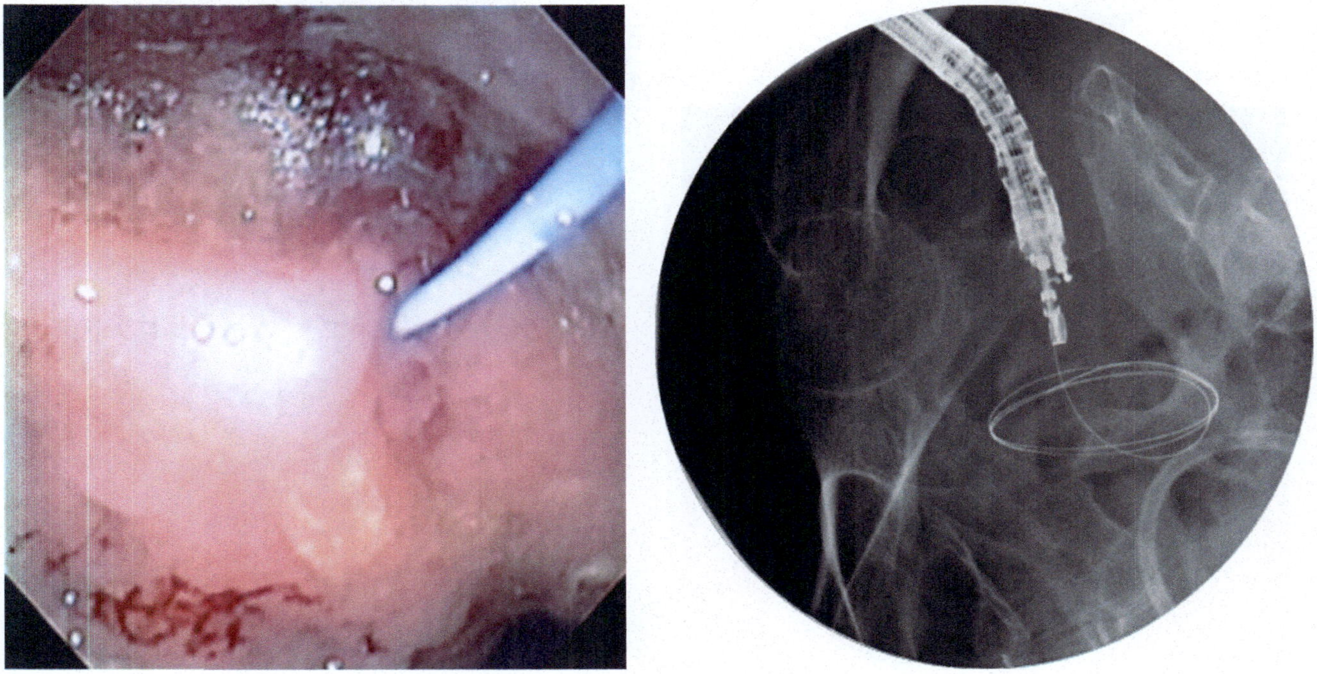

(a) (b)

Figure 38.3 A 0.035-inch guidewire is then coiled within the abscess cavity: (a) endoscopy view; (b) confirmed by fluoroscopy.

- A 0.035-inch guidewire is then passed via the 19-gauge needle and coiled within the abscess cavity (Figure 38.3).
- The transmural tract is then first dilated by passing a tapered-tip ERCP cannula (4.5/5.0 Fr) or a needle knife catheter through the working channel of the echoendoscope. The tract is further dilated using an 8–15 mm over-the-wire balloon (Figure 38.4). The presence of a large opening will facilitate better drainage of the abscess and provide easy access for future interventions.
- A 7 or 10 Fr double pigtail stent is then deployed over the guidewire into the abscess to establish complete drainage (Figure 38.5).
- In patients with pelvic abscesses measuring more than 8 cm in diameter or having thick content, a 10 Fr single pigtail drain may be placed in addition to the stent. To place a drain, guidewire (within cannula) is passed through the created opening, adjacent to the previously placed stent and then the drainage catheter is passed. The drain is secured to the gluteal region by application of tape. The drain is then flushed with 50 ml of normal saline, every four hours, until the abscess is completely evacuated.
- A CT scan of the pelvis is obtained at 48 hours to assess response to therapy. If the abscess has decreased in size by more than 50%, the drain is discontinued and the patient is discharged home. After obtaining a follow-up CT at two

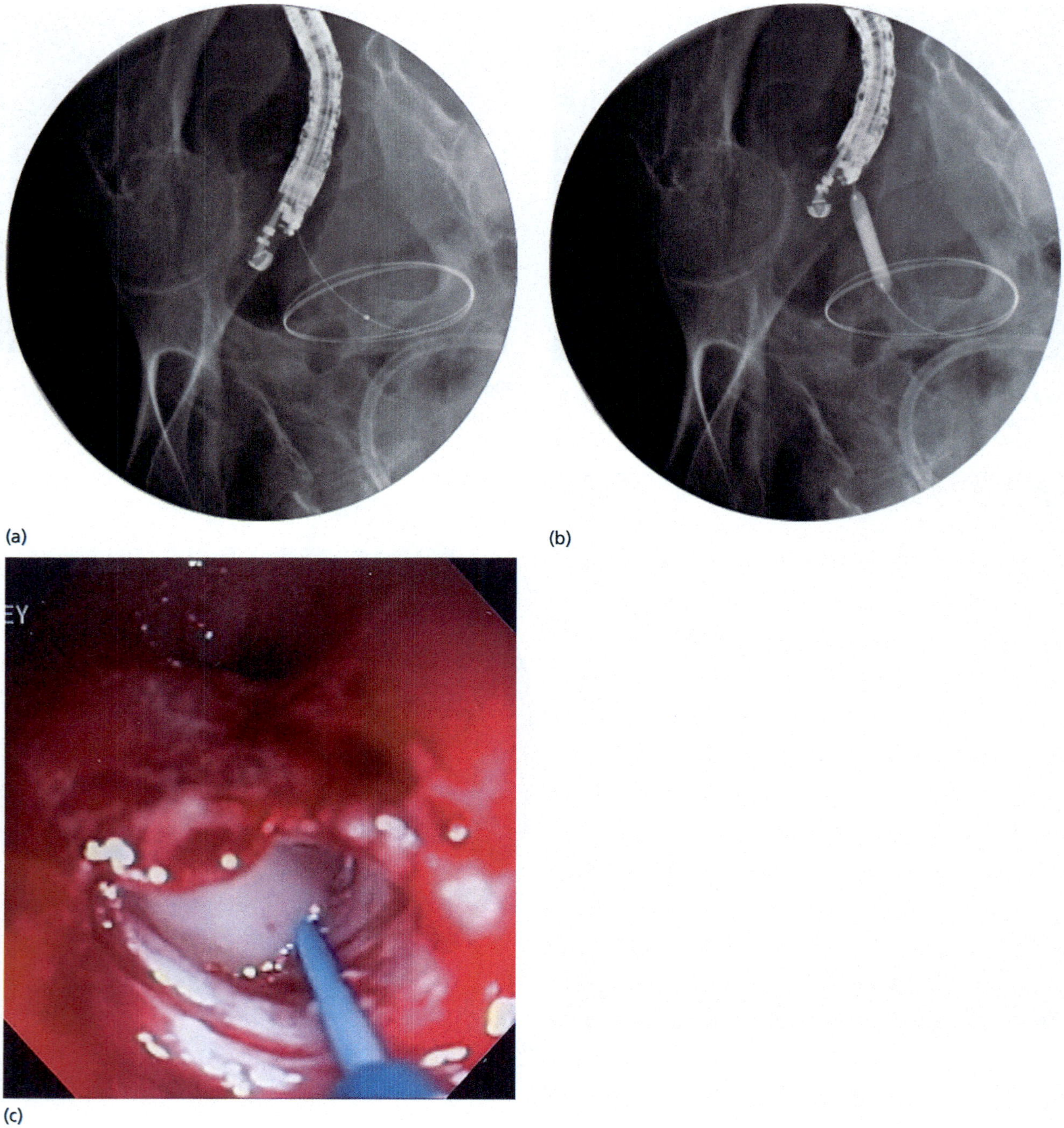

Figure 38.4 Fluoroscopy view revealing dilation of the tract using an endoscopic retrograde cholangiopancreatography (ERCP) cannula (a) and then an over-the-wire balloon dilator (b). Pus is seen to extrude following dilation of the transmural tract (c).

weeks to confirm complete resolution of the abscess, the transrectal stent is removed by sigmoidoscopy.

Clinical outcomes

In our experience with a carefully selected cohort of 25 consecutive patients, i.e. those with unilocular collections adjacent to the rectum or left colon, EUS-guided pelvic abscess drainage yielded a successful outcome in 96% of cases. No procedural complications were encountered and, unlike surgical or percutaneous techniques, patients were discharged home within two to three days following their procedures. In contrast to surgery and percutaneous techniques, EUS-guided drainage of pelvic abscess is less invasive, less costly, and is associated with minimal patient

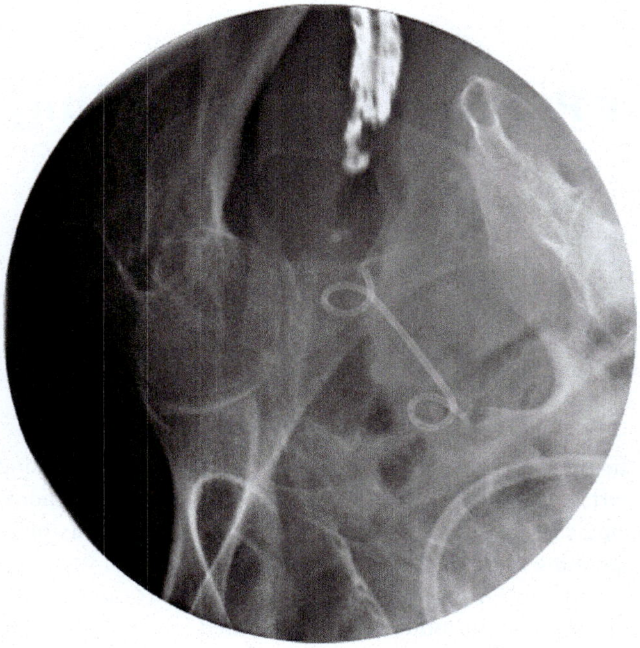

Figure 38.5 Fluoroscopic view revealing the presence of a stent within the pelvic abscess cavity.

discomfort. We recently compared the outcomes between transcolonic and transrectal drainage of pelvic abscesses in 38 patients and observed no difference in rates of technical success, treatment success, or complications between both approaches. However, when evaluated by etiology, treatment success for diverticular abscess was significantly lower when compared with other causes.

Technical limitations

Drainage of pelvic abscess cannot be undertaken when the wall of the abscess cavity is more than 20 mm from the EUS transducer. Also, the presence of multiple cavities in an abscess precludes successful drainage. It is important to carry out a helical CT scan before embarking on this procedure because poorly defined or multilocular fluid collections are not suitable for this non-surgical method of drainage. Also, stent deployment may not be possible in patients with pelvic abscesses that measure less than 4 cm in size. As the linear array echoendoscope can be advanced only up to 40 cm in the colon, only those fluid collections adjacent to the rectum or left colon can be drained using this technique. Perianal fluid collections are not suitable for EUS-guided drainage.

Conclusions

Endoscopic ultrasound-guided drainage can be an effective treatment modality for management of patients with abscesses or fluid collections in the pelvis that are within the reach of the echoendoscope. Comparative studies with other treatment modalities that include a larger number of patients will help identify cases that will benefit the most from this technique.

Chapter video clip

Video 38.1 The technique of EUS-guided pelvic abscess drainage. Source: Aloka.

39 How to do Doppler Probe EUS for Bleeding

Richard C.K. Wong
Case Western Reserve University and University Hospitals Case Medical Center, Cleveland, OH, USA

Background and equipment

Doppler ultrasound, particularly use of the endoscopic Doppler ultrasound (DopUS) probe, is quite different from traditional endoscopic ultrasound (EUS) and miniature EUS probes inasmuch that the currently available DopUS probe is non-imaging, the equipment is portable and significantly less expensive than EUS systems, and advanced endoscopic training in traditional EUS is not required. In addition, because the DopUS probe makes direct physical contact with the gastrointestinal (GI) tract lesion of interest, acoustic coupling with instilled water or with a water-filled balloon are not required. Signal output from the non-imaging DopUS probe system is in the form of an audible Doppler ultrasound signal with or without graphic display of the acoustic Doppler ultrasound waveform.

Within the last decade, two DopUS systems have been utilized in published studies: Endo-Dop (DWL GmbH, Singen, Germany) and VTI Endoscopic Doppler System (Vascular Technology Inc., Nashua, NH) (Figures 39.1 and 39.2). However, only the VTI system has received US Food and Drug Administration (FDA) clearance for use in GI endoscopy in the United States. Both systems are AC powered.

Practical application of DopUS probe

Advanced endoscopic training, detailed knowledge of EUS, or specific training in EUS is not required to use DopUS. The technique of DopUS can be readily acquired by most GI endoscopists in a relatively short time.

Modern DopUS probe systems utilize pulsed-wave ultrasound technology, which allows the endoscopist to vary scanning depth, to select the most appropriate depth for the specific bleeding lesion of interest, and to exclude deep serosal vessels ("innocent bystanders") that are not involved in the bleeding process. Available DopUS systems are small and portable, and can be easily placed on an emergency endoscopy cart for patients located in intensive care units or in operating rooms.

With current DopUS probe technology, a 16- or 20-MHz pulsed-wave ultrasound beam is emitted in a linear fashion from the distal tip of a small flexible probe that is passed down the accessory channel of a standard diagnostic (or therapeutic) forward-viewing (or side-viewing) endoscope to make direct physical contact with the GI tract lesion of interest. It is important to select the scanning depth based on the lesion of interest: shallow (0–1.5 mm) for peptic ulcers versus mid (0–4 mm) for varices. Depending on the manufacturer, DopUS probes are marketed either as disposable, single-use only, or reusable after gas sterilization or high-level liquid disinfection.

Preprocedure system check

Before each use, it is important to perform a preprocedure check to ensure that the DopUS system is functioning appropriately. This is done by first connecting the DopUS probe to the base unit, turning the power on, and tapping the distal probe tip gently with an ungloved finger. In an appropriately functioning system, a corresponding tapping sound should be heard. In units that allow for adjustment of sound volume, this should be kept at maximum. The preprocedure system check is then completed. Note that the system should be turned off before passing the probe through the accessory channel of the endoscope.

Doppler ultrasound signals

- Positive versus negative versus artifact:
  - Positive signal: a repetitive and similar audible and/or visual signal of at least three consecutive cycles duration.
  - Negative signal: absence of a positive signal.

Atlas of Endoscopic Ultrasonography, Second Edition. Edited by Frank Gress, Thomas Savides, Brenna Casey, and Everson L. A. Artifon.

Companion website: www.wiley.com/go/gress/atlas

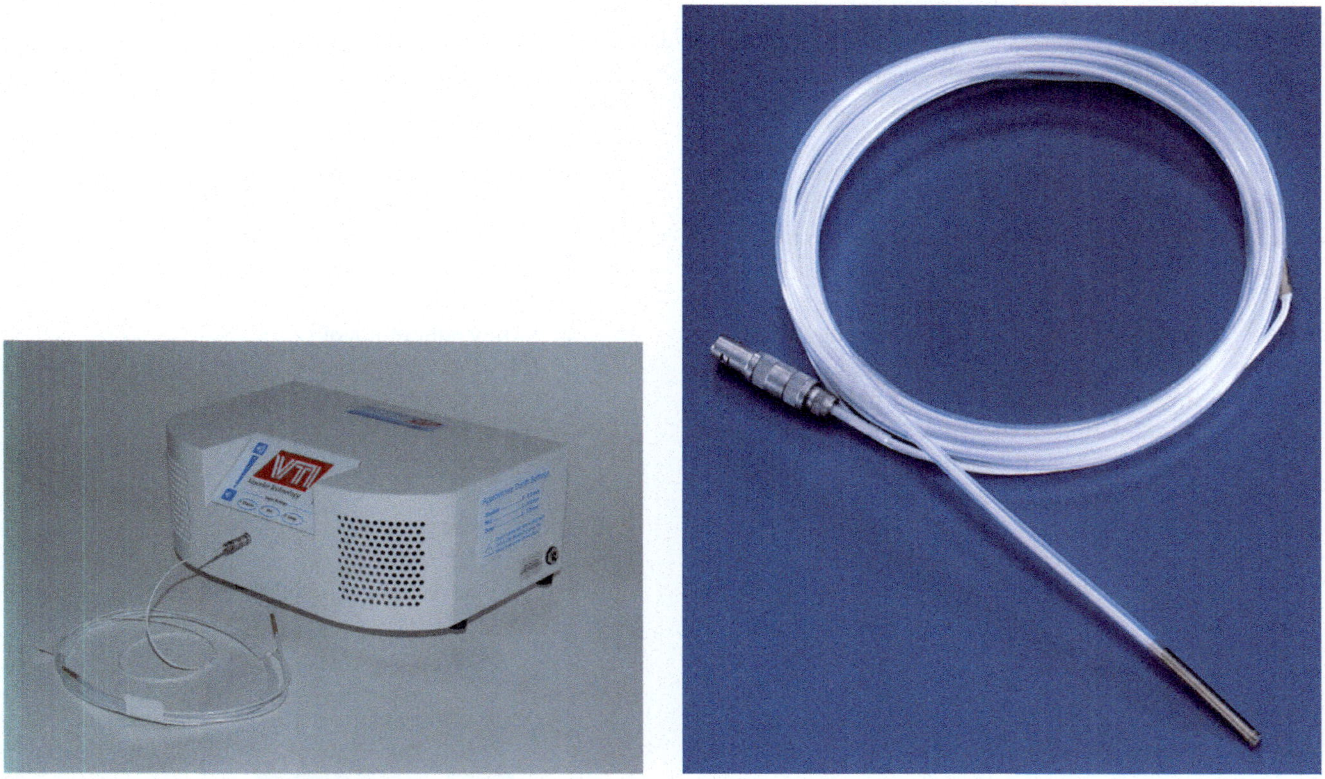

(a) (b)

Figure 39.1 VTI endoscopic Doppler system. (a) A 20-MHz pulsed-wave Doppler ultrasound system. Doppler ultrasound output signal: audible only. Weight: 1.18 kg. United States Food and Drug Administration (FDA) clearance: yes. (b) Doppler ultrasound probe: single-use, probe diameter 2.5 mm, lengths 165 cm and 245 cm. Source: reproduced by permission of Vascular Technology, Inc., Nashua, NH.

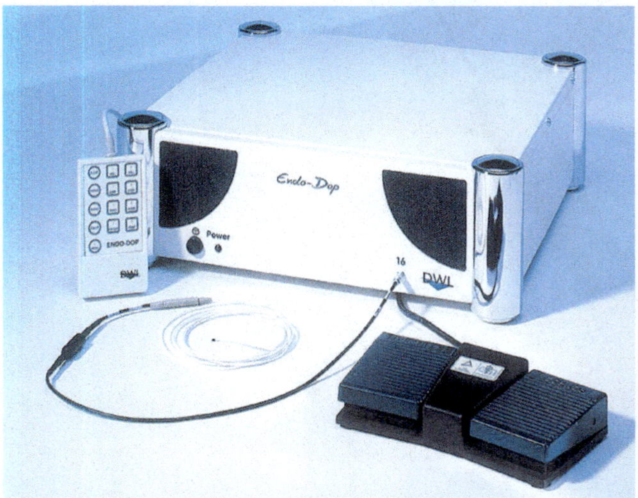

Figure 39.2 Endo-Dop, 16-MHz pulsed-wave, multigated Doppler ultrasound (DopUS) system with reusable DopUS probe and optional foot pedal. Doppler US output signal: visual and audible. Weight: 6.76 kg. United States Food and Drug Administration (FDA) clearance: no. Source: reproduced by permission of Elsevier.

  - Artifact signal: simple movement of the probe tip against mucosa will produce a false, artifact signal. This can be readily differentiated from a positive signal by the fact that physical movement is required. In addition, artifact signals can occur if the probe tip is placed in an area where there are naturally transmitted pulsations, e.g. transmitted cardiac pulsations in the fundus of the stomach.
- Arterial versus venous blood flow:
  - Arterial blood flow: spiking, high-pitch sound and/or waveform.
  - Venous blood flow: continuous, low-pitch sound and/or waveform.

Peptic ulcer (Figures 39.3–39.7)

- Irrigate the base of the ulcer with water to clear away any fibrinopurulent exudate.
- Position the DopUS probe in direct physical contact with the ulcer base using moderate pressure, at multiple points, including immediately adjacent to any stigmata of recent hemorrhage (SRH).

• The endoscopist should vary the angle of the probe with the ulcer base so as to minimize the chance of a false-negative Doppler signal. Note that a false-negative Doppler signal can occur if the ultrasound beam is directed at a right angle (90 degrees) to the subsurface blood vessel.

• Scanning depth: in peptic ulcer hemorrhage, the selection of scanning depth depends on whether there is increased physical distance between the ulcer base and the subsurface vessel of interest. For untreated ulcers, the scanning depth should be kept shallow (0–1.5 mm). For treated ulcers, selection of scanning depth depends on whether injection therapy has been performed and whether a subsurface cushion (or bleb) of injectate (fluid) is still present at the time of the DopUS examination. Thus, if injection therapy is performed alone (monotherapy), scanning depth should be increased to mid-range (0–4 mm) because of the existence of the subsurface fluid bleb. On the other hand, if dual combination therapy is performed (injection therapy first followed by thermal-contact therapy with a heat probe or bipolar probe), then the subsurface fluid bleb has been eliminated by the cratering effect of the thermal-contact treatment and scanning depth can be kept shallow (0–1.5 mm).

- Shallow (0–1.5 mm):
  a. Untreated peptic ulcer
  b. Injection followed by thermal-contact therapy
  c. Thermal-contact therapy alone
  d. Endoclip therapy alone.
- Mid (0–4 mm):
  a. Firmly adherent clot
  b. Injection therapy alone
  c. Injection followed by endoclip.
- Deep (0–7 mm):
  - Usually not needed.

Published studies

Published studies using the DopUS probe in acute peptic ulcer bleeding have demonstrated the following.

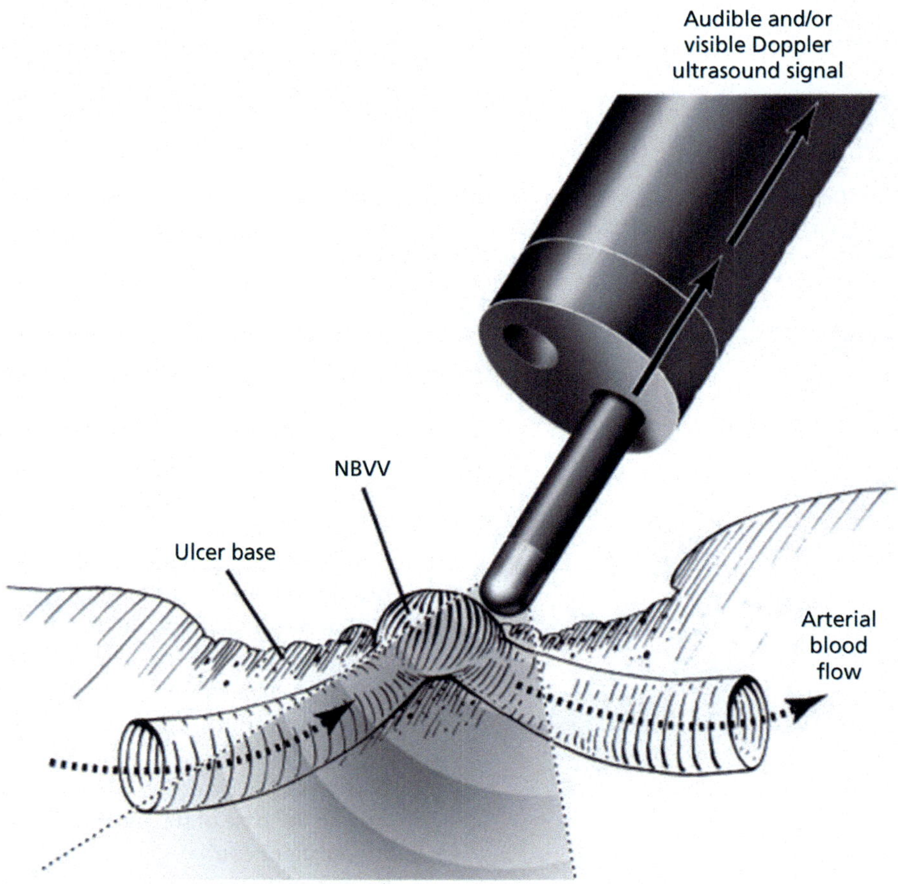

Figure 39.3 Illustration of a bleeding peptic ulcer with a non-bleeding visible vessel (NBVV) undergoing Doppler ultrasound (DopUS) examination using an endoscopic DopUS probe that was passed via the accessory channel of a standard endoscope. Source: Wong RCK. Risk stratification of nonvariceal UGI hemorrhage for the practicing endoscopist. *Tech Gastrointest Endosc* 2005;7(3):118–123. © 2005, Elsevier.

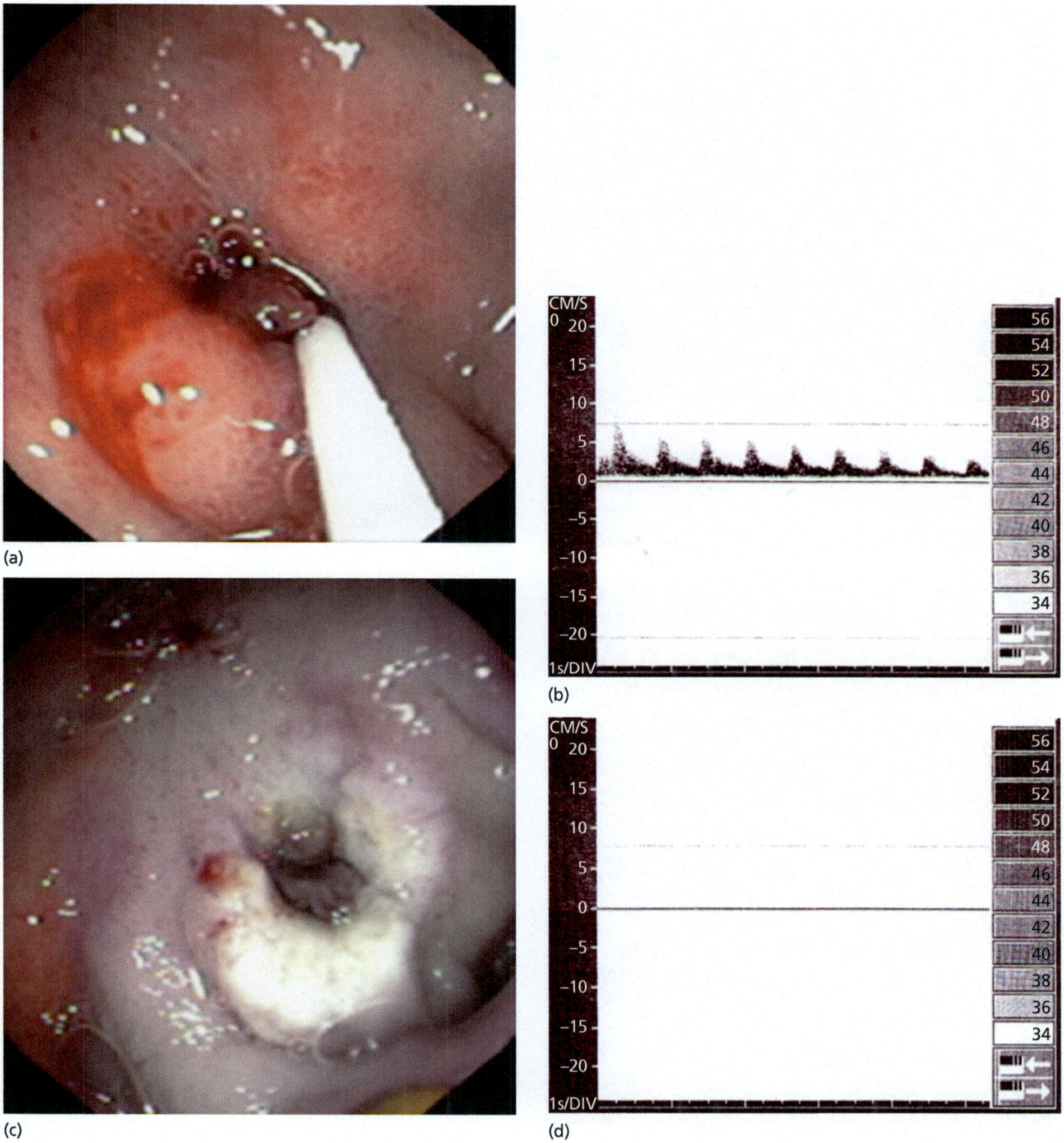

Figure 39.4 Doppler ultrasound (DopUS) in acute peptic ulcer bleeding. (a) Endoscopic image of a DopUS probe on a bleeding duodenal ulcer with a non-bleeding visible vessel: Doppler positive. (b) Visual graphic display of the corresponding positive DopUS signal: *y*-axis, frequency shift (kHz); *x*-axis, time (s). (c) Endoscopic image of the same ulcer after combination endoscopic therapy with epinephrine injection and heat probe: Doppler negative. (d) Visual graphic display of the corresponding negative DopUS signal. Source: (b, d) Wong RCK. Endoscopic Doppler US probe for acute peptic ulcer hemorrhage. *Gastrointest Endosc* 2004;60(5):804–812. © 2004, Elsevier.

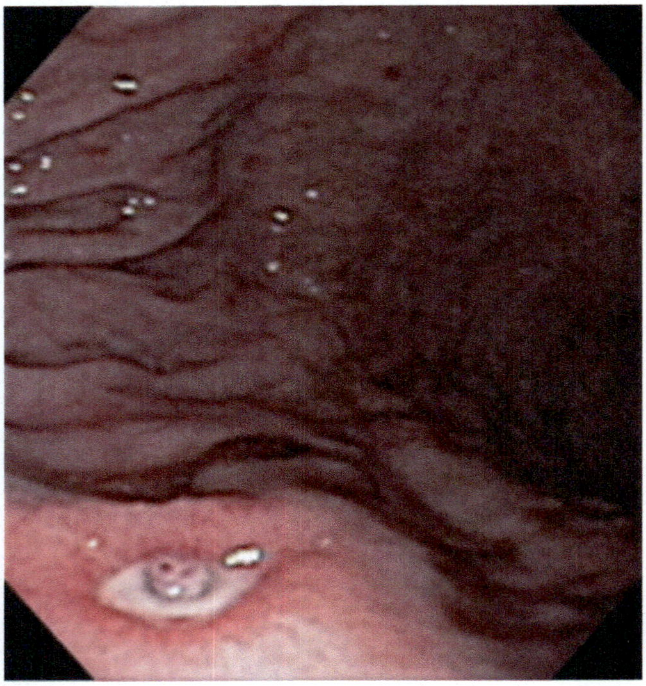

(a)

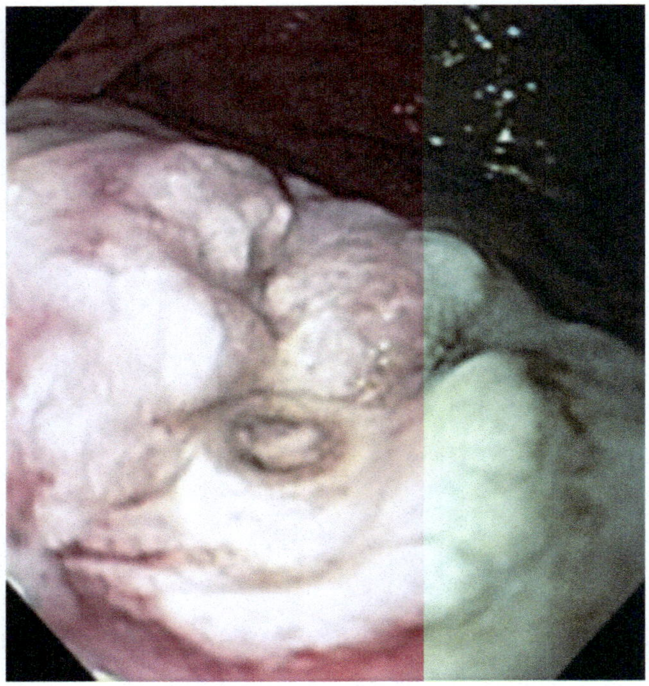

(b)

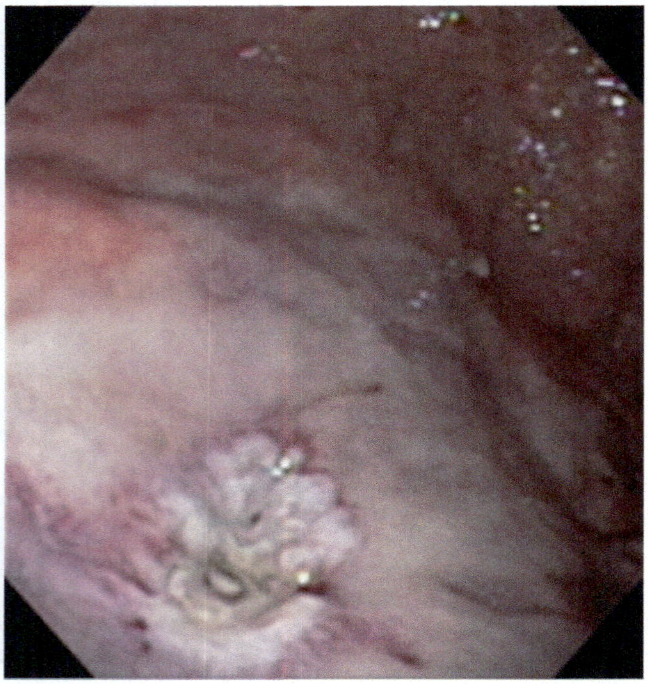

(c)

Figure 39.5 Doppler ultrasound-guided hemostasis in acute peptic ulcer bleeding. (a) Gastric ulcer with a non-bleeding visible vessel: Doppler positive. (b) Immediately following dual combination endoscopic therapy with epinephrine injection and heat probe: Doppler positive. (c) Targeted, additional heat probe application to location of positive Doppler signal: Doppler negative. No recurrent bleeding at 30 days.

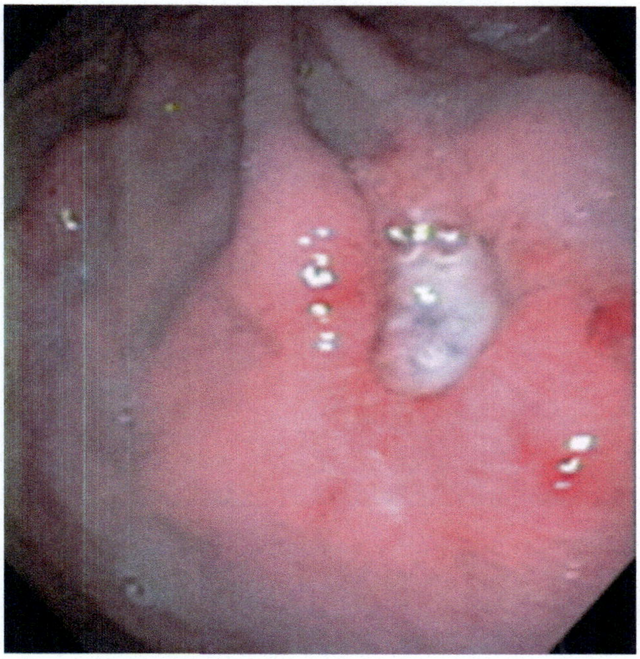

Figure 39.6 Atypical peptic ulcer bleeding: recurrent major bleeding from a gastric ulcer, clean base, without stigmata of recent hemorrhage (requiring a 7-unit blood transfusion in a healthy 23-year-old man). Doppler ultrasound (DopUS) localized a strongly positive arterial Doppler at the 11 o'clock position, targeted DopUS-guided hemostatic therapy was performed with no recurrent bleeding at 30 days.

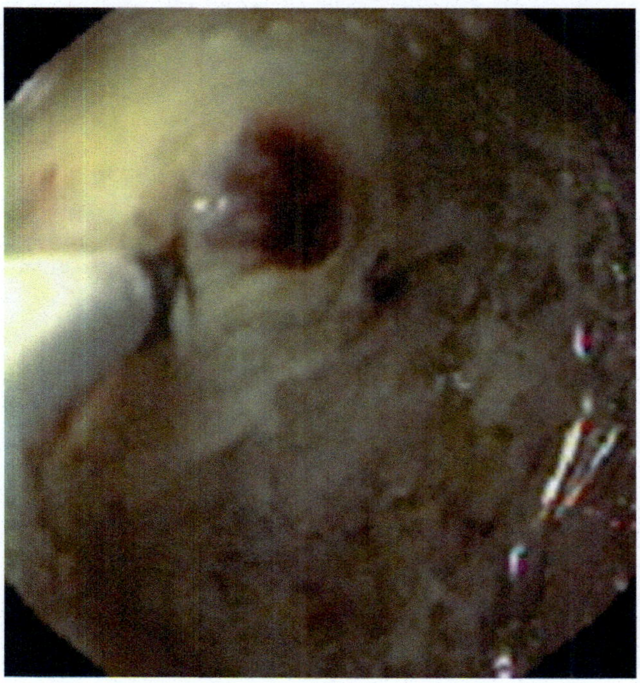

Figure 39.7 Doppler-negative non-bleeding visible vessel. Endoscopic image of a Doppler ultrasound probe being placed on an untreated bleeding duodenal ulcer.

Table 39.1 Correlation of endoscopic appearance of peptic or anastomotic ulcers with endoscopic Doppler ultrasound signal.

Endoscopic appearance	Doppler (+) (%)
Active bleeding (spurting)	100
Active bleeding (oozing)	60
Non-bleeding visible vessel	44
Adherent clot	14
Flat pigmented spot	9
Clean base	11

1. Recurrent bleeding is significantly more likely to occur in ulcers that are Doppler positive than in those that are Doppler negative.
2. Ulcers that remain Doppler positive immediately after endoscopic therapy are at significantly increased risk of recurrent bleeding than those where the Doppler signal is abolished.
3. Positive correlation exists between endoscopic SRH and Doppler signal (Table 39.1).

Clinical scenarios

Clinical scenarios where use of the endoscopic DopUS probe could be useful include the evaluation of uncertain visual SRH, in the assessment of adequacy of endoscopic hemostatic therapy, and in the evaluation of bleeding ulcers that behave functionally as high risk but which appear to be low risk by visual stigmata alone (e.g. recurrent bleeding from a clean-based ulcer or ulcer with flat pigmented spot).

Gastric varices versus thickened gastric folds versus gastrointestinal stromal tumor

(Figures 39.8 and 39.9)

- Place probe tip on lesion of interest using light pressure.
- Scanning depth: mid (0–4 mm).
- Vary incident angle.
  - Gastric varices: continuous, low-pitch sound and/or waveform. Consistency: soft.
  - Thickened gastric folds: no Doppler signal. Consistency: soft.
  - Gastrointestinal stromal tumor: ± Doppler signal, but only at base of lesion. Consistency: firm.
- DopUS probe-guided glue injection of bleeding gastric varices. Although there are reports of this technique being used, further studies are required to evaluate its clinical utility.

Miscellaneous disorders

DopUS probe has been used in the following disorders but further studies are required to evaluate clinical utility.

- Dieulafoy's lesion (Figures 39.10 and 39.11).
- Diverticular bleeding.
- Colonic polyps.
- Esophageal varices.

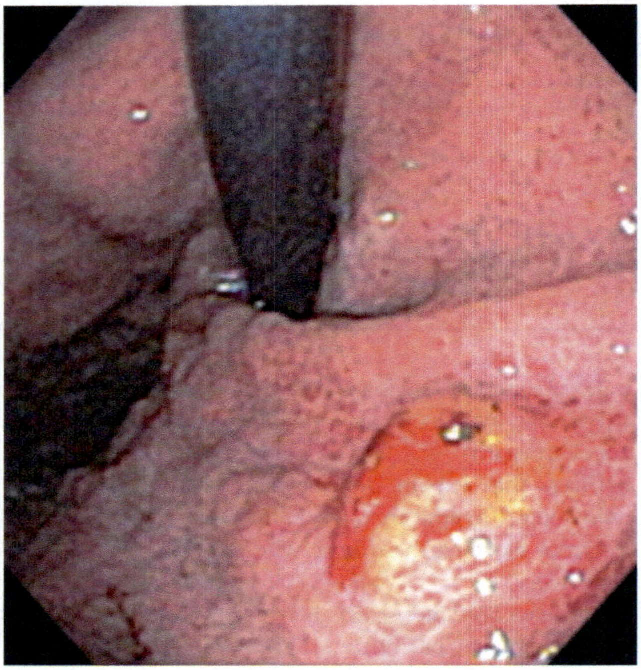

Figure 39.8 Atypical appearance of a bleeding gastric varix. Mild active oozing of blood from a single, small, yellowish submucosal lesion in the gastric fundus, Doppler positive. Source: reproduced by permission of Elsevier.

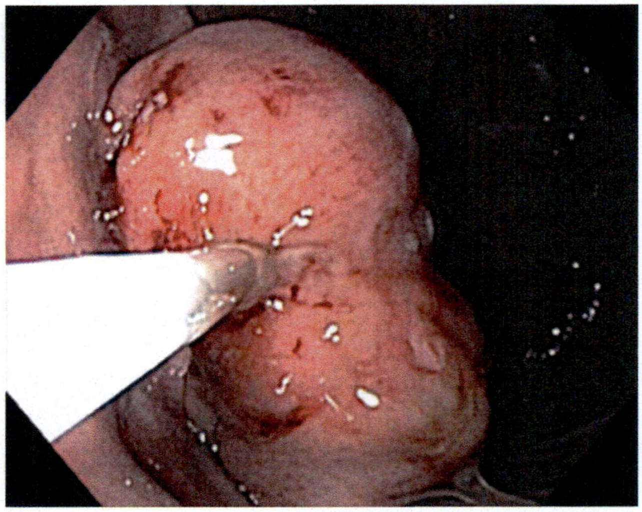

Figure 39.9 Doppler ultrasound examination of a gastrointestinal stromal tumor in the gastric fundus, Doppler negative. Source: reproduced by permission of Elsevier.

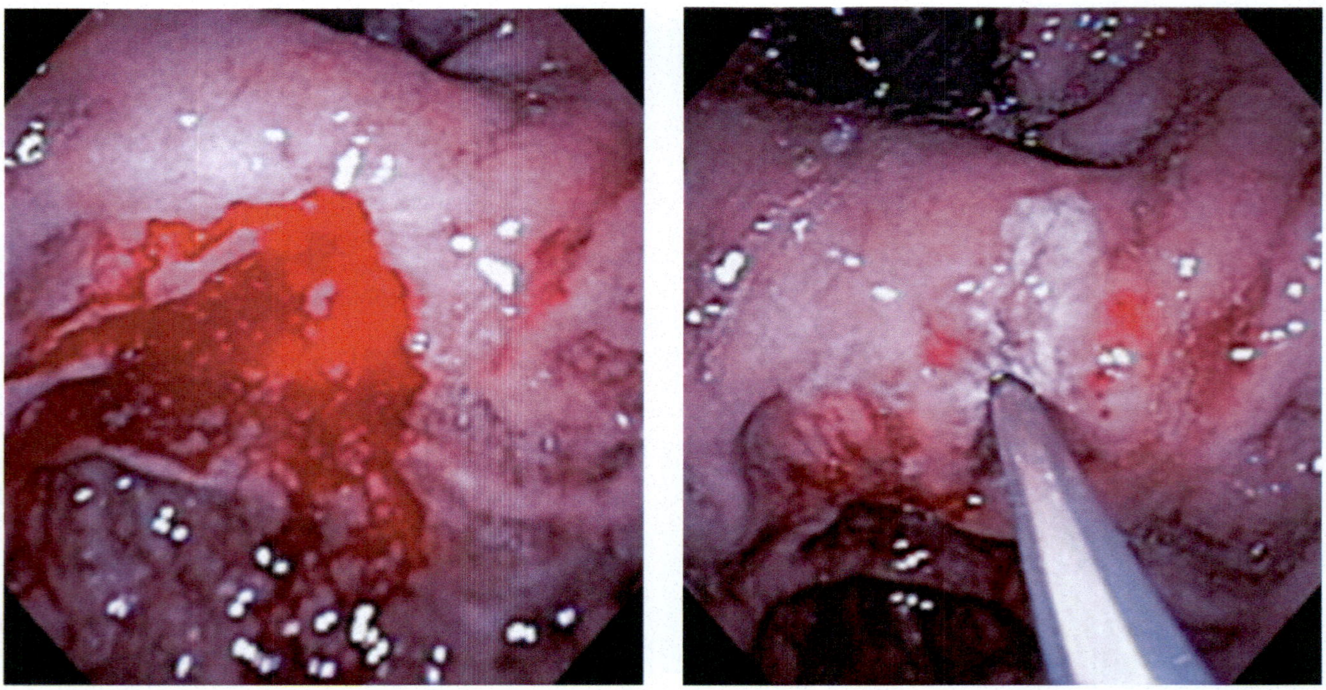

(a) (b)

Figure 39.10 Dieulafoy lesion in gastric cardia. (a) Active bleeding. (b) Doppler ultrasound probe examination immediately following dual combination hemostatic therapy.

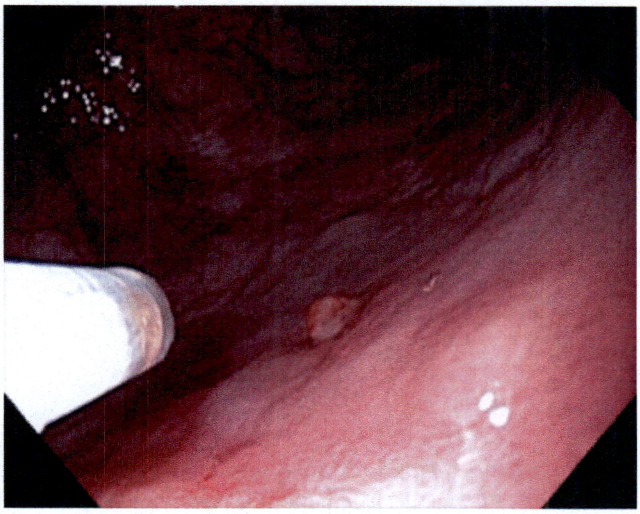

Figure 39.11 Dieulafoy lesion in rectum, Doppler with strong arterial signal.

- Major papilla before endoscopic retrograde cholangio-pancreatography (ERCP) with sphincterotomy.
- Post-endoscopic submucosal dissection (ESD) ulcer.

Conclusions

The endoscopic DopUS probe allows the endoscopist to determine the presence or absence of subsurface blood flow in bleeding lesions, to differentiate between arterial and venous blood flow, to estimate depth of the subsurface blood vessel, and to estimate location of the subsurface blood vessel. Being able to generate such a subsurface map of blood flow could potentially allow for precise targeting and titration of endoscopic hemostatic therapy based not on visual surface stigmata alone, but with additional knowledge of subsurface blood flow.

Conflicts of interest disclosure

The author has received research funding from Vascular Technology, Inc.

Chapter video clips

Video 39.1 Peptic ulcer bleeding.

Video 39.2 Gastric varices. Source: Aloka.

40 How to do Endoscopic Ultrasound-guided Portal Pressure Gradient Measurement

Rintaro Hashimoto and Kenneth J. Chang
University of California, Irvine, Orange, CA, USA

Introduction

Portal hypertension (PH) is a serious adverse event of liver cirrhosis. Clinically significant PH (>10 mmHg) predicts the development of esophageal varices bleeding and hepatocellular carcinoma. Portal venous pressure (PVP) accurately reflects the degree of PH and is the single best prognostic indicator in liver disease. The evaluation of PVP had been performed by an indirect measurement of the hepatic venous pressure gradient (HVPG), in which a catheter is inserted into the hepatic vein percutaneously via either the jugular or femoral vein. This technique requires skill and is not commonly performed. HVPG can be affected by hepatic tissue compliance. In addition, HVPG has been found to differ from PVP even among patients with the same pathogenesis. Recently, a simple novel technique for EUS-guided portal pressure gradient measurement (PPGM) using a compact manometer (Cook Medical, Bloomington, IN) (Figure 40.1) has been developed. This enables measurement of portal venous pressure with the manometer directly through the endoscopic ultrasound (EUS) needle. The time required for the procedure is short, under 30 minutes. EUS-guided liver biopsies can be performed at the same procedure.

Endoscopic ultrasound-guided PPGM technique

The EUS manometry apparatus used in our human study is a simple set-up that includes a 25-gauge fine needle aspiration (FNA) needle, noncompressible tubing, a compact digital manometer, and heparinized saline. The tubing is connected by a Luer lock to the distal port of the manometer while the heparinized saline is connected the proximal port. The end of the tubing is connected via a Luer lock to the inlet of the 25G needle. The patient is positioned supine and during EUS-guided pressure measurement reading, the manometer is placed at the patient's mid-axillary line (Figure 40.2). We prefer monitored anesthesia care or general anesthesia for this procedure.

The hepatic venous pressure is measured first. Of the hepatic veins, the middle hepatic vein is targeted most commonly because of its larger caliber and better alignment with the needle trajectory on linear EUS (Figure 40.3). Doppler flow is used to confirm the typical multiphasic waveform of hepatic venous flow (Figure 40.4). Using the 25G FNA needle, a transgastric transhepatic approach is used to puncture the hepatic vein. Approximately 0.5 ml of heparinized saline is used to flush the needle, which is visible on EUS,

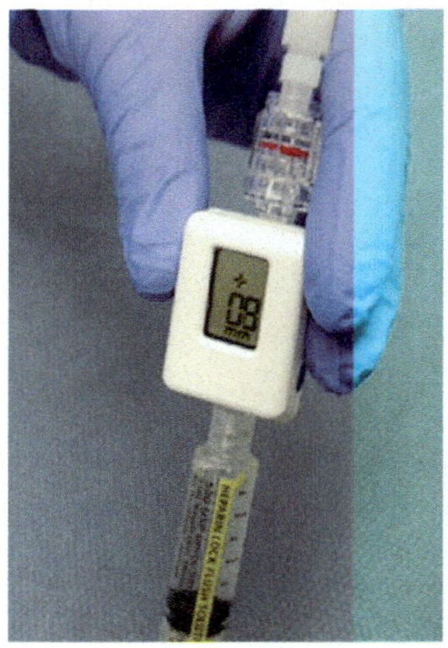

Figure 40.1 Compact manometer for EUS-guided portal pressure measurement. Source: Cook Medical, Bloomington, IN, USA.

Atlas of Endoscopic Ultrasonography, Second Edition. Edited by Frank Gress, Thomas Savides, Brenna Casey, and Everson L. A. Artifon.

Companion website: www.wiley.com/go/gress/atlas

confirming good position within the vessel. Following the flush, the pressure reading on the manometer will immediately increase and then decrease and equilibrate at a steady pressure, which is recorded. This measurement should be repeated a second and third time to minimize any error or fluctuation and to give a range of pressures from which to derive a mean pressure. The mean of the three pressures is then considered the hepatic vein pressure. The FNA needle is slowly withdrawn from the vein into the liver parenchyma and then back into the needle sheath, with Doppler flow on to ensure there is no flow within the needle tract.

The portal venous pressure is measured next, using the umbilical portion of the left portal vein. The pressure reading on the manometer will immediately increase and then decrease and equilibrate at a steady pressure, which is recorded (Figure 40.5). Doppler flow is used to confirm the typical venous hum of portal venous flow (Figure 40.6). This measurement should be repeated a second and third time. The mean of the three pressures is then considered the portal venous pressure. The FNA needle is slowly withdrawn from the vein into the liver parenchyma and then back into the needle sheath, with Doppler flow on to ensure there is no flow within the needle tract. The portal pressure gradient is calculated by subtracting the mean portal venous pressure from the mean hepatic venous pressure. The patient is recovered in a manner similar to that used for routine diagnostic EUS with FNA. Postprocedural antibiotics are usually given for three to five days after the procedure.

We have conducted animal studies in a pig model, with PH induced by dextran-40 administration, to investigate the feasibility of this compact manometer [1]. Correlations between EUS-guided and percutaneous pressure measurements were very strong, with r values in all vessels greater than or equal to 0.985. Our group has also performed the first prospective pilot study of EUS-guided PPGM in 28 human patients, with 100% technical success and no adverse events [2]. PPGM correlated well with clinical and endoscopic parameters, with significant differences in portal pressure gradient noted in patients who were high risk versus low risk for cirrhosis and in patients with esophageal varices,

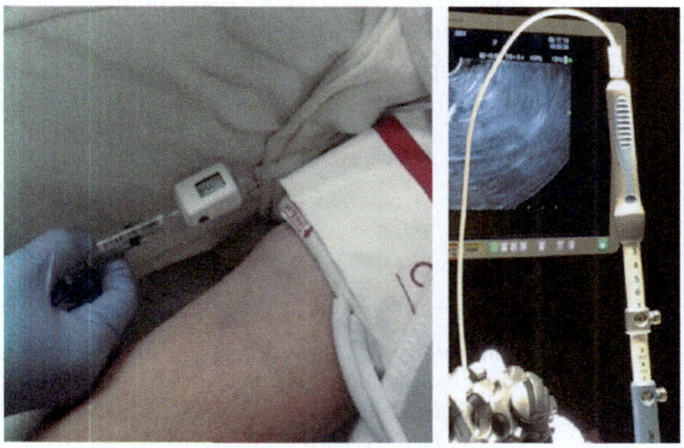

Figure 40.2 EUS-guided portal pressure measurement apparatus showing noncompressible tubing attached to the DNA needle inlet (*right*) and compact manometer being placed at the mid-axillary line of the patient (*left*).

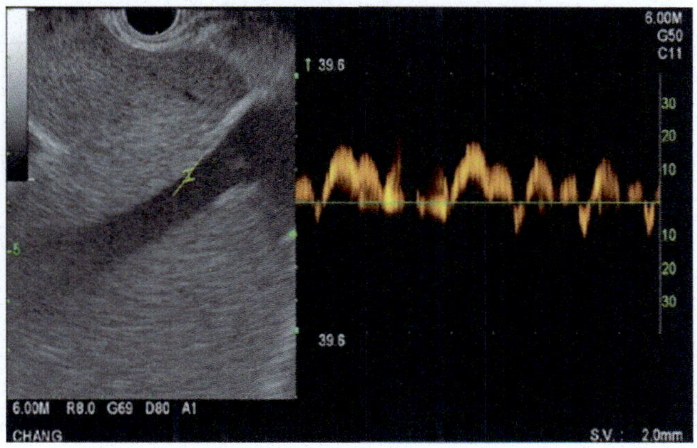

Figure 40.4 EUS Doppler flow image of the middle hepatic vein demonstrating multiphasic waveform.

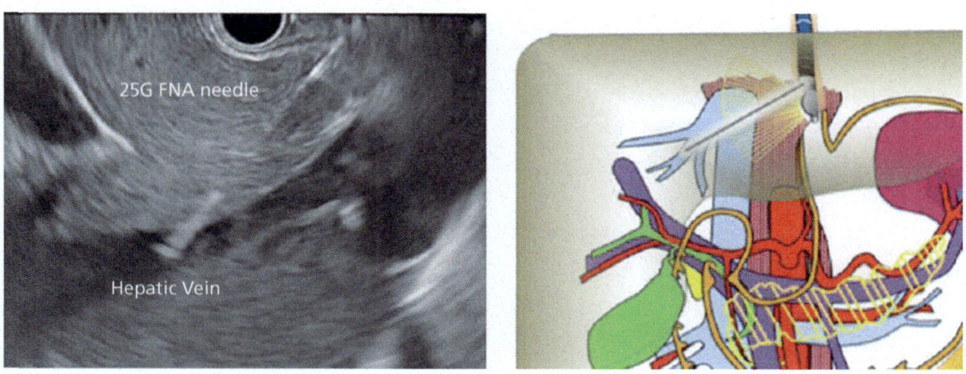

(a) (b)

Figure 40.3 EUS image (a) and schematic (b) of needle puncture of the middle hepatic vein with 25G FNA needle.

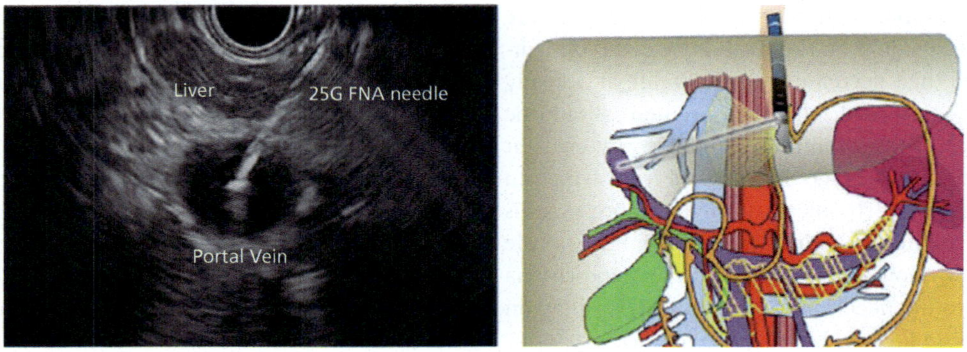

(a) (b)

Figure 40.5 EUS image (a) and schematic (b) of needle puncture of the left portal vein with 25G FNA needle.

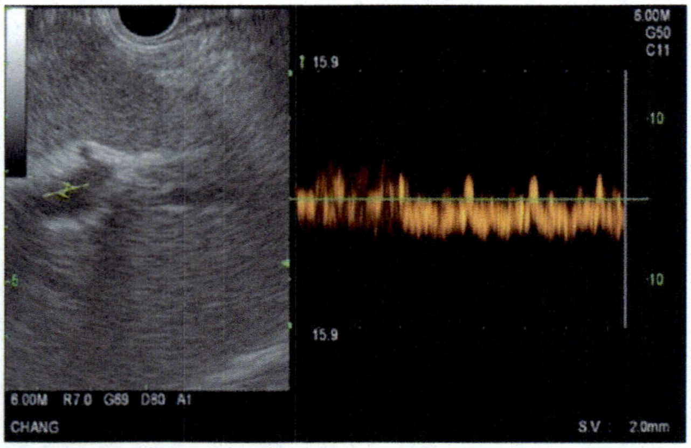

Figure 40.6 EUS Doppler flow image of the left portal vein demonstrating typical waveform.

portal hypertensive gastropathy, and thrombocytopenia relative to patients without these conditions. Recently, our prospective series has continued with data from 51 patients who underwent EUS-guided PPGM with 100% technical success and no adverse events [3]. The portal pressure gradient ranged from 0 to 27.3 mmHg and was significantly higher in patients with clinical features of cirrhosis (11.26 vs. 3.14 mmHg; *P* <0.001), endoscopic evidence of varices (14.94 vs. 4.09 mmHg; *P* <0.001), or portal hypertensive gastropathy (14.37 vs. 5.23 mmHg; *P* <0.001) and laboratory evidence of thrombocytopenia (10.91 vs. 4.81 mmHg; *P* <0.001). Minor discomfort was reported in three patients (6%), all of whom were managed with oral pain medication. In addition, most of the patients in this study underwent EUS-guided liver biopsies during the same procedure, suggesting that combining PPGM and liver biopsy in the same session should be safe.

References

1. Huang JY, Samarasena JB, Tsujino T, Chang KJ. EUS-guided portal pressure gradient measurement with a novel 25-gauge needle device versus standard transjugular approach: a comparison animal study. *Gastrointest Endosc* 2016;84:358–362.
2. Huang JY, Samarasena JB, Tsujino T, et al. EUS-guided portal pressure gradient measurement with a simple novel device: a human pilot study. *Gastrointest Endosc* 2017;85:996–1001.
3. Samarasena JB, Huang JY, Tsujino T, et al. EUS-guided portal pressure gradient measurement with a simple novel device: a human pilot study. *VideoGIE* 2018;3:361–363.

41 How to do Endoscopic Ultrasound-guided Liver Biopsy

David L. Diehl
Geisinger Medical Center and Geisinger Commonwealth School of Medicine, Danville, PA, USA

There remains an important role for liver biopsy in the current management of liver diseases despite advancements in non-invasive hepatic assessment [1–3]. Gastroenterologists are no longer trained in the technique of percutaneous liver biopsy, and this workload has largely gone to interventional radiology.

However, use of endoscopic ultrasound-guided liver biopsy (EUS-LB) is increasing, and has several advantages.

1. Tissue cores can be obtained from both lobes easily, decreasing sampling error.
2. Biopsies are done under real-time ultrasound guidance, potentially decreasing risk.
3. Patients are sedated for the procedure, increasing procedural comfort and decreasing anxiety.
4. If esophagogastroduodenoscopy or EUS is also required, a single procedure can be done, decreasing inconvenience and overall costs.

Comparison of tissue yields between percutaneous, transjugular, and EUS-guided routes has shown comparable tissue yields [4]. Use of newer core needles has further increased the tissue yields for EUS-LB.

Indications and contraindications

Indications for EUS-LB are broadly any patient who needs a liver biopsy and does not require a transjugular approach. If the patient requires endoscopy (e.g. to exclude varices, Barrett's surveillance or detection, evaluation of upper gastrointestinal symptoms) or EUS (evaluation of common bile duct, gallbladder, pancreas, or other EUS indication) in addition to a liver biopsy, then EUS-LB is highly efficient. Some patients require a sedated liver biopsy, for example anxious patients or children [5].

Absolute contraindications include coagulopathy, use of anticoagulants, and obvious cirrhosis, while ascites is a relative contraindication. We require a platelet count of 50×10^9/l or above and an international normalized ratio (INR) of less than 1.5. More recently, thromboelastography (TEG) has been used as a potentially better measure of the interaction of platelets with the entire coagulation cascade, and it is possible that patients with an elevated INR but normal TEG could safely undergo liver biopsy. However, there are no data on this at present.

EUS-LB technique

Identification of liver lobes

EUS-LB is performed with the curvilinear echoendoscope, which allows real-time monitoring of needle entry into the liver. The left hepatic lobe is found by identifying the liver from the proximal stomach (Figure 41.1). It is important to positively identify liver and distinguish it from the spleen, which is found in a similar location (Figure 41.2). In some cases, the echotexture of the liver and spleen can be similar. Confirmation of appropriate targeting of the left lobe of the liver is important to avoid inadvertent splenic puncture [6].

The right hepatic lobe is found by placing the tip of the EUS scope in the duodenal bulb and torquing counterclockwise until the large area of the right lobe is identified (Figure 41.3). For patients after gastric bypass, only the left lobe can be easily sampled.

Whether single lobe or bilobar liver biopsy should be done is a matter of debate. Some liver diseases can show heterogeneity in histologic findings between lobes, and bilobar biopsy may be favored to decrease sampling error. For non-alcoholic steatohepatitis, it has been our practice to sample both lobes [7].

Atlas of Endoscopic Ultrasonography, Second Edition. Edited by Frank Gress, Thomas Savides, Brenna Casey, and Everson L. A. Artifon.

Companion website: www.wiley.com/go/gress/atlas

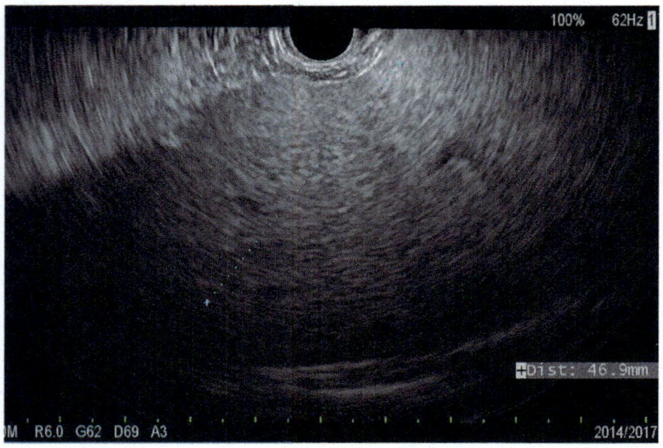

Figure 41.1 Visualization of the left hepatic lobe from the proximal stomach. The cursor shows the expected trajectory of the biopsy needle when obtaining the core specimen.

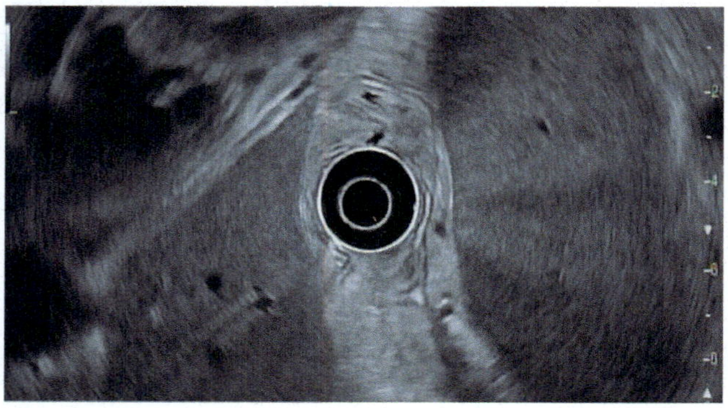

Figure 41.2 View of liver (on the left) and spleen (on the right) from the proximal stomach with the radial echoendoscope. In some cases, the spleen can be very prominent, and care must be taken to positively identify the left lobe of the liver and distinguish it from the spleen.

Needle selection

A 19G EUS needle provides the best tissue cores for pathologic interpretation (Figure 41.4). A 19G fine needle biopsy (FNB) needle has been shown to be better than a regular fine needle aspiration (FNA) needle [8] (Figures 41.5 and 41.6). Smaller, 22G FNB needles have been used for EUS-LB and often provide adequate specimens; however, the diameter of the cores is smaller and specimen fragmentation during processing has been noted [9].

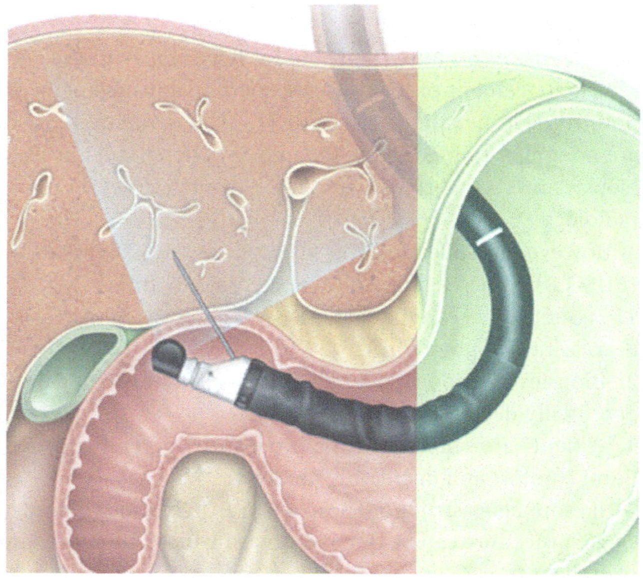

Figure 41.3 Right lobe biopsies are obtained with the echoendoscope tip placed in the duodenal bulb. Source: image used by permission of Boston Scientific.

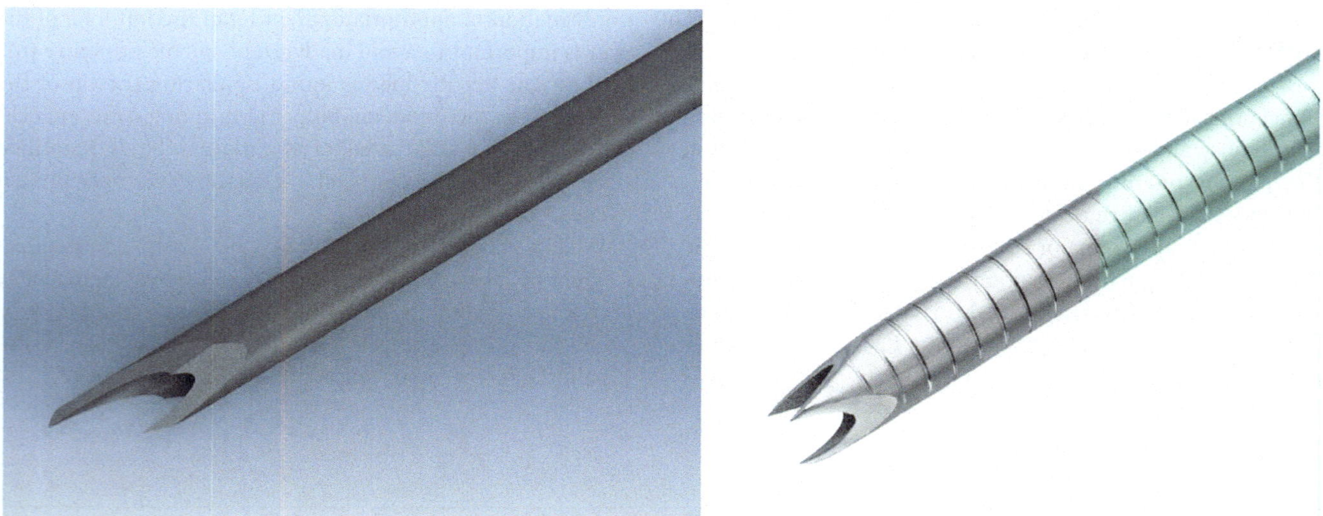

Figure 41.4 Close-up of the tips of the core needles used for EUS-LB: (*left*) SharkCore needle (Medtronic); (*right*) Acquire needle (Boston Scientific). Source: images used with permission of Boston Scientific and Medtronic.

Needle preparation

The wet suction technique is superior to dry suction for EUS-LB [10]. For wet suction, the stylet is removed and the needle lumen primed with saline or heparin flush prior to biopsy (Figure 41.7). The heparin flush decreases clogging of the needle lumen by blood and produces a less bloody tissue specimen [11]. This in turn leads to easier tissue handling by the pathology laboratory.

Needle technique

In the chosen lobe, a trajectory for needle passage is identified that does not include larger hepatic or portal vein branches. The longest trajectory of needle travel is sought, which is typically about 3–6 cm. The endoscopy assistant can hold the echoendoscope at the bite block, preventing "recoiling" of the echoendoscope during the needle throw. After a suitable trajectory is defined, the luminal wall is punctured and the needle positioned in the liver parenchyma.

The stopcock on the suction syringe is then turned to "on" (full suction). Three to-and-fro actuations of the needle are made into the liver [12]. The stopcock on the vacuum syringe is turned off prior to removing the needle from the parenchyma. The needle is then removed from the echoendoscope.

Specimen handling

The contents of the needle are expressed directly into a formalin cup by either stylet reinsertion or flushing the contents with saline or the heparin flush. Most, if not all, the specimen will be in the needle lumen, although if blood has entered the vacuum syringe, tissue may be found there as well.

We are currently utilizing a "tissue sieve" to separate tissue from blood (CoreCatcher; ProAct Ltd, Center Hall, PA) (Figure 41.8). Heparinization of the needle prevents formation of blood clots in the needle, which can be visualized as "blood noodles" in the formalin. When using the tissue filter, the needle contents are expressed first onto the sieve. The specimen is then rinsed gently with saline, which leaves only (or mainly) liver tissue on the sieve. This tissue is then placed into formalin (Figure 41.9).

The surgical pathology receiving laboratory is typically used to processing small specimens. The endosonographer should discuss EUS-LB with the pathologist to ensure optimal specimen handling. Excessive handling of the cores should be avoided to limit specimen fragmentation.

Postprocedure recovery after EUS-LB

We use a one-hour recovery period after EUS-LB, including for bilobar biopsies. Post-biopsy abdominal discomfort, if present, is typically easily controlled by a single dose of opiate analgesic (we usually use hydromorphone hydrochloride 0.5–1 mg).

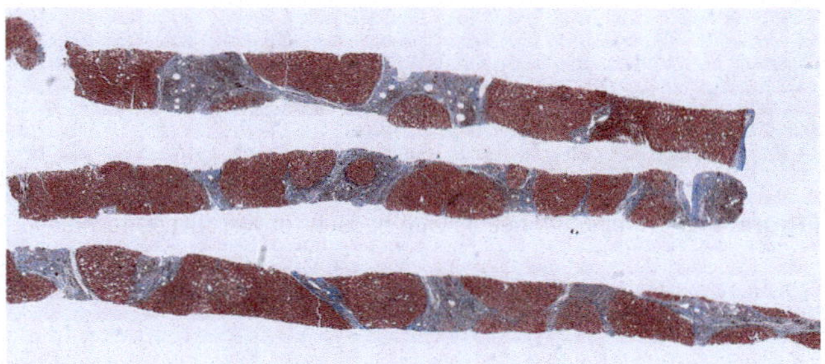

Figure 41.6 Excellent core of cirrhotic liver obtained with the 19G FNB needle.

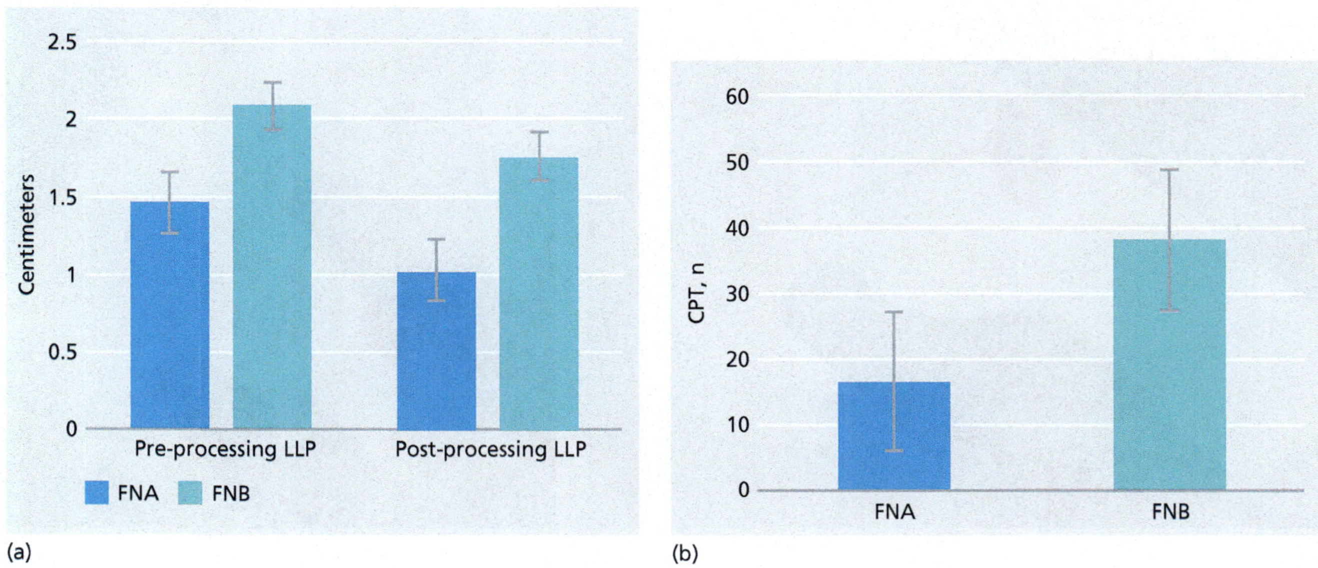

Figure 41.5 Comparison of a 19G FNB needle to 19G FNA needle in terms of (a) length of the longest piece (LLP) before and after histologic processing, and (b) total complete portal triad (CPT) count as shown in a recent prospective randomized trial [8].

Adverse effects

Adverse effects after EUS-LB are uncommon. An adverse effect unique to EUS-LB is inadvertent splenic puncture [6]. This can occur from misidentification of the left lobe of the liver and confusing it with the spleen (see Figure 41.2). Occasionally, the echotexture of the spleen and left lobe of the liver are remarkably similar.

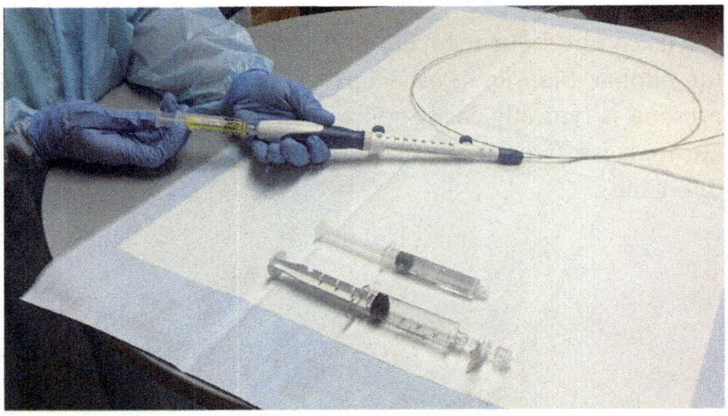

Figure 41.7 Priming the needle with heparin for wet suction technique.

Conclusions

EUS-LB is emerging as an important approach for obtaining excellent tissue cores from the liver. It has several advantages over other techniques and obviously is a more "humane" way of performing a liver biopsy. The safety

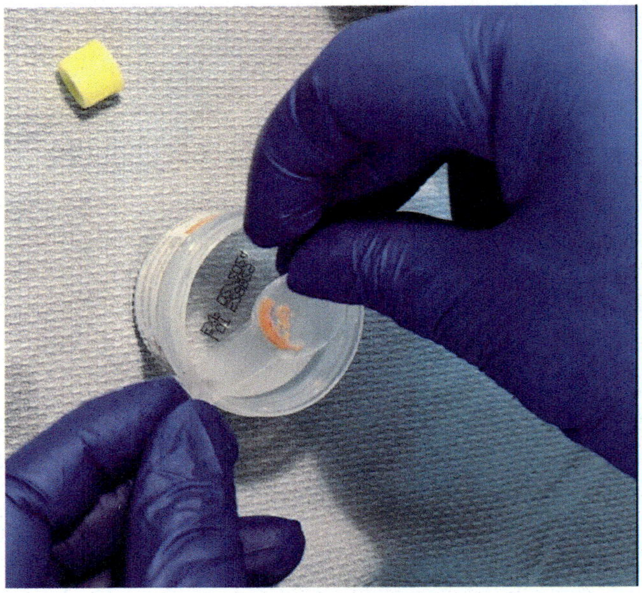

Figure 41.9 Long liver core is placed in formalin jar without excessive handling.

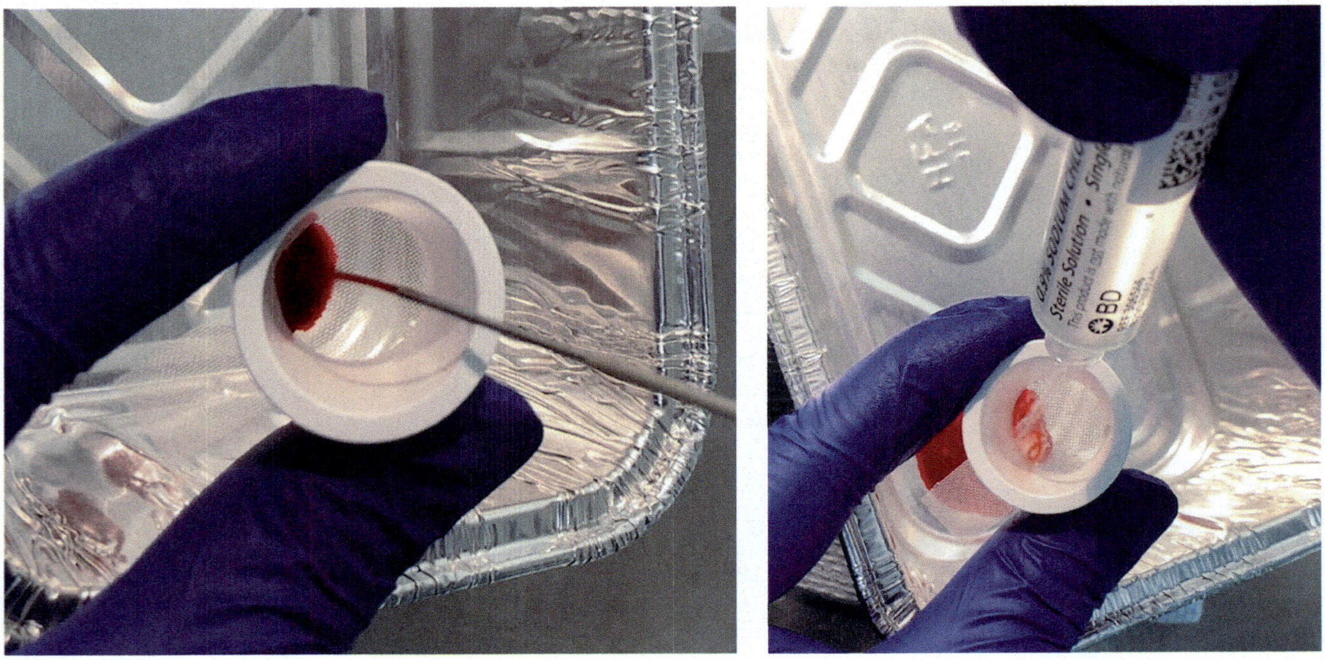

(a) (b)

Figure 41.8 (a) Use of tissue sieve (CoreCatcher; ProAct Ltd, Center Hall, PA) to collect specimen from biopsy needle. (b) Core sample is washed with saline to remove blood.

profile is excellent, although inadvertent splenic puncture, potentially leading to severe bleeding, is a complication unique to EUS-LB. It can be avoided by positive confirmation of the liver as the biopsy target (and not the spleen) prior to the biopsy.

There are a variety of techniques for accomplishing EUS-LB, including choice of needles. Use of wet suction provides the best results. Prospective randomized trials have confirmed the superiority of a 19G core needle (FNB) over a 19G FNA needle, and over a 22G FNB needle. However, if the FNB needle is not available, wet suction with the 19G FNA needle is a reasonable option.

Chapter video clip

Video 41.1 How to perform EUS-guided liver biopsy.

References

1. Rockey DC, Caldwell SH, Goodman ZD, et al. Liver biopsy. *Hepatology* 2009;49(3):1017–1044.
2. Caldwell S. Liver biopsy: the reports of its demise are greatly exaggerated. *Clin Transl Gastroenterol* 2016;7(5):e171.
3. Bravo AA, Sheth SG, Chopra S. Liver biopsy. *N Engl J Med* 2001;344(7):495–500.
4. Pineda JJ, Diehl DL, Miao CL, et al. EUS-guided liver biopsy provides diagnostic samples comparable with those via the percutaneous or transjugular route. *Gastrointest Endosc* 2016;83(2):360–365.
5. Johal AS, Maksimak MG, Diehl DL. Endoscopic ultrasound-guided liver biopsy in pediatric patients. *Endosc Ultrasound* 2014;3(3):191–194.
6. Diehl DL, Mehta M, Shafqet MA, et al. Splenic biopsy as an unintended consequence of EUS-guided liver biopsy: a cautionary tale. *Gastrointest Endosc* 2020;91(1):195–196.
7. Khurana S, Butt W, Khara HS, et al. Bi-lobar liver biopsy via EUS enhances the assessment of disease severity in patients with non-alcoholic steatohepatitis. *Hepatol Int* 2019;13(3):323–329.
8. Ching-Campanioni R, Diehl DL, Confer B, et al. A prospective randomized trial of 19-gauge (G) aspiration needle versus 19G core biopsy needle for endoscopic ultrasound guided liver biopsy. *Endoscopy* 2019;51(11):1059–1065.
9. Mok SR, Diehl DL, Johal AS, et al. Endoscopic ultrasound-guided biopsy in chronic liver disease: a randomized comparison of 19-G FNA and 22-G FNB needles. *Endosc Int Open* 2019;7(1):E62–E71.
10. Mok SR, Diehl DL, Johal AS, et al. A prospective pilot comparison of wet and dry heparinized suction for EUS-guided liver biopsy (with videos). *Gastrointest Endosc* 2018;88(6):919–925.
11. Diehl DL, Mok SR, Khara HS. Heparin priming of EUS-FNA needles does not adversely affect tissue cytology or immunohistochemical staining. *Endosc Int Open* 2018;6(3):E356–E362.
12. Ching-Companioni R, Johal AS, Confer B. One versus three needle actuations for EUS-guided liver biopsy: a prospective randomized trial: Fellows-in-Training Award (Interventional Endoscopy Category). *Am J Gastroenterol* 2018;113:S420.

42 How to do EUS-guided Treatment of Gastric Varices

Dalton Marques Chaves and Filipe Tomishige Chaves
Gastrointestinal Endoscopy Unit, University of Sao Paulo, Sao Paulo-Brazil

Introduction

Since the initial description of the *N*-butyl-2-cyanoacrylate injection by Sohendra in 1986 for treatment of bleeding gastric varices, it is still considered the standard treatment for this type of varix, despite the significant incidence of adverse events. More recently, endoscopic ultrasound (EUS)-guided treatment using cyanoacrylate or coil has showed itself a secure and efficient method, with the advantage of allowing the precise injection of cyanoacrylate into the vessel lumen, even in cases with blood in the gastric lumen. Furthermore, it is also possible to confirm varix obliteration and evaluate recurrences with the Doppler system.

In 2007, Romero-Castro et al. described for the first time the echoguided treatment of gastric varices by injection of cyanoacrylate directly into the varix, with 100% eradication efficiency. However, this method did not decrease the risk of embolism when compared with the normal endoscopic technique, with an incidence of up to 50%.

Because of the risk of embolism with cyanoacrylate, the treatment of gastric varices with coil has become an interesting option. These coils, already in use for endovascular therapy, are composed of synthetic fibers connected to a metallic wire that, when released into the bloodstream, may lead to thrombosis. The size of coil to be employed is selected according to the varix diameter. In 2010, Romero-Castro et al. described for the first time the use of coil in the treatment of gastric varices, treating four patients with success. However, due to the high number of coils necessary for the treatment, cost has been a limitation.

In 2011, Binmoeller et al. reported on the successful use of the echoguided technique combining coil and cyanoacrylate. The goal of this combination is to cause the synthetic fiber coils to retain the glue, lowering the risk of embolism and reducing the necessary volume of cyanoacrylate and number of coils. In a prospective randomized study, we compared echoguided treatment (coil plus cyanoacrylate) and conventional cyanoacrylate technique. The volume of cyanoacrylate used in the combined technique was lower (1.4 vs. 3.0 ml), as was the incidence of pulmonary embolism diagnosed by chest computed tomography (25% vs. 50%).

A systematic review by McCarty et al. in 2019 that analyzed the three types of echoguided treatment (isolated cyanoacrylate, isolated coil, and coil plus cyanoacrylate combination) suggests that combined treatment is the best option.

Technique (Video 42.1)

The steps involved in performing echoguided treatment using coil and cyanoacrylate are as follows.

1. Insert echoendoscope with patient under sedation. If patient is in poor condition, we recommend anesthesia with orotracheal intubation.

2. On rear view, with endoscopic imaging, we identify the varix to be treated (Figure 42.1).

3. On rectified position, move the endoscope to the proximal one-third of the stomach and inject about 50 ml of water into the gastric lumen.

4. Move the endoscopic probe on to the greater curvature of the gastric fundus, looking to identify the varix under water seal.

5. Evaluate the echoendoscopic aspect of the gastric varix (Figures 42.2 and 42.3).

6. Determine the best path to perform echoguided puncture (transgastrically or transesophageally).

7. Identify the widest vascular caliber inside the varix for coil delivery.

Atlas of Endoscopic Ultrasonography, Second Edition. Edited by Frank Gress, Thomas Savides, Brenna Casey, and Everson L. A. Artifon.

Companion website: www.wiley.com/go/gress/atlas

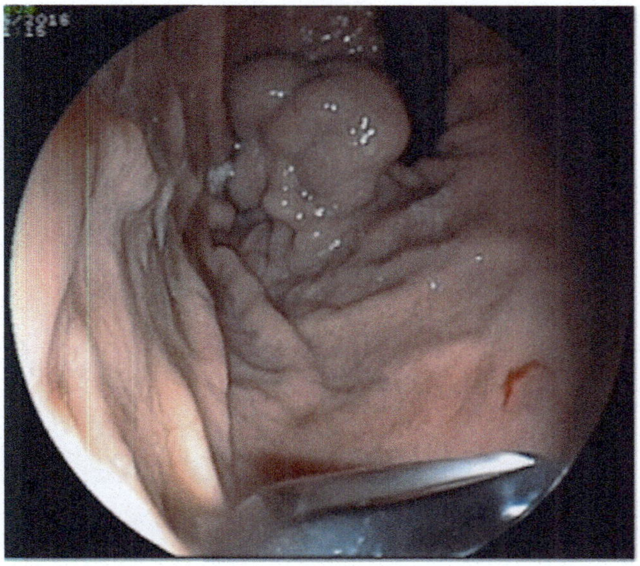

Figure 42.1 Endoscopic imaging of gastric varix.

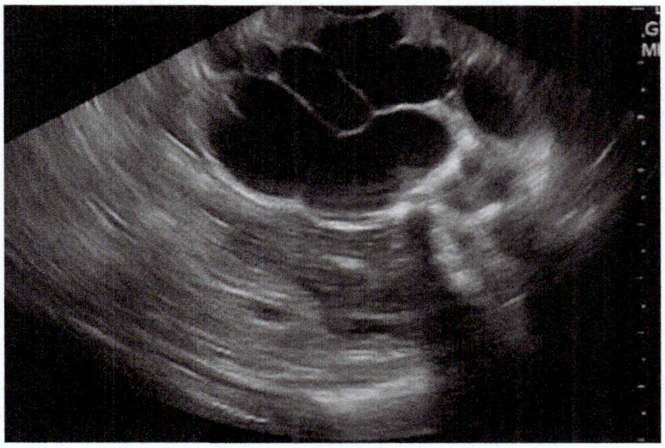

Figure 42.2 Gastric varix seen by endoscopic ultrasonography.

8. Choose the coil size to be used (Embolization Coil, Cook Medical or Interlock, Boston Scientific), not larger than the widest vascular caliber previously chosen.

9. Insertion of 19G puncture needle in the echoendoscope channel.

10. Perform varix puncture under echoendoscopic view (Figure 42.4).

11. Remove stylet from needle.

12. Inject 2 ml of distillated water through needle, checking the position of the needle in the varix.

13. Place coil inside the needle and push it with stylet until coil is delivered inside the varix.

14. Withdraw the stylet from the needle.

15. Inject 3 ml of distilled water through the needle.

16. Fill needle with mixture of 0.5 ml *N*-butyl-2-cyanoacrylate (Histoacryl) and Lipiodol, at a ratio of 1 : 1.

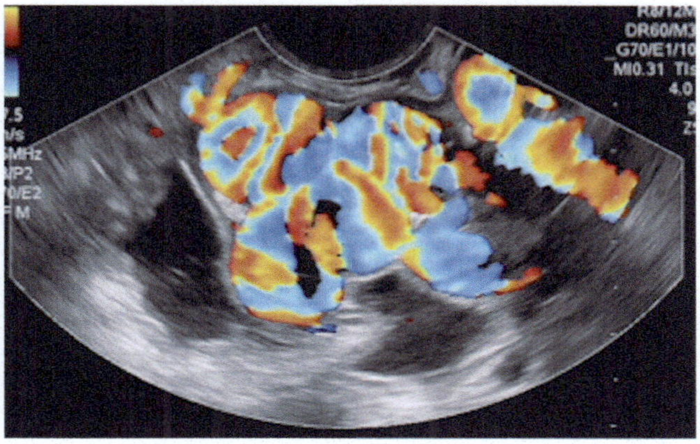

Figure 42.3 Gastric varix seen with color Doppler.

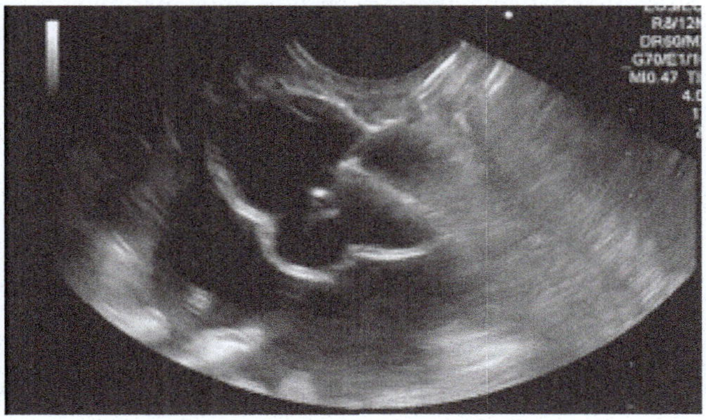

Figure 42.4 Needle inside the varix.

17. Inject 3 ml of distilled water over 30–40 seconds and remove needle while maintaining continuous infusion of distilled water.

18. Next, confirm the absence of blood flow inside the varix (Figures 42.5 and 42.6).

19. We have been using only one coil and 0.5 ml of Histoacryl per session. In cases where immediate occlusion of the varix is less than 50%, we suggest that a new puncture is undertaken immediately.

20. Perform control echoendoscopy in 30 days.

21. In cases of varix flow persistence, we recommend a new session.

Complicatons

The combined echoguided treatment (coil plus cyanoacrylate) for gastric varices has been shown to be efficient and safe, with technical and clinical success rates of 96–100%. The incidence of side effects varies between 0 and 25%. Pulmonary embolism is the main complication, despite most cases being asymptomatic. In 2016, Baht et al. described a case of symptomatic pulmonary embolism among 152 treated

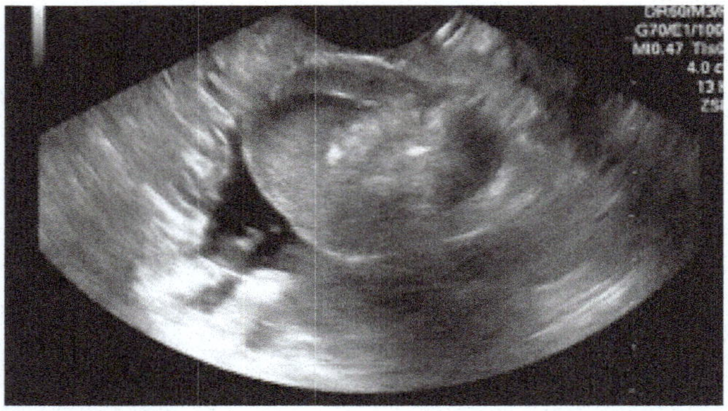

Figure 42.5 Obliterated varix right after treatment.

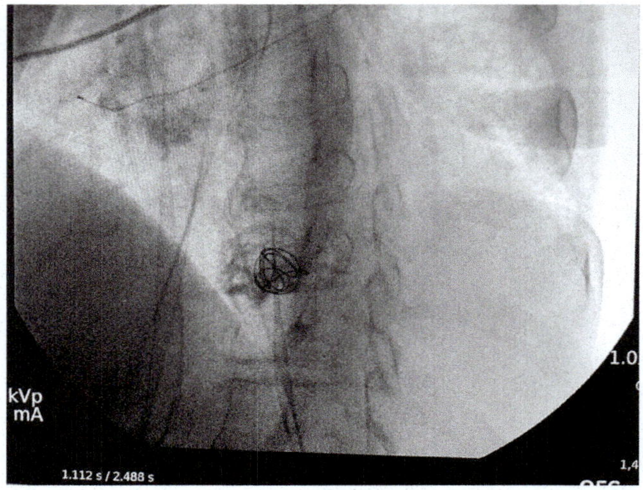

Figure 42.6 Radiographic image of the coil inside the varix.

patients. In our study in 2019, when performing chest CT on all treated patients, the incidence of pulmonary embolism caused by Histoacryl was 25%, with all of them being asymptomatic. Most patients have received only one coil and one Histoacryl ampoule (0.5 ml). The success rate after only one treatment session was 73.4% of treated cases. Treatment was repeated if necessary only after 30 days, which is sufficient time for the thrombosis to consolidate. Abdominal pain has also been reported in up to 25% of cases, fever in up to 3%, and minor delayed upper gastrointestinal bleeding from coil/glue extrusion in 3%.

Chapter video clip

Video 42.1 Ultrasound-guided treatment of gastric varix.

43

How to do EUS-guided Arterial Embolization

Marc Barthet and Jean-Michel Gonzalez
Digestive endoscopy and gastroenterology department, North Hospital, Marseille, France

Background

Recent developments in therapeutic endoscopic ultrasound (EUS) have opened up new fields and EUS-guided sclerotherapy and embolization for gastrointestinal bleeding represents a possible new therapeutic approach [1–3]. In approximately 10–15% of cases, conventional endoscopy is insufficient and leads to early recurrence of bleeding [4]. To date, a limited number of human studies with small patient cohorts [1–3] have been reported in the literature, with 13 series including at least 242 patients having been published [3]. Nevertheless, the effectiveness and possible complications of the EUS-guided vascular approach in the treatment of refractory gastrointestinal bleeding have been poorly assessed in the literature [5–15].

Most of the cases with recurrent bleeding of gastric or peri-anastomotic varices have been treated with injection of polidocanol or cyanoacrylate, with a satisfactory final success rate [8,11,13,15]. More recently, EUS-guided vascular embolization with microcoils has been advocated as decreasing the risk of pulmonary embolism [12,15]. Some rare cases of ulcerations or ulcerations related to a gastrointestinal stromal tumor (GIST) have also been treated using this approach [5,8,14]. Three cases of pseudoaneurysm treated with injection of cyanoacrylate under EUS guidance have been reported, with success in all cases [8,13,14].

The potential limitations of this new application of therapeutic EUS are numerous [1–3,5–15] and include the limited visual field of the scope, the risk of damaging the operating channel, and the risk of induced infections and pulmonary embolism.

Technique

All procedures were performed on hemodynamically stable patients who received systemic antibiotic prophylaxis (2 g of amoxicillin and clavulanate) 30 minutes before the procedure. Proton pump inhibitor infusion was administered over one week. Patients were maintained under general anesthesia in the operating room, with X-ray control. Following conventional endoscopy, a linear endoscope with a large working channel (3.8 mm; Pentax UTK, Japan) with Doppler-enhanced EUS was used. The procedure involved the puncture of the target vessel with a 19-gauge needle (EchoTip; Cook, Winston Salem, NC), followed by the injection of a combination of cyanoacrylate and Lipiodol (2 ml) under direct visualization. The combination of cyanoacrylate glue and Lipiodol was used in both patients since microcoil embolization was not available in our hospital. Doppler monitoring was performed at the end of the procedure to ensure the disappearance of the Doppler signal.

Technical illustration in two cases

The first patient (Figure 43.1) was an 83-year-old man presenting with recurrent hematemesis and melena. Endoscopy showed a huge gastric cancer located to the lesser curve and computed tomography (CT) showed multiple liver metastases. The lesion was a large, deeply excavated ulcer measuring at least 3 cm. He underwent two attempts of conventional hemostatic endoscopic treatment with either coagulation or clips. As he was unfit for surgery, it was decided to perform EUS-guided vascular treatment. After endoscopic assessment of the tumor ulceration directly with the EUS scope, the gastric lumen was suctioned until all the air was completely removed (Video 43.1). EUS assessment was cautiously performed until the feeding artery of the tumor could be observed. The vessel was targeted with a 19G needle under Doppler control. The combination of Lipiodol (1 ml) and cyanoacrylate (1 ml) was injected directly into the vessel, followed by injection of 2 ml of pure Lipiodol to rinse the content of the 19G needle. Complete disappearence of the Doppler signal was checked at the end of the procedure.

Atlas of Endoscopic Ultrasonography, Second Edition. Edited by Frank Gress, Thomas Savides, Brenna Casey, and Everson L. A. Artifon.

Companion website: www.wiley.com/go/gress/atlas

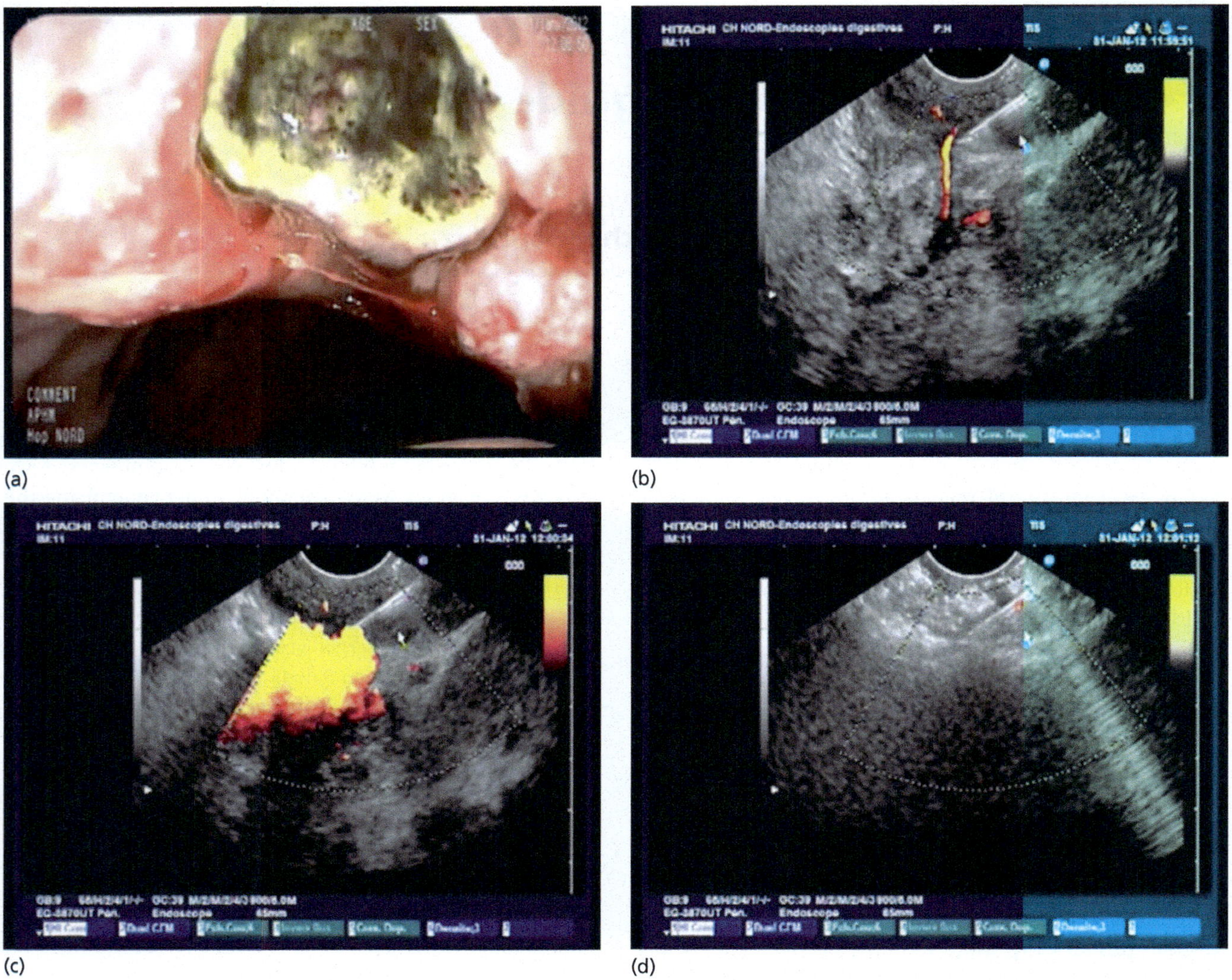

Figure 43.1 Patient 1 with refractory bleeding due to gastric cancer. (a) Bleeding gastric cancer to the lesser curve. (b) Feeding artery with 19G needle in close contact. (c) Injection of combination of Lipiodol and cyanoacrylate glue. (d) Disappearence of the Doppler signal.

The second patient (Figure 43.2) was a 48-year-old man with early alcoholic chronic pancreatitis without calcifications. It was his second attack of acute pancreatitis, diagnosed as necrotizing acute pancreatitis. The patient was hospitalized in the intensive care unit and at day 4, a massive bleeding occurred. At endoscopy, no mucosal lesion could be demonstrated but CT scan showed a pseudoaneurysm located to the head of the pancreas. Once haemodynamic stability was achieved, EUS-guided vascular treatment was indicated. EUS located the pseudoaneurysm in the head of the pancreas (Video 43.2). The pancreatic artery within the pseudoaneurysm was targeted with ultrasound and Doppler and a 19G needle was advanced cautiously into the artery lumen. The mixture of Lipiodol and cyanoacrylate glue was injected, followed by 2 ml of pure Lipiodol. X-ray control showed partial reflux in the gastroduodenal artery and then the hepatic artery but without any clinical or biological consequences.

Postprocedural management and complications

Patients were allowed to eat again from three days after the procedure. Clinical and laboratory evaluations were performed daily for one week, with CT scans performed within the first week post procedure. CT scan in the second patient showed complete occlusion of the pseudoaneurysm, highlighted by the Lipiodol injection.

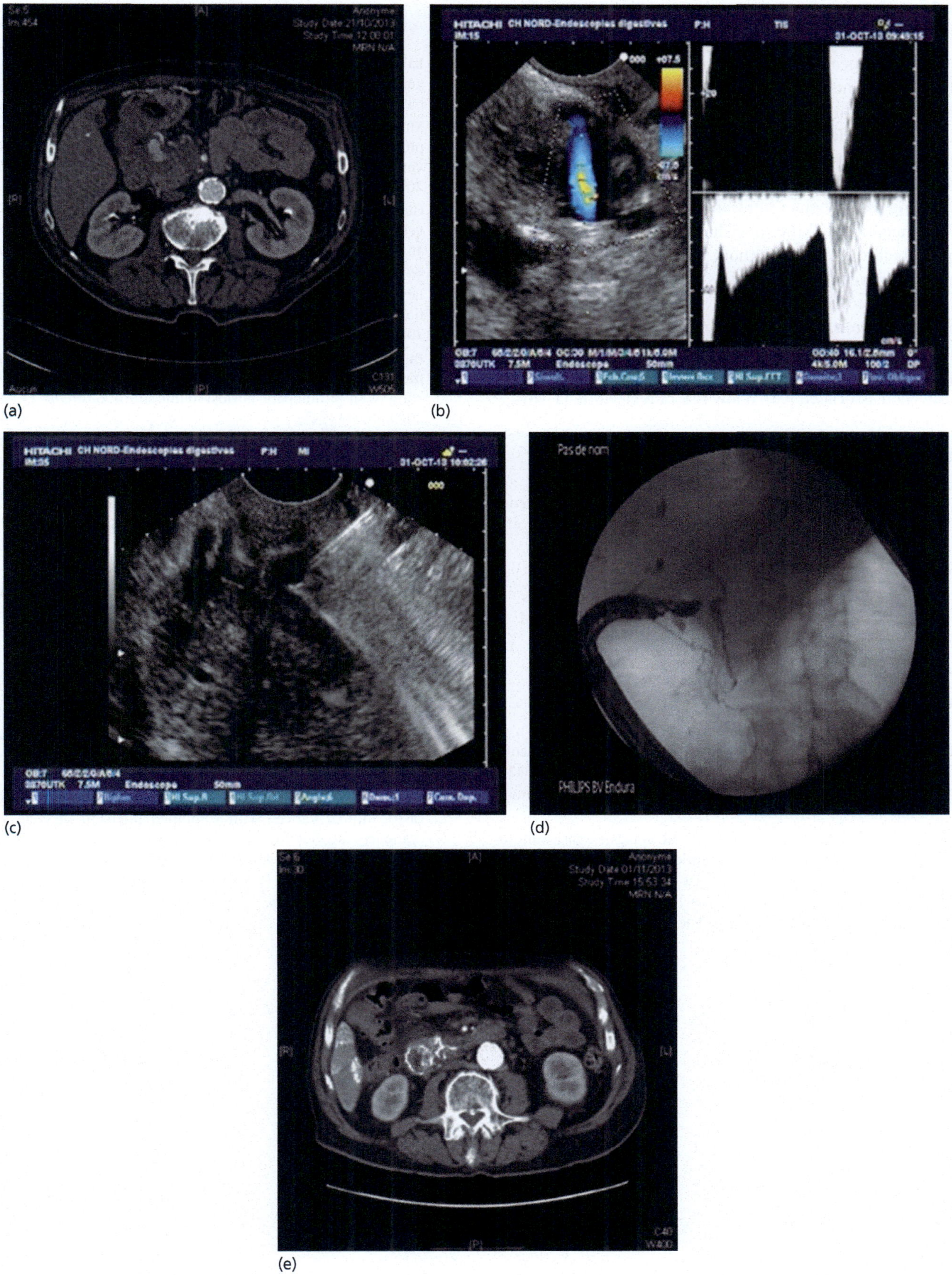

Figure 43.2 Patient 2 with bleeding pseudoaneurysm located to the pancreatic head. (a) CT scan of the pseudoaneurysm in the pancreatic head. (b) EUS view with Doppler. (c) Insertion of 19G needle inside the pseudoaneurysm. (d) Injection of combination of Lipiodol and cyanoacrylate glue under X-ray control. (e) Postoperative CT scan showing efficient embolization of the pseudoaneurysm.

No recurrence of bleeding occurred during the follow-up of these patients. No infection nor liver damage occurred based on clinical and biological examinations.

There were few complications in most of the series, in which the patients received antibiotic prophylaxis [1–3,5–15]. At the time of each intervention, the target vessel was identified using color Doppler ultrasound and then punctured with a 19G needle. In all the procedures, it was possible to inject the embolization agent without damage to the EUS equipment. We observed that if the loss of Doppler signal within the target vessel could be confirmed at the end of the procedure, there was no recurrence of hemorrhage, as shown in seven of our eight patients [1]. The absence of a Doppler ultrasound signal after endoscopic treatment of bleeding ulcers has previously been associated with a low risk of rebleeding [1,16].

Chapter video clips

Video 43.1 Arterial embolization of a feeding vessel in a patient with gastric cancer and refractory bleeding. Source: Hitachi Ltd.

Video 43.2 Arterial embolization in a patient with pseudoaneurysm located in the head of the pancreas after acute necrotizing pancreatitis. Source: Hitachi Ltd.

References

1. Gonzalez JM, Giacino C, Pioche M, et al. EUS-guided vascular therapies: is it safe and effective? *Endoscopy* 2012;44:539–542.
2. Siddiqui UM, Levy MJ. EUS-guided transluminal interventions. *Gastroenterology* 2018;154:1911–1924.
3. Dain D, Thosani N, Shingal S, et al. EUS-assisted gastrointestinal hemostasis: an evolving technique. *Ther Adv Gastroenterol* 2016;9:635–647.
4. Laine L. Endoscopic therapy for bleeding ulcers: room for improvement. *Gastrointest Endosc* 2003;57:557–560.
5. Law R, Fujii L, Wong Kee Song LM, et al. Efficacy of EUS-guided hemostatic interventions for resistant non-variceal bleedings. *Clin Gastroenterol Hepatol* 2014;13:808–812.
6. Magno P, Ko CW, Buscaglia JM, et al. EUS-guided angiography: a novel approach to diagnostic and therapeutic interventions in the vascular system. *Gastrointest Endosc* 2007;66:587–591.
7. Giday SA, Clarke JO, Buscaglia JM, et al. EUS-guided portal vein catheterization: a promising novel approach for portal angiography and portal vein pressure measurements. *Gastrointest Endosc* 2008;67:338–342.
8. Levy MJ, Chak A. EUS 2008 working group document: evaluation of EUS-guided vascular therapy. *Gastrointest Endosc* 2009;69(2 Suppl):S37–S42.
9. Buscaglia JM, Dray X, Shin EJ, et al. A new alternative for a transjugular intrahepatic portosystemic shunt: EUS-guided creation of an intrahepatic portosystemic shunt. *Gastrointest Endosc* 2009;69:941–947.
10. Fockens P, Meenan J, Van Dullemen HM, et al. Dieulafoy's disease: endosonographic detection and endosonography-guided treatment. *Gastrointest Endosc* 1996;44:437–442.
11. Romero-Castro R, Pellicer-Bautista FJ, Jimenez-Saenz M, et al. EUS-guided injection of cyanoacrylate in perforating feeding veins in gastric varices: results in 5 cases. *Gastrointest Endosc* 2007;66:402–407.
12. Levy MJ, Wong Kee Song LM, Kendrick ML, et al. EUS-guided coil embolization for refractory ectopic variceal bleeding. *Gastrointest Endosc* 2008;67:572–574.
13. Gonzales JM, Ezzedine S, Vitton V, et al. Endoscopic ultrasound treatment of vascular complications in acute pancreatitis. *Endoscopy* 2009;41:721–724.
14. Levy MJ, Wong Kee Song LM, Farnell MB, et al. Endoscopic ultrasound (EUS)-guided angiotherapy of refractory gastrointestinal bleeding. *Am J Gastroenterol* 2008;103: 352–359.
15. Baht Y, Weilert F, Freidrick R, et al. EUS-guided treatment of gastric fundal varices with combined injection of coils and cyanoacrylate glue: a large U.S. experience over 6 years (with Video). *Gastrointest Endosc* 2016;83:1164–1172.
16. Wong RC. Endoscopic Doppler US probe for acute peptic ulcer hemorrhage. *Gastrointest Endosc* 2004;60:804–812.

44

How to do EUS-guided Radiofrequency Ablation of Pancreatic Neuroendocrine Tumors

Marc Barthet, Mohamed Gasmi, and Jean-Michel Gonzalez
Digestive endoscopy and gastroenterology department, North Hospital, Marseille, France

Introduction

EUS-guided radiofrequency ablation (RFA) has recently emerged as a new technique for pancreatic tumor ablation, mostly neuroendocrine tumors (NETs), pancreatic cystic neoplasm (PCN), or pancreatic adenocarcinoma. NETs are probably an indication of choice for EUS-guided RFA. NETs are mostly non-functional and do not induce secretory disorder [1]. Once their nature is yielded by diagnostic tests such as EUS-guided fine needle aspiration (FNA), incidental nonfunctional NETs currently lead to management difficulties when their largest diameter is less than 2 cm [2–4]. In patients with tumors ranging in size from 1 to 2 cm, therapeutic surgical choices could be challenged by EUS-guided treatment [5–7]. An interesting alternative to surgery could be destruction with endoscopic RFA [8–11].

About five series have been published including NETs or PCNs, most of them being retrospective or including only few patients [12–16]. In addition, the follow-up of the patients in these series is short, less than 13 months [12–16]. The short-term efficacy in these series ranges between 71.4 and 100% for NETs, but the long-term outcome and risk of recurrence are still unknown [12–16]. Despite these interesting results regarding short-term efficacy, surgery remains the treatment of choice in the absence of long-term follow-up and randomized series. However, with regard to the results of surgical resection of benign tumors, the mortality rate is 3–14% and morbidity rate 15–30%, compared to no mortality and morbidity of 3–10% [17,18].

Studies assessing the results of EUS-guided RFA were conducted between 2015 and 2019 [12–16]. Of these, three were prospective studies with a follow-up ranging from six months to one year [12,14,15]. Our team conducted a multicenter prospective study between February 2015 and February 2017 with a one-year follow-up [14]; recently, the long-term outcome of these patients with follow-up at three to five years became available.

Methods for EUS-guided RFA

Technique

Endoscopic examination should be performed with an EUS therapeutic scope. In the case of NETs, the operative needle can be used directly.

EUS-RFA can be performed with a 19G RFA needle (Starmed, Taewong, Korea) applying a 50-W current under continuance mode setting until reaching 100 Ω impedance (appearance of white bubbles) and not exceeding 500 Ω. RFA was stopped either when the ultrasound operator saw white bubbles alongside the needle and outside the targeted lesions or when the impedance exceeded 100 Ω. RFA duration was usually 15–45 seconds. One to three shots can be performed during the same session: one shot for pancreatic NETs (pNETs) of 1 cm; three shots for pNETs of 15–20 mm. Normally, operators should not exceed three shots because of the risk of further complications such as pancreatitis or ductal damage (biliary or pancreatic), mainly if the lesion is located in the head of the pancreas. Another device is also available: a thin radiofrequency probe that can be introduced into the lumen of a 19G FNA needle and ejected from the needle tip for application of radiofrequency abaltion (Habib™ EndoHPB probe, Boston Scientific, Marlborough, MA). With this device, white bubbles due to thermic injury are often difficult to see.

The use of contrast-enhanced harmonic (CEH)-EUS is recommended before and after applying EUS-guided RFA (Figure 44.1). A recent series in 19 patients with solid abdominal tumors demonstrated the usefulness of targeting EUS-guided RFA using CEH-EUS findings [19]. As pNETs are

Atlas of Endoscopic Ultrasonography, Second Edition. Edited by Frank Gress, Thomas Savides, Brenna Casey, and Everson L. A. Artifon.

Companion website: www.wiley.com/go/gress/atlas

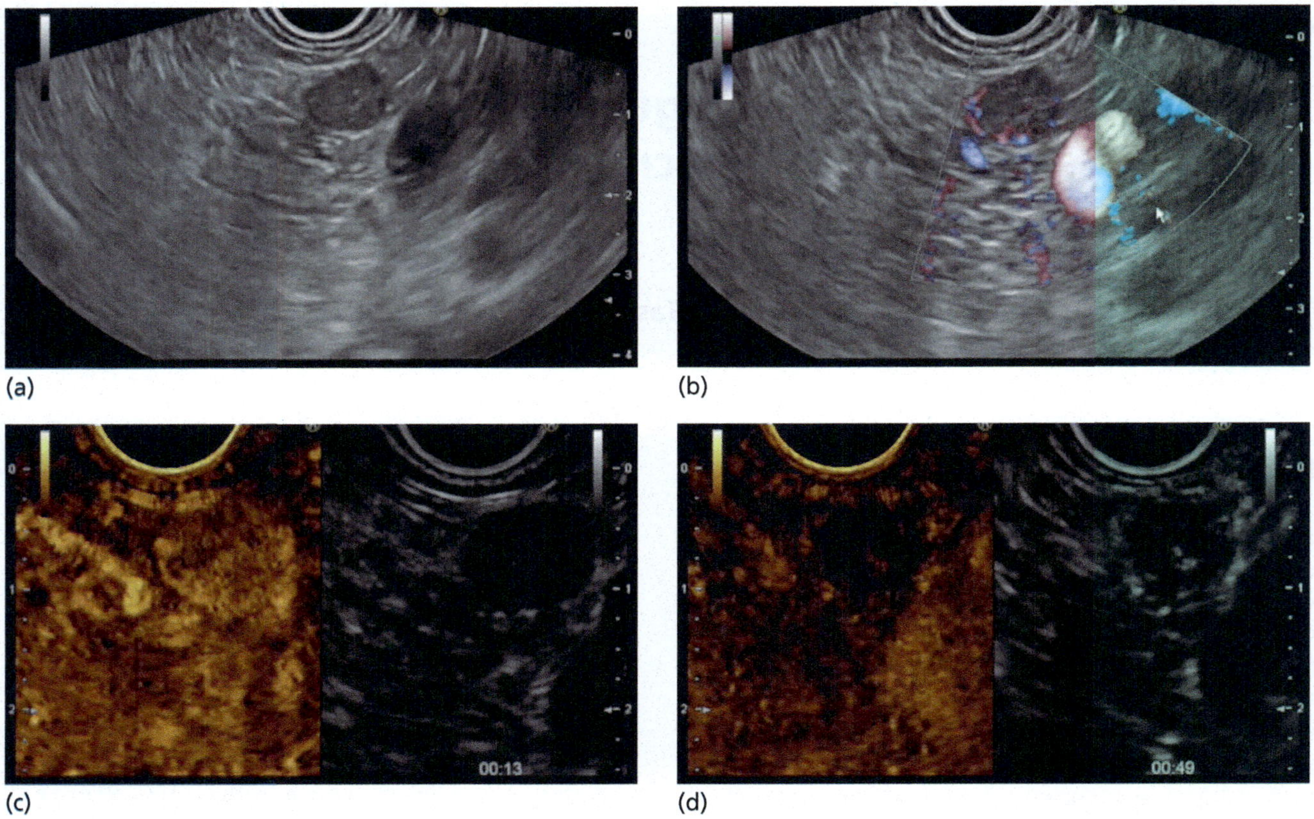

Figure 44.1 EUS-guided RFA with contrast enhancement control for NET located in the body of the pancreas. (a) EUS view of NET located in the body of the pancreas, 11 mm size, homogeneous. (b) EUS view of NET with fine Doppler showing peripheral arterial vascularization. (c) CEH-EUS view of NET showing early hyperenhancement. (d) Immediate CEH-EUS view of NET after EUS-RFA showing no more enhancement of the treated NET.

usually hypervascularized, CEH-EUS allows targeting of the RFA application. Particularly in large pNETs close to 2 cm in size, areas of sustained hypervascularization could persist despite multiple shots, which should not exceed three attempts (unpublished data). In such cases, postoperative CEH-EUS may allow any remaining vascularized areas to be targeted for a subsequent shot.

Prophylaxis for complications

Prophylaxis should be instituted to prevent acute pancreatitis, infection, and perforation [14]. Rectal diclofenac was used, as recommended before endoscopic retrograde cholangiopancreatography (ERCP), to prevent post-endoscopic pancreatitis. Antibiotic prophylaxis (2 g of amoxicillin and clavulanic acid intravenously) was used to prevent infection. Suctioning the main fluid content in cases of pancreatic cystic neoplasm was performed before RFA in order to avoid excessive transmission of radiofrequency current into the liquid component.

Indications

Starting with EUS-guided RFA for pNETs, only patients unfit for surgery were selected for EUS-guided RFA [5,7,8–16]. International recommendations (European NET guidelines and the revised NCCN guidelines) suggest follow-up for pNETs under 1 cm and surgery for pNETs over 2 cm because of the high risk of lymph node and distant metastasis [20–22]. However the management of pNETs ranging between 1 and 2 cm in size is debated. The balance between the spontaneous risk of lymphatic or metastatic spreading (up to 28%) and the morbidity and mortality of surgery (10–30%) should be considered [17,18,20–22]. As the morbidity of EUS-guided RFA is low (3–10%), it is increasingly accepted that it should be indicated for lesions ranging between 1 and 2 cm in size [5–7,11–16].

If the indications for EUS-guided RFA should be restricted to pNET diameters of 1–2 cm, the pathology should be assessed before any EUS-guided management. Only pNETs belonging to grade 1 of the World Health Organization (WHO) classification should be treated with EUS management, since grade 2 or 3 pNETs lead to excessive risk for lymph node or metastatic spreading. The accuracy of FNA for grading using the WHO classification seems to be accurate in more than 75% of cases [23].

Therefore only patients with grade 1 pNETs of 1–2 cm should be considered for EUS-guided RFA.

Results for EUS-guided RFA studies

Overall results

An increasing number of studies have evaluated EUS-guided RFA for treating premalignant pancreatic tumors (i.e. NETs), but most of them either include a small number of patients or are retrospective [12–16]. Five series studying EUS-guided RFA of NETs have been published [16–20], three of them being prospective and including one to twelve patients [12–16,24,25]. Even though the efficacy for NETs is 71.4–100% and for PCNs 48.4–65%, the long-term results are still unknown and we cannot rule out the risk of recurrences or an unfavorable outcome such as early malignancy [18,24–26].

With regard to efficacy, promising initial results using the dedicated cooling needle or Habib probe in the treatment of pNETs have been shown in short series (3 to 30 patients of a total of 51 patients) [12–16]. Interestingly, in one series comprising three functional NETs (insulinomas), rapid symptomatic and biological improvement occurred within two days following the procedure, with sustained results at two years follow-up [13]. With regard to the efficacy of treatment for pNETs, one series found complete resolution in 70–85% at one year follow-up despite an incomplete significant response in 70% at six months follow-up [14,16]. Some delayed response could occur after six months follow-up, probably due to stimulation of immune responses [14].

The overall morbidity rate in the largest prospective series was three cases (10%) [14]. In two of the cases, the morbidity was due to acute pancreatitis with early infection in one, and perforation of adjacent jejunum in the other. After modifying the study protocol to reduce the risk of pancreatitis, infection or damage to adjacent organs in cystic lesions, only one case occurred (3.5%). This was an obstructive pancreatitis due to fistulization of an NET within the main pancreatic duct; the case was successfully treated by ERCP, including pancreatic sphincterotomy and stenting. One year later, all these three patients were doing well with no tumor present. Very few data about the safety of the technique can be found in the articles about EUS-guided RFA in PCN [12–16]. Pai et al. [12] applied EUS-guided RFA using the Habib probe in six PCNs (four mucinous cystadenomas, one intraductal papillary mucinous neoplasm [IPMN], and one cystic NET) and two patients experienced transient mild pain that resolved within three days [12].

Results of long-term follow-up

In all the published series, the longest follow-up was 13 months [12–16]. Long-term data from the largest prospective series including 30 patients have been presented recently [14, and unpublished data].

A total of 12 patients had 14 pNETs, the series comprising seven males (58%) and five females, with a mean age of 59.9 years (range 45–77 years). All NETs were well differenciated and non-functional and belonged to OMS grade 1 classification, associated in one case with multiple endocrine neoplasia (MEN) type 1. The mean size of the NETs was 13.1 mm (range 10–20 mm), with three located in the head, six in the body, and five in the tail of the pancreas.

Patients were followed for at least three years (mean 45.6 months), the last patient being included in February 2017; mean age at the end of follow-up was 62.5 years (range 52–87 years). The mean duration of follow-up was 42.9 months (range 36–53 months). Two males (aged 52–77 years) died during follow-up at 42 months from causes other than the inclusion criteria: one patient who had MEN-1 and NET committed suicide; the other, originally treated with EUS-guided RFA for an IPMN located in the head of the pancreas and who had no cystic lesions in the tail of the pancreas, developed cancer in the tail of the pancreas.

At one-year follow-up, 12 NETs (85.7%) had completely disappeared or exhibited necrosis. Two were considered failures. At the end of follow-up (45.6 months), 12 NETs had completely disappeared. One of the patients exhibited a small hyperechoic scar at six months' follow-up, with no contrast enhancement on computed tomography (CT) and EUS and negative FNA. The scar remained stable from 6 to 41 months of follow-up. Another patient, initially considered a failure at one year because the cystic lesion located in the tail of the pancreas still measured 20 mm, exhibited no contrast enhancement on EUS. At the end of follow-up (53 months), the lesion disappeared completely on CT scan and EUS.

There were two failures, of whom one was a recurrence after disappearance at one year and another had persistent disease at one-year follow-up.

1. A 73-year-old male patient. The lesion was located in the body of the pancreas and measured 18 mm at inclusion. At six months the lesion measured 13 mm, but at one year the lesion could not be found and treatment was considered a success. At the end of follow-up (42 months), the lesion again measured 16 mm on EUS with no enhancement on CEH-EUS. FNA showed well-differentiated neuroendocrine cells (G1 in the WHO classification).

2. A 65-year-old female patient. The lesion was located in the body of the pancreas and measured 19 mm at inclusion. She was considered a failure at one year, the lesion measuring 12 mm at six months and 16 mm at one year. She received a second session of EUS-RFA at 23 months, and the size of the lesion decreased to 13 mm. Unfortunately, she developed asymptomatic liver metastases at 36 months, with positron emission tomography (PET) identifying intense uptake on liver metastases and pancreatic tail. The patient is doing well and receives somatostatin therapy. Pathological re-examination of the first FNA corrected the WHO classification from G1 to G2.

With regard to the RFA indications for NETs, the long-term results of EUS-guided RFA in the 14 lesions in 12 patients appeared to be stable, with 85.7% success at one year and at the end of follow-up. In fact, despite these stable results, there was one late response and one late recurrence. In one case considered a failure at one year, the tumor disappeared completely at 53 months follow-up. It was a 20-mm lesion located in the tail of the pancreas that completely disappeared at one year on CEH-EUS. This delayed success may be related to activated immune responses related to RFA [14]. Conversely, an 18-mm NET located in the body of the pancreas seemed to disappear at one year after its size decreased to 13 mm at six months but it reoccurred at 42 months' follow-up, measuring 16 mm. No enhancement on CEH-EUS could be demonstrated but EUS-FNA showed well-differentiated endocrine cells belonging to a G1 WHO classification. We have no clear explanation for this late and benign recurrence. Although the protocol of this study specified only one RFA shot of 50 W not exceeding 100 Ω, we now apply one to three shots depending on the results of immediate CEH-EUS. After considering the complete diffusion of the white bubbles into the volume of the tumor, we controlled by CEH-EUS. In cases of persistent contrast enhancement, we added a targeted RFA shot. The same approach has been promoted by other authors [22,24,25]. A recent series of 19 patients with solid abdominal tumor demonstrated the usefulness of targeting EUS-guided RFA with CEH-EUS findings [22]. Unfortunately, one case showed an unfavorable outcome, with metastatic spreading in a 65-year-old female. The lesion was located in the body of the pancreas. measuring 19 mm at inclusion with a G1 WHO classification at FNA. She was considered a failure at one year, with a 12-mm lesion at six months and a 16-mm lesion at one year. She received a second session of EUS-RFA at 23 months, the size of the lesion decreasing to 13 mm. She developed asymptomatic liver metastases at 36 months, with PET scan identifying an intense uptake on liver metastases and pancreatic tail. The patient is doing well and receives somatostatin therapy. As we did not understand the metastatic outcome, we requested a pathological re-examination of the first FNA, and this corrected the WHO classification from G1 to G2. It has been shown in the literature that the accuracy of FNA for an adequate WHO classification is not complete, ranging from 74 to 87.5% [23]. This could explain the discrepancy between the two pathological results, emphasizing that long-term follow-up is always required, and in case of failure at one year surgery should be recommended, despite one delayed healing case occurring after one year follow-up. In this series, in the event of RFA failure the risk of unfavorable and metastatic outcome is 50%. Nevertheless, in our case, the patient was not operable, leading to a second RFA session at two years' follow-up and discovery of metastatic liver spreading at 36 months. The risk of developing further malignancy during the follow-up of NETs larger than 2 cm has been estimated to be up to 27.3% for lymph nodes and 9% for metastases [27]. The European NET guidelines and the revised NCCN guidelines suggest surveillance for lesions under 2 cm (and no more surgery) [20–22]. Pancreatic surgery for NETs is associated with a mortality rate of 3–6% and morbidity rate of 14–58%, mainly due to pancreatic fistula [17]. In the same systematic review, the five-year overall survival and disease-specific survival were, respectively, 85% and 93%. A randomized series comparing surgical resection and EUS-guided RFA should be conducted.

Conclusion

EUS-RFA management of pNETs is associated with an efficient long-term outcome, with size ranging between 1 and 2 cm and grade 1 WHO classification. Complete disappearance of NETs occurs in 85.7% of cases, with morbidity lower than 10%.

Conflicts of interest disclosure

Marc Barthet received a research grant from Boston Scientific (endoscopic gastrojejunal anastomosis).

Chapter video clips

Video 44.1 EUS-guided RFA for NET located in the body of the pancreas with microbubbles contrast enhancement

Video 44.2 EUS-guided RFA for NET located in the uncinate process with fine doppler assessment

References

1. Lee DW, Kim MK, Kim HG. Diagnosis of pancreatic neuroendocrine tumors. *Clin Endosc* 2017;50:537–545.
2. Sachs T, Pratt WB, Callery MP, et al. The incidental asymptomatic pancreatic lesion: nuisance or threat? *J Gastrointest Surg* 2009;13:405–415.
3. Strosberg JR, Cheema A, Weber J, et al. Prognostic validity of a novel American Joint Committee on Cancer Staging Classification for pancreatic neuroendocrine tumors. *J Clin Oncol* 2011;29:3044–3049.
4. Metz DC, Jensen RT. Gastrointestinal neuroendocrine tumors: pancreatic endocrine tumors. *Gastroenterology* 2008;135:1469–1492.
5. Finks JF, Osborne NH, Birkmeyer JD. Trends in hospital volume and operative mortality for high-risk surgery. *N Engl J Med* 2011;364:2128–2137.
6. Lakhtakia S. Therapy of pancreatic neuroendocrine tumors: fine needle intervention including ethanol and radiofrequency ablation. *Clin Endosc* 2017;50:546–551.
7. Chennat J. Current status of endoscopic ultrasound guided ablation techniques. *Gastroenterology* 2011;140:1403–1409.
8. Lakhtakia S, Seo D-W. Endoscopic ultrasonography-guided tumor ablation. *Dig Endosc* 2017;29:486–494.
9. Zacharoulis D, Lazoura O, Rountas C, et al. Experimental animal study of a novel radiofrequency endovascular occlusion device. *Am J Surg* 2011;202:103–109.

10. Sethi A, Ellrichmann M, Dhar S, et al. Endoscopic ultrasound-guided lymph node ablation with a novel radiofrequency ablation probe: feasibility study in an acute porcine model. *Endoscopy* 2014;46:411–415.
11. Kim HJ, Seo D-W, Hassanuddin A, et al. EUS-guided radiofrequency ablation of the porcine pancreas. *Gastrointest Endosc* 2012;76:1039–1043.
12. Pai M, Habib N, Senturk H, et al. Endoscopic ultrasound guided radiofrequency ablation for pancreatic cystic neoplasms and neuroendocrine tumors. *World J Gastrointest Surg* 2015;7:52–59.
13. Lakhtakia S, Ramchandani M, Galasso D, et al. EUS-guided radiofrequency ablation for management of pancreatic insulinoma by using a novel needle electrode (with videos). *Gastrointest Endosc* 2016;83:234–239.
14. Barthet M, Giovannini M, Lesavre N, et al. Endoscopic ultrasound guided radiofrequency ablation for pancreatic neuroendocrine tumors and pancreatic cystic neoplasms: a prospective multicenter study. *Endoscopy* 2019;51:836–842.
15. Choi JHS, Song TJ, Park DH, et al. Endoscopic ultrasound-guided radiofrequency ablation for management of benign solid pancreatic tumors. *Endoscopy* 2018;50:1099–1104.
16. Oleinikov KD, Epshtein J, Benson A, et al. Endoscopic ultrasound-guided radiofrequency ablation: a new therapeutic approach for pancreatic neuroendocrine tumors. *J Clin Endocrinol Metab* 2019;104:2637–2647.
17. Jilesen APJ, Van Eijck CHJ, in't Hof KH, et al. Postoperative complications, in-hospital mortality and 5-year survival after surgical resection for patients with a pancreatic neuroendocrine tumor: a systematic review. *World J Surg* 2016;40: 729–748.
18. Feng Q, Li C, Zhang S, et al. Recurrence and survival after surgery for pancreatic cancer with or without pancreatitis. *World J Gastroenterol* 2019;25:6006–6015.
19. Choi JH, Seo DW, Song TJ, et al. Utility of contrast-enhanced harmonic endoscopic ultrasound for the guidance and monitoring of endoscopic radiofrequency ablation. *Gut Liver* 2020;14(6):826–832.
20. Falconi M, Eriksson B, Kaltsas G, et al. ENETS consensus guidelines update for the managementof patients with pancreatic functional neuroendocrine tumors and pancreatic non-functional neuroendocrine tumors. *Neuroendocrinology* 2016;103: 153–171.
21. Teo RYA, Teo TZ, Tai DWM, et al. Systematic review of current prognostication systems for pancreatic neuroendocrine neoplasms. *Surgery* 2019;165:672–685.
22. Choi JH, Choi YH, Kang J, et al. Natural history of small pancreatic lesions suspected to be non-functioning pancreatic neuroendocrine tumors. *Pancreas* 2018;47:1358–1364.
23. Sugimoto M, Takagi T, Hikichi T, et al. Efficacy of endoscopic ultrasonography-guided fine needle aspiration for pancreatic neuroendocrine tumor grading. *World J Gastroenterol* 2015;21:8818–8124.
24. Rimbas M, Horumba M, Rizzatti G, et al. Interventional endoscopic ultrasound for pancreatic neuroendocrine neoplasms. Dig Endosc 2020;32(7):1031–1041.
25. Larghi A, Rizzatti G, Rimbas M, et al. Endoscopic ultrasound-guided radiofrequency ablation as an alternative to surgery for pancreatic neuroendocrine neoplasms: who should we treat? *Endosc Ultrasound* 2019;8:220–226.
26. Canakis A, Law R, Baron T. An updated review on ablative treatment of pancreatic cystic lesions. *Gastrointest Endosc* 2020;91:520–526.
27. Lombardi M, De Lio N, Funel M, et al. Prognostic factors for pancreatic neuroendocrine neoplasms (pNET) and the risk of small non-functional pNET. *J Endocrinol Invest* 2015;38: 605–613.

45 How to do EUS Pancreatic Duct Access and Drainage

Alberto Larghi[1], Mihai Rimbaş[2], and Mauricio K. Minata[3]

[1] Digestive Endoscopy Unit, Fondazione Policlinico A. Gemelli IRCCS, Rome, Italy

[2] Department of Gastroenterology, Colentina Clinical Hospital; Internal Medicine Department, Carol Davila University of Medicine, Bucharest, Romania

[3] Digestive Endoscopy Unit, University of São Paulo, SP, Brazil

Introduction

In recent years, technological advancements in endoscopy have allowed minimally invasive interventions to the pancreatic and biliary ductal systems. Endoscopic retrograde cholangiopancreatography (ERCP) is considered a first-line treatment for main pancreatic duct (MPD) strictures, disruption or obstruction. However, even in expert referral centers, in around 10% of patients ERCP may be impossible due to surgically altered anatomy, or may fail due to inaccessible papilla, tight MPD strictures, pancreatic duct disruption, or other technical and anatomic conditions.

Endoscopic ultrasound (EUS) grants access to a wide variety of procedures. Since the initial description of EUS-assisted pancreatography by Harada in 1995 and Wiersema in 1996, the procedure has continued to evolve so that even EUS-guided MPD access and drainage has been performed. Despite the high level of difficulty and very selective indications, EUS-guided pancreatic duct drainage (EUS-PDD) is a powerful tool when ERCP is impossible or fails.

Indications

At present, the generally accepted indications for EUS-PDD include the following.

- Symptomatic obstruction of the MPD after failed ERCP and cancer excluded.
- Symptomatic ductal stones after failed extracorporeal shock wave lithotripsy (ESWL) and standard ERCP.
- Symptomatic obstruction of the MPD in patients with inaccessible papilla in the presence of postsurgical anatomy (gastrectomy, Roux-en-Y anastomosis, post-Whipple procedure).
- Disconnected pancreatic tail syndrome.

Contraindications

General contraindications for therapeutic endoscopy apply also to EUS-PDD. The other contraindications that must be considered include:

- hemodynamic instability
- severe thrombocytopenia (platelet count $<50 \times 10^9$/l)
- uncorrectable coagulopathy (INR >1.5)
- inability to localize the MPD
- intervening structures, in particular vessels
- multiple MPD strictures.

Before the procedure

The procedure should be performed with the patient under general anesthesia. Prophylactic intravenous antibiotics should be administered before EUS-PDD, and the procedure should be performed using a therapeutic channel echoendoscope utilizing CO_2 insufflation. Patient positioning is also important, since the prone position allows easier recognition of the MPD under fluoroscopy guidance.

Techniques for drainage

EUS-PDD can be performed as an anterograde, retrograde, or rendezvous procedure (Figure 45.1). The terms "anterograde" and "retrograde" refer to the direction of stent insertion and drainage. In the anterograde approach, the stent insertion is in the ampulla direction, whereas the retrograde drainage moves toward a caudal path. The MPD can be accessed by the transgastric, transduodenal, or transenteric approach.

Atlas of Endoscopic Ultrasonography, Second Edition. Edited by Frank Gress, Thomas Savides, Brenna Casey, and Everson L. A. Artifon.

Companion website: www.wiley.com/go/gress/atlas

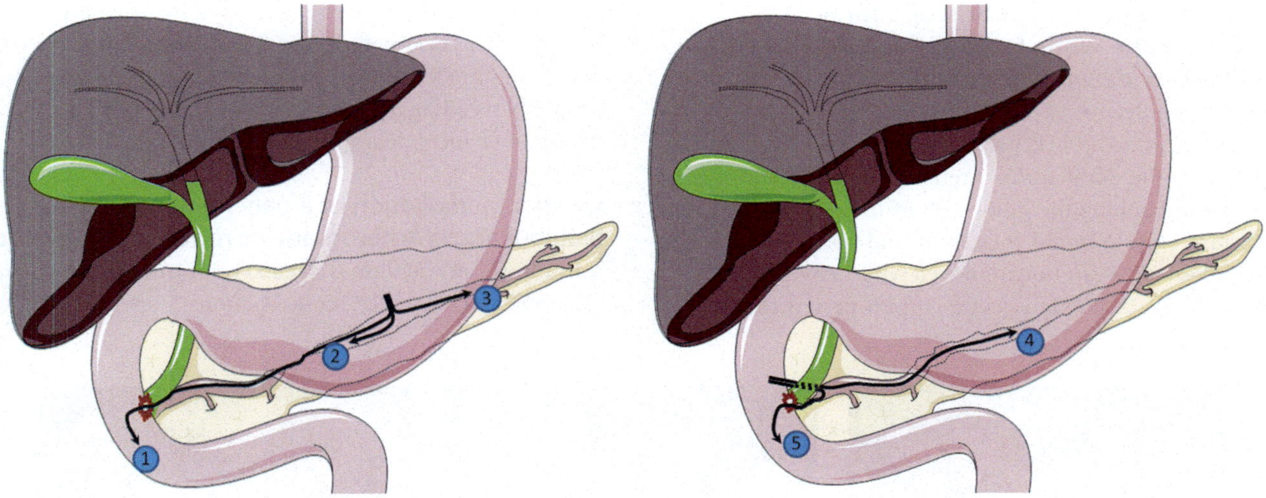

Figure 45.1 Access points and routes for EUS-PDD: 1, transgastric rendezvous; 2, transgastric MPD access for antegrade stenting; 3, transgastric MPD access for retrograde stenting; 4, transduodenal MPD access for retrograde stenting; 5, transduodenal rendezvous. Source: Rimbas M, Larghi A. Endoscopic ultrasonography-guided techniques for accessing and draining the biliary system and the pancreatic duct. *Gastrointest Endosc Clin North Am* 2017;27:681–705. © 2017, Elsevier.

The procedural steps are very similar to those commonly performed for EUS-guided biliary drainage. However, EUS-PDD is definitely more demanding and challenging than EUS-guided biliary drainage, mainly because the stability of the echoendoscope in the stomach is relatively low and it does not allow application of forces on the different endoscopic accessories that are being used during the procedure.

Needle puncture

First, four variables must be considered in every procedure:

- distance between the EUS transducer and MPD
- stability of the scope
- degree of MPD dilation
- presence of chronic pancreatitis.

The long scope position with the tip of the echoendoscope in the distal antrum, pyloric ring or duodenal bulb allows better stability and facilitates stent manipulation. The access site for performing puncture should take into consideration the shortest distance between the transducer and the MPD, maximal scope stability, absence of interposed vessels, and angle for tract dilation and stent deployment.

To access the MPD, the 19-gauge fine needle aspiration (FNA) needle is generally utilized since it allows the use of larger-diameter guidewires that guarantee better stability during stent deployment. Accessing a non-dilated MPD or traversing a large amount of fibrotic parenchyma can be very challenging. In these cases, puncture can be facilitated using a number of tricks.

- A puncture deeper than the level of the pancreatic duct could be done followed by withdrawal of the needle until it reaches the duct lumen.
- Stylet is removed to increase needle flexibility and maneuverability.
- Use smaller (22-gauge) needles to obtain the initial access to the duct.

If antegrade stenting is planned, the MPD is ideally accessed in the body/tail region in order to direct the guidewire towards the head of the pancreas, while for retrograde stenting the MPD is optimally accessed at the head with the guidewire directed toward the tail region. Positioning the long axis of the needle as parallel as possible with the direction of the pancreatic duct offers a larger target area and facilitates insertion of guidewire, dilation devices, and stents.

Once the needle is inside the MPD, aspiration of pancreatic juice is recommended and then the pancreatogram is performed under fluoroscopic control with a limited quantity of contrast injection.

Guidewire insertion and manipulation

The guidewire size should be chosen, considering especially the stiffness and ability to traverse tight strictures. Rendezvous procedures often require the use of a hydrophilic guidewire (e.g. 0.025 or 0.035-inch Visiglide, Olympus Corp.; Glidewire, Jagwire, Boston Scientific; 0.032-inch Radifocus, Terumo).

Thinner guidewires (0.021 or 0.018 inch) that can work with a 22-gauge needle are useful for passing tortuous or tight strictures, but are less visible fluoroscopically, kink very easily, lack stiffness, and may render exchange of accessories difficult. Therefore they should be exchanged for larger and stiffer wires once passed through the stricture. The guidewire should be advanced, looping or coiling distally as many times as possible. However, thicker guidewires may peel during to-and-fro manipulation after puncture.

Exchange of the echoendoscope for a duodenoscope while leaving the guidewire in place (Rendezvous technique)

Once the guidewire is placed through the stomach or the duodenum into the MPD and can be advanced across the papilla into the duodenum, a rendezvous procedure can be performed. Looping the guidewire in the small bowel is an important step to avoid migration and loss of access. The echoendoscope is carefully removed while leaving the guidewire in place. A duodenoscope is then passed next to the papilla where the guidewire is grasped by using a snare or a biopsy forceps and withdrawn through the accessory channel of the duodenoscope, thus gaining retrograde access to the MPD to complete the procedure as a standard endoscopic retrograde pancreatography (ERP) (Figure 45.2).

Creation and dilation of a pancreatic–enteric fistulous tract (Anterograde or retrograde technique)

A fistulous tract dilation is needed prior to stenting. It can be performed with hydrostatic balloons, tapered catheters,

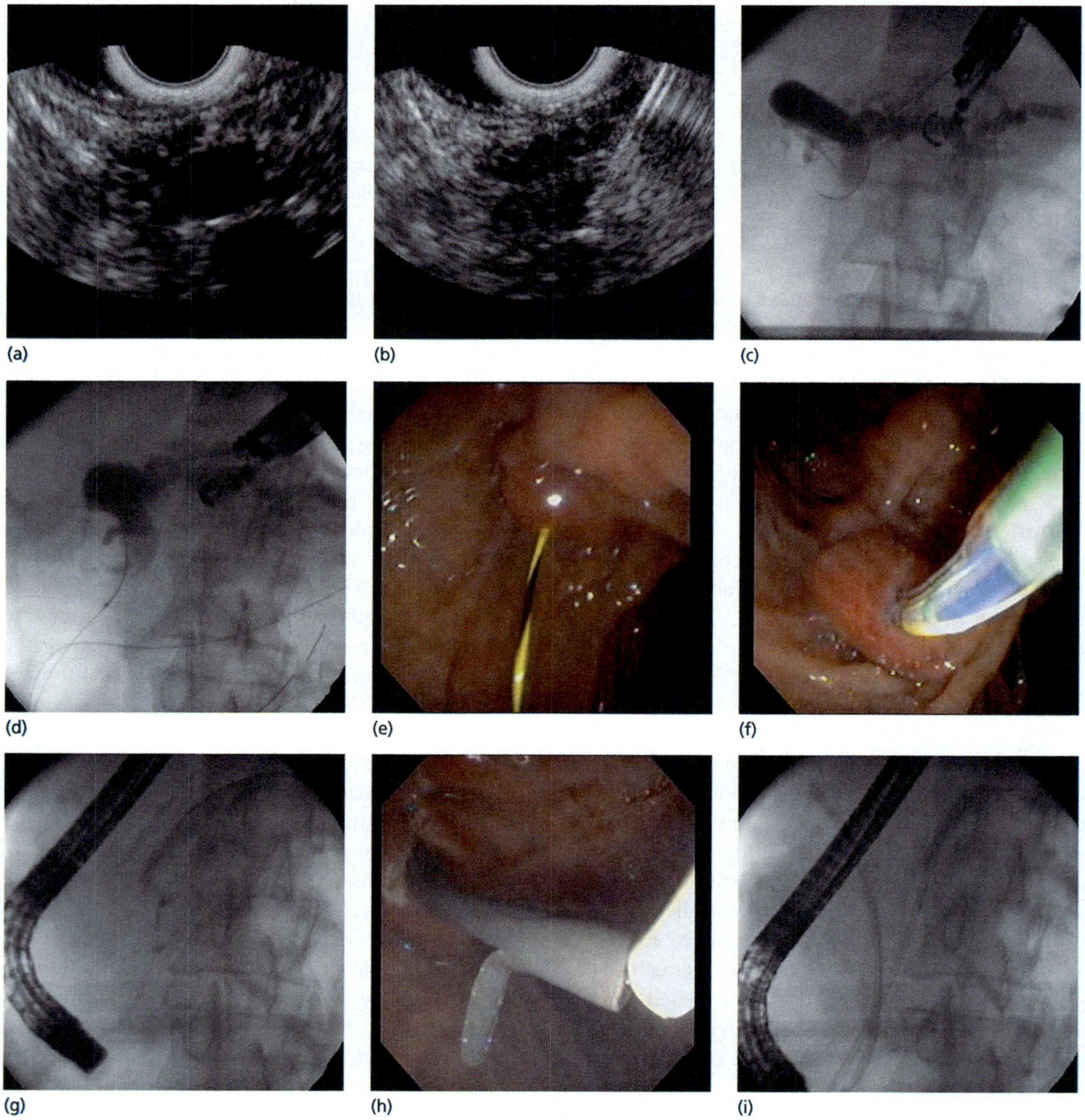

Figure 45.2 Transgastric EUS-guided rendezvous for MPD drainage. (a) Dilated MPD at the level of the pancreatic body. (b) Puncture of the MPD with a 19-gauge needle. (c) Pancreatogram showing a dilated MPD. (d) Guidewire looping in the small bowel. (e) Duodenoscope view of the papilla with the previously placed guidewire. (f) Access of the MPD over the guidewire. (g) Fluoroscopic view of the MPD plastic stent insertion. (h) Endoscopic view of the MPD plastic stent insertion. (i) Fluoroscopy view at the end of the procedure during which drainage of the bile duct was also performed.

cannulas, and diathermy catheters. Dilation of the tract using balloons or dilation catheters can be difficult given the often-hardened pancreatic parenchyma in cases of chronic pancreatitis. An alternative option is the use of cautery-assisted devices (diathermy catheters or needle knifes) with a short burst of pure cut current for tract dissection and fistula creation (Figure 45.3). Recently, a fine-gauge electrocautery dilator with a 3-Fr metallic tip has been developed and tested, which may avoid the excessive use of diathermy (Figure 45.4).

The use of non-cautery-assisted devices may increase the risk of bleeding, perforation, and leaks. On the other hand, the use of diathermy may increase the risk of pancreatitis due to the cautery effect. To date, there is a lack of comparative studies evaluating the ideal tract dilation technique. Regardless of personal choice in deciding which equipment to use, continuous EUS and fluoroscopic imaging are very useful at this stage to maintain a stable scope position.

Placement of a transpapillary or transmural stent (not needed for rendezvous cases)

Once proper dilation is attained, placement of a transpapillary or transmural stent can be accomplished under continuous fluoroscopy with endoscopic control. Plastic stents (straight, single or double pigtail) or self-expanding metal stents (SEMS) can be used for EUS-PDD. Standard plastic stents are suitable, preferably with retrievable features to avoid stent migration into the abdominal cavity.

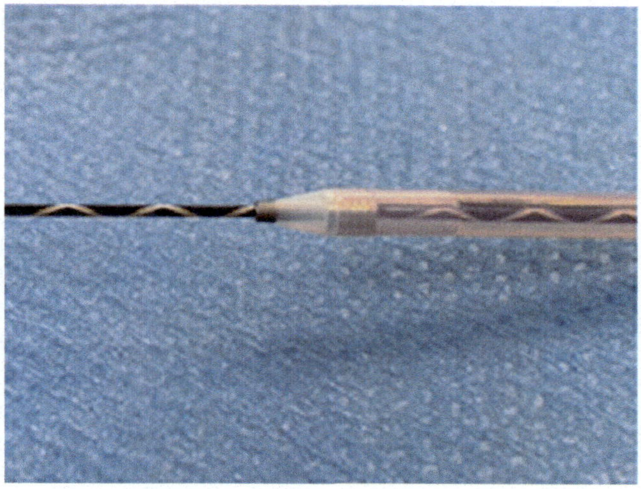

Figure 45.4 The novel wire-guided fine-gauge electrocautery dilator, with a distal metal tip 3-Fr dilator (Fine025; Medico's Hirata Inc., Osaka, Japan). Source: reproduced with permission from Ogura T, Yamada M, Higuchi K. Reintervention after deployment of several metal stents using novel fine-gauge electrocautery dilator. *Dig Endosc* 2019;31:467.

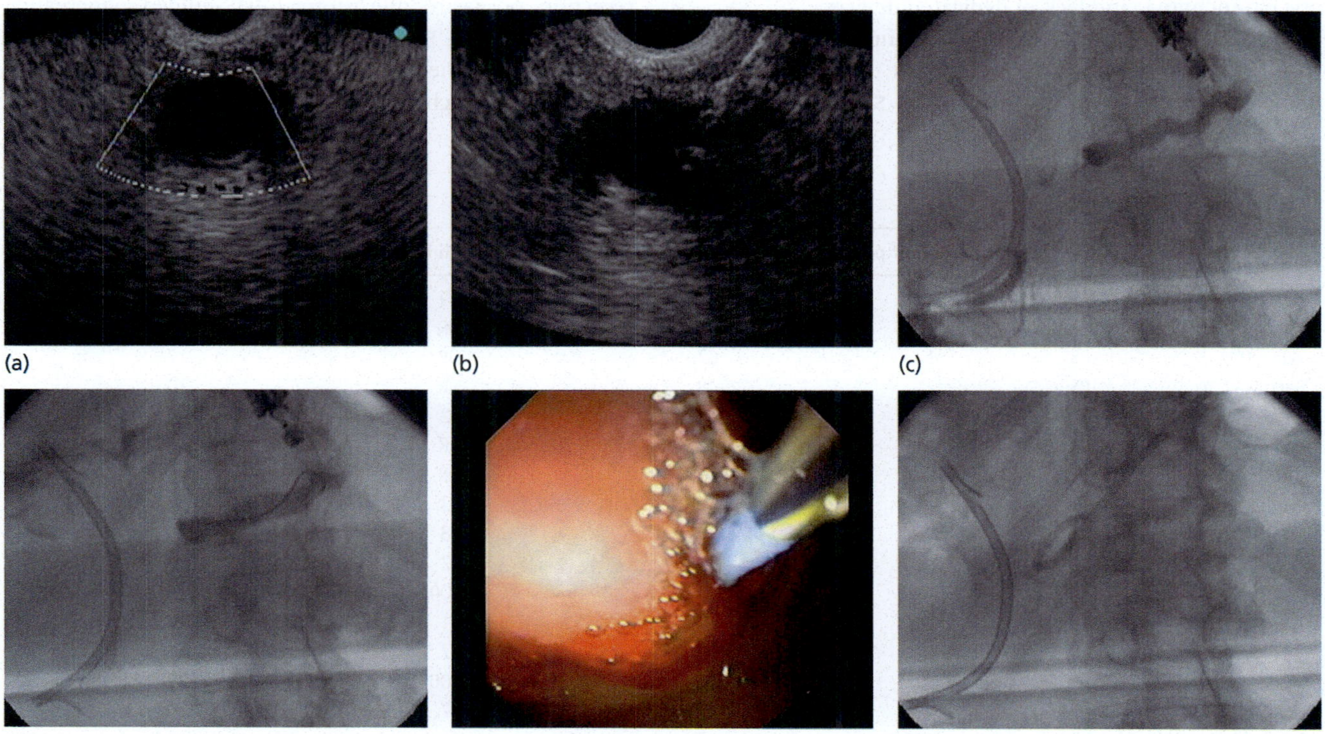

(a) (b) (c) (d) (e) (f)

Figure 45.3 Transgastric EUS-PDD. (a) Dilated MPD at the level of the pancreatic body/tail. (b) Puncture of the MPD with a 19-gauge needle. (c) Pancreatogram showing stricture of the MPD with upstream dilatation. (d) Guidewire looping in the MPD. (e) Creation of a fistulous tract between the stomach and the MPD by using a needle knife. (f) EUS-PDD with placement of a plastic double pigtail stent.

There is a lack of specific devices for EUS-PDD, except for a dedicated plastic stent. Fully covered SEMS and lumen-apposing fully covered SEMS have also been reported to be effective, once the fear of blocking side-branch pancreatic ducts has been overcome or the duct is sufficiently dilated. Currently, there is no consensus on the most suitable stent for EUS-PDD.

Outcomes

Most of the available studies on EUS-PDD are retrospective, with no randomized controlled trials available. Results of all the relevant published studies with at least 10 patients enrolled are shown in Table 45.1. The mean pooled technical and clinical success rates in these 16 studies are 80% and 84%, respectively, with a 17% complications rate.

A recent review of the literature reported pooled adverse events of 18%, including abdominal pain, bleeding, acute pancreatitis, perforation, pancreatic abscess formation, shaving of the guidewire coating, fever, pneumoperitoneum, pseudocyst, pseudocyst with aneurysm, and perigastric fluid collection. Considering the most recent and largest series published, EUS-PDD has a failure rate around 10% and a rate of adverse events above 10%. Potentially contributing factors for procedure failure include small MPD diameter, unsuccessful manipulation of the guidewire, fibrotic pancreatic parenchyma, and lack of dedicated devices.

There is a lack of long-term follow-up of patients who have undergone EUS-PDD. At present, endoscopic treatment should be repeated if necessary. Stent revisions for plastic stents should be performed approximately two to three months after the index procedure. If stent dysfunction occurs, exchange should be performed if the patient is symptomatic or the MPD is dilated on imaging studies. Serial dilations and repeated stent exchanges are often required for fistula maturation until stents can be removed.

No data on the long-term management of fully covered SEMS in this clinical scenario are available. In the two largest series published so far, 94 and 80 patients were reported over a 12- and 10-year period, thus indicating that the number of patients who require this procedure is limited. This suggests that EUS-PDD should be also limited to very few highly expert centers.

Algorithm

Based on our experience, we propose a treatment algorithm for performing EUS-guided PDD (Figure 45.5). Excluding patients with disconnected MPD, for whom a pancreatico-gastrostomy should be performed, the first step is the evaluation of accessibility of the papilla. A rendezvous procedure should be first attempted when the papilla is endoscopically accessible. When the papilla cannot be reached, the decision of which approach should be used may be guided by patient anatomy. If the pancreas is in situ and the patient has undergone previous Roux-en-Y reconstruction, Billroth II gastric resection or gastroenterostomy, EUS-guided pancreatico-gastrostomy or EUS-guided pancreatico-duodenostomy should be performed. Antegrade internal drainage should be the approach of choice in patients with previous Whipple

Table 45.1 Outcomes of EUS-PDD.

Study	Design	No. of patients	Technical success (%)	Clinical success (%)	Complications (%)
Tessier, 2007	RS	36	92	69	14
Kahaleh, 2007	PS	12	83	NR	17
Will, 2007	PS	12	67	NR	17
Barkay, 2010	RS	21	48	NR	10
Ergun, 2011	RS	20	90	72	10
Shah, 2012	RS	22	86	NR	18
Villa, 2012	RS	19	58	NR	26
Kurihara, 2013	RS	14	93	93	7
Fujii, 2013	RS	45	73	78	6
Will, 2015	RS	83	63	82	22
Oh, 2016	RS	25	100	100	20
Tyberg, 2017	PS	80	89	81	20
Chen, 2017	RS	40	92.5	87.5	35
Matsunami, 2018	PS	30	100	100	23.3
Uchida, 2018	RS	15	86.6	92.3	26.7
Dalal, 2019	RS	44	88.6	81.8	22.7
Total		518	80	84	17

RS, retrospective study; PS, prospective study; NR, not reported.

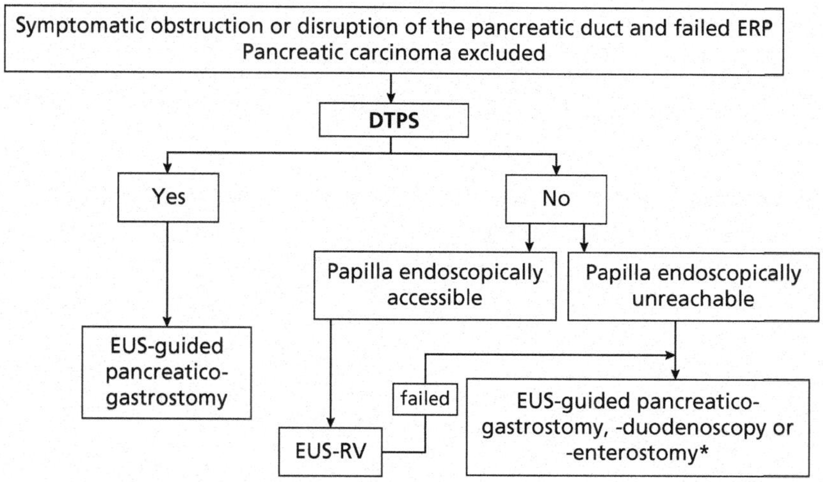

Figure 45.5 Algorithm for EUS-PDD. *, depending on the anatomic conditions and possible EUS approach to the MPD. DTPA, disconnected pancreatic tail syndrome; ERP, endoscopic retrograde pancreatography; EUS-RV, EUS-guided rendezvous.

procedure or pancreatico-jejunostomy with suspected anastomotic stenosis.

Controversies and future directions

The available evidence on EUS-guided pancreatic duct drainage indicates that the procedure has very selective indications, is technically extremely challenging, and can be associated with a considerable rate of adverse events.

In order to improve technical success and limit complications, adequate devices facilitating access and drainage are urgently required. A major concern about the development of this technique is that the number of cases per year per experienced center is too low to allow the technique to be accurately evaluated and compared in prospective studies. Moreover, it might be of limited interest for accessory companies to put great efforts into the development of dedicated accessories for the performance of EUS-PDD.

46 How to do EUS Gallbladder Drainage

Shannon Melissa Chan and Anthony Yuen Bun Teoh
Department of Surgery, Prince of Wales Hospital, The Chinese University of Hong Kong, Shatin, Hong Kong

Introduction

Acute cholecystitis has been managed with laparoscopic cholecystectomy in surgically fit patients. In patients who are high-risk surgical candidates, percutaneous transhepatic gallbladder drainage (PT-GBD) has traditionally been the treatment of choice [1,2]. In recent years, internal drainage of the gallbladder using an endoscopic ultrasound-guided transmural approach has emerged as a feasible and safe alternative [3–5]. Technical and clinical success were achieved in 95.3% and 90.8% of patients, respectively [6]. The technique was first described in 2007 [7]. In initial studies, the gallbladder was drained with transmural nasobiliary drainage tubes or plastic stents [8,9]. In recent years, the development of lumen-apposing metal stents (LAMS) has gained widespread popularity due to the ease of deployment and lower concern for bile leakage [3,5,10]. LAMS also allows for subsequent advanced procedures such as stone removal [11]. According to the latest Tokyo Guidelines 2018, endoscopic ultrasound-guided gallbladder drainage (EUS-GBD) could be considered an alternative in high-volume centers when performed by skilled endoscopists [12]. Certain technical aspects and controversies with EUS-GBD are discussed in this chapter.

Background concept

The gallbladder can be drained with the EUS transmural approach via the antrum or duodenum. In other words, a cholecystogastric or cholecystoduodenal anastomosis is being created endoscopically. However, the gallbladder and the antrum or duodenum are inherently separate organs that are not adhered to each other. Therefore, there is a risk of stent migration, bile leakage, and pneumoperitoneum. Therefore, the puncture site and choice of stent determine the integrity of the anastomosis, and thus the success of the procedure.

Choice of stents: metal stents versus plastic stents

Initial studies reported the use of EUS-guided insertion of nasocholecystic drains [8,9]. A cholecystogram was performed 48–72 hours later after sepsis subsided, and the nasocholecystic drain was exchanged for a double pigtail or was removed. When compared to PT-GBD, EUS-GBD with nasocholecystic drain showed similar rates of technical (97% vs. 97%) and clinical (100% vs. 96%) success [13]. The median postprocedure pain score was significantly lower after EUS-GBD than after PT-GBD [13]. This may be preferable in patients in whom cholecystectomy is contemplated in the future. However, plastic stents are easily occluded due to the narrow lumen. Fully covered self-expandable metal stents have a larger lumen than plastic double pigtail stents. However, they are not designed for transluminal drainage and do not have tissue apposition ability. Thus, they are prone to stent migration and may result in leakage and peritonitis.

LAMS were designed for transluminal drainage. All LAMS presently available on the market are initially intended for drainage of pancreatic fluid collections. They were designed with properties of tissue apposition and a large lumen to prevent stent occlusion. They are made of braided nitinol mesh with widely flared or dumbbell-shaped flanges. All models are also covered with silicone membrane. Covered stents help to prevent leakage of air and bile. The silicone lining also impedes tissue ingrowth, making LAMS easily removable when needed [14]. LAMS that are currently available in the market are listed in Table 46.1. The larger lumens of LAMS allow for quick and effective drainage of infectious

Atlas of Endoscopic Ultrasonography, Second Edition. Edited by Frank Gress, Thomas Savides, Brenna Casey, and Everson L. A. Artifon.

Companion website: www.wiley.com/go/gress/atlas

Table 46.1 Currently available LAMS on the market.

Stent	Brand	Introducer diameter (Fr)	Internal diameter (mm)	Flange diameter (mm)	Saddle length (mm)	Cautery tip delivery system available
Axios	Boston Scientific	10.8	10/15/20	21/24/29	10/10/10	Yes
Spaxus	Taewoong	10	10/16	23/25/31	20	Yes
Hanarostent	M.I.Tech	10.5	10/12/14 16	22/24/26/28	10/30	No

material and allows for further transluminal interventions via the stent in the gallbladder. A range of different diagnostic and interventional procedures through the stent, such as magnifying endoscopy, laser lithotripsy and basket mechanical lithotripsy for stone clearance, have also been reported in the gallbladder [11].

Several studies comparing EUS-GBD and PT-GBD have been published [15–18]. The two procedures have similar rates of technical (EUS-GBD 85.7–96.6% vs. PT-GBD 99–100%) and clinical success (EUS-GBD 89.8–95% vs. PT-GBD 86–94.9%) [15,16,18]. PT-GBD has been shown to be associated with more adverse events and more unplanned admissions [16], and also to have a higher need for reintervention [15]. In addition, a meta-analysis that included five comparative studies (206 patients in the EUS-GBD group vs. 289 patients in the PT-GBD group) concluded that EUS-GBD had fewer adverse events than PT-GBD (odds ratio [OR] 0.43, 95% confidence interval [CI] 0.18–1.00; $P = 0.05$; $I^2 = 66\%$), shorter hospital stays with pooled standard mean difference of −2.53 (95% CI −4.28 to −0.78; $P = 0.005$; $I^2 = 98\%$), and required significantly fewer reinterventions (OR 0.16, 95% CI 0.04–0.042; $P < 0.001$; $I^2 = 32\%$) resulting in significantly fewer unplanned readmissions (OR 0.16, 95% CI 0.05–0.53; $P = 0.003$; $I^2 = 79\%$) [19].

EUS-GBD with LAMS

LAMS can be inserted by delivery systems that are with or without cautery enhanced tip. For LAMS without a cautery tip, the conventional method of EUS-guided insertion is required. The procedure is as follows.

1. The gallbladder is identified using a linear echoendoscope. A suitable puncture site without intervening blood vessels is then located in the gastric antrum or the duodenum. According to published data, there is no difference between the efficacy and adverse events of the procedure when the puncture site is in the gastric antrum or duodenum [16,20]. However, there are several practical reasons to consider.

a. By anatomy, the duodenal bulb is much closer to the gallbladder when compared with the antrum. This may potentially decrease the tension of the stent, thus causing less buried stent syndrome and stent migration.

b. The risk of food reflux into the gallbladder, especially in large-calibre metal stents, is lower with the transduodenal approach.

c. There is some suggestion that cholecystectomy after EUS-GBD may be less technically demanding via the trangastric approach, since repair of the gastric wall is safer and easier than repair of the duodenal wall. However, a comparative study did not show any significant difference [21].

Thus, these points should be considered when deciding on the site for drainage of the gallbladder.

2. The gallbladder is punctured with a 19-gauge needle, and the position is confirmed by the aspiration of bile or contrast injection and visualized using fluoroscopy (Figure 46.1). Most of the time, aspiration of bile is adequate to confirm the position. The injection of contrast will double confirm the position but may induce flare-up of sepsis and should be minimized (Figure 46.2). The forward-viewing echoendoscope can also be used if there is difficulty passing the linear echoendoscope into the duodenum (Figure 46.3).

3. A 0.025- or 0.035-inch guidewire is then passed through the needle and looped within the gallbladder (Figure 46.4).

4. The next step is track dilatation. This can be performed with either the cautery or non-cautery devices. For the cautery devices, there is the option of a 6-Fr or 8.5-Fr cystotome (EndoFlex, GmbH, Voerde, Germany). In centers where the cystotome is not available, the needle knife can be used.

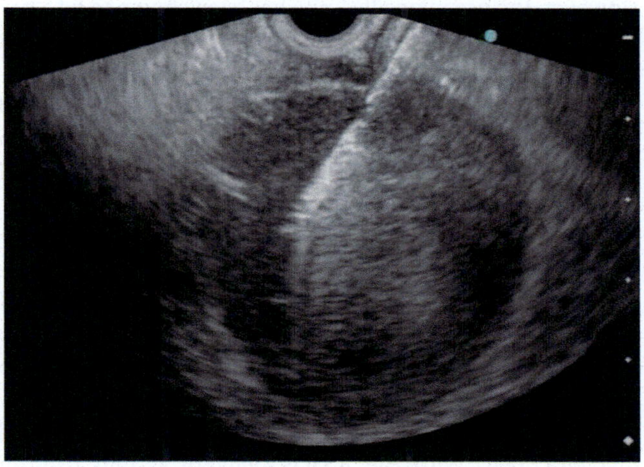

Figure 46.1 Puncture of gallbladder with 19-gauge needle with linear echoendoscope.

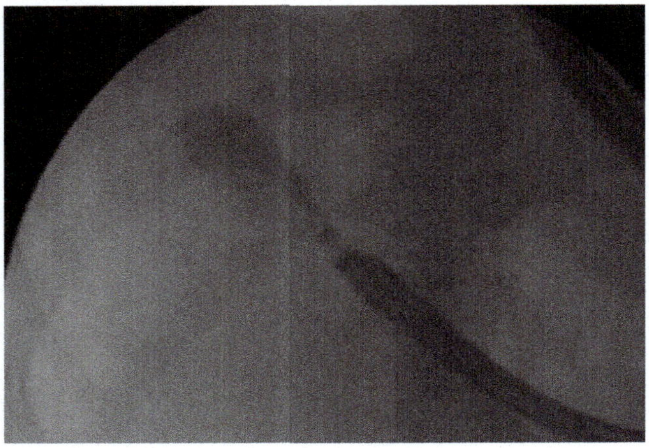

Figure 46.2 Contrast injection within the gallbladder.

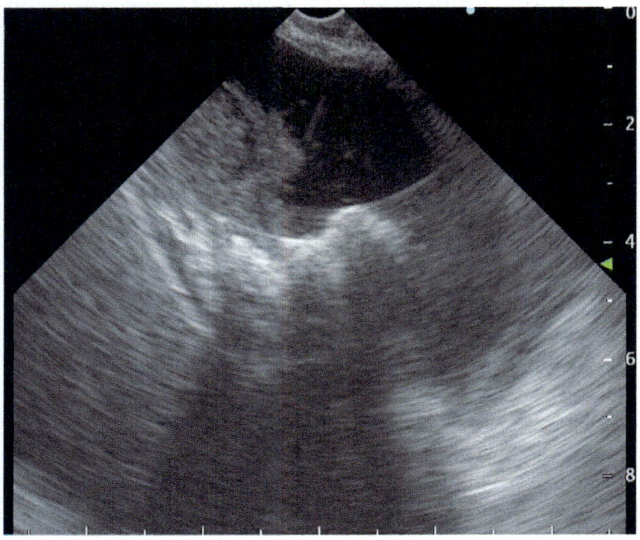

Figure 46.3 Puncturing of gallbladder with forward-viewing echoendoscope.

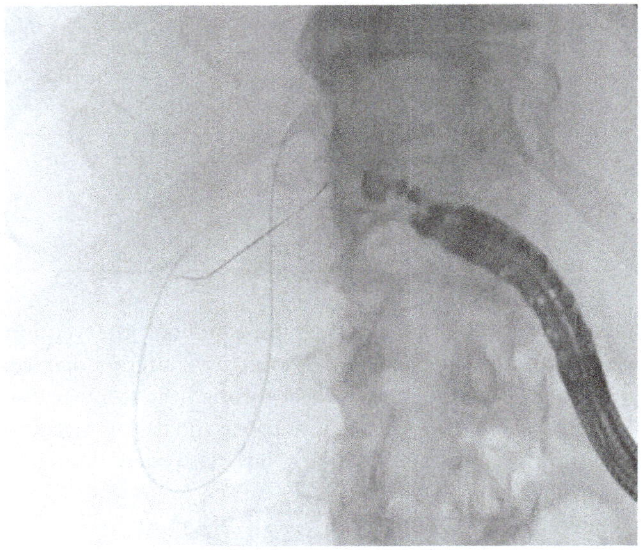

Figure 46.4 Looping of guidewire within the gallbladder.

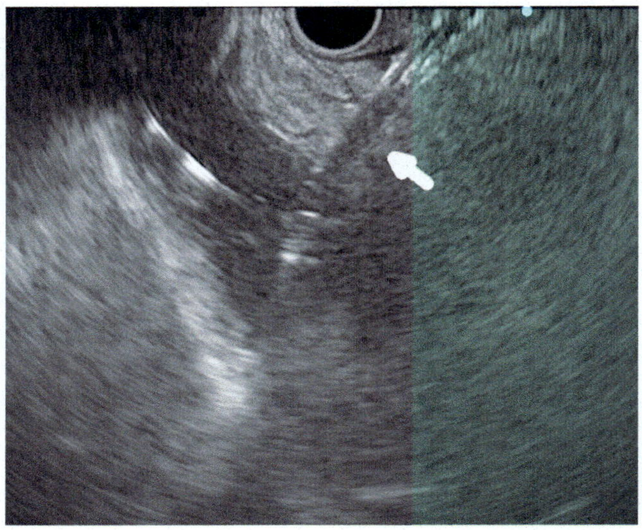

Figure 46.5 Tract dilatation with 4-mm biliary balloon (EUS view).

However, the use of needle knife has been shown to be a risk factor for developing adverse events in a small cohort study [22]. The track can subsequently be dilated with a 4-mm biliary balloon (Figure 46.5). In our center, our usual practice is to dilate the tract with 6-Fr cystotome, then 4-mm biliary balloon. To avoid bile leakage, the delivery system of LAMS should be made ready before the balloon is deflated.

5. The delivery system for the LAMS is then inserted. The distal flange is deployed under EUS or fluoroscopic guidance (Figure 46.6). Once the distal flange is deployed, the delivery system is pulled back with gentle tension to appose the two organs. The proximal flange can then be deployed using two methods: (i) endoscopic visualization or (ii) within the endoscope channel. Endoscopic visualization was the method first described. With the AXIOS delivery system (Boston Scientific, Marlborough, MA), a "black mark" would be visualized endoscopically upon right torque of the scope (Figure 46.7). Once the black mark is seen, the proximal flange can be deployed under endoscopic guidance. For the deployment in channel method, the delivery system is pulled back gently until a slight distortion of the stent is seen on EUS view. Then the rest of the stent is completely deployed within the channel. A right torque is then applied and the stent gradually pushed out of the channel. The stent will be seen deploying in the endoscopic view (Figure 46.8).

6. The dilatation of the stent with balloon dilators to facilitate drainage is optional. However, the stent does fully expand the next day even without dilatation. The insertion of double pigtail stents through the LAMS is also optional. The rationale behind use of these stents includes avoiding blockage of LAMS by gallstones/debris, and facilitating salvage of the fistula tract in case of stent migration [23].

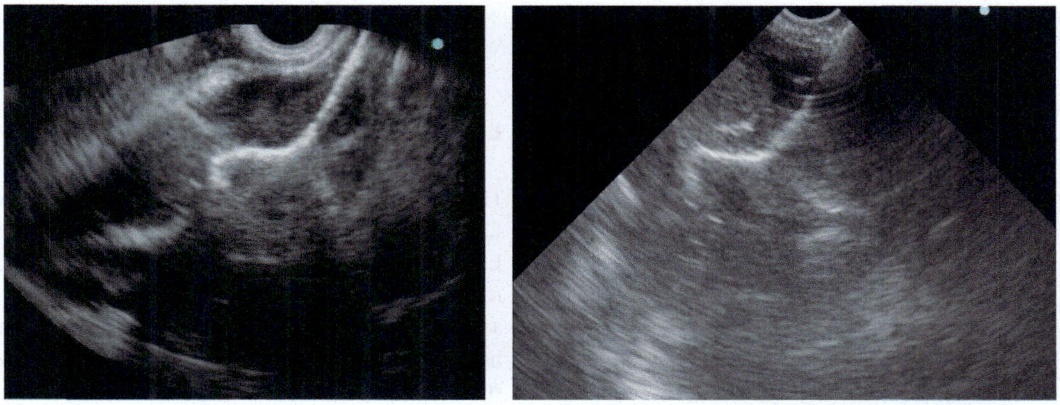

(a) (b)

Figure 46.6 (a) Distal flange of AXIOS stent deployed under EUS guidance. (b) Distal flange of SPAXUS stent deployed with forward-viewing echoendoscope with EUS guidance.

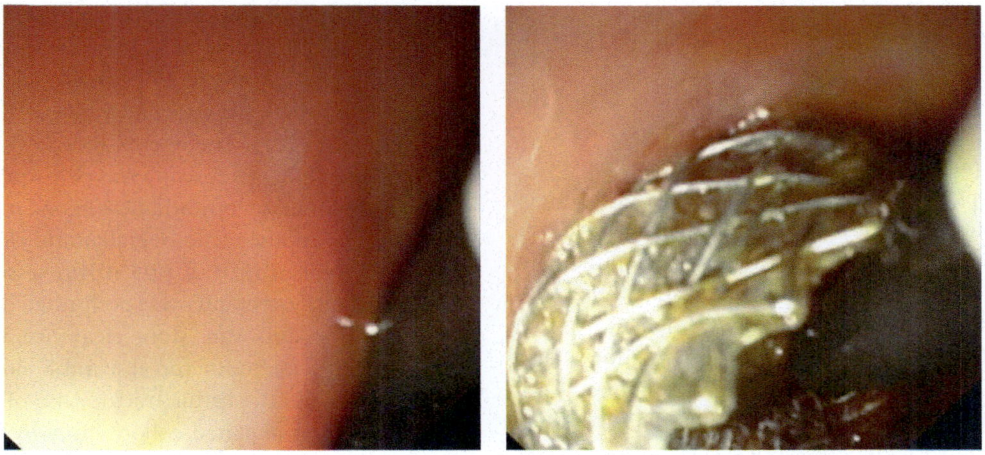

(a) (b)

Figure 46.7 (a) Luminal view of "black mark" with the AXIOS stent. Once the black mark is seen, the proximal flange can be deployed. (b) Luminal view after proximal flange deployed.

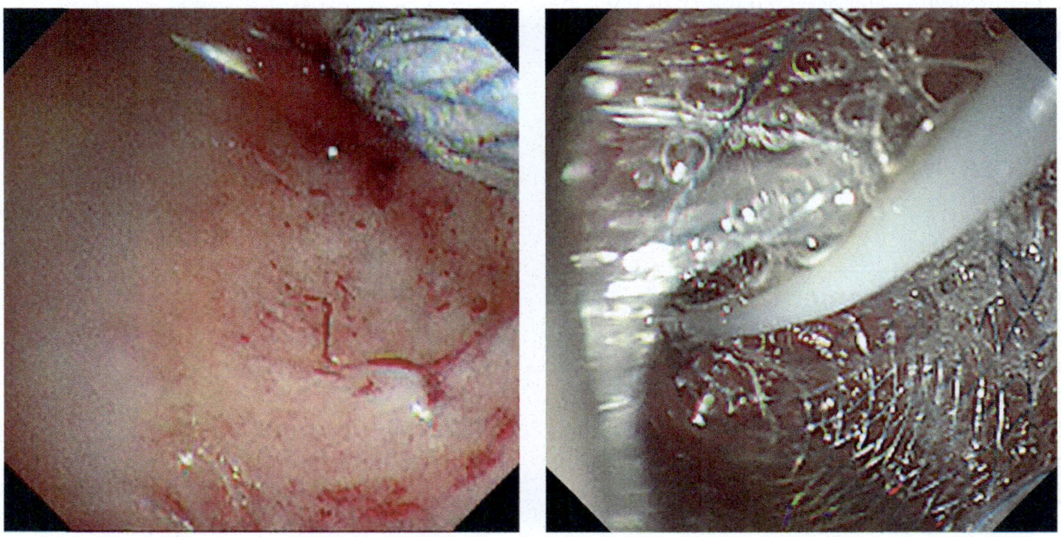

(a) (b)

Figure 46.8 (a) Luminal view with SPAXUS stent using the deployment-in-channel technique. The proximal end of stent has been fully deployed within the channel and the stent gradually pushed out under luminal view. (b) Luminal view of the SPAXUS stent after deployment of the proximal stent.

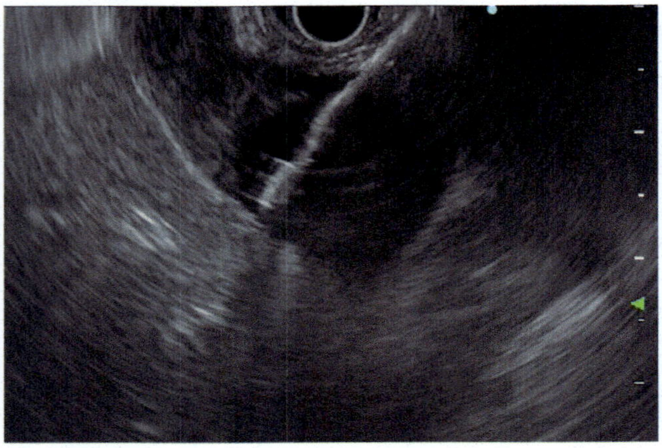

Figure 46.9 Direct puncture with the Hot AXIOS into the gallbladder.

However, the use of these double pigtail stents has yet to be proven to improve outcomes.

For delivery systems equipped with a cautery tip, the direct puncture method is used. This method simplifies the procedure by avoiding multiple over-the-wire exchanges.

1. The initial steps are identical to those for the non-cautery device. A suitable puncture site is first located in the gastric antrum or the duodenum. The gallbladder can be punctured with a 19-gauge needle with guidewire inserted first and exchanged for the cautery-equipped AXIOS delivery system (Boston Scientific, Marlborough, MA). This method is also referred to as the hybrid free-hand technique [20]. Alternatively, the gallbladder can be punctured directly with the cautery-equipped AXIOS delivery system (Figure 46.9). The hybrid technique allows for diagnostic aspiration and the insertion of guidewire to secure the fistula tract before introduction of the stent. Theoretically, the presence of a guidewire would prevent cautery-related injury to the contralateral wall of the gallbladder. This could also potentially reduce rates of stent misdeployment and allows for salvage procedures such as insertion of additional stents in case misdeployment occurs.

2. The distal and proximal flanges are deployed as in the non-cautery method.

Postprocedural management

Patients should be monitored after the procedure for relief of sepsis. Oral diet can be resumed next day if sepsis subsides. If a positive response is not present within 48–72 hours, patients should be reassessed for potential complications of acute cholecystitis, such as gangrenous cholecystitis or perforation. It could also be secondary from complications of the procedure. Computed tomography should be performed when in doubt. Common causes include flare-up of sepsis and blockage of the stent by stones, which may be treated with insertion of a double pigtail stent within the LAMS with a forward-viewing endoscope.

Long-term management

There is still no consensus on management of gallstones and LAMS after EUS-GBD. The main concerns about keeping the LAMS long term are stent erosion causing bleeding and stent migration. Choi et al. reported a 7.1% adverse event rate at a median follow-up of 275 days. Two patients had asymptomatic distal stent migration and two acute cholecystitis with stent occlusion. The cumulative stent patency rate was 86% [24]. Walter et al. also reported no adverse events after a median follow-up of 364 days [25]. However, there are also proponents of stone removal and subsequent stent removal. With EUS-GBD performed with LAMS, a forward-viewing endoscope can be inserted via the stent into the gallbladder. This allows a wide range of advanced diagnostic and therapeutic procedures. In a retrospective cohort performed at our center, there were 25 patients with 29 cholecystoscopies performed [11]. The overall technical success rate was 93.1%. Magnifying endoscopy was performed in 10 patients, confocal endomicroscopy and EUS in one patient, and endocytoscopy in another. The overall stone clearance rate was 88% after a mean (SD) of 1.25 (0.46) sessions of cholecystoscopy. Cholecystography was performed in 11 patients and all were successful. After stone clearance, the LAMSs were removed with rat tooth forceps and a double pigtail was inserted to retain the fistula tract in case of future cholecystitis. In the case-matched cohort study by Teoh et al. [16], cholecystoscopy was performed one to three months after LAMS insertion for stone clearance. The procedure was repeated until all stones were cleared and the metal stent removed. The stents would be kept in situ if the patient refused repeat endoscopy or was unfit to proceed to further interventions. A total of 17 out of 59 patients had their stents removed and the rate of recurrent cholecystitis was 0%. In a recent review article by Ogura et al., the authors suggested that permanent stent placement may be suitable for patients with shorter expected survival in order to avoid repeated endoscopic procedures. In patients with longer expected survival, stent removal may be more suitable to reduce stent-related complications [26].

Conclusion

EUS-GBD is emerging as a promising alternative to PT-GBD, especially in patients unfit for surgery. The procedure is associated with high technical and clinical success rates, with a low adverse event rate. Since this procedure is relatively new, the published data on technical aspects are based mostly on personal experience and preference. The optimal technique has yet to be determined with further studies.

References

1. Glenn F. Cholecystostomy in the high risk patient with biliary tract disease. *Ann Surg* 1977;185:185–191.
2. McGillicuddy EA, Schuster KM, Barre K, et al. Non-operative management of acute cholecystitis in the elderly. *Br J Surg* 2012;99:1254–1261.
3. Teoh AY, Binmoeller KF, Lau JY. Single-step EUS-guided puncture and delivery of a lumen-apposing stent for gallbladder drainage using a novel cautery-tipped stent delivery system. *Gastrointest Endosc* 2014;80:1171.
4. Itoi T, Sofuni A, Itokawa F, et al. Endoscopic transpapillary gallbladder drainage in patients with acute cholecystitis in whom percutaneous transhepatic approach is contraindicated or anatomically impossible (with video). *Gastrointest Endosc* 2008;68: 455–460.
5. de la Serna-Higuera C, Perez-Miranda M, Gil-Simon P, et al. EUS-guided transenteric gallbladder drainage with a new fistula-forming, lumen-apposing metal stent. *Gastrointest Endosc* 2013;77:303–308.
6. Teoh AY, Perez-Miranda M, Kunda R, et al. Outcomes of an international multicenter registry on EUS-guided gallbladder drainage in patients at high risk for cholecystectomy. *Endosc Int Open* 2019;7:E964–E973.
7. Baron TH, Topazian MD. Endoscopic transduodenal drainage of the gallbladder: implications for endoluminal treatment of gallbladder disease. *Gastrointest Endosc* 2007;65:735–737.
8. Lee SS, Park DH, Hwang CY, et al. EUS-guided transmural cholecystostomy as rescue management for acute cholecystitis in elderly or high-risk patients: a prospective feasibility study. *Gastrointest Endosc* 2007;66:1008–1012.
9. Kwan V, Eisendrath P, Antaki F, et al. EUS-guided cholecystenterostomy: a new technique (with videos). *Gastrointest Endosc* 2007;66:582–586.
10. Jang JW, Lee SS, Park DH, et al. Feasibility and safety of EUS-guided transgastric/transduodenal gallbladder drainage with single-step placement of a modified covered self-expandable metal stent in patients unsuitable for cholecystectomy. *Gastrointest Endosc* 2011;74:176–181.
11. Chan SM, Teoh AYB, Yip HC, et al. Feasibility of per-oral cholecystoscopy and advanced gallbladder interventions after EUS-guided gallbladder stenting (with video). *Gastrointest Endosc* 2017;85:1225–1232.
12. Mori Y, Itoi T, Baron TH, et al. Tokyo Guidelines 2018: management strategies for gallbladder drainage in patients with acute cholecystitis (with videos). *J Hepatobiliary Pancreat Sci* 2018;25:87–95.
13. Jang JW, Lee SS, Song TJ, et al. Endoscopic ultrasound-guided transmural and percutaneous transhepatic gallbladder drainage are comparable for acute cholecystitis. *Gastroenterology* 2012;142:805–811.
14. Stier MW, Waxman I. Lumen-apposing metal stents: which one and why? *Gastrointest Endosc Clin North Am* 2018;28:207–217.
15. Tyberg A, Saumoy M, Sequeiros EV, et al. EUS-guided versus percutaneous gallbladder drainage: isn't it time to convert? *J Clin Gastroenterol* 2018;52:79–84.
16. Teoh AYB, Serna C, Penas I, et al. Endoscopic ultrasound-guided gallbladder drainage reduces adverse events compared with percutaneous cholecystostomy in patients who are unfit for cholecystectomy. *Endoscopy* 2017;49:130–138.
17. Irani S, Ngamruengphong S, Teoh A, et al. Similar efficacies of endoscopic ultrasound gallbladder drainage with a lumen-apposing metal stent versus percutaneous transhepatic gallbladder drainage for acute cholecystitis. *Clin Gastroenterol Hepatol* 2017;15:738–745.
18. Choi JH, Kim HW, Lee JC, et al. Percutaneous transhepatic versus EUS-guided gallbladder drainage for malignant cystic duct obstruction. *Gastrointest Endosc* 2017;85:357–364.
19. Luk SW, Irani S, Krishnamoorthi R, et al. Endoscopic ultrasound-guided gallbladder drainage versus percutaneous cholecystostomy for high risk surgical patients with acute cholecystitis: a systematic review and meta-analysis. *Endoscopy* 2019;51(8):722–732.
20. Perez-Miranda M. Technical considerations in EUS-guided gallbladder drainage. *Endosc Ultrasound* 2018;7:79–82.
21. Saumoy M, Tyberg A, Brown E, et al. Successful cholecystectomy after endoscopic ultrasound gallbladder drainage compared with percutaneous cholecystostomy, can it be done? *J Clin Gastroenterol* 2019;53:231–235.
22. Park DH, Jang JW, Lee SS, et al. EUS-guided biliary drainage with transluminal stenting after failed ERCP: predictors of adverse events and long-term results. *Gastrointest Endosc* 2011;74:1276–1284.
23. Irani S, Kozarek RA. The buried lumen-apposing metal stent: is this a stent problem, a location problem, or both? *VideoGIE* 2016;1:25–26.
24. Choi JH, Lee SS, Choi JH, et al. Long-term outcomes after endoscopic ultrasonography-guided gallbladder drainage for acute cholecystitis. *Endoscopy* 2014;46:656–661.
25. Walter D, Teoh AY, Itoi T, et al. EUS-guided gall bladder drainage with a lumen-apposing metal stent: a prospective long-term evaluation. *Gut* 2016;65:6–8.
26. Ogura T, Higuchi K. Endoscopic ultrasound-guided gallbladder drainage: current status and future prospects. *Dig Endosc* 2019;31(Suppl 1):55–64.

47 How to do an EUS-guided Gastrojejunostomy

Sohini Sameera and Michel Kahaleh
Rutgers Robert Wood Johnson Medical School, New Brunswick, NJ, USA

Introduction

Gastric outlet obstruction (GOO) is a common complication of gastrointestinal malignancies and inflammatory processes; it can lead to significant weight loss and nutritional deficiencies [1,2]. The current standard of care for treating GOO is surgical gastrojejunostomy; however, invasive intervention can be challenging in this patient population due to chronic malnourishment. The procedure itself carries a high complication rate that approaches more than 40% [1,2]. In addition, other adverse events associated with surgical bypass, such as delayed gastric emptying, prolonged hospital stays and overall increased cost, lead clinicians away from this treatment route. Endoscopic ultrasound-guided gastrojejunal bypass (EUSGJ) has emerged as a minimally invasive alternative and may improve quality of life, especially in high-risk surgical candidates.

When comparing EUSGJ with surgical gastrojejunostomy, results regarding technical success tend to vary; one study found the technical success rate significantly higher in the surgical cohort while another study found no difference [3,4]. Furthermore, the rate of adverse events has been shown to be significantly lower in the EUSGJ cohort [4]. A meta-analysis demonstrated the immediate safety and efficacy of EUSGJ as between 88 and 95%, with a pooled clinical success rate of 90% [5]. Finally, one study determined a significant difference between patients' ability to eat before and after the EUSGJ, indicating great potential for clinical use [6]. Although there is a need for more data prior to endorsing EUSGJ as standard of care for GOO, the early results are promising and suggest that the procedure is safe and efficacious.

Technique (Video 47.1)

EUSGJ was first introduced by Fritscher-Ravens et al. in 2003; it has since been studied and various techniques have been proposed [7]. However, it is only when lumen-apposing metal stents (LAMS) arrived that the procedure became more widespread [8]. Initially performed over a wire targeting a loop of bowel inflated with saline injection, the development of cautery-enhanced LAMS (Hot AXIOS™, Boston Scientific, Natick, MA) made the procedure faster and easier to perform [2,8,9].

After identification of a loop of bowel appropriately distended by placement of a nasojejunal catheter or direct injection of contrast into the targeted lumen (Figure 47.1), a cautery-enhanced LAMS is advanced through the stomach into the small bowel lumen. The first flange of the LAMS is then deployed, allowing the endoscopist to approximate the small bowel to the stomach (Figure 47.2) before deploying the second flange into the stomach (Figures 47.3 and 47.4).

Complications

A commonly reported complication is stent misplacement. A case series examining international centers reported adverse events in 3 of 26 patients (11.5%) [8]. Two of these patients had stent misplacement, one of whom developed fulminant peritonitis. This patient, who had a long-standing history of malignancy with peritoneal carcinomatosis, died the day after EUSGJ. In another case series by Itoi et al., 2 of 20 of patients (10%) experienced stent misplacement, which was quickly corrected with stent removal and conservative management [6]. Other less common complications include postprocedural pain, bleeding, and perforation. One patient in the Tyberg et al. study [8] experienced postprocedural pain and ultimately underwent a surgical gastrojejunostomy while another patient required a transfusion for failed LAMS placement without fistula closure.

Atlas of Endoscopic Ultrasonography, Second Edition. Edited by Frank Gress, Thomas Savides, Brenna Casey, and Everson L. A. Artifon.

Companion website: www.wiley.com/go/gress/atlas

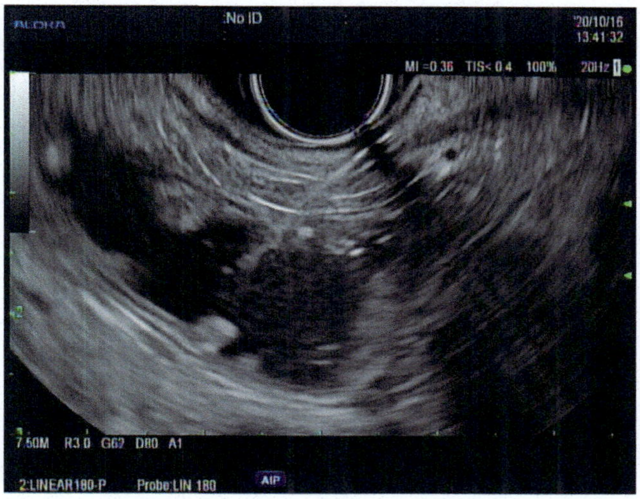

Figure 47.1 Puncture of the targeted bowel under endosonography. Source: Aloka.

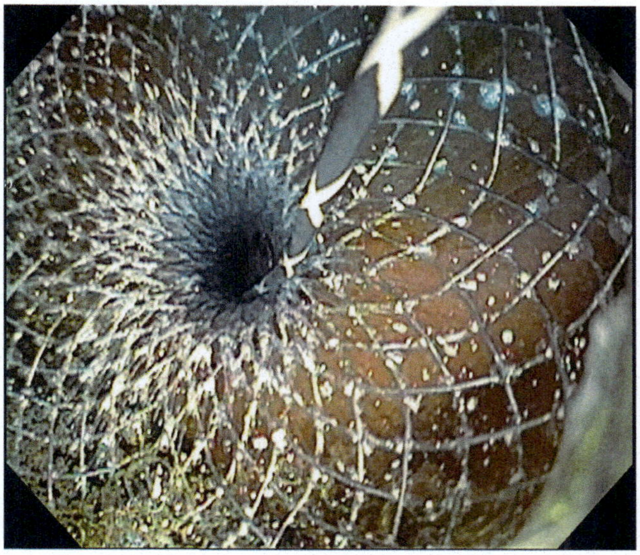

Figure 47.2 Deployment of the lumen-apposing metal stent into the small bowel and connected to the stomach.

Chapter video clip

Video 47.1 How to do an EUS-guided gastrojejunostomy.

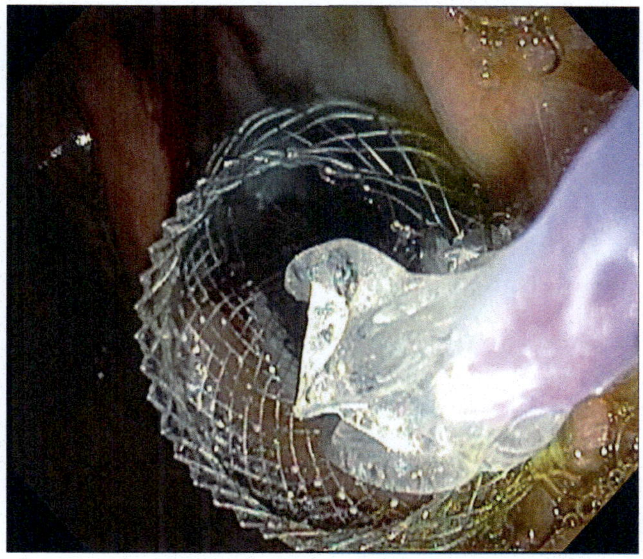

Figure 47.3 Balloon dilatation of the lumen-apposing metal stent.

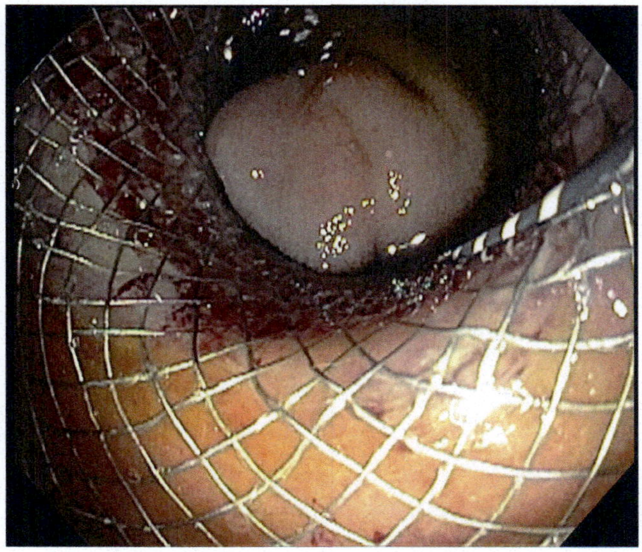

Figure 47.4 Visualization of the bowel through the fully distended lumen-apposing metal stent.

References

1. Khashab M, Alawad AS, Shin EJ, et al. Enteral stenting versus gastrojejunostomy for palliation of malignant gastric outlet obstruction. *Surg Endosc* 2013;27:2068–2075.
2. Itoi T, Baron TH, Khashab MA, et al. Technical review of endoscopic ultrasonography-guided gastroenterostomy in 2017. *Dig Endosc* 2017;29:495–502.
3. Khashab MA, Messallam AA, Penas I, et al. International multicenter comparative trial of transluminal EUS-guided biliary drainage via hepatogastrostomy vs. choledochoduodenostomy approaches. *Endosc Int Open* 2016;4:E175–E181.
4. Perez-Miranda M, Tyberg A, Poletto D, et al. EUS-guided gastrojejunostomy versus laparoscopic gastrojejunostomy: an international collaborative study. *J Clin Gastroenterol* 2017;51: 896–899.
5. McCarty TR, Garg R, Thompson CC, Rustagi T. Efficacy and safety of EUS-guided gastroenterostomy for benign and malignant gastric outlet obstruction: a systematic review and meta-analysis. *Endosc Int Open* 2019;7:E1474–E1482.

6. Itoi T, Ishii K, Ikeuchi N, et al. Prospective evaluation of endoscopic ultrasonography-guided double-balloon-occluded gastrojejunostomy bypass (EPASS) for malignant gastric outlet obstruction. *Gut* 2016;65:193–195.
7. Fritscher-Ravens A, Mosse CA, Mukherjee D, et al. Transluminal endosurgery: single lumen access anastomotic device for flexible endoscopy. *Gastrointest Endosc* 2003;58:585–591.
8. Tyberg A, Perez-Miranda M, Sanchez-Ocana R, et al. Endoscopic ultrasound-guided gastrojejunostomy with a lumen-apposing metal stent: a multicenter, international experience. *Endosc Int Open* 2016;4:E276–E281.
9. Chen YI, Kunda R, Storm AC, et al. EUS-guided gastroenterostomy: a multicenter study comparing the direct and balloon-assisted techniques. *Gastrointest Endosc* 2018;87:1215–1221.

48 How to do EUS Elastography

Julio Iglesias-Garcia, Jose Lariño-Noia, Daniel de la Iglesia-García, and J. Enrique Dominguez-Muñoz

Department of Gastroenterology and Hepatology, Health Research Institute, University Hospital of Santiago de Compostela, Santiago de Compostela, Spain

Introduction

The introduction of endoscopic ultrasound (EUS) in clinical practice is an important advancement in the management of a wide variety of diseases. EUS has been demonstrated to have significantly changed the diagnosis and/or management in up to 25–50% of cases. Nevertheless, an accurate diagnosis cannot always be determined using only conventional B-mode EUS imaging. However, in 80–95% of cases, EUS-guided tissue acquisition can provide a definitive diagnosis, but there remain a few cases which require efforts to increase this diagnostic yield. Hence, new methods have been warranted, allowing for a more accurate but still noninvasive characterization of lesions, limiting the need for EUS-guided tissue sampling and guided biopsies of areas with the highest suspicion of malignancy in cases where tissue sampling is still necessary. Among them, EUS-guided elastography has arisen as a very promising technique.

Elastography is a novel technique for tissue characterization, providing a noninvasive method for the evaluation of the mechanical properties of different tissues, in this case tissue stiffness. Elastography has emerged from the development of the fremitus technique in breast ultrasonography, which demonstrates that healthy breast tissue vibrates more than solid malignant lesions, despite their isoechoic appearance under B-mode ultrasound. It is well known that inflammatory processes and neoplastic infiltration induce changes in normal tissue structure, thus causing a change in its elasticity, becoming harder or softer. This is a qualitative method for evaluating tissue stiffness based on external or internal generated force, which in EUS is based on the internal force concept. The measurement algorithm is based on the extended combined autocorrelation method. It is based on stiff tissues presenting lower strain so that they deform less under compression when compared with soft tissues. With strain elastography, the compression-induced tissue deformations within a region of interest (ROI) are assessed in a comparative fashion and are visualized using a transparent color overlay on the B-mode image.

As previously described, several different diseases, including cancer, can induce alterations in tissue stiffness. In this chapter we focus on how to perform an EUS-guided elastography study, and briefly mention the main indications of this method, according to the clinical evidence.

Technique

Before describing the method, we need to initially emphasize that no specific preparation of the patient is needed for performing EUS-guided elastography. Patient positioning does not differ from that required for the performance of a standard EUS exploration.

Elastography evaluates stiffness through the application of slight compression, using the tip of the scope (ultrasound part), to the targeted tissue (lesion) and recording the resulting tissue displacement from the region evaluated. Basically, elastography relies on the quantification of the compression-induced deformation of the structures in the B-mode image using the degree of deformation as an indicator of tissue stiffness. During EUS, together with the compression performed by the tip of the scope, we also use the physiologic vascular pulsations and respiratory movements to obtain important additional vibration and compressions necessary for the study. Small structural deformations will be caused by compression and be detected on the B-mode image, so that the strain is smaller in hard tissues than in soft tissues. To optimize and have confidence in the evaluation, large blood vessels should be avoided because movement of blood produces an artificially large displacement or softness. A ROI is used to define an area in a similar way to Doppler evaluation

Atlas of Endoscopic Ultrasonography, Second Edition. Edited by Frank Gress, Thomas Savides, Brenna Casey, and Everson L. A. Artifon.

Companion website: www.wiley.com/go/gress/atlas

(Figure 48.1). As described previously, little compression is necessary because the regular pressure variation from the pulsation of adjacent vessels is sufficient. The size of the ROI is crucial because it needs to be sufficiently large to include both the pathologic tissue and surrounding normal tissue as reference (Figure 48.2). The best image quality has been documented when the area under study covers 25–50% of the ROI. At this point, there are two different

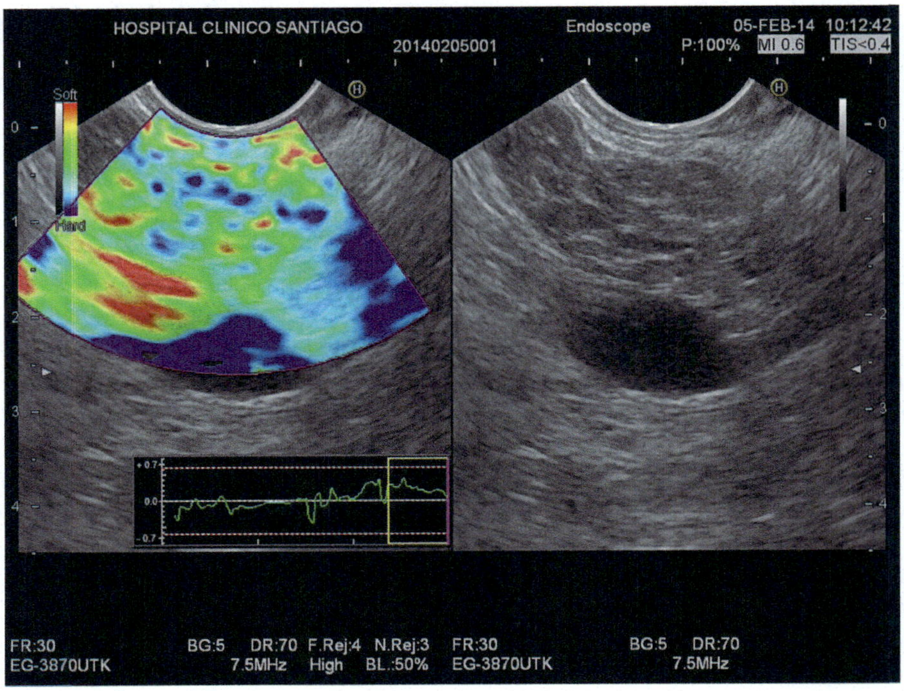

Figure 48.1 Standard EUS elastographic image. A ROI is used to define the area of interest in a similar way to Doppler evaluation. Both B-mode and the elastographic image can be seen on the screen.

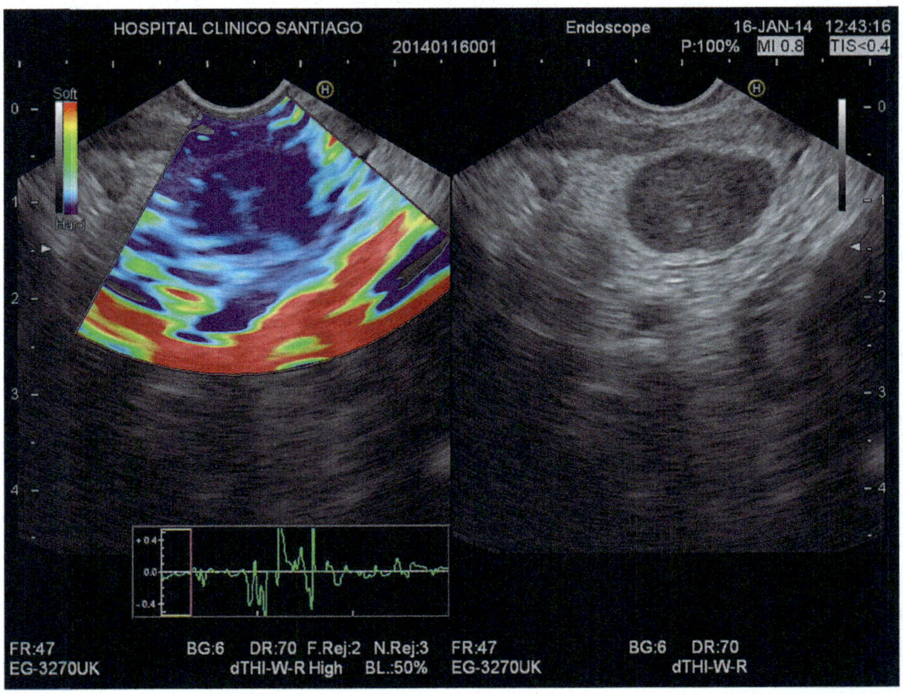

Figure 48.2 EUS-guided elastography of a malignant lymph node. This image emphasizes the size of the ROI, with the lesion covering 25–50% of the ROI.

Table 48.1 Elastographic pattern classification.

Color and pattern	Stiffness	Malignancy
Homogeneous blue predominant	Hard	Yes
Heterogeneous blue predominant (Figure 48.3)	Hard	Yes
Heterogeneous green predominant (Figure 48.4)	Intermediate	No
Homogeneous green predominant (Figure 48.5)	Soft	No
Heterogeneous green and blue without predominant color	Intermediate hard	Undetermined

options for EUS-guided elastography: qualitative and quantitative evaluation. We describe both methodologies.

Qualitative elastography

Qualitative elasticity (on a scale of 1–255) is depicted using a color map (red, green, and blue), wherein hard tissue is shown in dark blue, tissue with intermediate hardness in green, medium soft tissue in yellow, and soft tissue in red. The elastography pattern is demonstrated by superimposing the color pattern on a conventional B-mode picture. Usually, a two-panel image is used for presentation, including the conventional gray-scale B-mode image and the elastographic image, which represents different elasticity values marked with different colors, resulting in different elastographic patterns.

Table 48.1 shows the elastographic pattern classification.

Quantitative elastography

Currently, there are two different methods allowing a quantitative elastographic evaluation: the strain ratio and the strain histogram.

Strain ratio

Strain ratio calculations are based on standard qualitative EUS elastography data. Two different areas (A and B) are selected for quantitative elastographic analysis. Area A is selected so that it includes as much of the target lesion as possible without including the surrounding tissues. Area B is selected within a soft (red) reference area outside the target lesion, preferably the gut wall. The strain ratio is calculated as the quotient of B/A. However, the color map is just a guide because the ratio is calculated using raw strain data and does not depend on the color map display. A presumption of this method is that the investigated disease does not significantly alter the hardness of the reference connective or fat tissues. Figure 48.3 shows an example of a malignant pancreatic tumor, whereas Figure 48.4 shows a mass forming chronic pancreatitis. Figure 48.5 shows an example of a normal pancreas.

Strain histogram

Strain histogram is based on the qualitative EUS elastography data for a manually selected ROI within the standard elastography image. For the measurement, the largest measurement box that touches the inside boundary of the lesion within the ROI must be selected. The *x*-axis in the strain histogram represents the elasticity, from 0 (hardest) to 255 (softest), of the tissue. This method analyzes the range and distribution of strains within a large ROI. It shows several key parameters, such as mean strain, standard deviation, percent of area (blue), and complexity (relation of circumference to area of blue patches). Figure 48.3 shows an example of a malignant pancreatic tumor, while Figure 48.5 shows an example of a normal pancreas.

Table 48.2 shows the elastographic values on quantitative evaluation.

Indications

The use of EUS-guided elastography has grown since it was first demonstrated to be useful for several indications. Elastography is an excellent method in the field of pancreatic diseases, particularly in the differential diagnosis of solid pancreatic lesions, with sensitivities reported as close to 100% and specificities ranging between 65 and 90%. A recent indication is in the evaluation of patients with suspected chronic pancreatitis, providing an opportunity to evaluate pancreatic fibrosis in support of the diagnosis. This technique also has a role in the evaluation of lymph nodes, mainly for determining the probability of malignancy (Figures 48.6 and 48.7). In this setting, the diagnostic yield of elastography can reach values of 80–90%. There are emerging indications for EUS-guided elastography, such as the evaluation of liver lesions, subepithelial lesions (Figure 48.8), and left adrenal gland masses (Figure 48.9).

Complications

There are no specific complications related to EUS-guided elastography for any indication, apart from those related to the EUS procedure itself.

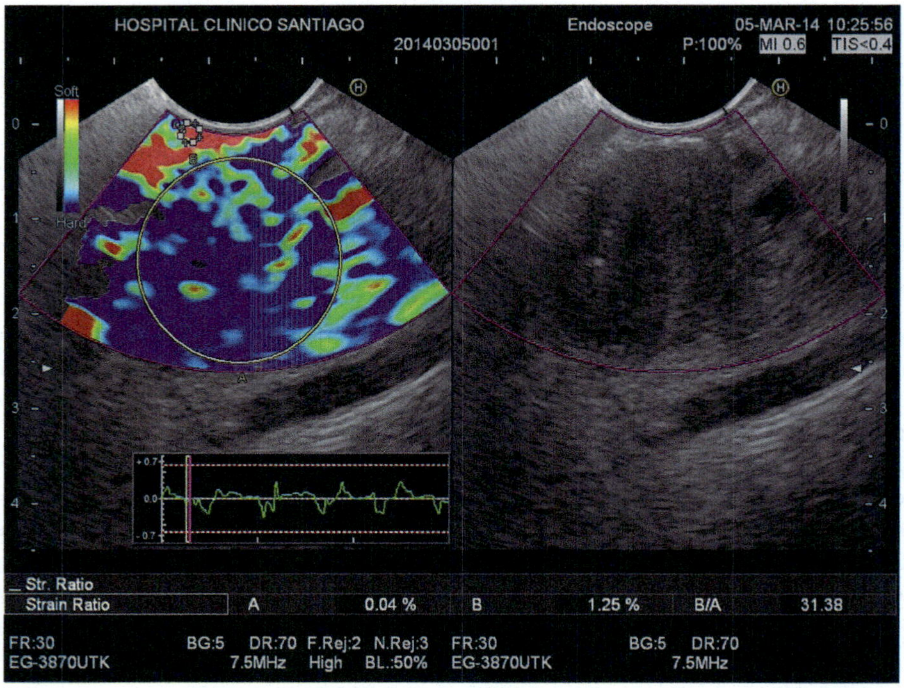

(a)

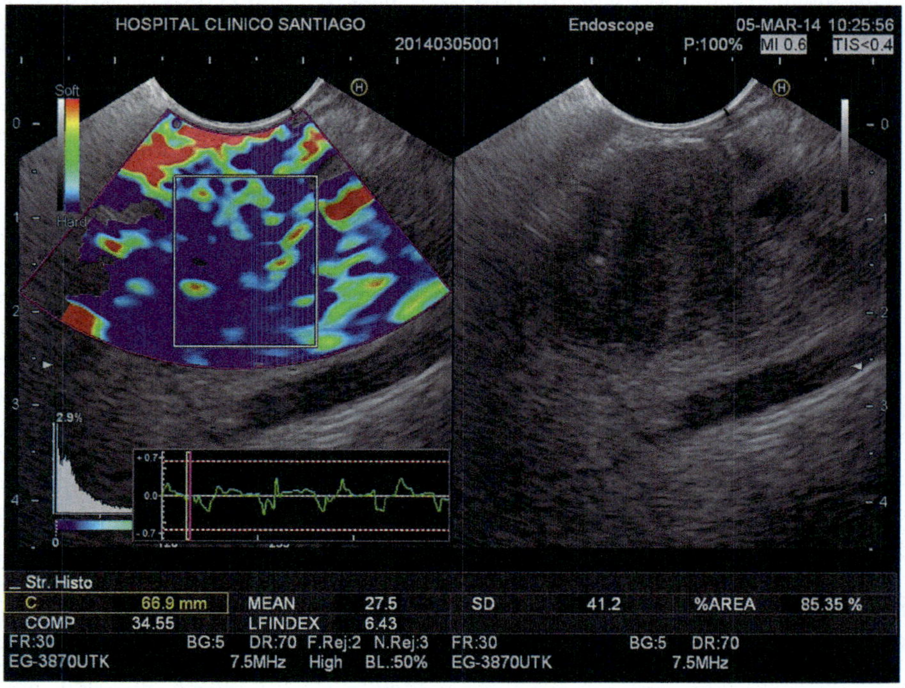

(b)

Figure 48.3 Pancreatic adenocarcinoma displaying a predominantly heterogeneous blue pattern, with a strain ratio higher than 10 (a) and a strain histogram lower than 50 (b).

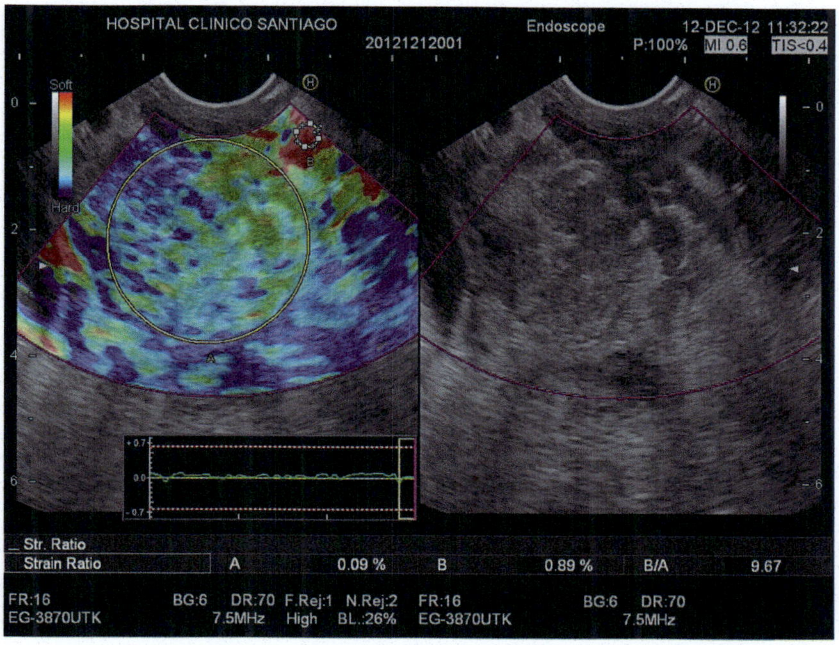

Figure 48.4 Mass forming chronic pancreatitis displaying a predominantly heterogeneous green pattern, and a strain ratio below 10.

Further reading

Dietrich CF, Jenssen C, Arcidiacono PG, et al. Endoscopic ultrasound: elastographic lymph node evaluation. *Endosc Ultrasound* 2015;4(3):176–90.

Dietrich CF, Bibby E, Jenssen C, et al. EUS elastography: how to do it? *Endosc Ultrasound* 2018;7(1):20–28.

Dietrich CF, Burmeister S, Hollerbach S, et al. Do we need elastography for EUS? *Endosc Ultrasound* 2020;9(5):284–290.

Iglesias-Garcia J, Larino-Noia J, Abdulkader I, et al. Quantitative endoscopic ultrasound elastography: an accurate method for the differentiation of solid pancreatic masses. *Gastroenterology* 2010;139(4):1172–1180.

Iglesias-García J, Lariño-Noia J, Domínguez-Muñoz JE. New imaging techniques: endoscopic ultrasound-guided elastography. *Gastrointest Endosc Clin North Am* 2017;27(4):551–567.

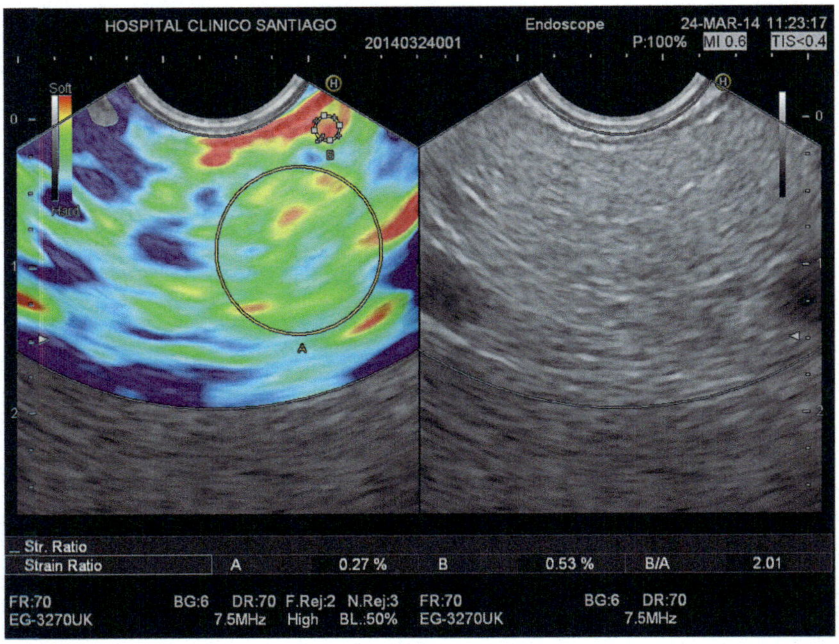

(a)

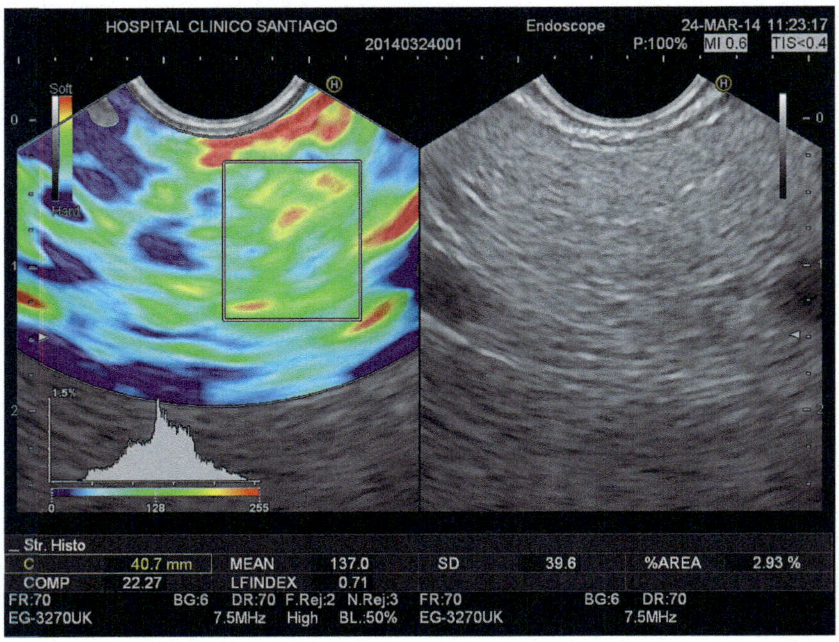

(b)

Figure 48.5 EUS-guided elastography from normal pancreas showing a predominantly homogeneous green pattern, with a low strain (a) and high values on strain histogram (b). These are the typical patterns of benign diseases.

Table 48.2 Elastographic quantitative evaluation.

Strain ratio	Strain histogram	Malignancy
>10	<50	Yes
<10	>50	No

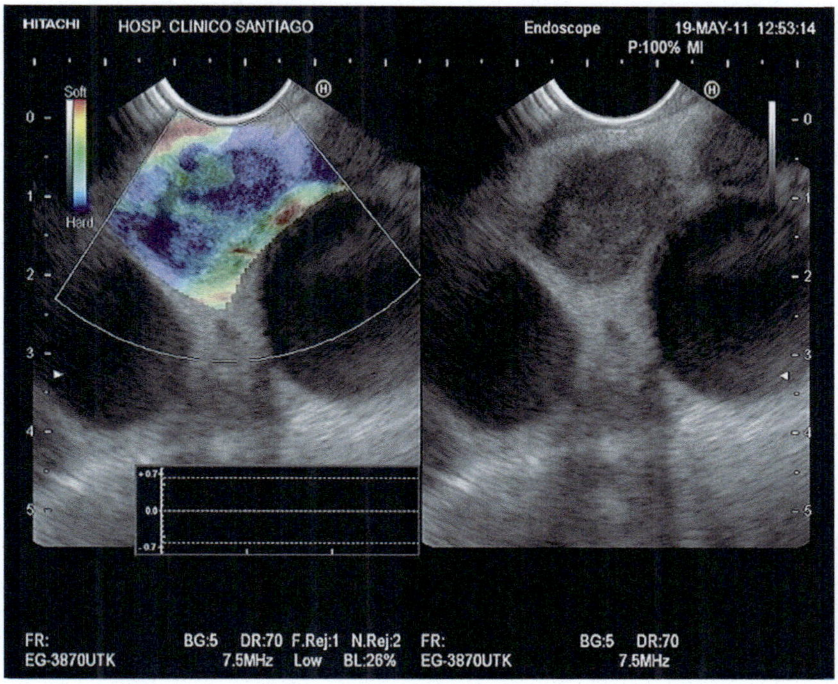

Figure 48.6 EUS-guided elastography displaying a blue pattern in a metastatic lymph node, in the setting of a patient with a gastric cancer.

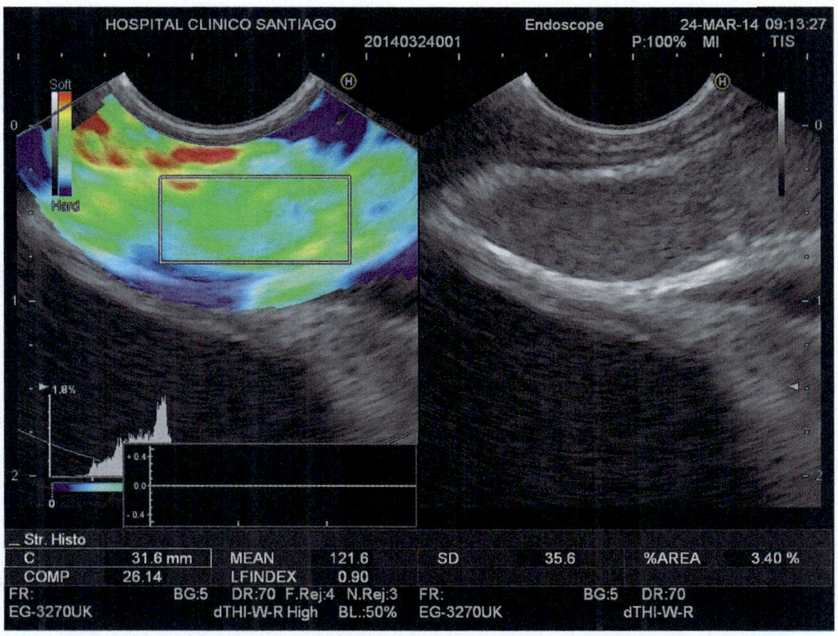

Figure 48.7 EUS-guided elastography of a typical benign lymph node.

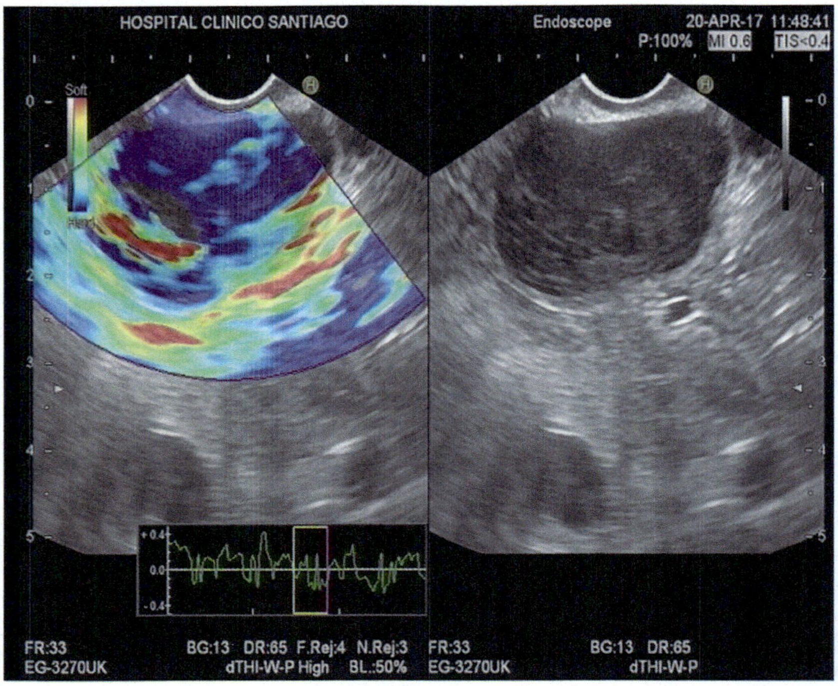

Figure 48.8 Elastographic evaluation of a subepithelial lesion showing a heterogeneous blue pattern. Lesion eventually diagnosed as a gastrointestinal stromal cell tumor.

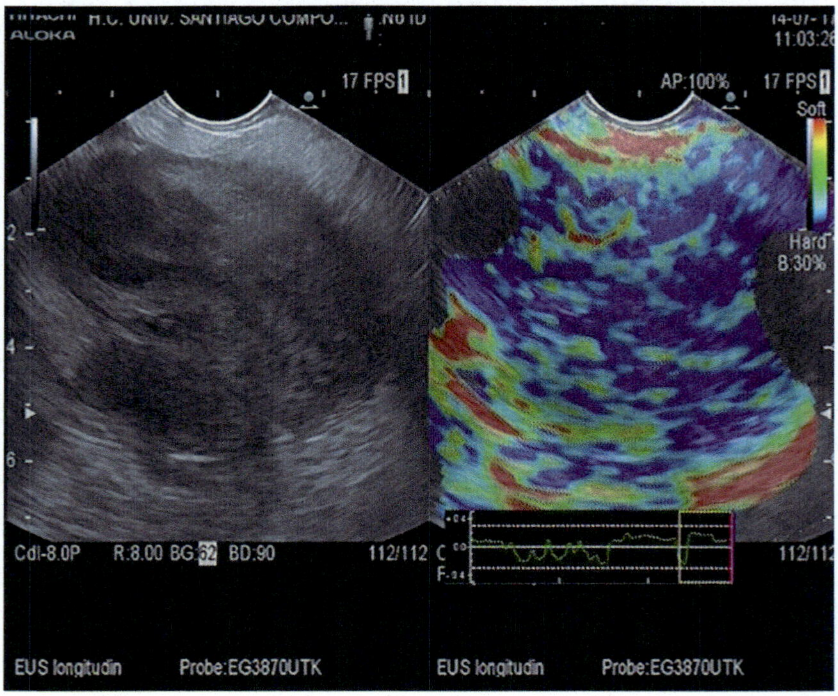

Figure 48.9 Metastatic lesion on left adrenal gland, from a lung cancer, displaying a heterogeneous blue pattern at elastography.

49 How to do Contrast-enhanced EUS

Yasunobu Yamashita and Masayuki Kitano
Second Department of Internal Medicine, Wakayama Medical University, Wakayama, Japan

Introduction

Endoscopic ultrasonography (EUS) is considered one of the most reliable and efficient diagnostic modalities for digestive diseases, since it demonstrates better outcomes than other modalities with regard to spatial resolution. However, one of its primary limitations is differential diagnosis, which particularly focuses on vascularity to characterize digestive diseases. To address this issue, a number of studies have employed contrast-enhanced harmonic EUS (CH-EUS) to diagnose digestive diseases.

Principle of CH-EUS

Contrast harmonic imaging is based on the following principle: upon exposure to the ultrasound beams, microbubbles in the contrast agent either disrupt or resonate and subsequently release several harmonic signals. Exposure to ultrasound waves leads to the production of harmonic components in tissues and microbubbles that are integer multiples of the fundamental frequency; furthermore, microbubbles generate higher harmonic content than tissues. Selectively depicting the second harmonic component facilitates a better visualization of signals from microbubbles than those from the tissue (Figure 49.1). Therefore, this technology can detect signals without Doppler-related artifacts from microbubbles in vessels that demonstrate extremely slow flow rates and is used to successfully characterize vascularity.

Critical points for performing CH-EUS

Figure 49.2 demonstrates the impact of exposure to ultrasound beams on microbubble behavior, according to a mechanical index (MI). A dual screen with fundamental B-mode and CH-EUS images should be displayed. The CH-EUS echo image should be dark enough to permit the visualization of the few signals from the tissue, before administering the contrast agent. The focal point should be set at the bottom of the target lesion. Before performing CH-EUS, the target lesion should be imaged as close as possible, since ultrasound beam penetration via CH-EUS is inferior to that with fundamental B-mode. A bolus injection of contrast agent (Sonazoid, 15 ml/kg body weight; Sonovue, 2.4–4.8 ml per patient; Definity, 10 ml/kg body weight) is administered through a peripheral vein. Signals from the contrast agent appear after 10–15 seconds and peak at approximately 20 seconds (Figure 49.3).

Characterizing a lesion involves classifying the enhancement patterns of the surrounding tissue into four patterns (avascular, hypovascular, isovascular, and hypervascular) (Figure 49.4). Additionally, enhancement patterns observed in the tumor are classified as either homogeneous (uniform enhancement of the entire tumor) or inhomogeneous enhancement (tumor enhanced at different levels) (Figure 49.5).

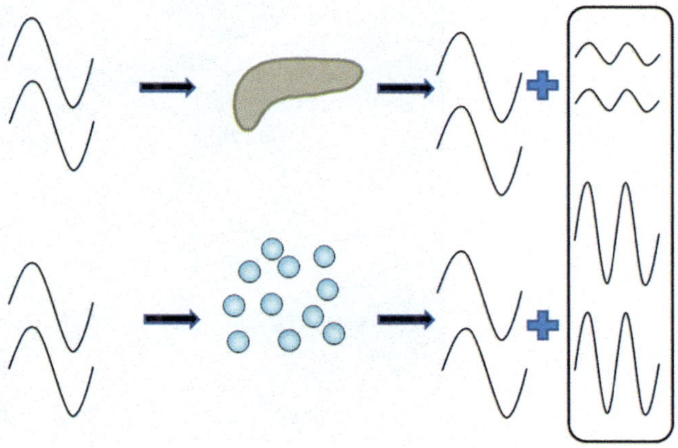

Figure 49.1 Principle of contrast harmonic imaging.

Atlas of Endoscopic Ultrasonography, Second Edition. Edited by Frank Gress, Thomas Savides, Brenna Casey, and Everson L. A. Artifon.

Companion website: www.wiley.com/go/gress/atlas

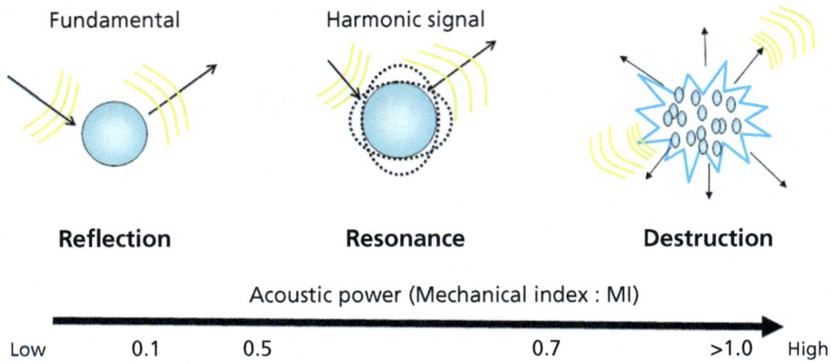

Figure 49.2 Behavior of microbubbles when exposed to ultrasound beams based on the mechanical index.

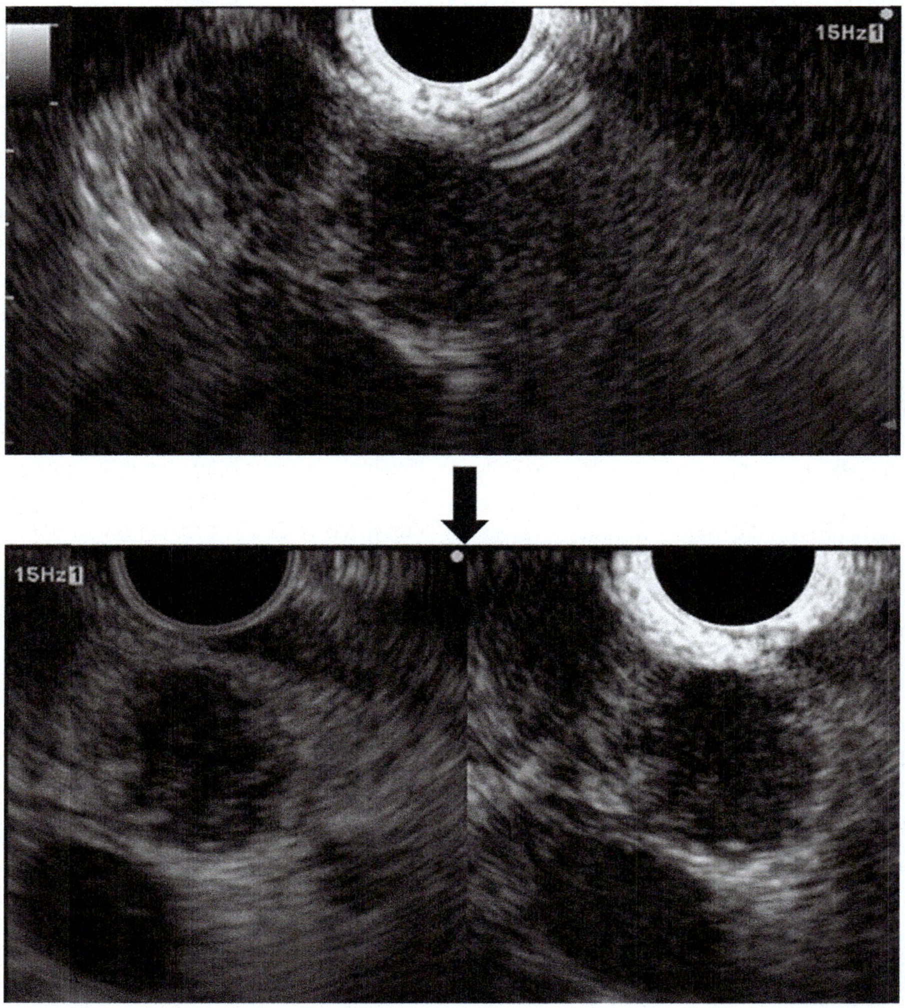

Figure 49.3 Contrast-enhanced endoscopic ultrasonography (CH-EUS) procedures. 1, Both fundamental B-mode and CH-EUS images are displayed on the dual screen. 2, Echo image of CH-EUS (*right*) is dark enough to facilitate visualization of small amounts of signal from the tissue. 3, The focal point (arrowhead) is set at the bottom of the screen. 4, The mechanical index (MI) (yellow box) is set at 0.2–0.4. 5, A bolus injection of contrast agent is administered through a peripheral vein. 6, In the pancreas, signals from the contrast agent appear approximately 10 seconds after administering the contrast agent, which allows visualization of the detailed structure of vessels (arrowhead). Here, an extremely small cyst in the pancreatic parenchyma is identified as a non-enhancement lesion (arrow).

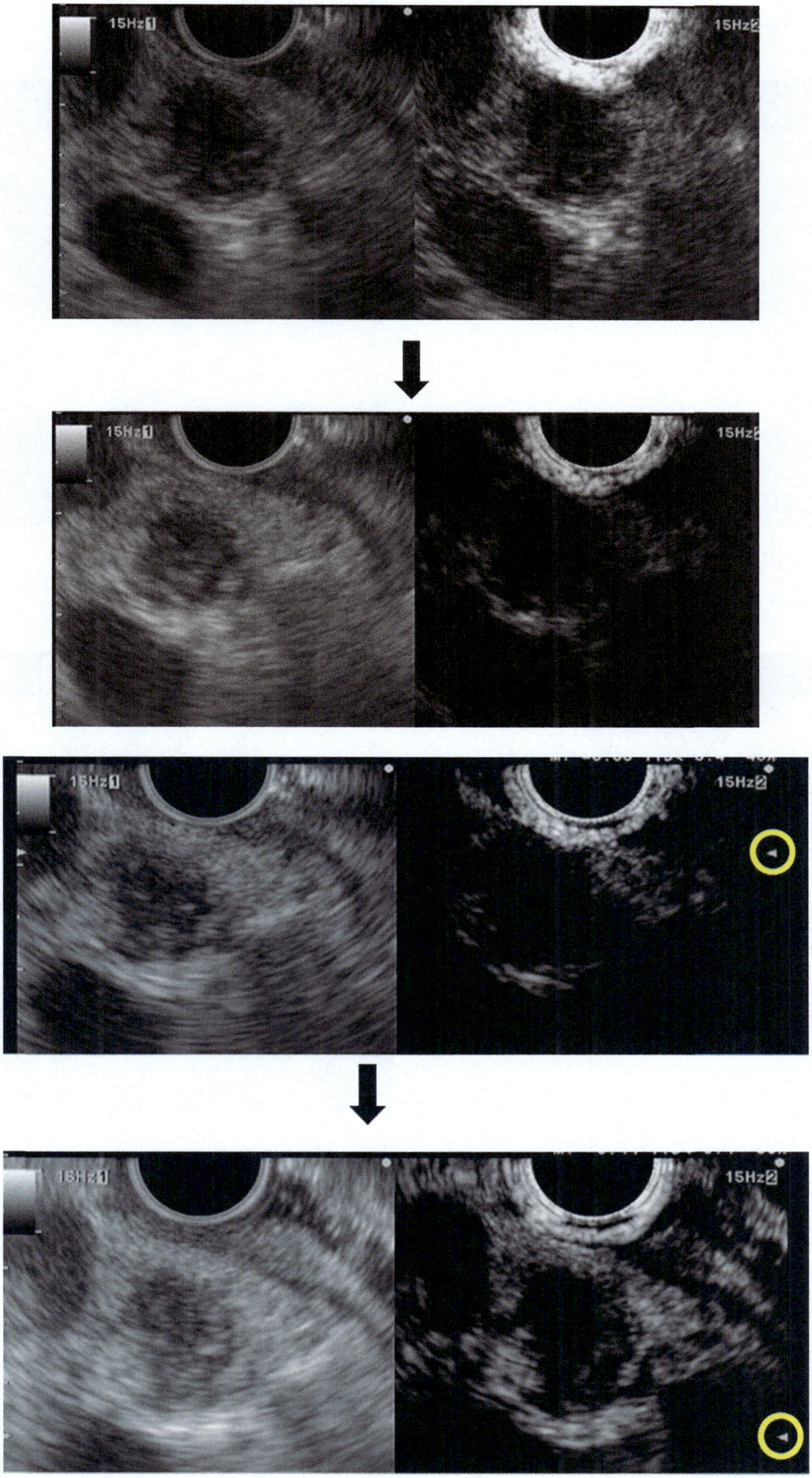

Figure 49.3 (Continued)

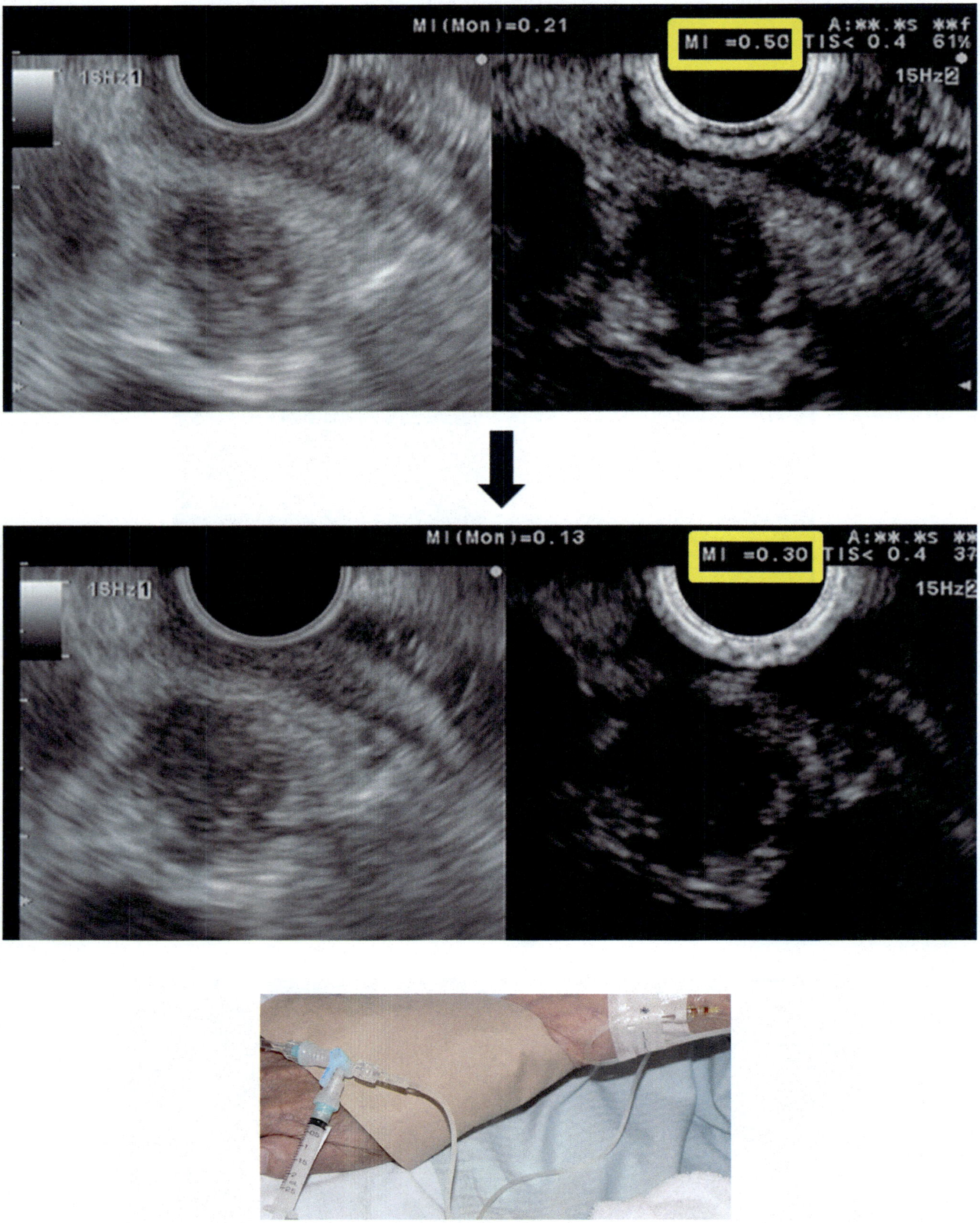

Figure 49.3 (Continued)

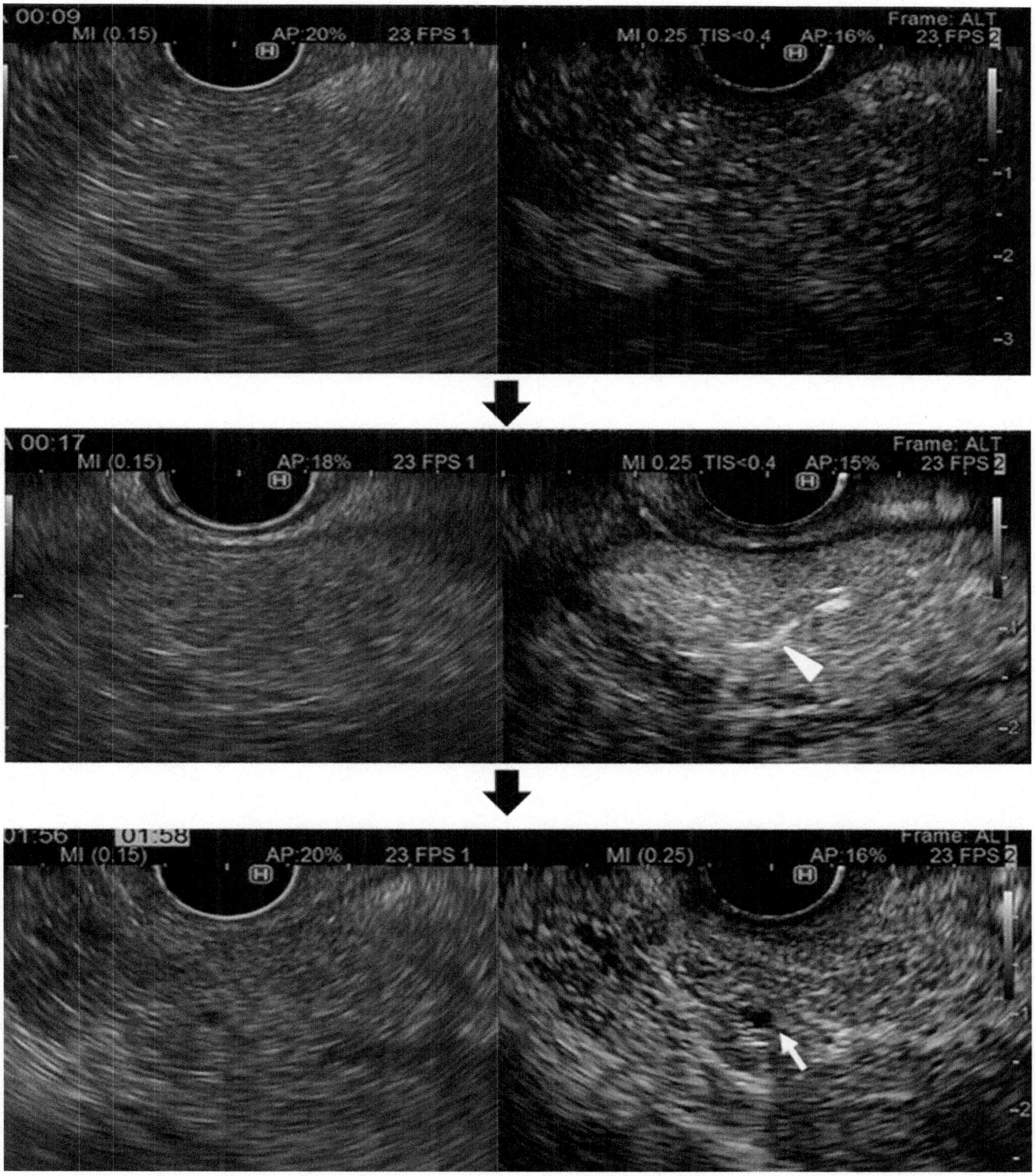

Figure 49.3 (Continued)

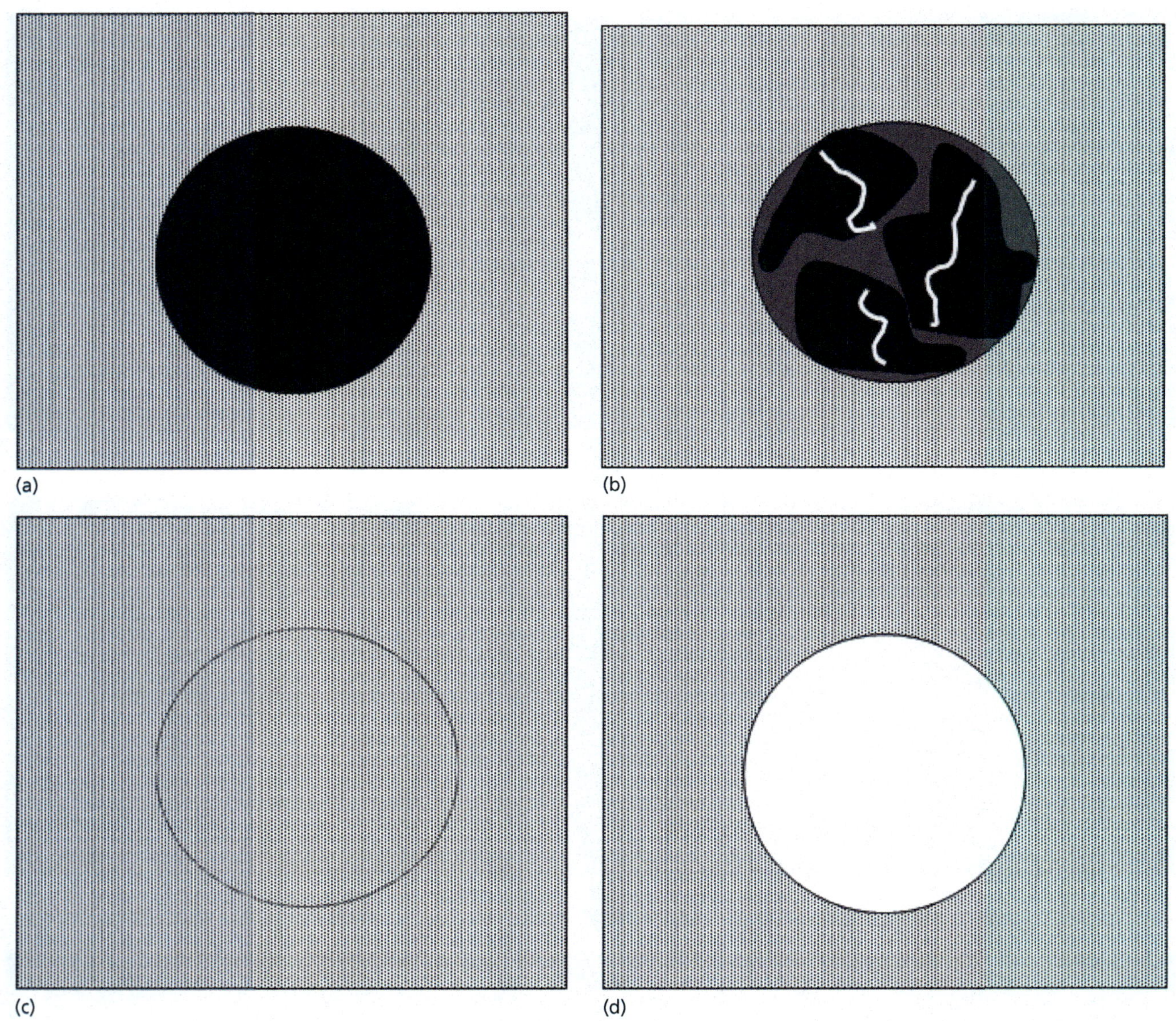

Figure 49.4 Contrast-enhanced pattern compared to the surrounding tissue: (a) non-enhancement; (b) hypo-enhancement; (c) iso-enhancement; (d) hyper-enhancement.

Advantages of CH-EUS compared to other contrast-enhanced modalities

CH-EUS primarily offers three advantages over other imaging methods.

First, it can detect signals from microbubbles in vessels with extremely low flow rates without Doppler-related artifacts, when compared with contrast-enhanced color and power Doppler EUS. Second, CH-EUS is better than contrast-enhanced magnetic resonance imaging (MRI) and computed tomography (CT) for patients demonstrating contraindications for contrast materials, including renal failure or contrast allergy, even though contrast agent-associated adverse reactions are rare in humans. Third, CH-EUS allows real-time dynamic imaging and repeated examinations.

Advantages of CH-EUS compared to conventional EUS

CH-EUS is superior to conventional EUS in the following three ways. First, it is often difficult to perform differential diagnoses of a digestive disease using EUS, since most solid lesions present as a hypoechoic mass. However, CH-EUS can characterize solid lesions via contrast enhancement. Second, CH-EUS is better at detecting isoechoic lesions than EUS as it

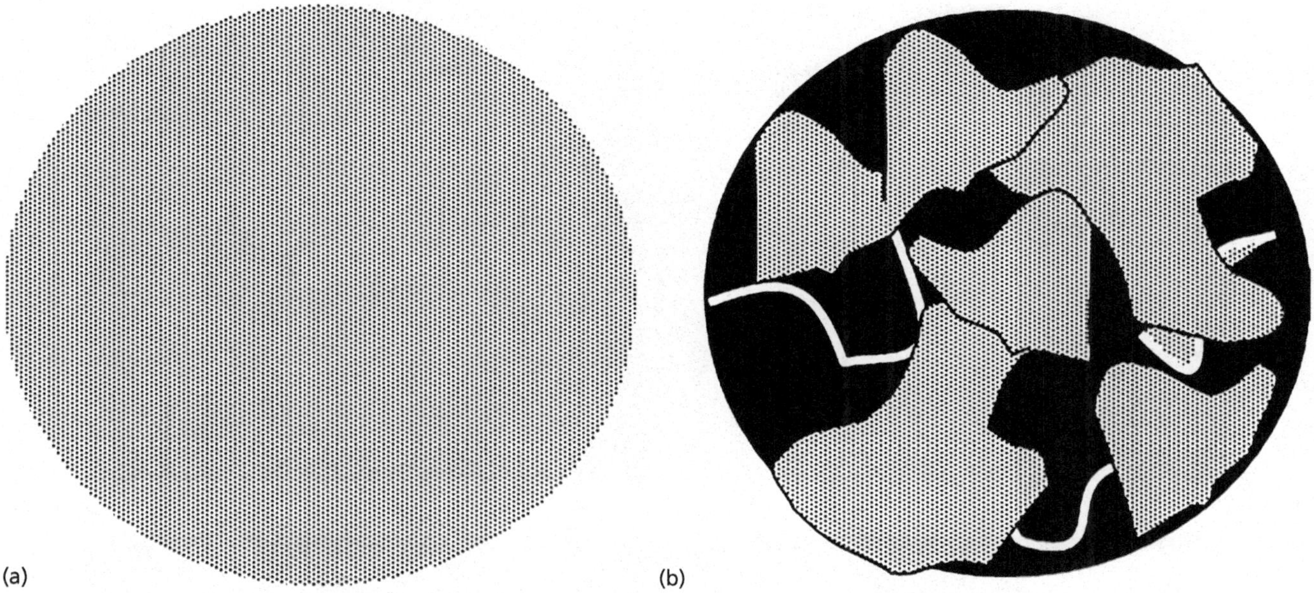

Figure 49.5 Comparison of contrast-enhanced patterns in the lesion: (a) homogeneous enhancement; (b) heterogeneous enhancement.

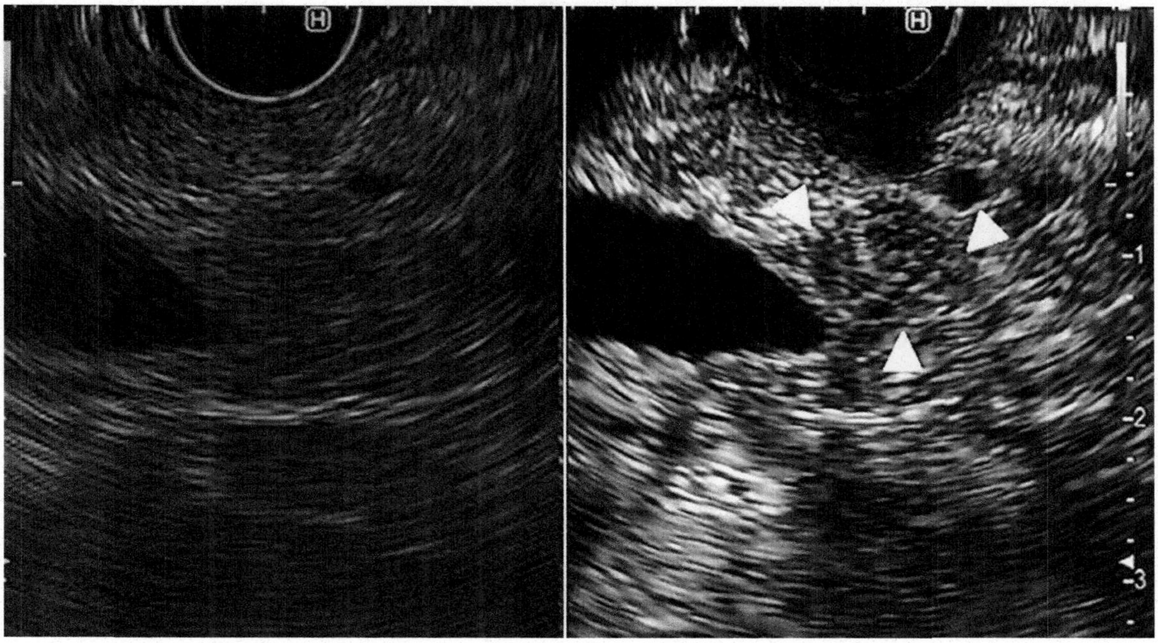

Figure 49.6 Detecting a lesion via contrast-enhanced endoscopic ultrasonography. The image on the left does not show the presence of any lesions via conventional EUS. However, a hypo-enhancement lesion is clearly visible in contrast-enhanced endoscopic ultrasonography (CH-EUS) (*right*).

employs contrast enhancement to identify the lesion margin (Figure 49.6). Third, it is a distinct possibility that EUS may not always be able to distinguish between a tumor and sludge (or mucous clot), even though the decision to consider surgical intervention depends on the presence or absence of tumor. Alternatively, CH-EUS can discriminate a tumor from a mucous clot (or sludge) using contrast enhancement (Figure 49.7).

Evaluation of CH-EUS image for lesions in different organs

Solid pancreatic lesions

Since most pancreatic solid lesions present as a hypoechoic mass, it is often difficult to characterize them using EUS. Alternatively, CH-EUS can be employed to differentiate them using the enhancement pattern. CH-EUS images char-

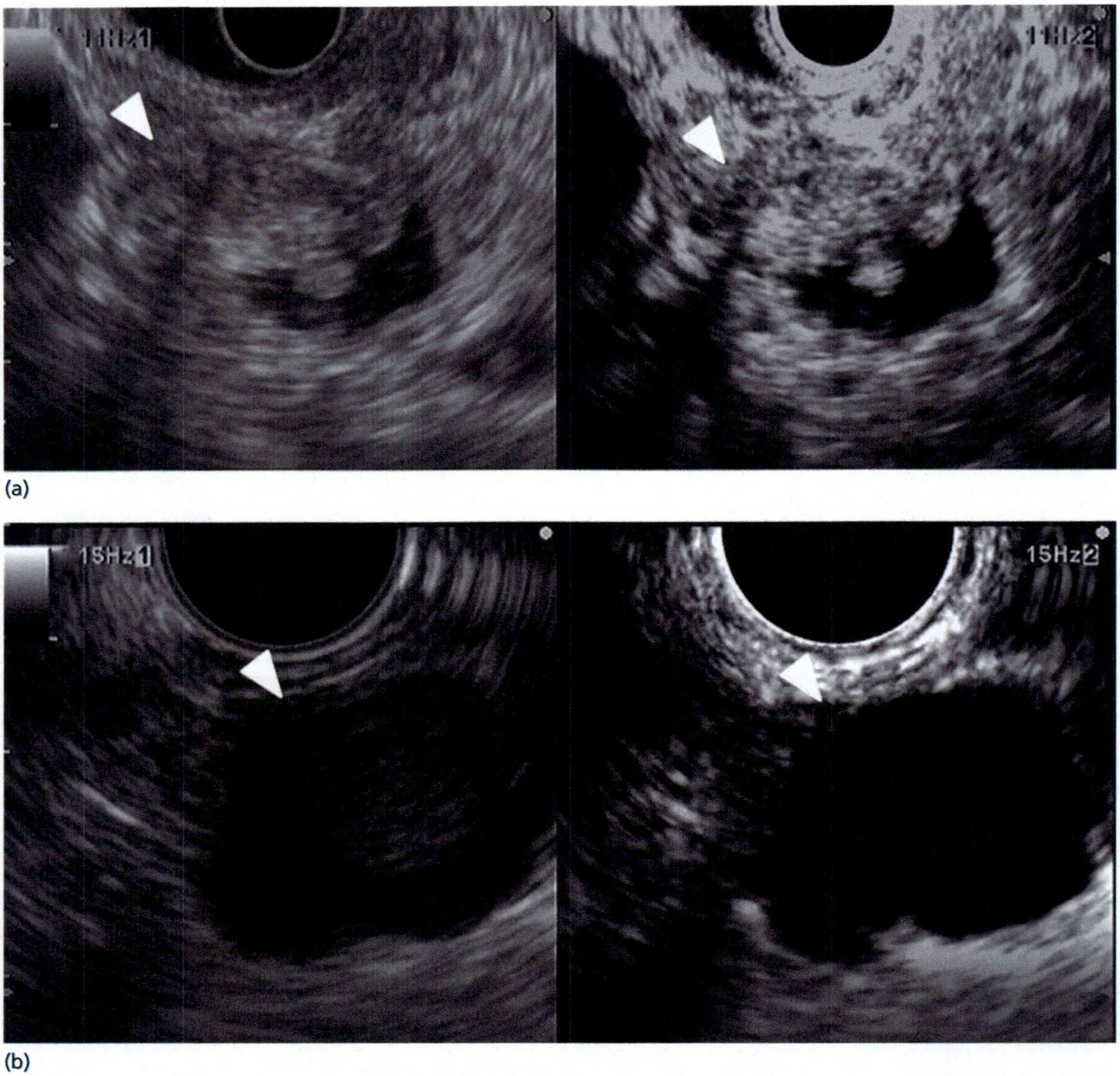

Figure 49.7 Distinguishing a mural nodule from a mucous clot using contrast-enhanced endoscopic ultrasonography (CH-EUS). (a) Representative case of mural nodule: identification of a hyperechoic mural lesion (arrowhead) using conventional EUS (*left*). CH-EUS (*right*) detects the presence of vascularity in the mural lesion (arrowhead). (b) A representative case of mucous clot: conventional EUS (*left*) reveals a hyperechoic mural lesion (arrowhead). CH-EUS (*right*) reveals no vascularity in the mural lesion (arrowhead).

acterized pancreatic cancers, inflammatory masses, and neuroendocrine tumors as hypovascular (Figure 49.8a), isovascular (Figure 49.8b), and hypervascular (Figure 49.8c), respectively.

Pancreatic cyst

EUS often fails to distinguish between a mural nodule and mucous clot in intraductal papillary mucinous neoplasm (IPMN), although the presence or absence of mural nodules is one of the important factors that influence decisions regarding surgical intervention for IPMNs. Alternatively, CH-EUS is able to discriminate mural nodule from mucous clot via contrast enhancement (Figure 49.7).

Subepithelial lesions

Gastrointestinal stromal tumors (GISTs) demonstrate a low to high range of malignant potential. Although it is difficult to characterize the malignant degree of GIST using EUS, CH-EUS can be used to do the same by investigating the presence or absence of an intratumoral vessel (Figure 49.9).

Lymph node

It is often difficult to characterize lymph node swellings using EUS, even though nodal staging is important for determining the appropriate treatment strategy for cancer (Figure 49.10a). Alternatively, CH-EUS is able to distinguish malignant from benign lymph nodes using contrast enhancement with enhancement pattern (Figure 49.10b).

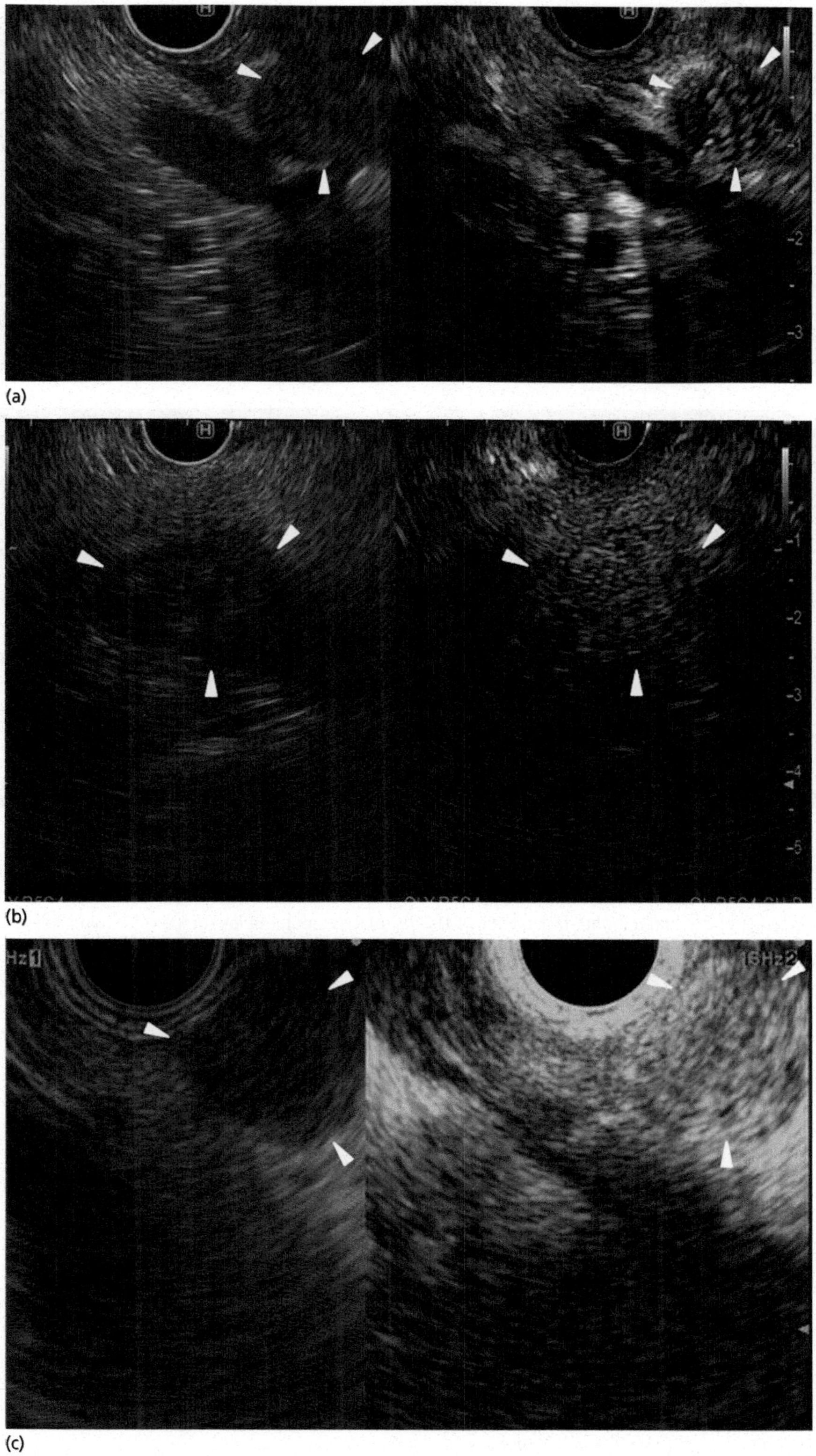

Figure 49.8 Typical contrast-enhanced endoscopic ultrasonography (CH-EUS) findings of hypoechoic pancreatic solid lesions, which are detected using conventional EUS. (a) Representative case of pancreatic cancer: CH-EUS image (*right*) shows that the lesion (arrowheads) has a lower echo signal intensity than that of the surrounding pancreatic tissue. (b) Representative case of an inflammatory mass: CH-EUS (*right*) demonstrates that the lesions (arrowheads) have a higher isointense echo signal than that of the surrounding pancreatic tissue. (c) Representative case of a neuroendocrine tumor: CH-EUS (*right*) demonstrates that the lesions (arrowheads) have a higher echo signal intensity than that of the surrounding pancreatic tissue.

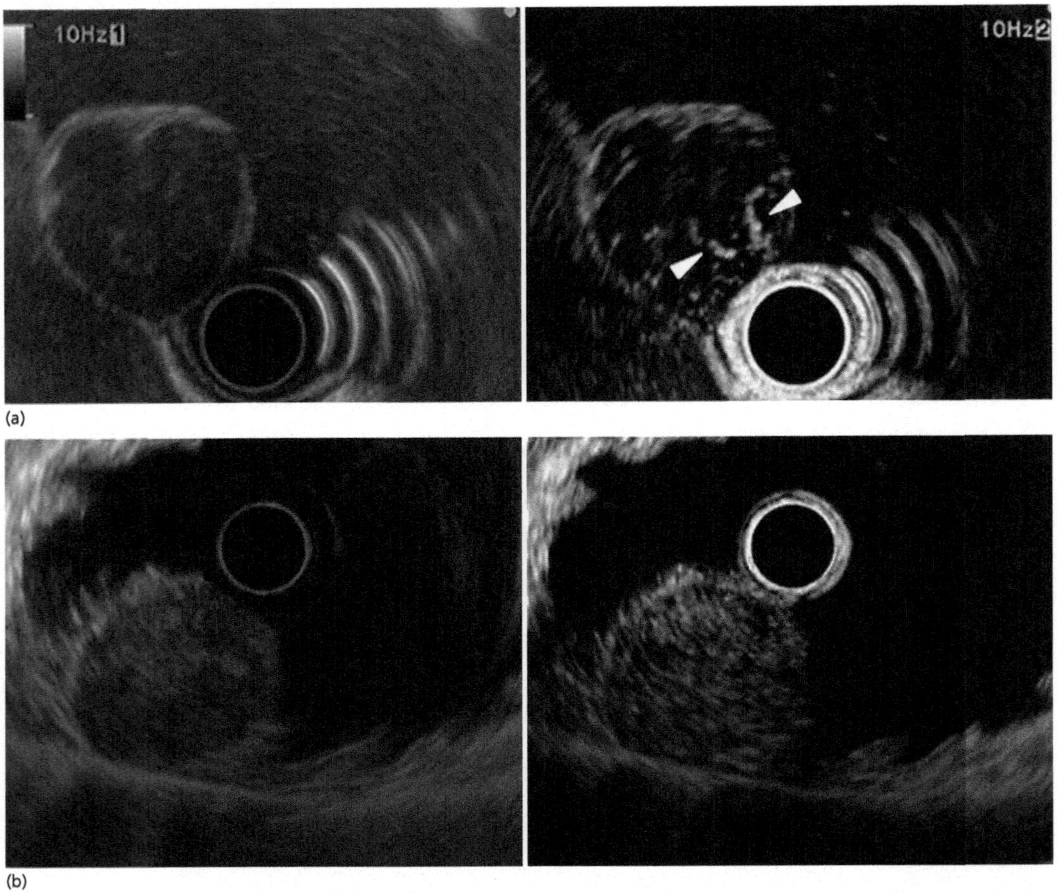

Figure 49.9 Contrast-enhanced endoscopic ultrasonography (CH-EUS) for gastrointestinal stromal tumor (GIST). (a) Representative high-grade GIST: using conventional EUS (*left*) to detect GIST as a low echoic lesion. Detection of irregular subepithelial intratumoral vessels (arrowhead), emanating from the peripheral part within the tumor to the center of the tumor (*right*), facilitated by CH-EUS. (b) Representative low-grade GIST: using conventional EUS (*left*) to detect GIST as a low echoic lesion. Detecting a homogeneous enhanced tumor without depiction of intratumoral irregular vessels using CH-EUS (*right*).

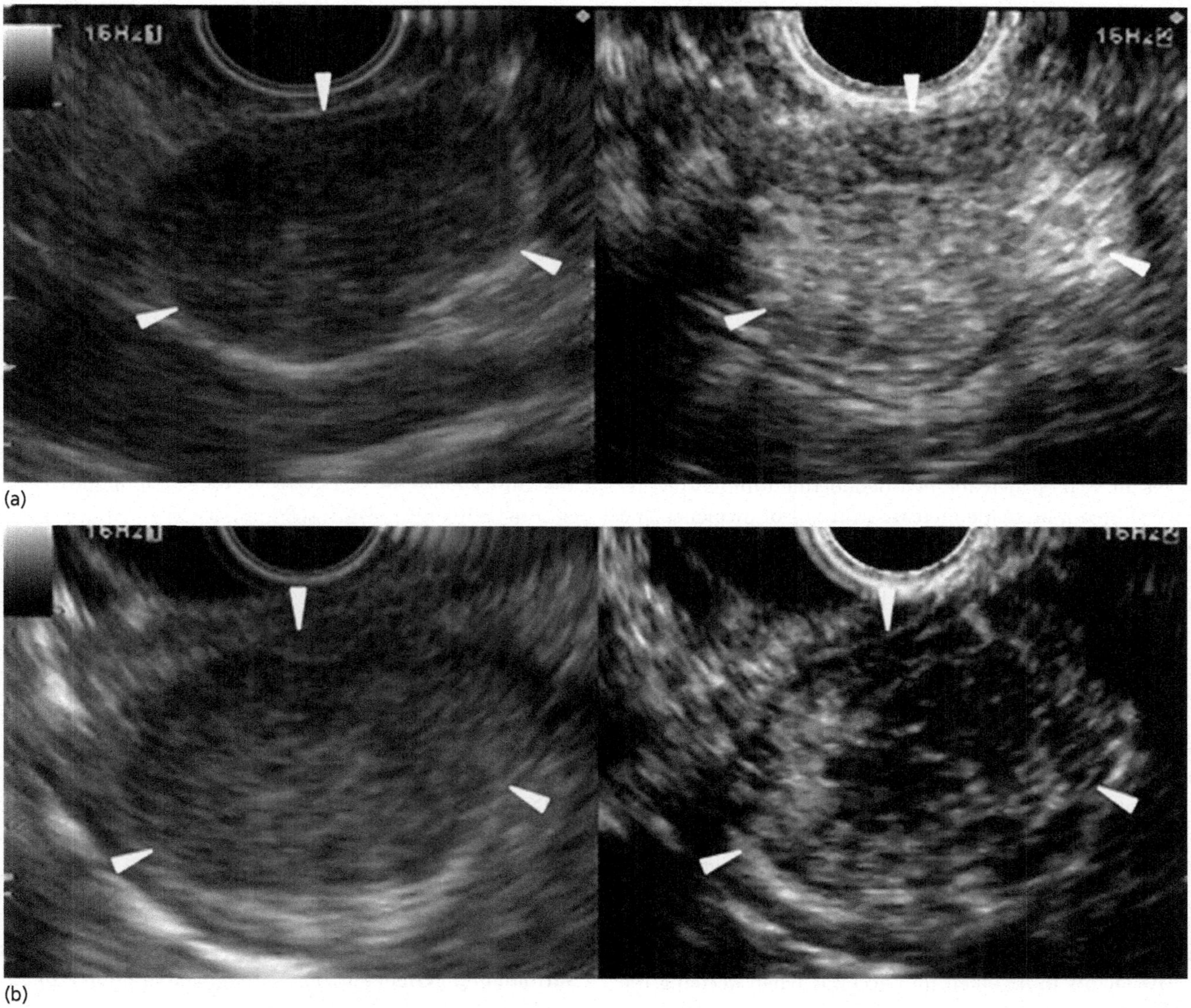

Figure 49.10 Distinguishing malignant from benign lymph nodes in contrast-enhanced endoscopic ultrasonography (CH-EUS). (a) Representative case of a benign lymph node: conventional EUS (*left*) shows low echoic lymph node (arrowheads). CH-EUS (*right*) reveals homogeneous enhancement in the lymph node (arrowheads). (b) Representative case of malignant lymph node: conventional EUS (*left*) shows low echoic lymph node (arrowheads). CH-EUS (*right*) reveals heterogeneous enhancement with avascular area in the lymph node (arrowheads).

50 How to do EUS-guided Ablation of Pancreatic Neurendocrine Tumors

Sabrina Gloria Giulia Testoni, Gemma Rossi, Livia Archibugi, and Paolo Giorgio Arcidiacono

San Raffaele Scientific Institute IRCCS, Vita-Salute San Raffaele University, Milan, Italy

Introduction and indications

In recent years pancreatic neuroendocrine tumors (pNETs) have shown a dramatic increase in terms of incidence and prevalence, especially since the widespread use of imaging studies and their better resolution. pNETs are classified mostly for the ability to secrete hormones and cause a specific syndrome (functional, F-pNETs, with gastrinoma and insulinoma being the most frequent) or not (non-functional, NF-pNETs), and for the expression of Ki-67.

Despite the prominent role of surgery as curative treatment, the complications of pancreatic surgery in this type of disease remain frequent: Jilesen and colleagues reported pancreatic fistula in 14–58% of the cases, delayed gastric emptying in 15–18%, postoperative bleeding in 1–7%, and in-hospital mortality in 4–6%, depending on the type of surgical resection. It is therefore intuitive how minimally invasive locoregional ablative techniques under endoscopic ultrasound (EUS) guidance can have a prominent role.

The factors to be taken into account when deciding the management of the patient with pNET are either patient related (comorbidities, risk of postoperative complications, life expectancy, risk of postoperative endocrine and exocrine insufficiency) or pNET related (F vs. NF, stage, number of lesions, size, grading, location of the lesion), which are also strictly linked to the known risk of progression.

It is therefore intuitive to consider ablation of localized lesions with a risk of progression or unfavorable outcome (F-pNETs, lesions >2 cm, high Ki-67 index) but at high risk of perioperative/postoperative complications. ENETS guidelines from 2016 reported the possibility of locoregional ablation of localized insulinomas that were not candidates for surgery, despite little evidence. Exclusion of lymph nodes, liver, and other distant metastases is of paramount importance when enrolling a patient for locoregional ablation.

For F-pNETs the goal is to induce necrosis of as many cells as possible in order to reduce the secretion of hormones and therefore abolish the related syndrome. For other pNETs and in other situations (MEN-1, NF-pNETs, etc.), there are currently no indications.

Techniques

The two main techniques currently under evaluation for EUS-guided ablation of p-NETs are radiofrequency ablation and ethanol injection.

EUS-guided radiofrequency ablation

Radiofrequency ablation (RFA) works at high temperatures (60 and 100°C), inducing thermally irreversible cellular damage on target tissues, with eventual cellular apoptosis and coagulative necrosis. The ablated area after RFA shows three well-recognized zones: a central coagulative necrosis, a surrounding peripheral zone with sublethal injury, and an external healthy surrounding zone.

Despite numerous clinical oncologic applications (liver, kidney and prostate gland cancers and metastasis), RFA of pancreatic tumors has always been regarded with reluctance by clinicians for fear of serious adverse events (such as pancreatitis, perforation, peritonitis, and adjacent structural injury). However, EUS-guided RFA could provide undoubted advantages in pancreatic tumor ablation, i.e. real-time imaging and monitoring during treatment, the ability to reach extremely distant anatomic areas, and minimally invasive technique.

Technical aspects of EUS-guided RFA

Two EUS-guided RFA monopolar (requiring grounding pads) systems are available on the market.

Atlas of Endoscopic Ultrasonography, Second Edition. Edited by Frank Gress, Thomas Savides, Brenna Casey, and Everson L. A. Artifon.

Companion website: www.wiley.com/go/gress/atlas

EUS RFA System (STARmed, Goyang, South Korea) (Figure 50.1)

The equipment is composed of an 18- or 19-gauge needle (EUSRA) inserted in the echoendoscope operative channel (length 140 cm, monopolar electrode located on the distal part, available in lengths of 5, 10, 15, 20, 25, and 30 mm), a radiofrequency generator (VIVA, STARmed) releasing the energy, and a peristaltic pump connected to the needle, which is cooled and internally perfused by circulating chilled saline solution during the ablation to avoid tissue charring (and maximizing ablation volume). Ablation power can be set on the generator, and tissue impedance and current are continuously monitored: the system can automatically modulate the power during the ablation if tissue impedance quickly increases or can eventually stop if the impedance (and temperature) rises beyond safety thresholds (impedance ≥500 Ω; temperature >100°C).

Habib™ EUS RFA (EMcision Ltd, London, UK)

The equipment is composed of a 1-Fr wire (0.33 mm, 0.013 inch) catheter (length 190 cm, electrode located on the distal part) that can be inserted in a standard 19- or 22-gauge EUS needle (with stylet removed), a RITA generator (electrosurgical RF generator) releasing the energy and monitoring the temperature in real time, and a remote foot pedal for hands-free and device activation.

Both systems do not have specific ablation settings (power, time) for treating pancreatic solid lesions such as pNETs. Previous experiences has shown heterogeneity in ablation settings (power and time) and results, with no procedure standardization (Table 50.1).

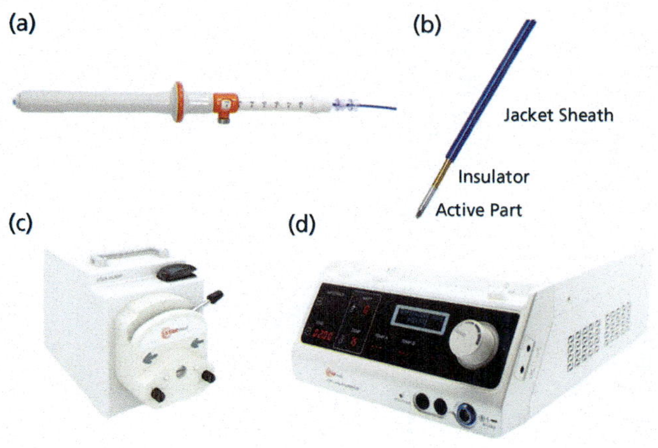

Figure 50.1 EUS-RFA radiofrequency system. a) EUSRA (STARmed, Goyang, South Korea) needle (sizes 18 or 19-gauge). (b) EUSRA needle tip: terminal part is the "active part" (electrode), available in sizes of 5, 10, 15, 20, 25, and 30 mm. (c) Peristaltic pump connected to the needle, cooled and internally perfused by circulating chilled (0°C) saline solution in order to avoid tissue charring. (d) VIVA radiofrequency generator (STARmed). Source: (a–d) STARmed, Seoul, South Korea.

Figures 50.2–50.4 and Videos 50.1 and 50.2 show an EUS-guided RFA procedure for the treatment of a symptomatic pancreatic tail insulinoma; Figures 50.2 and 50.3 and Video 50.1 show diagnostic evaluation before RFA while Figure 50.4 and Video 50.2 show the appearance of the lesion during the RFA procedure. Patient showed relief of symptoms.

EUS-guided ethanol injection

EUS-guided ethanol injection (EI) was first successfully used by Jurgensen and colleagues in 2006 for ablation of F-pNETs (insulinoma). Ethanol is a low-viscosity sclerosing agent able to induce cell lysis, denaturation of proteins and vascular occlusion, leading to coagulative necrosis and cell death. Subsequently, EUS-guided EI was proposed also for treatment of NF-pNETs in patients not eligible for surgical resection, and various small case series and case reports have been published.

However, with a median follow-up of 20 months (range 2–48 months), the reported outcomes were heterogeneous, with cases where morphologic disappearance of pNET, clinical complete resolution and biochemical normalization were achieved even after only one EI session, and other cases where only a partial response was obtained or there was tumor size reduction only after multiple sessions or injection of large volumes of alcohol leading to a high rate of postprocedural pancreatitis.

In fact, this technique is not free from adverse events, with some graded as severe. Among complications reported in the literature are cases of moderate-graded acute pancreatitis, necrotizing acute pancreatitis, fever, and duodenal wall ulceration. Ethanol volumes in excess of 2 ml and concentration above 98% were most associated with the occurrence of pancreatitis.

Technical aspects of EUS-guided EI

This therapeutic technique is performed using a 22- or 25-gauge EUS-FNA needle that is inserted into the pNET, not extending beyond the tumor margins. Needles with multiple side holes are not indicated for EI. Subsequently, a small amount of ethanol is injected inside the pNET, in varying concentrations (40–98%) and volumes (0.1–8 ml) depending on the size of the lesions. If necessary, as for larger lesions, additional injections can be performed during needle withdrawal. Before needle removal, it may be held within the lesion for a short time (approximately 60 seconds) in order to minimize the tracking of ethanol into peripheral normal pancreatic tissue.

Depending on tumor size and the degree of spread of ethanol during intratumoral perfusion, multiple injections at different lesion sites may be performed during the same session until the tumor is entirely covered by a hyperechoic "cloud" that visibly expands within the tumor under EUS guidance. The injection should be stopped if the hyperechoic

Table 50.1 EUS-guided radiofrequency ablation for treatment of pNETs: literature review.

Study	N	Indication	Patient selection	Device	Thermokinetics	Size (mm)	Outcome	Complications
Rossi et al. (2014)	1	pNET	Refusing or unfit for surgery	Habib EUS-RFA catheter, Emcision Ltd, London	10–15 W	16	Complete radiologic ablation	None
Lakhtakia et al. (2015)	3	F-pNETs	Unfit for surgery	EUSRA RF electrode; STARmed, Goyang, Korea	50 W	17.7	Symptom resolution	None
Armellini et al. (2015)	1	pNET	Refusing surgery	EUSRA RF electrode; STARmed, Goyang, Korea	NA	20	Complete radiologic ablation	None
Pai et al. (2015)	2	NF-pNETs	NA	Habib EUS-RFA catheter, Emcision Ltd, London	20 W	27.5	Change in vascularity and central necrosis	None
Waung et al. (2016)	1	F-pNET	Failure of medical therapy, unfit for surgery	Habib EUS-RFA catheter, Emcision Ltd, London	10 W	18	Complete radiologic ablation Symptom resolution	None
Bas-Cutrina et al. (2017)	1	F-pNET	Unfit for surgery	Habib EUS-RFA catheter, Emcision Ltd, London	10 W	10	Complete radiologic ablation Symptom resolution	None
Choi et al. (2018)	8	1 F-pNET 7 NF-pNETs	Unfit for surgery	EUSRA RF electrode; STARmed, Goyang, Korea	50 W	20	Complete radiologic ablation	1 abdominal pain, 1 pancreatitis
Barthet et al. (2018)	14	NF-pNETs	pNET <2 cm, patient unfit or refusing surgery	EUSRA RF electrode; STARmed, Goyang, Korea	50 W	13.1	Complete radiologic ablation	1 mild pancreatitis

NA, not available.

"cloud" extends up to the tumor's border to prevent leakage of ethanol beyond the tumor.

Multiple sessions of EUS-guided EI can also be performed if the pNET persists morphologically on imaging controls or symptoms related to F-pNET are still present. Up to three sessions have been reported, with rates of tumor ablation varying from 54% after one session to 62% after two sessions.

In order to avoid procedure-related adverse events if the pNET is close to a vessel or the main pancreatic duct, it has been proposed that an ethanol volume equivalent to half or one-third of the calculated tumor volume is injected. Recently, EUS-EI combined with Lipiodol, an iodized poppy seed oil, was used successfully in treatment of pNETs of less than 2 cm (22-gauge needle, mean 1.9 sessions per patient and 1.6 sessions per tumor, median mixture volume per session of 1.1 ml, 99% ethanol), obtaining complete ablation in 45% and 60% of tumors after one and two sessions, respectively,with occurrence of mild to moderate pancreatitis in 3.2% of cases.

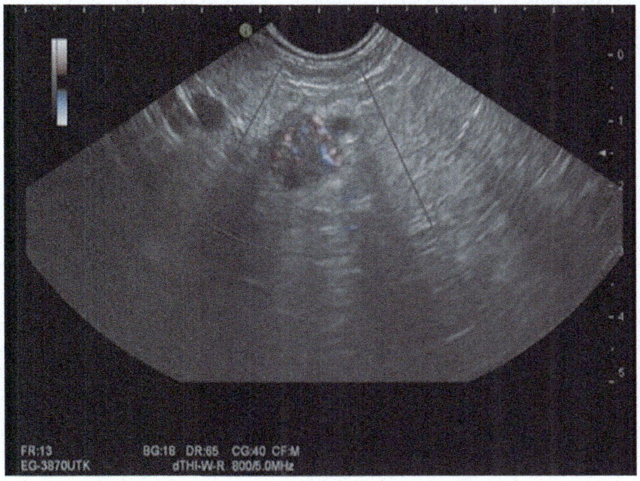

Figure 50.2 EUS-guided radiofrequency ablation of a pancreatic tail symptomatic insulinoma: Doppler evaluation.

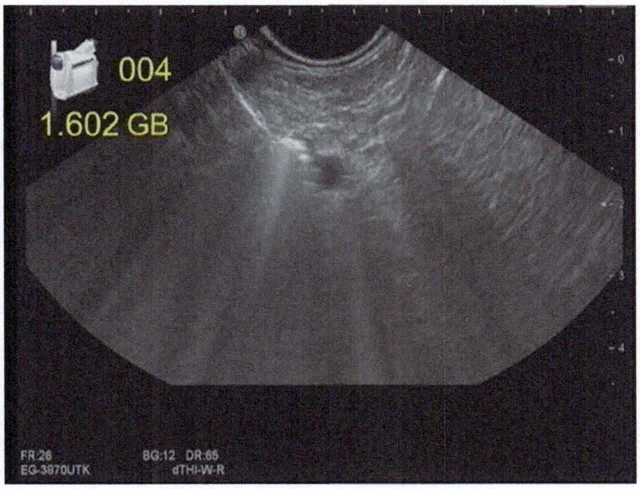

Figure 50.4 EUS-guided radiofrequency ablation of a pancreatic tail symptomatic insulinoma: EUS aspect of the insulinoma after ablation showing a hyperechoic area covering the center of the lesion.

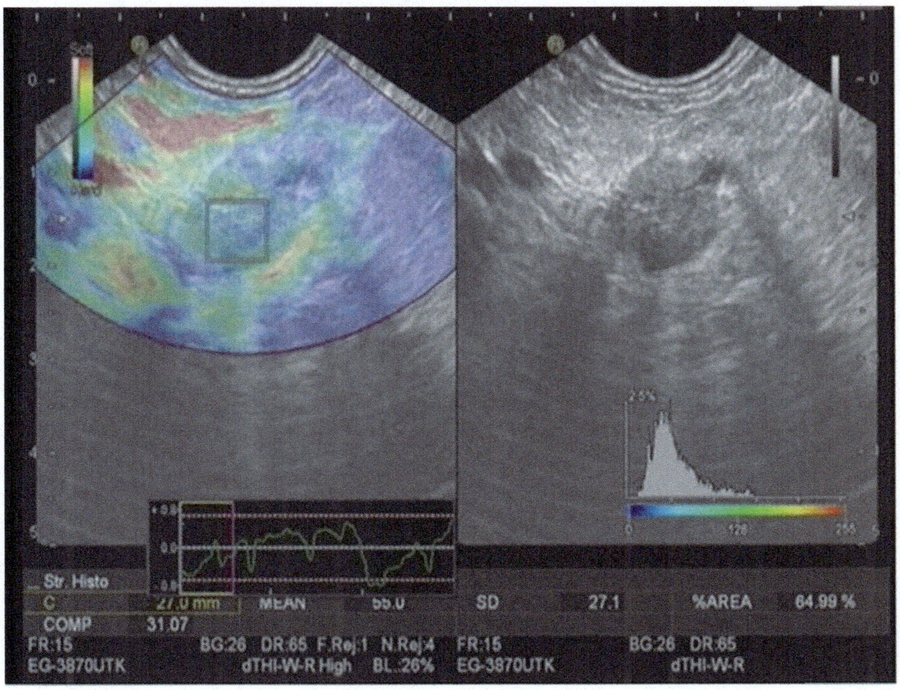

Figure 50.3 EUS-guided radiofrequency ablation of a pancreatic tail symptomatic insulinoma: elastography evaluation.

Technical variables reported in different case series and case reports vary widely, and include the needle type and caliber, volume injected, concentration of alcohol, and techniques to minimize the risk of pancreatitis (Table 50.2). Therefore, further studies with technical refinements, larger sample population, and long-term follow-up are needed in order to standardize the technical methodology and reduce the reported high rate of postprocedural pancreatitis, and to prove the efficacy of this technique.

Conclusion and future perspectives

While for F-pNETs it is intuitive how ablative techniques could become a standard of care, for NF-pNETs this is still under debate, especially since it is not entirely clear yet which tumors will progress and which will not. The answer will be reached once new studies regarding both ablative techniques and the actual risk of progression for small NF-pNETs have been published.

The hope is that, in the future, the low risk of complications of such procedures (compared to surgery) and the high rate of success of EUS-guided ablative procedures will make them a possible first-line therapeutic method for pNETs at high risk of unfavorable outcome, once solid reliable evidence is obtained.

Chapter video clips

Video 50.1 Contrast enhancement evaluation of the insulinoma before EUS-guided radiofrequency ablation (a millimetric avascular part inside the lesion is visible). Source: Hitachi Ltd.

Video 50.2 EUS-guided RFA of the pancreatic tail insulinoma with EUS-RFA radiofrequency system, with four different RFA applications in order to cover the whole lesion volume. Source: Hitachi Ltd.

Table 50.2 EUS-guided ethanol injection for treatment of pNETs: literature review.

Study	N	Indication	Size, mm (mean, range)	Needle, gauge	Alcohol,volume (range) and concentration	*N* sessions (mean, range)	Complications	Outcome
Jurgensen et al. (2006)	1	Insulinoma	13	22	8 ml 95%	1	Mild acute pancreatitis	Morphologic, clinical and biochemical resolution
Muscatiello et al. (2008)	1	2 NF-pNETs	9 (7–11)	NA	2 ml 40%	2	Pancreatitis, pancreatic necrotic lesion requiring laparascopic necrosectomy	Morphologic resolution
Deprez et al. (2008)	1	Insulinoma	17	21.25	3.5 ml 98%	1	Mild acute pancreatitis, duodenal wall hematoma and ulceration	Morphologic, clinical and biochemical resolution
Vleggaar et al. (2011)	1	Insulinoma	9	25	0.3 ml 96%	1	None	Size reduced, asymptomatic
Levy et al. (2012)	5	Insulinoma	15 (8–21)	22, 25	0.8 (0.12–3.0) ml 95–99%	2.3 (1–3), 3 injections per session (2–5)	None	60% clinical resolution
Schnack et al. (2012)	1	Insulinoma	6	NA	3.5 ml 98%	1	Mild acute pancreatitis	Clinical resolution
Lee et al. (2013)	1	Multiple insulinoma	11 (7–17)	22	1.3 (1–2) ml 95%	1	None	Clinical resolution
Bor et al. (2014)	1	Insulinoma	11	22	3 ml 95%	1	Abdominal pain	Clinical resolution
Quin et al. (2014)	4	Insulinoma	9.3 (5.4–11.8)	25	0.39 (0.25–0.5) ml 95%	1	None	Morphologic and clinical resolution
Yang et al. (2015)	4	Insulinoma	NA	22	3.1 (0.5–7.0) ml 98%	1.25 (1–2)	None	75% clinical resolution
Teoh et al. (2015)	1	NF-pNET	10	22	1 ml 100%	1	None	Partial morphologic response
Park et al. (2015)	11	10 NF-pNETs 4 Insulinoma	12.2 (8–19)	22	0.5–3.8 ml 99%	1 (11 lesions) 3 (3 lesions)	Mild acute pancreatitis (3), abdominal pain (1)	54% morphologic resolution, 61% clinical resolution
Paik et al. (2016)	8	2 NF-pNETs, 3 insulinoma, 1 gastrinoma, 1 SPN	15 (7–29)	19, 20, 22	2.8 (1.2–10.5) ml 99%	1	Severe acute pancreatitis (1), fever (1), abdominal pain (2)	75% morphologic and clinical resolution, 25% partial response
Trikudanathan et al. (2016)	1	Insulinoma	14	NA	1 ml 99%	1	None	Clinical resolution
Armellini et al. (2016)	1	NF-pNET	22	25	1.7 ml 95%	3	Mild acute pancreatitis (2)	Morphologic resolution
Dabkowski et al. (2017)	1	Insulinoma	15	22	1.5 (1–2) ml 96%	2	None	Morphologic and clinical resolution
Luo et al. (2017)	1	Insulinoma	27	19	1.5 ml 99%	1	Abdominal pain	Partial clinical response
Choi et al. (2018)	33	39 NF-pNETs, 1 insulinoma	11 (7–20)	22	(0.8–1.9) ml 99% + Lipiodol (1 : 1 ratio)	1.9 per patient, 1.6 per tumor	Mild acute pancreatitis (1), moderate acute pancreatitis (1)	60% complete ablation, clinical resolution
Burghardt et al. (2018)	1	Insulinoma	16	NA	1 ml 96%	1	None	Clinical resolution

NA, not available; SPN, solid pseudopapillary neoplasm.

51 How to do EUS-guided Needle Confocal Laser Endomicroscopy of Pancreatic Cysts

Prashant Bhenswala[1] and Frank G. Gress[2]

[1] Department of Medicine, Mount Sinai South Nassau Hospital, Oceanside, NY, USA
[2] Department of Medicine, Division of Gastroenterology and Hepatology, Icahn School of Medicine at Mount Sinai and Mount Sinai South Nassau Hospital, Oceanside, NY, USA

Confocal laser endomicroscopy (CLE) is a relatively new technology that uses laser endomicroscopy in combination with fluorescein administered intravenously to image gastrointestinal (GI) structures. The technique for imaging the GI tract uses a catheter to deliver the confocal laser beam to achieve high magnification of cellular and subcellular structures in the GI tract. There have been several GI applications of CLE described, including identifying dysplasia in Barrett's esophagus, detection of early gastric cancer, identifying dysplasia associated with inflammatory bowel disease, and diagnosing early cancer in colon polyps.

Endoscopic ultrasound (EUS)-guided needle-based confocal laser endomicroscopy (nCLE) is a novel technique that uses EUS to guide a very small CLE probe through a 19-gauge EUS needle. The ability to place a CLE probe into pancreatic cysts and solid lesions within the pancreas has changed the way we manage these lesions and has aided in their diagnosis.

Currently, less invasive modalities utilized for management of pancreatic cysts are favored and the addition of CLE to EUS further conveys the versatility and importance of this technique. EUS itself plays a significant role in the management of pancreatic cysts as it allows direct visualization of the cystic or solid lesions within the pancreas. Additionally, accurate measurements of the cysts or lesions provide a means for tailored approaches to ensure improved outcomes and resolution. Difficulty in differentiating various pathologies within the pancreas is a common occurrence. Intraductal papillary mucinous neoplasms (IPMNs) can be challenging to discern from pancreatic cystic lesions without the use of EUS-guided techniques.

Since pancreatic cysts are easily visualized with EUS and cysts can be sampled using EUS fine needle aspiration (FNA), the same technique can be applied for performing nCLE of the cyst. Prior to beginning the procedure, prophylactic intravenous antibiotics are administered to prevent cyst infection. The next step is insertion of a needle, usually a 19-gauge, into a pancreatic cyst under real-time EUS guidance and the nCLE probe is then advanced under continued EUS guidance into the pancreatic cyst. Once images are obtained and a potential diagnosis rendered, the nCLE probe is withdrawn and the cyst is aspirated. Collected fluid is then analyzed for amylase, tumor markers such as carcinoembryonic antigen (CEA), mutations in tumor suppressor genes (loss of heterozygosity), oncogene point mutations, and also sent for cytology. Complications have been recently reported with this technique, including pancreatitis in 2.9%, intracystic hemorrhage in 0.7%, infection in 1.5%, and reactions to fluorescein in 1.5%.

In addition, another potential resource if needed is the ability to biopsy a focal area of the cyst wall using small-caliber biopsy forceps (Moray Micro Forceps; US Endoscopy, Mentor, OH; Figure 51.1) which can be inserted through the FNA needle channel to obtain additional biopsies.

There have been a number of studies published demonstrating the ability of nCLE to differentiate pancreatic cysts into mucinous cysts, i.e. IPMNs and mucinous cystic neoplasms (MCNs), non-mucinous cysts (i.e. serous cystadenoma, pseudocyst) or solid lesions with a cystic component (i.e. neuroendocrine tumors). Studies support a role for nCLE in differentiating benign serous cystadenomas, and improving the diagnostic yield of serous cystic neoplasms with high interobserver agreement therefore avoiding unnecessary surgery in this subset of patients. Furthermore, recent data suggests that nCLE may detect dysplasia in IPMN.

Atlas of Endoscopic Ultrasonography, Second Edition. Edited by Frank Gress, Thomas Savides, Brenna Casey, and Everson L. A. Artifon.

Companion website: www.wiley.com/go/gress/atlas

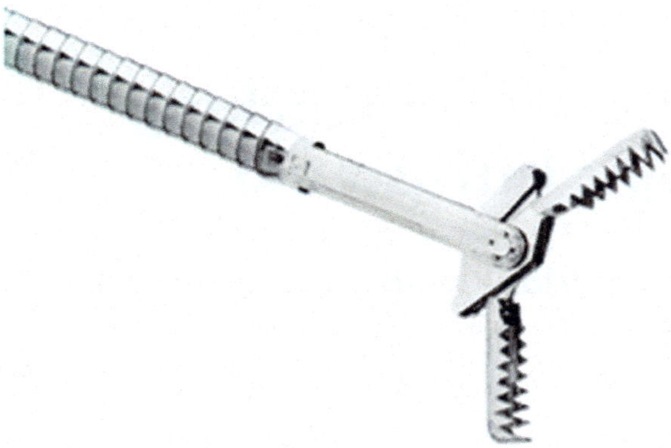

Figure 51.1 Moray micro forceps. Source: STERIS.

Confocal laser endomicroscopy technique

The nCLE probes have a diameter small enough to be passed through EUS-FNA 19-gauge needles in the operating channel of a standard endoscope as described in Figure 51.2. The nCLE probe was designed to be inserted through a 19-gauge EUS needle into pancreatic cysts. The probes can be used up to 10 times after sterilization as per the manufacturer's guidelines.

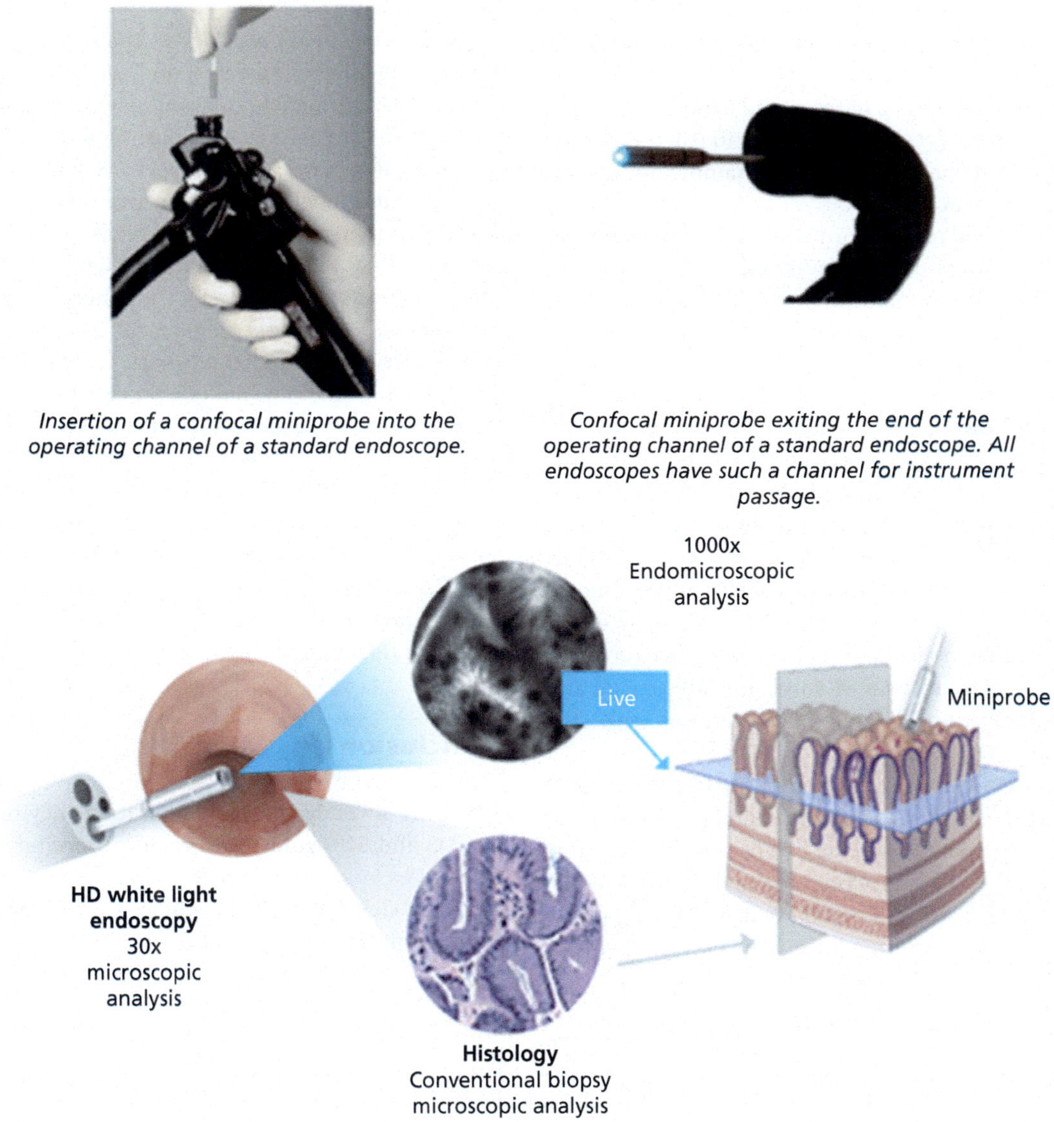

Figure 51.2 Overview of nCLE technique. Source: Mauna Kea Technologies.

52 How to use ex vivo Models in Teaching Therapeutic Endoscopic Ultrasound

Spencer Cheng, Mauricio K. Minata, Carlos K. Furuya, and Edson Ide
Department of Gastroenterology, Gastrointestinal Endoscopy Unit, University of São Paulo, São Paulo, Brazil

Introduction

Learning endoscopic ultrasound (EUS) can be challenging since it is one of the most difficult endoscopic techniques. Generally, a long learning curve is necessary to master EUS. A variety of strategies have been developed to improve mastery of EUS, respecting the principle of achieving a high level of expertise without causing harm to the patient. There is a necessity to develop experimental models to teach EUS considering the great demand for learning, training and testing new techniques and accessories.

Currently available models for EUS training include computer-based simulators, tabletop phantom models, ex vivo models, and live animal models. In this chapter, we cover topics concerning ex vivo models.

Ex vivo models

The EASIE model was the first and most widely used as the basis for all current ex vivo models employed for training of endoscopic therapeutic techniques. Later, the EUS RK model was developed, based on improvements in the EASIE model by adding miscellaneous substance molds to simulate extraparietal lesions. This model has become a reference for training EUS puncture techniques of subepithelial, hepatic and lymph node lesions, and drainage of collections with self-expanding metal or plastic stents.

Further progress was made when the use of animal models showed a good correlation with human anatomy for EUS. Artifon et al. adapted porcine ex vivo models for training EUS puncture with good acceptance and reproducibility. The study of anatomy with EUS and the diagnosis and puncture of lesions can be performed using the extracted viscera consisting of esophagus, stomach, duodenum, jejunum, liver, and gallbladder, fixed in a box (Figure 52.1). Vascular structures can be simulated using a segment of small bowel filled with water and positioned near the stomach of ex vivo models (Figure 52.2).

Very simple materials, such as chicken tenderloin, grapes, spleen, omentum fragments, and gel, can be used to create models. These models can simulate lymph nodes, hepatic nodules and subepithelial lesions (Figures 52.3 and 52.4).

Some other simple, fast, inexpensive and easily reproduced experimental models have been described for simulation of pancreatic pseudocysts and fluid collections. Cysts can be simulated with a porcine bladder filled with ultrasound gel and the model used to practice EUS fine needle aspiration (FNA) and pseudocyst drainage (Figures 52.5 and 52.6). These models are very good simulations with regard to the visual and perceptual realities for multiple procedures in a single model, it being easy to create various sizes, positions and types of lesions, and allowing good current transmission useful in the use of accessories such as cystotomes.

Another advantage of ex vivo models is the wide variety of structures and therapeutic situations that can be simulated. Small bowel filled with gel can be used to simulate a dilated hepatocholedochus (Figure 52.7) and EUS biliary drainage (Figure 52.8).

Conclusion

There are several learning models for achieving competency in EUS and EUS-guided therapeutic procedures. The advantages of ex vivo models are low cost, easy reproduction, possibility of development of a wide variety of models and good correlation with real-life procedures.

Atlas of Endoscopic Ultrasonography, Second Edition. Edited by Frank Gress, Thomas Savides, Brenna Casey, and Everson L. A. Artifon.

Companion website: www.wiley.com/go/gress/atlas

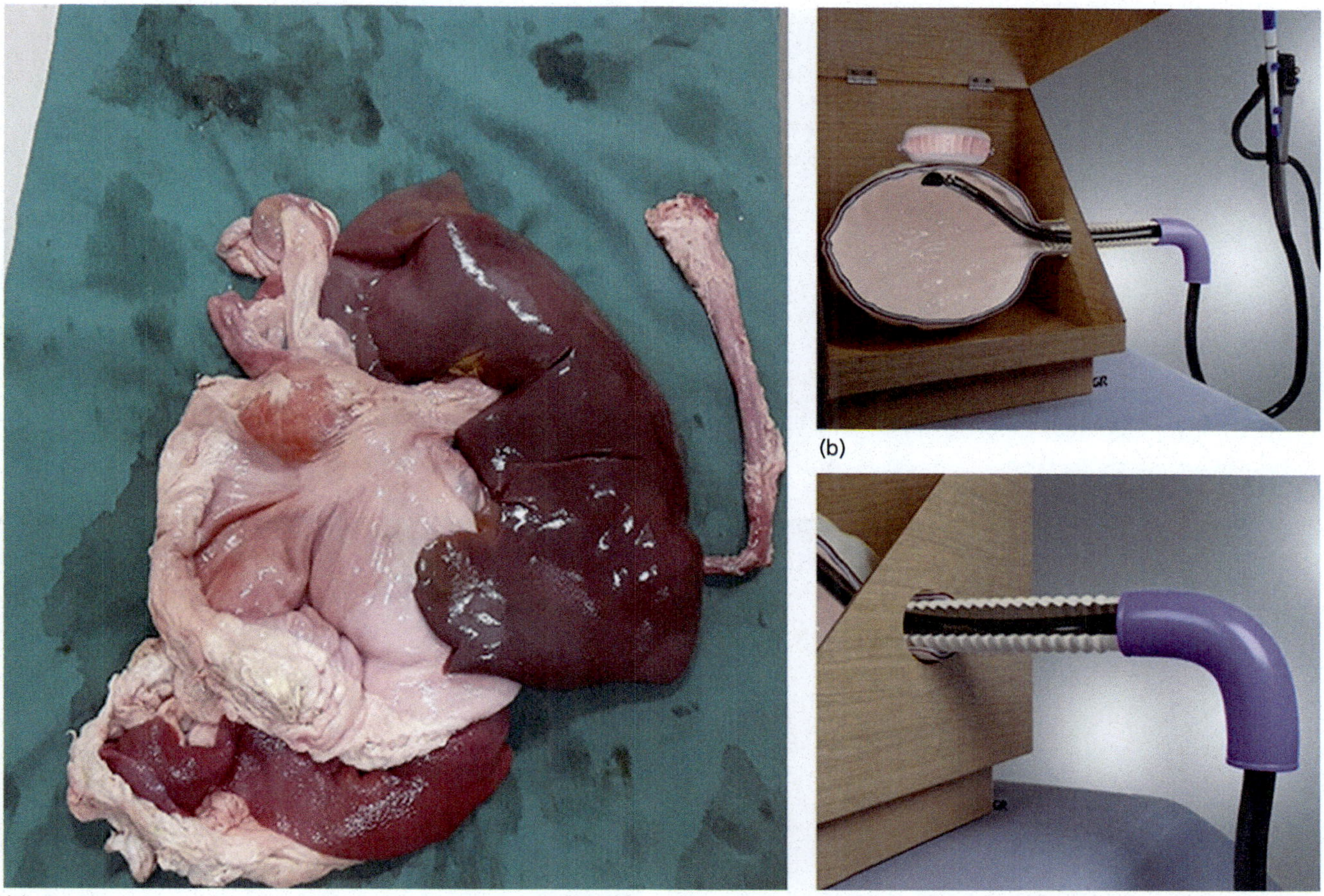

(a) (b) (c)

Figure 52.1 (a) Dissected specimen: esophagus, stomach, duodenum, pancreas, liver and gallbladder. The organs are positioned in their original positions with the use of clamps. (b) Dissected specimen is fixed in a specially prepared box. (c) The plastic duct allows the echoendoscope to pass easily.

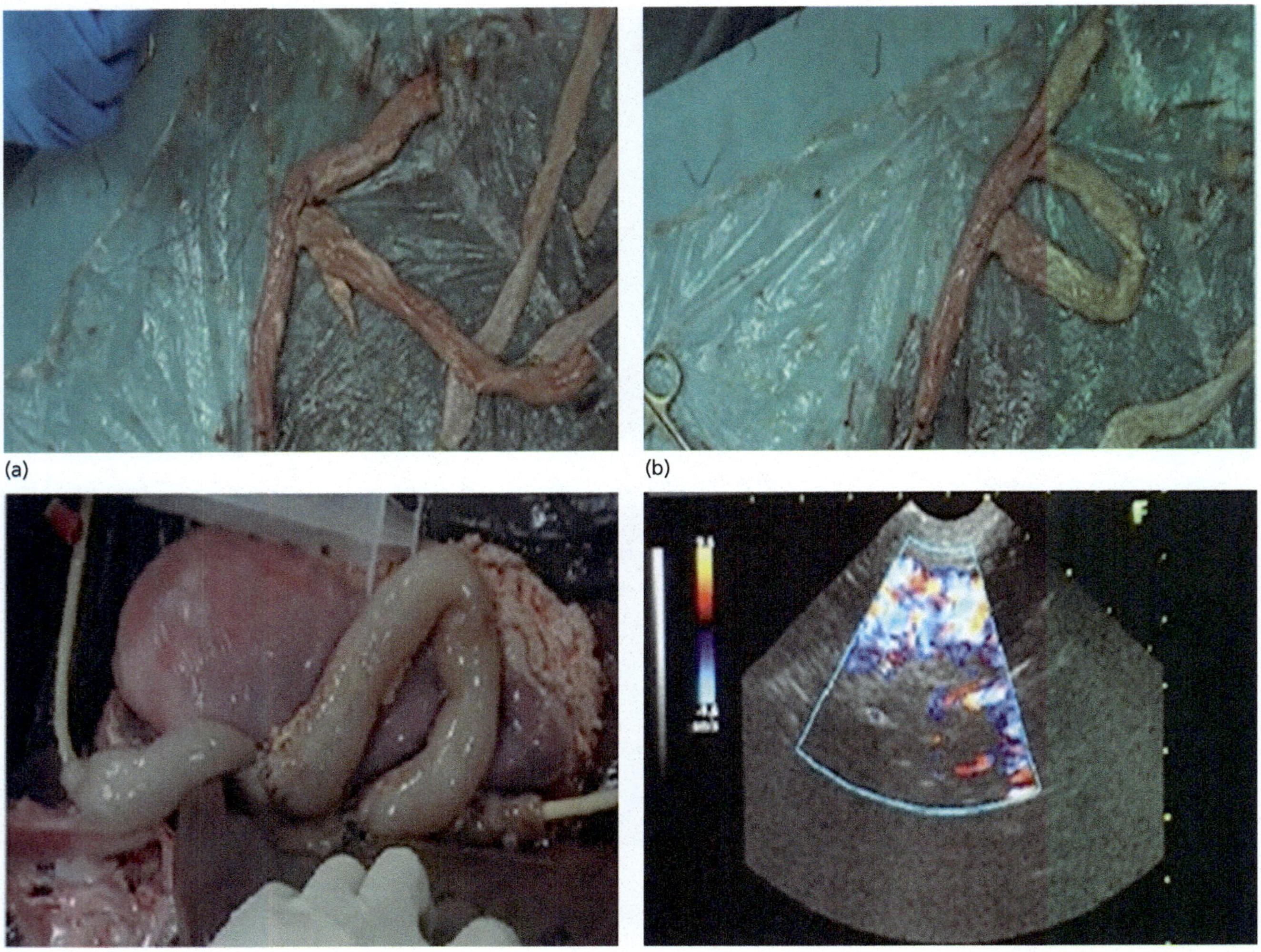

(a) (b) (c) (d)

Figure 52.2 Vascular simulation of aorta and use of the color Doppler feature. A 30-cm segment of small bowel is filled with water and at each end a 20-Fr Foley tube and a 60-ml syringe coupled to pass water from one end to the other, simulating blood flow. The model was then positioned near the posterior wall of the stomach and the color Doppler effect was obtained with manipulation of the syringe plungers. (a) Small bowel segments attached to simulate celiac and upper mesenteric trunk. (b) Final model. (c) Position of the model on the posterior wall of the stomach. (d) EUS view of Doppler effect.

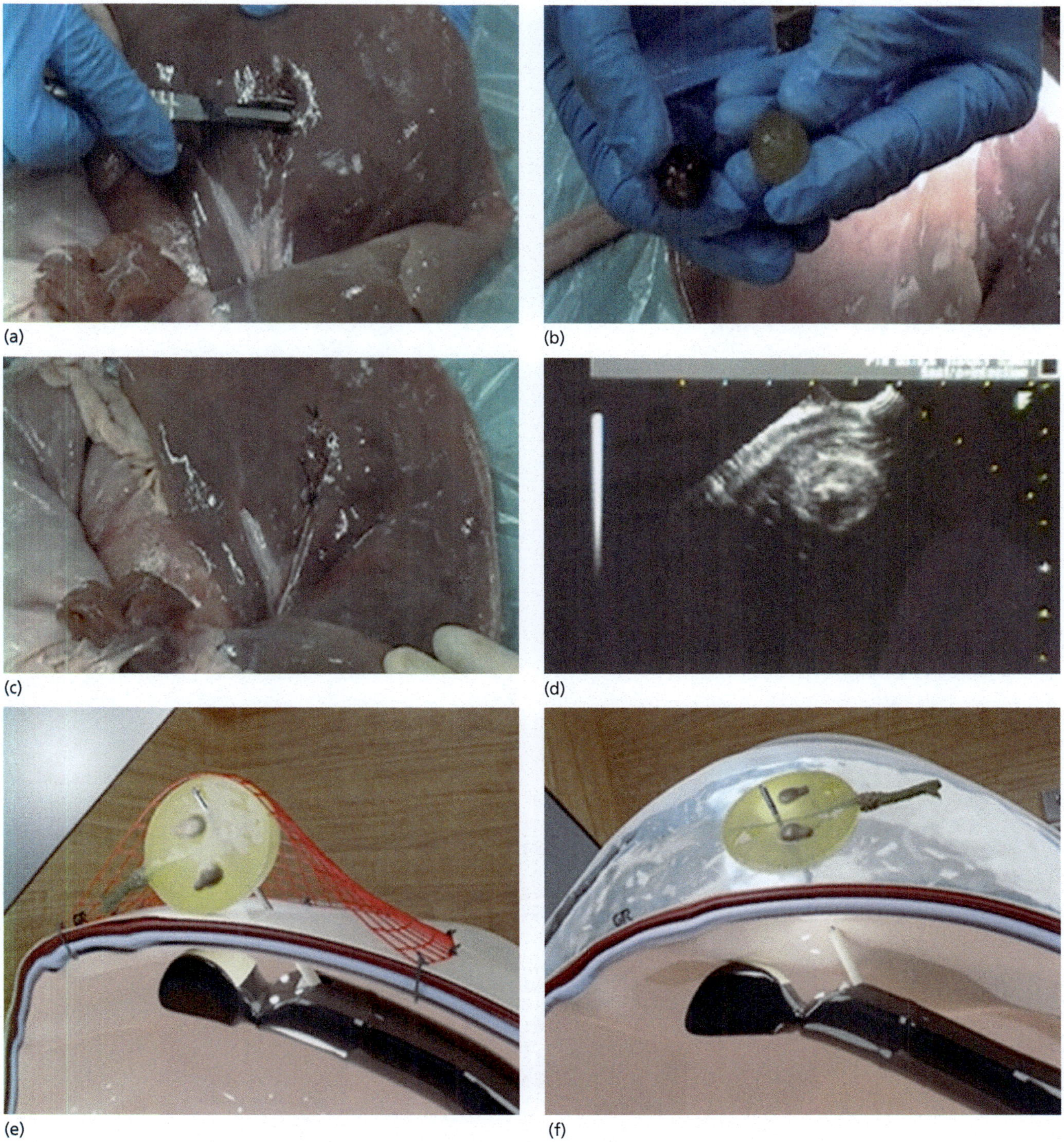

Figure 52.3 Simulation of hepatic nodules and lymph nodes. (a) Incision in the liver and preparation to implant a nodule (grape) in the liver parenchyma. (b) Seedless/skinless grape. (c) Nodule implanted and incision closed with 2-0 cotton stitches. (d) EUS image of liver-implanted grape. (e, f) Grape fixed outside the stomach with a mesh or gel bag simulating a lymph node as an ex vivo model for EUS-FNA.

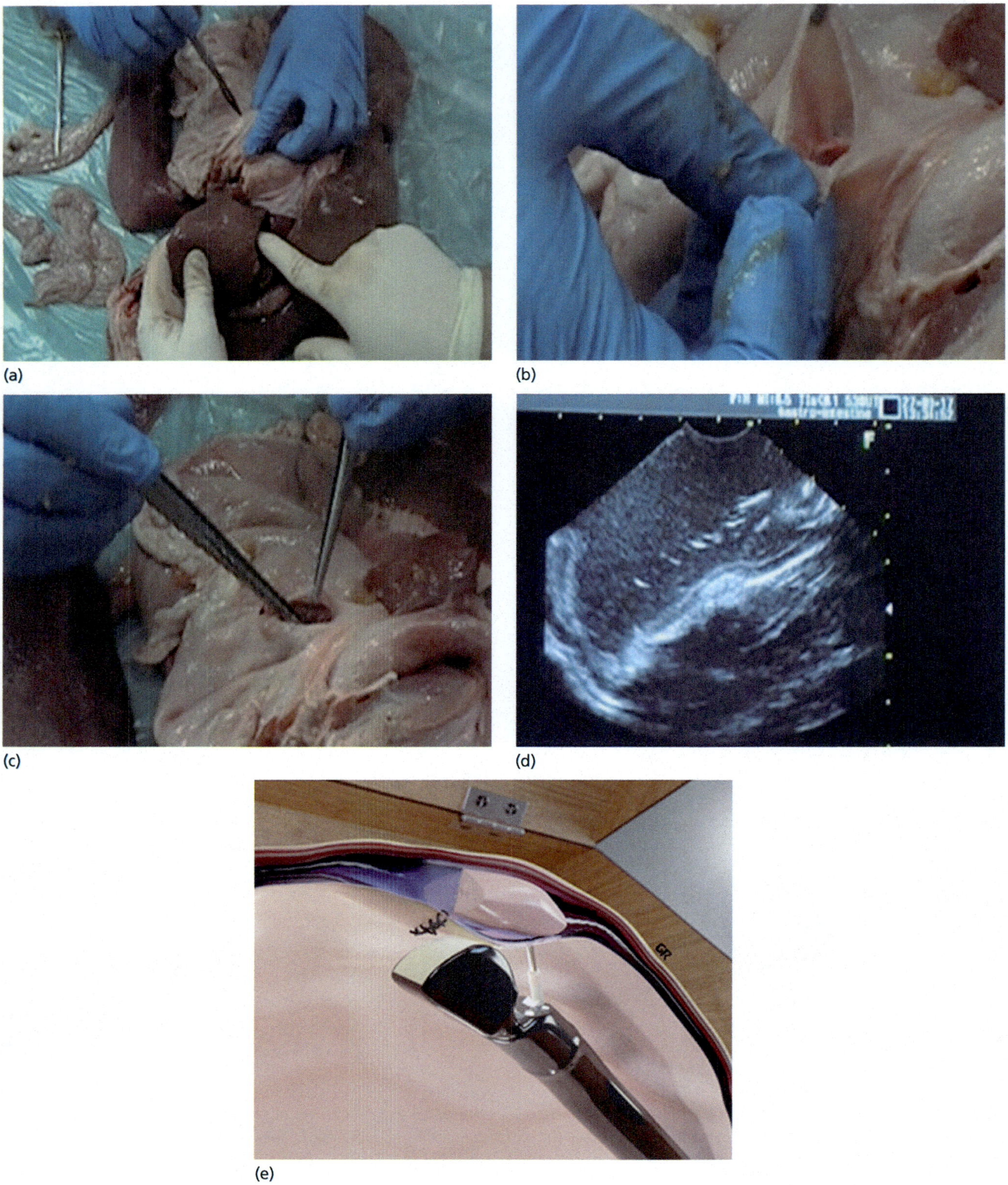

Figure 52.4 Simulation of subepithelial lesions. (a) Serous and muscle layer incision and submucosal space dissection. (b) Dissected submucosal space. (c) Implantation of a piece of spleen or chicken tenderloin to simulate a solid lesion. (d) EUS image of a subepithelial lesion. (e) ex vivo model for EUS-FNA.

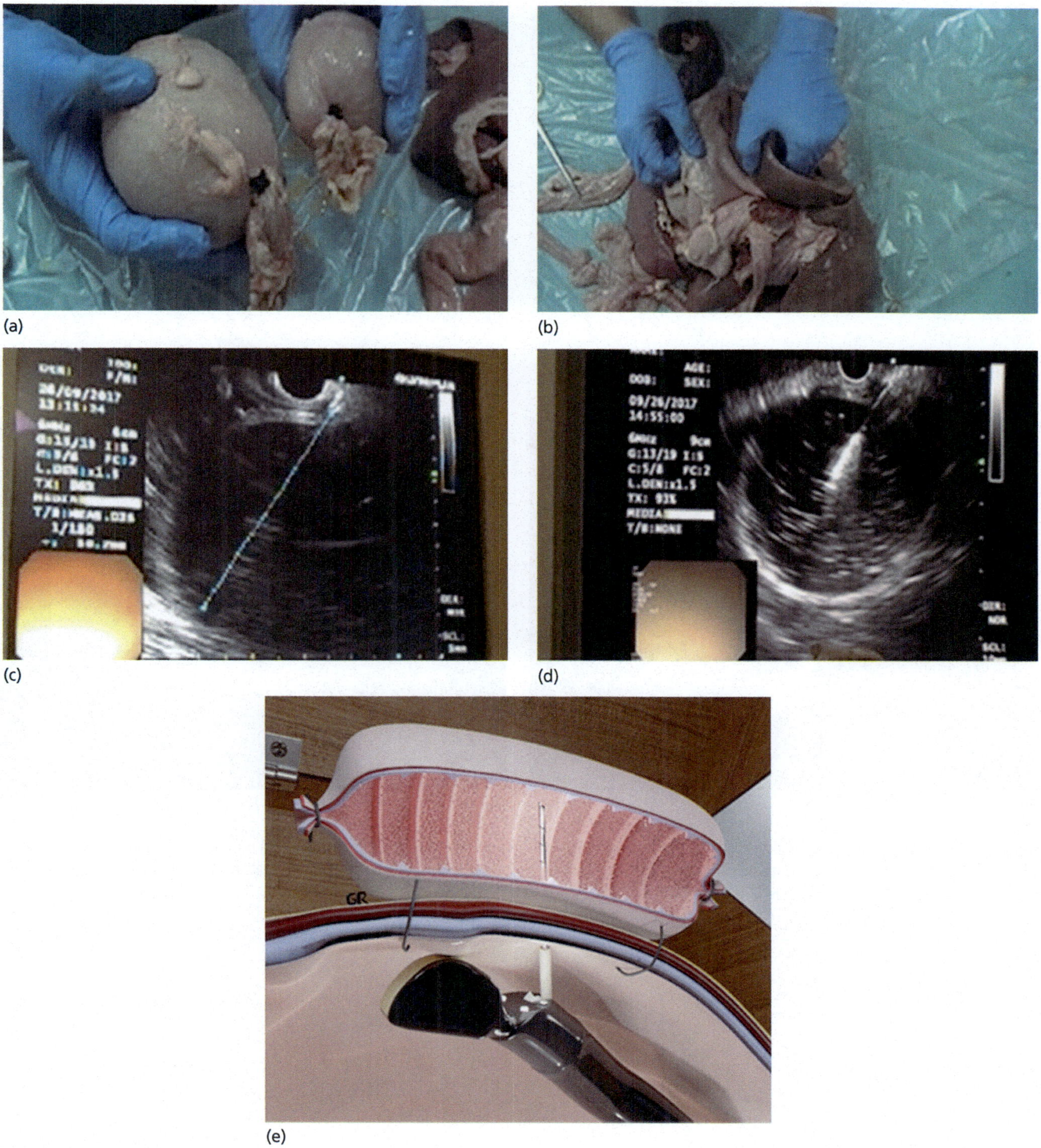

Figure 52.5 Ex vivo model for EUS-FNA of cystic lesions. The cysts were created with porcine bladder or bowel segment filled with ultrasound gel and placed adjacent to the gastric wall. (a) Gel-filled porcine bladder. (b) Positioning the bladder adjacent to the gastric wall. (c) EUS image measuring cyst size. (d) EUS image of FNA. (e) Illustration of a gel-filled intestinal segment fixed outside the stomach simulating a pseudocyst.

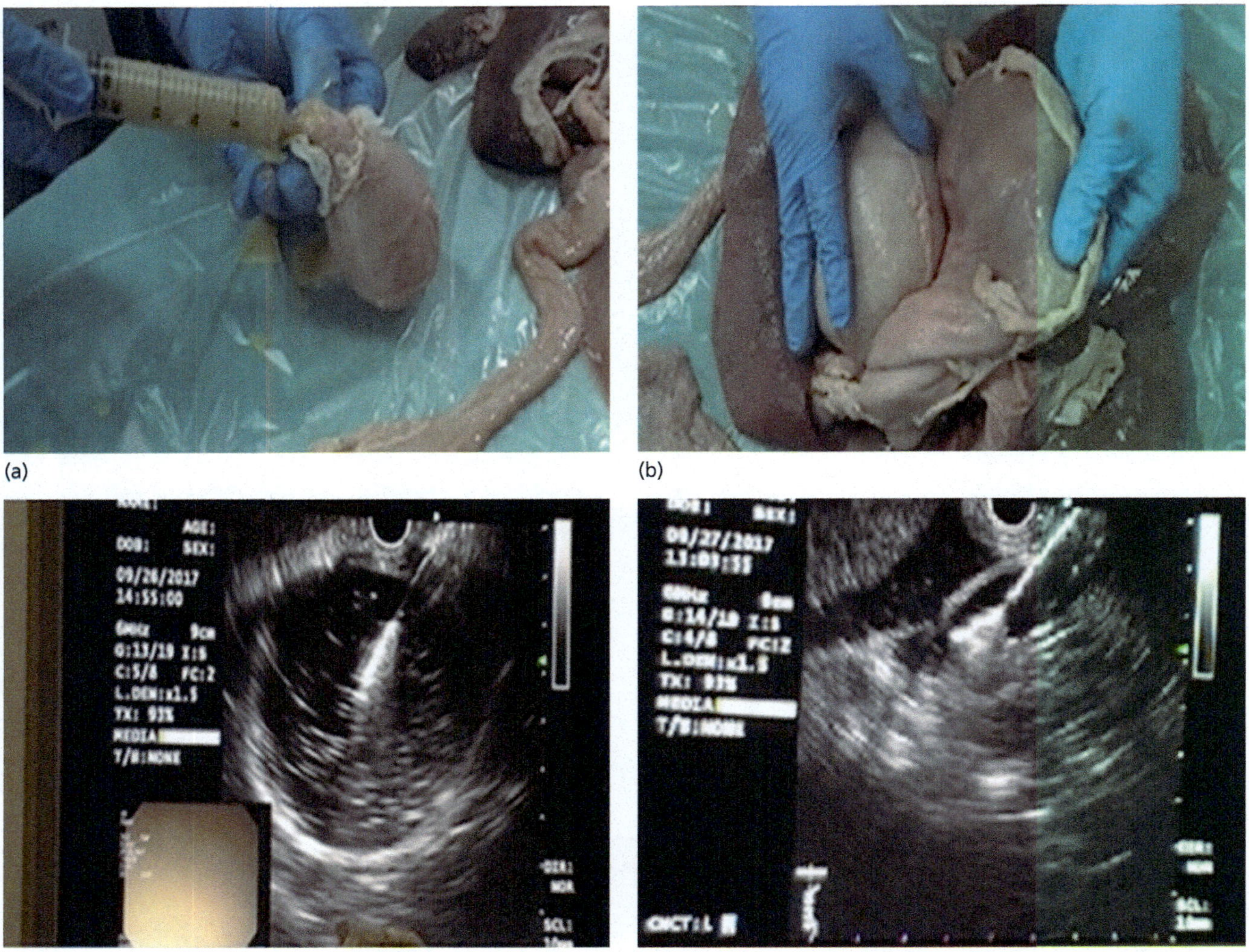

(a) (b) (c) (d)

Figure 52.6 Ex vivo model for pseudocyst drainage. The pseudocysts were created by filling porcine bladder with a mixture of ultrasound gel, milk and soluble coffee and then placed on the retrogastric wall. (a) Porcine bladder filled with a mixture of gel, coffee and milk. (b) Positioning of the pseudocyst in the gastric wall. (c) EUS-guided puncture of the pseudocyst. (d) EUS image of stent deployment.

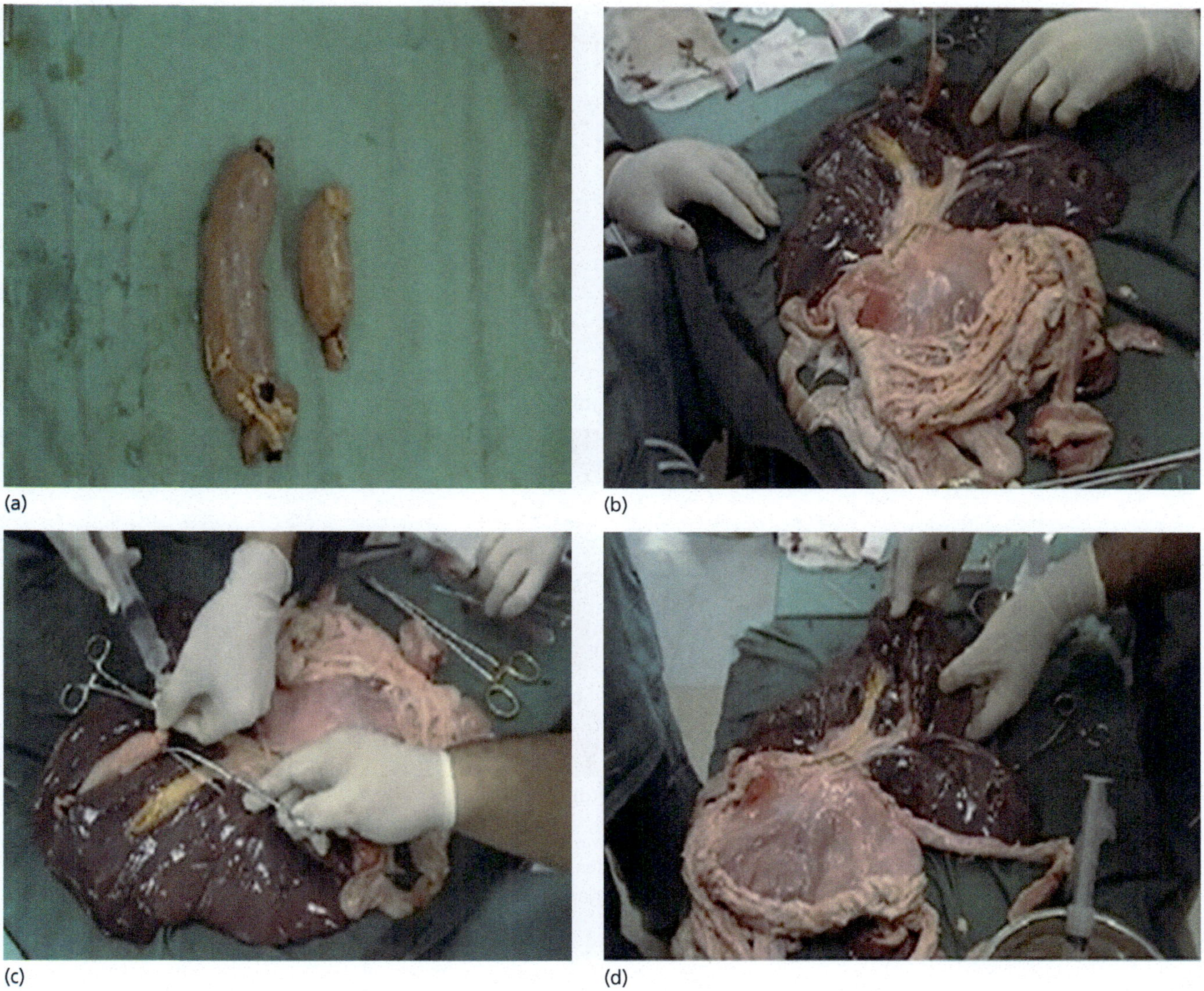

Figure 52.7 Ex vivo model for dilated hepatocholedochus evaluation. The hepatocholedochus was made from a 15-cm small bowel segment filled with water and ultrasound gel, then positioned in the hepatic hilum and fixed with 2-0 cotton sutures. (a) Simulation of dilated hepatocholedochus with small bowel segments filled with gel and water. (b, c) Dilated hepatocholedochus implantation site. (d) Final model.

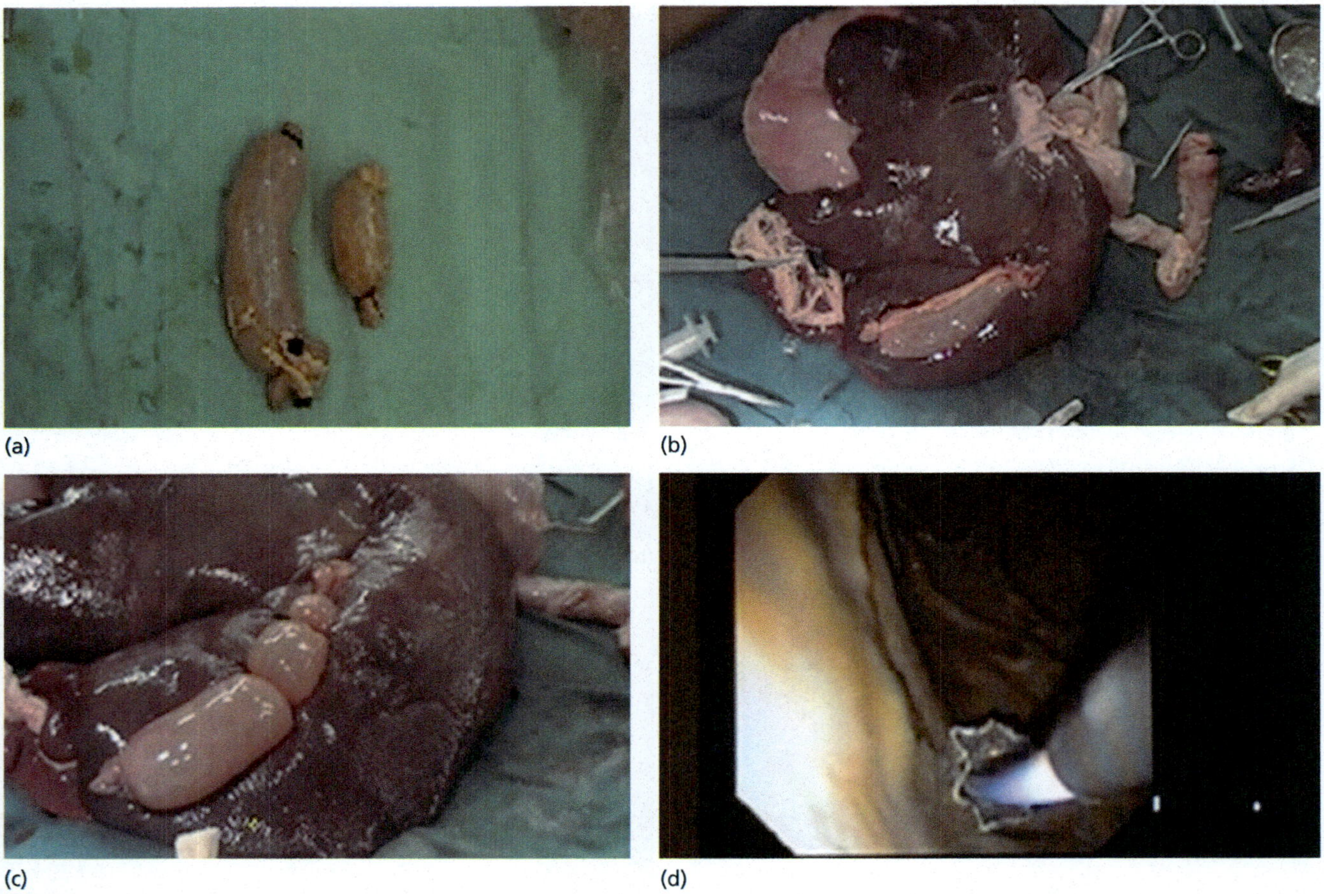

Figure 52.8 Ex vivo model for EUS biliary drainage. The dilated biliary tract was made in the same fashion as the hepatocholedochus model and then positioned on the lower border of the left hepatic lobe and fixed with 2-0 cotton stitches. (a) Small bowel segments filled with gel and water to simulate dilated intrahepatic biliary tract. (b, c) Small bowel segment positioned on porcine specimen. (d) Endoscopic view of self-expanding metal stent release.

53 How to do Endoscopic Necrosectomy

Wilson T. Kwong
University of California San Diego Health Sciences, La Jolla, CA, USA

Introduction

Endoscopic management of necrotizing pancreatitis is now first-line management in centers with the appropriate expertise. Minimally invasive approaches to treating necrotizing pancreatitis including percutaneous and endoscopic drainage have a lower mortality compared to open surgical necrosectomy [1,2]. Randomized controlled trials have recently demonstrated similar outcomes between surgical step-up therapy with percutaneous drainage and endoscopic drainage followed by endoscopic necrosectomy, with fewer adverse effects including lower rates of fistula with the endoscopic approach [3]. Published series report success rates for endoscopic necrosectomy of 84–91% in resolving walled-off pancreatic necrosis [4–6]. Endoscopic necrosectomy requires the creation of a cystgastrostomy or cystenterostomy to access a walled-off pancreatic collection. A gastroscope is then inserted directly into the walled-off necrosis and necrotic debris is subsequently debrided and removed from the necrotic collection. Endoscopic necrosectomy is indicated when patients have persistent sepsis despite cystgastrostomy/cystenterostomy or percutaneous drainage and antibiotics. Patient who have failure to thrive, weight loss, or persistent abdominal pain despite drainage may also benefit from endoscopic necrosectomy. However, in patients improving after endoscopic or percutaneous drainage, endoscopic necrosectomy is not mandatory and may not be necessary. Based on prospective trials, necrosectomy will be necessary in about two-thirds of patients after initial drainage [3].

Preprocedure assessment

Prior to endoscopic drainage and subsequent necrosectomy, a thorough preoperative assessment should be performed. Checking for coagulopathy with international normalized ratio (INR) should be performed and corrected with vitamin K and fresh frozen plasma as appropriate. Anticoagulants and antiplatelet agents with the exception of aspirin should be ideally held as endoscopic drainage and necrosectomy are high risk for bleeding. Contrast-enhanced computed tomography (CT) with arterial and venous phases should be performed to evaluate for pseudoaneurysms and varices which can form secondary to portal and splenic vein thromboses. Pseudoaneurysms should be embolized prior to necrosectomy. Perigastric and abdominal varices are not an absolute contraindication to necrosectomy but great care should be taken to avoid these vessels and the operator should have sufficient experience to recognize these vessels during the procedure (Figure 53.1). The CT scan should be reviewed by the endoscopist to assess the optimal site for drainage, assess if multiple sites of drainage should be performed for walled-off collections that may not communicate,

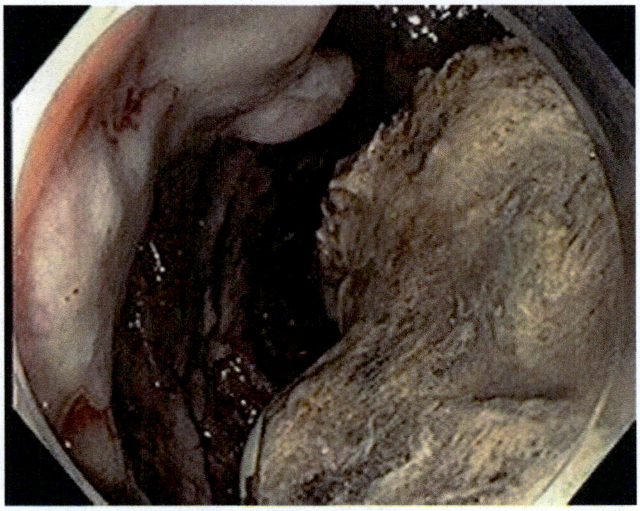

Figure 53.1 There is a perigastric varix present within the wall of a necrotic collection (top left of image).

Atlas of Endoscopic Ultrasonography, Second Edition. Edited by Frank Gress, Thomas Savides, Brenna Casey, and Everson L. A. Artifon.

Companion website: www.wiley.com/go/gress/atlas

and ensure the collections are sufficiently close enough for drainage, ideally 10 mm or less from the chosen site of drainage in the upper gastrointestinal tract.

EUS evaluation of walled-off pancreatic necrosis

Evaluation of walled-off pancreatic necrosis is preferably imaged with a linear echoendoscope as this is the scope that will be used to perform endoscopic drainage. Collections in the lesser sac will be visible from the stomach while necrotic collections in the right lower quadrant may be visualized from the first, second, or third portions of the duodenum. Walled-off necroses are generally heterogeneous collections consisting of anechoic fluid portions mixed with hyperechoic or isoechoic irregular solid debris of varying sizes (Figure 53.2). Collections with a large amount of solid debris may have extensive shadowing that may prevent ultrasound visualization of deeper portions of the necrotic collection beyond the debris. Blood products and clot within the collection can have a similar appearance to necrosis and cannot be reliably distinguished from necrosis alone based on endoscopic ultrasound (EUS) appearance (Figure 53.3). If clinical suspicion is high for hemorrhage into the collection, EUS aspiration of the collection immediately prior to drainage can be performed to assess for blood. Doppler ultrasound should also be performed around the collection to assess for any vessels within the gastric or duodenal wall and also varices or vessels surrounding the collection. If there are varices or large vessels around the collection, one should try to select a site of drainage further away from these vessels if possible and proceed with necrosectomy with greater caution.

Access creation: cystgastrostomy or cystenterostomy

Specifics of cystgastrostomy and cystenterostomy are covered in Chapter 33. The CT should be reviewed and a general location chosen that allows as direct route as possible for endoscopic access to the walled-off necrosis. For

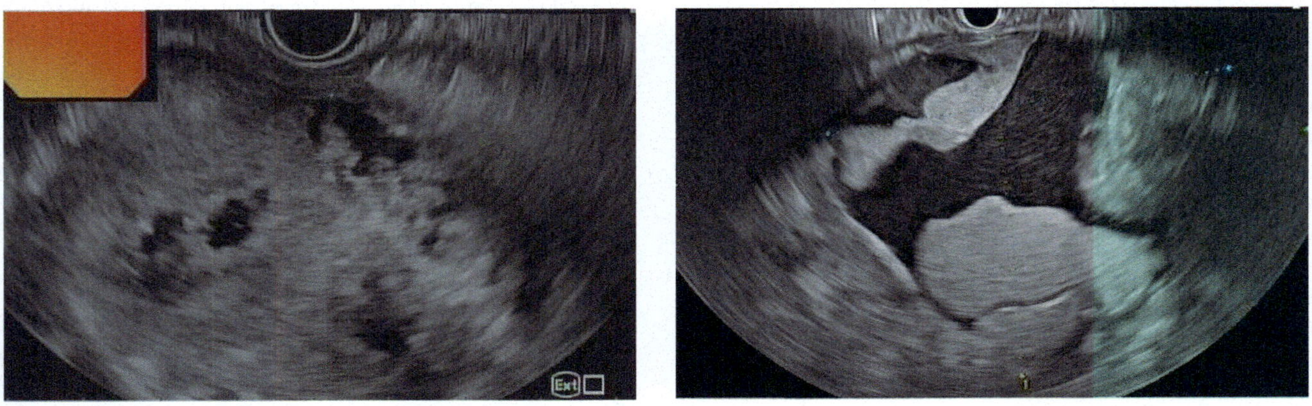

(a) (b)

Figure 53.2 (a, b) Hyperechoic and isoechoic solid necrosis within necrotic collections.

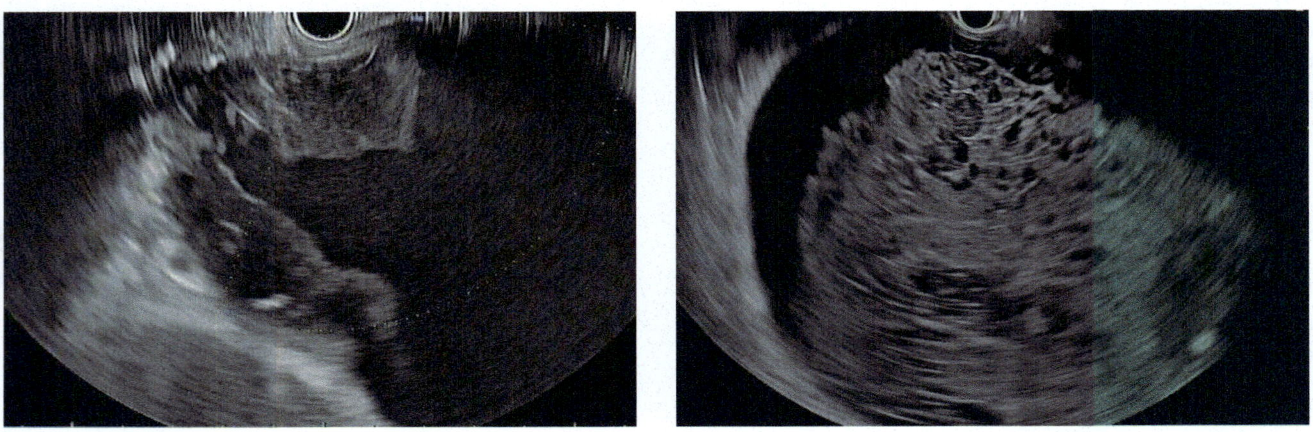

(a) (b)

Figure 53.3 (a, b) Clots and blood products within a peripancreatic collection which can have similar appearance to solid necrosis.

necrotic collections within the lesser sac, access in the proximal stomach usually allows a direct route for the endoscope without looping of the scope. This will help facilitate endoscopic necrosectomy, increase maneuverability within the necrotic collection, and allow the endoscope to go in and out of the collection as easily as possible. Endoscopic cystgastrostomy or cystenterostomy with a lumen-apposing metal stent (LAMS) allows for immediate necrosectomy after placement in patients whose clinical status requires this (Figure 53.4). The LAMS creates a more stable connection after initial tract creation, though perforation of the tract and dislodgement remain possible. Cystgastrostomy or cystenteroscopy with double pigtail stents do not allow for immediate necrosectomy as the tract is fresh and unstable; attempted insertion of an endoscope through this new tract has a high risk of perforation. Access creation using a metal biliary stent does not have a lumen caliber large enough to accommodate an endoscope and also does not allow for immediate necrosectomy. If the patient can wait for elective necrosectomy, the cystgastrostomy tract may be mature anywhere between one and two weeks and waiting at least two weeks is advisable. At that time the pigtail and metal biliary stents may be removed and the tract dilated with a controlled radial expansion balloon to 15 mm or more to allow for endoscope advancement into the collection. If a LAMS is in place then the scope may be inserted directly through the LAMS without removal. If the patient has a very large necrotic collection or multiple collections which do not communicate, then multiple cystgastrostomies or cystenterostomies may be necessary to achieve complete drainage (Figure 53.5).

Necrosectomy tools and technique

A diagnostic or a therapeutic gastroscope are both acceptable for endoscopic necrosectomy. The therapeutic scope has the advantage of better suctioning but is also thicker and results in decreased maneuverability within the collection. Carbon dioxide insufflation instead of air is mandatory to prevent complications including air embolus; fatalities during endoscopic necrosectomy have been reported as a result of air emboli [4]. Necrosectomy involves a combination of breaking up pieces of necrosis into smaller pieces and/or removing the necrosis from the collection and into the stomach/small bowel. Although there are no dedicated accessories for necrosectomy, forceps, snares, retrieval nets, and biliary stone extraction baskets are commonly used for necrosectomy and are effective for cutting necrosis into smaller pieces. Retrieval nets and snares can be used to remove larger loose pieces of necrosis from the collection and left in the stomach (Figure 53.6).

The necrotic collection is generally large with plenty of working space soon after drainage. However, on subsequent procedures with the passage of the time, the necrotic collection shrinks which then leaves much less space to work. Care must be taken not to perforate the walls of the collection during necrosectomy. When working space is limited, it is of benefit to use smaller snares, baskets, and nets as it will allow more control and precision during necrosectomy. The endoscopist should have a clear view of the working field at all times and make a careful assessment for any surrounding vessels. Prior to cutting with accessories, the endoscopist should have a clear view of what is grasped to avoid bleeding. In general, it may be safer to start necrosectomy from the center of the collection as there are likely to be more vessels running along the walls of the collection and this also

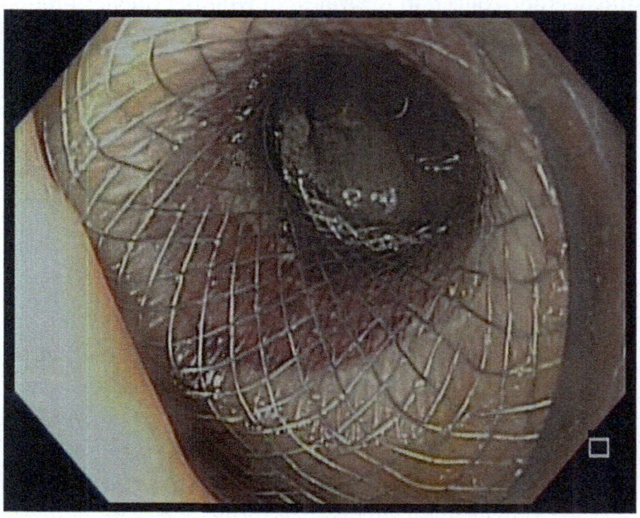

Figure 53.4 Lumen-apposing metal stent placed for cystgastrostomy.

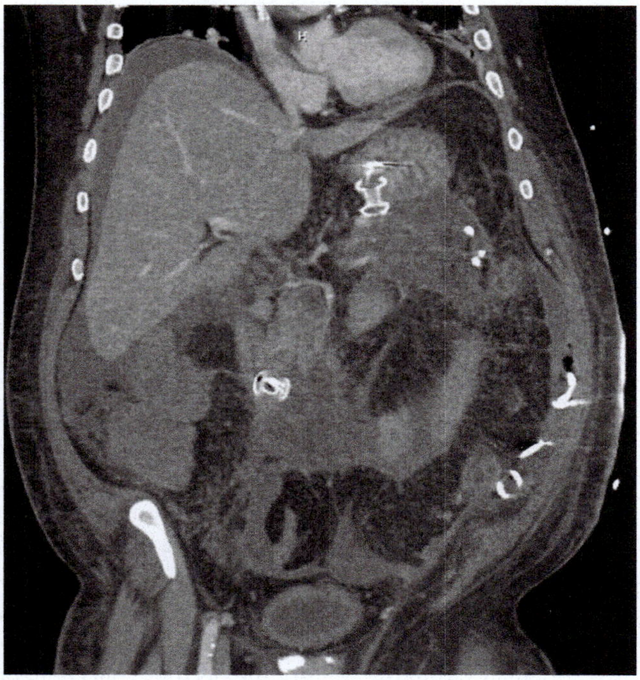

Figure 53.5 CT scan demonstrates two LAMS stents from the stomach and duodenum to drain two necrotic collections.

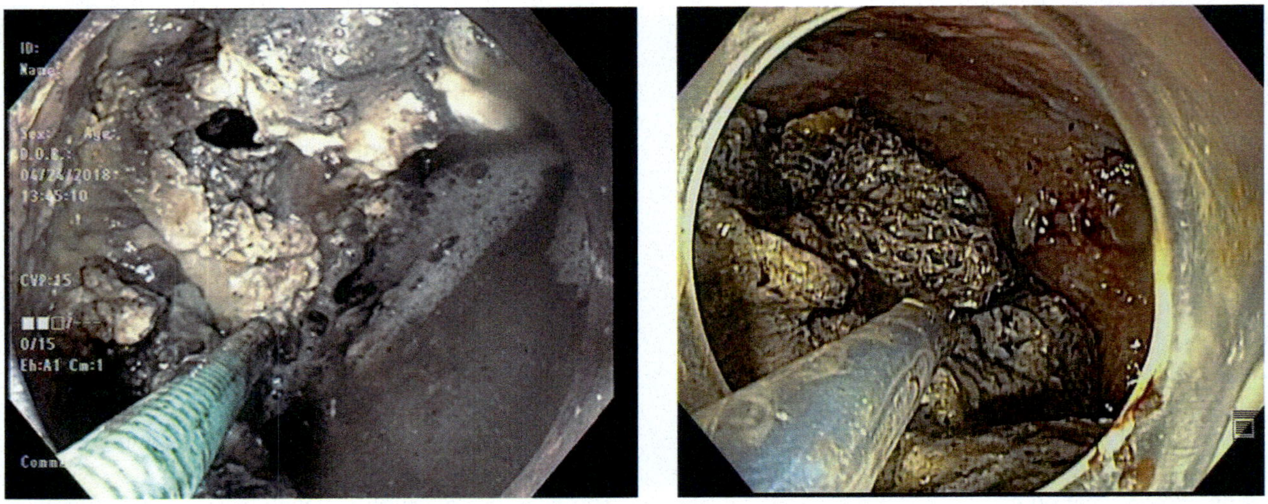

(a) (b)

Figure 53.6 (a, b) Endoscopic necrosectomy with rat tooth forceps and retrieval net.

allows more room for expansion of snare, basket, and nets. If the view is suboptimal then irrigation, suctioning, change of scope positioning, increasing the brightness on the video processor, or cleaning of the lens should be performed to optimize views. A cap or distal attachment on the scope may also help optimize views during necrosectomy. In cases with extensive necrosectomy, multiple sessions days to weeks apart are often necessary to completely clear the necrosis. If necrosectomy is incomplete, pigtail stents or LAMS should be left in place to ensure ongoing drainage and preserve access for future necrosectomy.

Complication management

Bleeding

Prospective trials and retrospective series of endoscopic necrosectomy report bleeding complications requiring intervention in approximately 20% of patients [3,4,6]. Most cases of bleeding were managed endoscopically but some patients required angiographic embolization or surgical management and a few fatalities related to massive bleeding have been reported. Bleeding may occur from gastric vessels from the cystgastrostomy tract, varices surrounding the necrotic collection, pseudoaneurysms, and branches of the splenic artery. Any of these vessels can be traumatized or lacerated as a result of endoscopic necrosectomy. For necrotic collections located in the lesser sac, bleeding is often from branches of the splenic artery. If bleeding is not severe, endoscopic evaluation can be considered. Bleeding from vessels in the stomach or cystgastrostomy tract can sometimes be managed with clip placement. However, if bleeding is brisk, originates from the walls of the necrotic collection, or the patient is unstable, then interventional radiology and surgical consultation should be obtained simultaneously. If the patient is felt to be stable for imaging, CT angiography can be considered to determine approach of hemostasis.

Perforation

Perforation can occur at the site of cystgastrostomy or at one of the walls of the necrotic collection as a result of endoscopic necrosectomy with or without dilation of the cystgastrostomy tract. Patients generally present within a day of necrosectomy with symptoms of pain and signs of sepsis. Emergent CT scan is indicated to assess these patients for perforation and will demonstrate localized or diffuse pneumoperitoneum and possible free abdominal fluid (Figure 53.7). If the patient does not demonstrate peritonitis, then emergent endoscopic management may avoid surgery. Management of diffuse peritonitis should be surgical. Endoscopic management involves preventing further spillage of gastrointestinal contents into the peritoneal cavity and necrotic collection regardless of whether the perforation is in the cystgastrostomy tract or the walls of the necrotic collection. The cystgastrostomy tract should be closed, preferably with over-the-scope clips or endoscopic suturing (Figure 53.8). If there is residual necrosis at the time of endoscopic closure, then an alternative means of drainage such as percutaneous drainage or repeat endoscopic drainage can be considered in the near future.

Infection

Signs of sepsis or worsening infection can be seen with introduction of gastrointestinal bacteria into the necrotic collection, occlusion of cystgastrostomy stents, or suboptimal drainage of a large necrotic collection. Sepsis and superinfection can be seen within a day of endoscopic cystgastrostomy or later. Management involves restoring adequate drainage and removing infected necrosis. After fluid resuscitation and

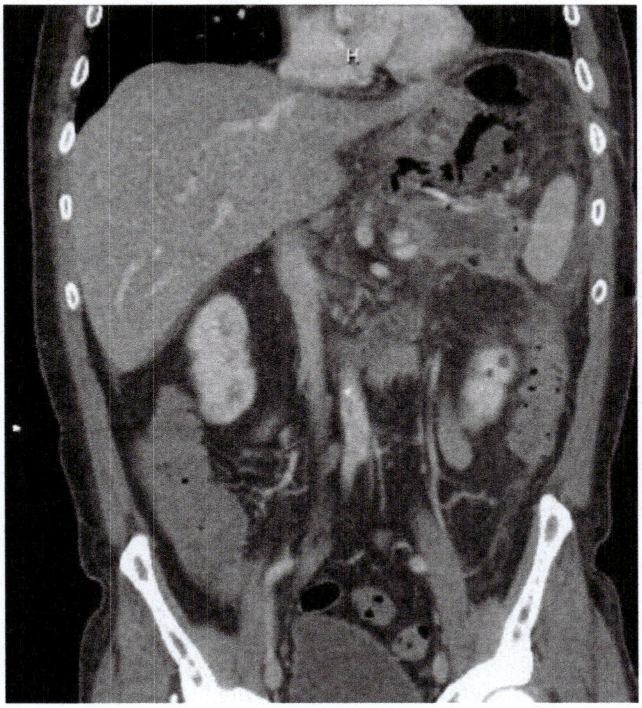

Figure 53.7 CT scan shows local pneumoperitoneum around the cystastrostomy site as a result of leak from the cystgastrostomy tract after necrosectomy.

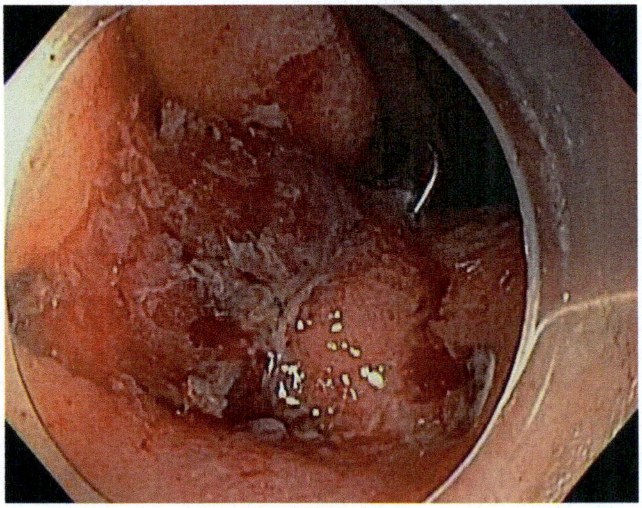

Figure 53.8 Over-the-scope clip placement for closure of cystgasatrostomy site to manage tract leak.

administration of antibiotics, endoscopic assessment for source control should be performed. Endoscopic techniques include unclogging/replacing occluded stents, further endoscopic necrosectomy to remove infected necrosis, and lavage of purulent fluid and debris (Figure 53.9). If endoscopic control of infection is inadequate or more distant areas of infection cannot be accessed, then adjunctive percutaneous drainage can be considered.

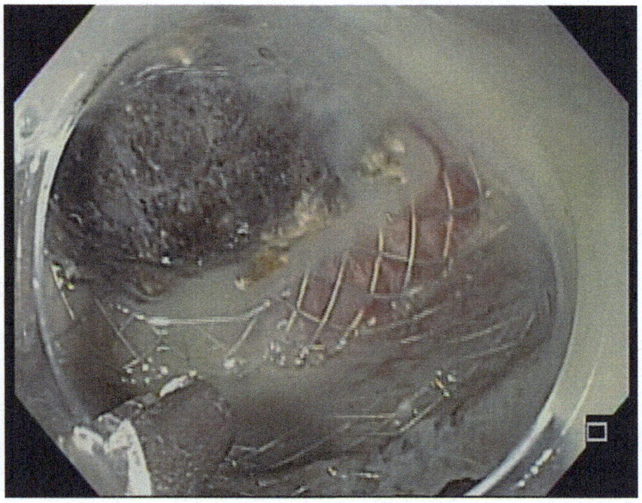

Figure 53.9 Purulence and infection as a result of occlusion of LAMS cystgastrostomy.

Conclusion

In experienced hands, endoscopic drainage followed by endoscopic necrosectomy is highly effective in resolving walled-off necrosis, with lower complication rates compared to surgical approaches. Endoscopic necrosectomy is not mandatory in all cases of walled-off necrosis. In patients who require drainage, a methodical and meticulous approach can help minimize the risk of complications. When complications do arise, it is important to recognize them immediately and intervene which may allow the patient to avoid surgery.

References

1 van Brunschot S, Hollemans RA, Bakker OJ, et al. Minimally invasive and endoscopic versus open necrosectomy for necrotising pancreatitis: a pooled analysis of individual data for 1980 patients. *Gut* 2018;67(4):697–706.

2. van Santvoort HC, Besselink MG, Bakker OJ, et al. A step-up approach or open necrosectomy for necrotizing pancreatitis. *N Engl J Med* 2010;362(16):1491–1502.

3. van Brunschot S, van Grinsven J, van Santvoort HC, et al. Endoscopic or surgical step-up approach for infected necrotising pancreatitis: a multicentre randomised trial. *Lancet* 2018;391(10115):51–58.

4. Seifert H, Biermer M, Schmitt W, et al. Transluminal endoscopic necrosectomy after acute pancreatitis: a multicentre study with long-term follow-up (the GEPARD Study). *Gut* 2009;58(9):1260–1266.

5. Gardner TB, Chahal P, Papachristou GI, et al. A comparison of direct endoscopic necrosectomy with transmural endoscopic drainage for the treatment of walled-off pancreatic necrosis. *Gastrointest Endosc* 2009;69(6):1085–1094.

6. Gardner TB, Coelho-Prabhu N, Gordon SR, et al. Direct endoscopic necrosectomy for the treatment of walled-off pancreatic necrosis: results from a multicenter U.S. series. *Gastrointest Endosc* 2011;73(4):718–726.

54 How to Perform Pancreatic Mass Fine Needle Biopsy

Ahmad Najdat Bazarbashi and Linda S. Lee
Division of Gastroenterology, Hepatology and Endoscopy, Brigham and Women's Hospital, Harvard Medical School, Boston, MA, USA

Introduction

The differential diagnosis for pancreatic masses is broad, ranging from benign to malignant lesions such as autoimmune pancreatitis and pancreatic adenocarcinoma. Therefore, many pancreatic masses seen on radiology imaging require biopsy, and endoscopic ultrasound (EUS) has emerged as the premier diagnostic modality for safely acquiring tissue. EUS provides real-time information about details of the mass, including its size, shape, border, content, echogenicity, and impact on surrounding structures, and assesses for locoregional spread. EUS-guided tissue sampling occurs via fine needle aspiration (FNA) or fine needle biopsy (FNB). FNA uses a hollow needle and provides cellular material for cytology, while FNB needles provide core tissue samples for architectural analysis (Figure 54.1). The first FNB needle called TruCut needle (Cook Medical, Bloomington, IN) was 19G. Now core biopsy needles are available as 19G, 22G, and 25G with different tip designs, although whether one configuration is superior remains to be determined. Fork-tip FNB needles may improve diagnostic yield, but further studies are needed. Compared to FNA, FNB increases histological yield and sufficient tissue for tumor genotyping with fewer passes needed for diagnosis, eliminates need for rapid on-site evaluation (ROSE), and may improve diagnostic accuracy in solid pancreatic masses. When lymphoma, sarcoidosis, or autoimmune pancreatitis are in the differential diagnosis, core biopsies should be obtained. Reassuringly, both FNA and FNB have low risk of complications, including 1–2% risk of pancreatitis.

Before EUS, history and physical examination should focus on symptoms related to the mass and risk factors for a pancreatic mass including history of autoimmune diseases, smoking and alcohol intake, and family history of pancreatic cancer. Platelet count and international normalized ratio (INR) should be obtained if there is concern for high risk of bleeding. Anticoagulation should be held after discussion with the prescribing clinician. Endosonographers must carefully review cross-sectional imaging to understand the patient's anatomy, location of the mass, presence of potential metastatic disease and to anticipate potential difficulties in finding and sampling the mass. Informed consent from the patient should review the nature of the procedure, risks, benefits and alternatives. Risks to highlight include bleeding, abdominal pain, pancreatitis, and perforation. Patients should be informed of potential issues including, for example, possible difficulties in accessing and obtaining biopsies from uncinate process masses. Anesthesia rather than intravenous conscious sedation may be associated with improved diagnostic yield.

Technique (Video 54.1)

Esophagogastroduodenoscopy (EGD) often precedes EUS to ensure there are no anatomical abnormalities that may interfere with advancing the echoendoscope or visualizing the pancreas and surrounding structures and not infrequently reveals unexpected findings. Once EGD is completed, the echoendoscope is passed into the stomach and duodenum. Linear echoendoscope should be used rather than radial echoendoscope since it allows tissue acquisition. EUS examination begins with evaluating for potential locoregional spread of disease to areas such as the liver or celiac region (Figure 54.2). FNA/FNB of lymphadenopathy and metastases to surrounding structures should be performed to confirm metastatic disease. From the stomach, the pancreas can be located by rotating 180 degrees from the thickest portion of the left lobe of the liver or by following the superior mesenteric artery to the body of the pancreas. The genu, body and tail of pancreas (Figure 54.3) can be evaluated from the transgastric station, while the head and

Atlas of Endoscopic Ultrasonography, Second Edition. Edited by Frank Gress, Thomas Savides, Brenna Casey, and Everson L. A. Artifon.

Companion website: www.wiley.com/go/gress/atlas

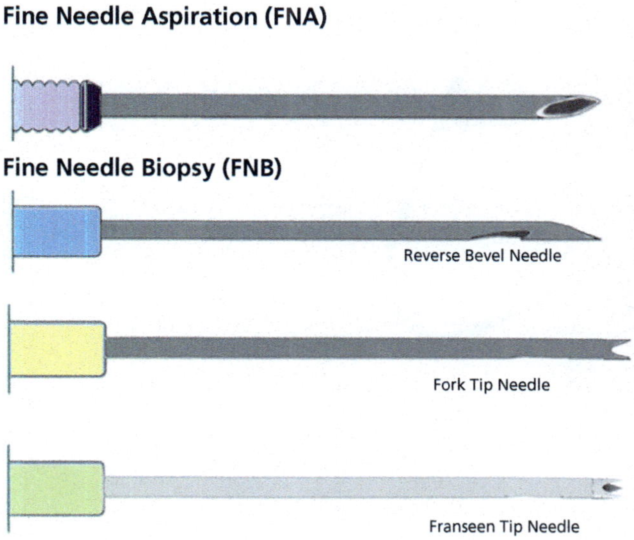

Figure 54.1 Fine needle aspiration versus fine needle biopsy needles.

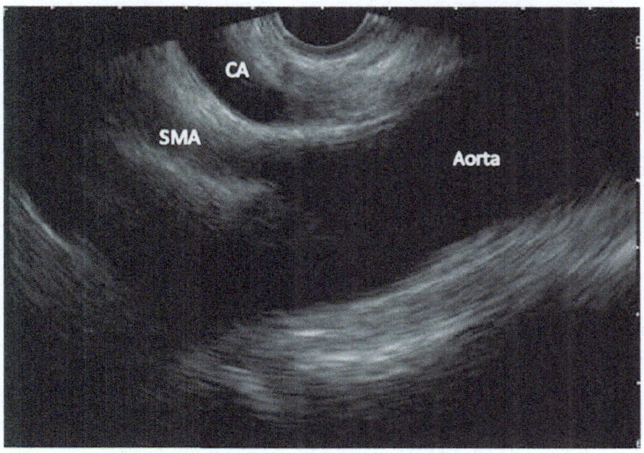

Figure 54.2 EUS of aorta, celiac artery (CA) and superior mesenteric artery (SMA). Source: Frank G. Gress.

uncinate process are usually seen from the transduodenal station (Figure 54.4).

Pancreatic masses usually appear hypoechoic and may be homogeneous or heterogeneous with regular or irregular borders (Figure 54.5). Once the location of the mass is confirmed, it is ideally placed near the 6 o'clock position as close to the tip of the echoendoscope as possible using the large dial. Doppler imaging ensures blood vessels are not in the path of needle insertion (Figure 54.6). For FNB, 22G and 25G needles are often used while 19G needles are usually not necessary and are more difficult to advance forward in the duodenum. FNB needles made of nitinol (Acquire 19G, Boston Scientific, Marlborough, MA and SharkCore 19G, Medtronic, Sunnyvale, CA) may be more flexible and easier to use in these torqued angulated positions. After removing the biopsy cap, the needle device is advanced down the accessory channel and locked onto the Luer lock at the accessory channel port. The large and small dials on the echoendoscope should be locked to ensure that slight movements or deviations during needle advancement are minimized. The position of the sheath can be adjusted using the bottom slider on the needle handle (Figure 54.7), which allows use of the various needles with the different brands of echoendoscopes. Once the sheath is visible, the sheath adjusting knob should be locked, and for some FNB needles the stylet is pulled back slightly to expose the needle. How far to advance the needle can be estimated by measuring the distance from the tip of the echoendoscope to the mass, and the adjustable needle knob near the top of the needle handle (Figure 54.7) should be locked in position accordingly to prevent accidentally advancing the needle too far. Then the needle is slowly advanced out of the sheath until it nears the gastric or duodenal wall. If the needle does not move easily, it should not be forced out as this could damage the echoendoscope; instead, reposition the echoendoscope and unlock the dials before trying to advance the needle. After using Doppler to ensure lack of blood vessels in the path of the needle and the elevator to adjust the angle of needle entry, the needle is advanced with a rapid, strong thrust to penetrate through the posterior gastric or duodenal wall into the pancreatic mass (Figure 54.8). The stylet is pushed back in to expel any gastric or duodenal wall tissue that may have been captured; however, whether a stylet is used for subsequent passes does not affect diagnostic yield. It serves to stiffen the needle and may help the assistant expel tissue from the needle. Application of some type of suction may increase diagnostic yield. Options include the stylet slow-pull technique where the assistant slowly and continuously pulls back on the stylet as the endosonographer moves the needle back and forth within the mass, vacuum syringe with a 10-ml syringe attached to the top of the needle handle, or wet suction where the needle is filled with saline before attaching the vacuum syringe. The latter two suction techniques require complete removal of the stylet first. If specimens

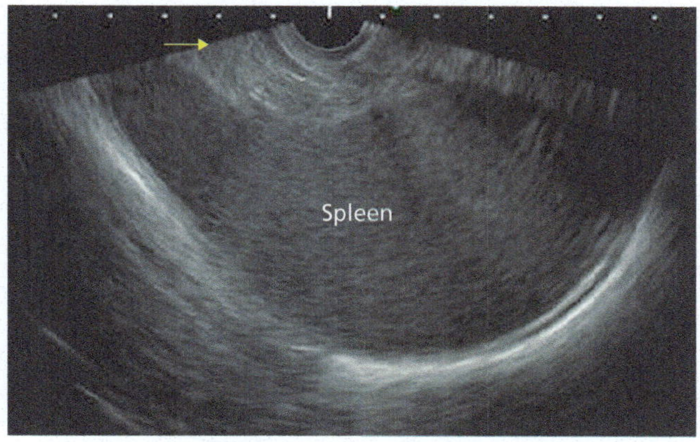

Figure 54.3 Tail of pancreas (yellow arrow) and spleen. Source: Frank G. Gress.

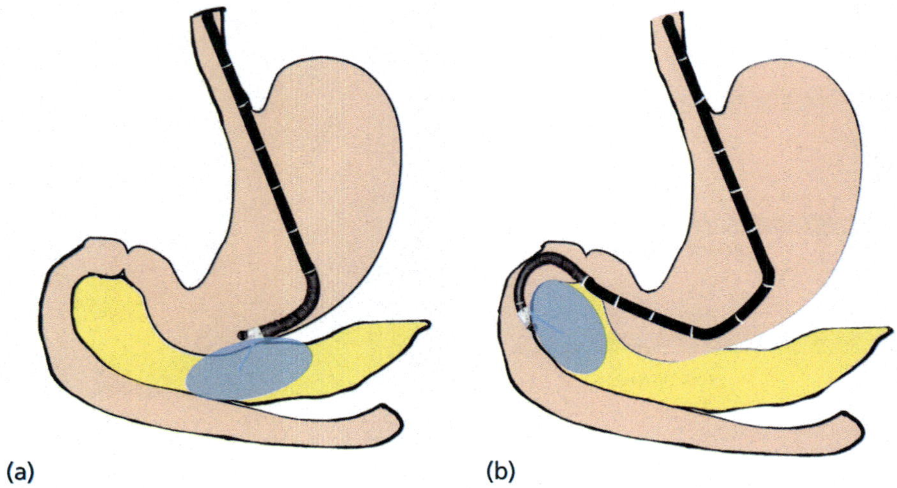

Figure 54.4 EUS-guided (a) transgastric and (b) transduodenal pancreatic tissue acquisition.

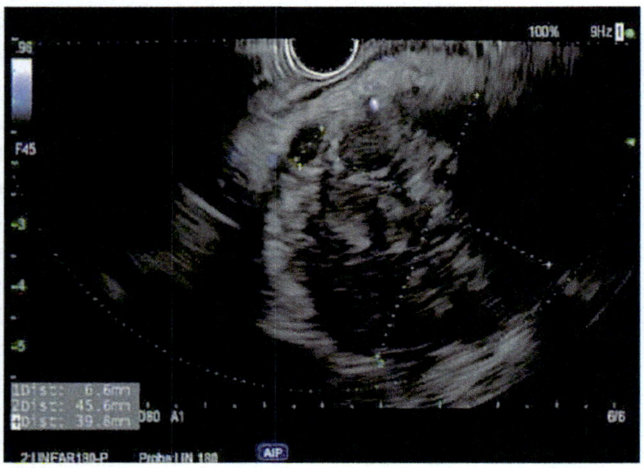

Figure 54.5 Large heterogeneous well-defined pancreatic head mass. Source: Frank G. Gress.

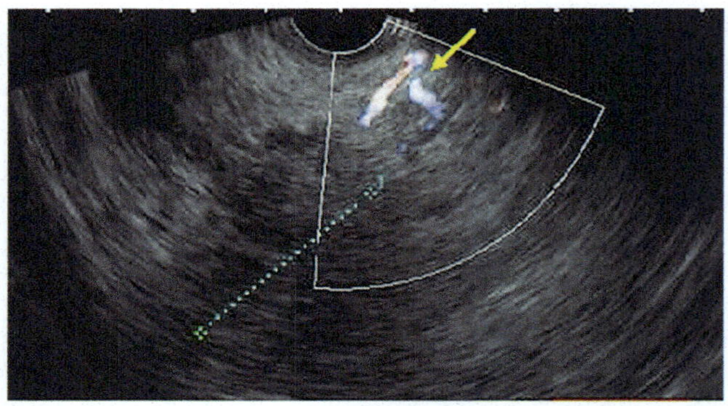

Figure 54.6 Vessels (yellow arrow) in path of FNB needle to pancreatic mass. Source: Frank G. Gress.

appear bloody, no suction can be used. Typically, the needle is moved back and forth within the mass about 10–15 times although fewer movements may be needed with FNB needles. The needle trajectory should be adjusted by using the elevator and/or large dial to "fan" the needle throughout the mass to increase diagnostic yield (Figure 54.9). The needle tip should always be visualized.

Once FNB is complete, the suction stopcock should be turned off with or without removing the syringe before the needle is withdrawn to avoid contaminating the collected specimen. The fully withdrawn needle locked in position is then completely removed from the echoendoscope. The assistant expels the tissue from the needle into a collection container using the stylet or air from the vacuum syringe. Macroscopic evaluation of the tissue to confirm presence of visible pale cores of tissue is associated with histological diagnosis (Figure 54.10). When FNB is compared with FNA plus ROSE, diagnostic yield is comparable. If ROSE is not used, two to three separate FNB passes are recommended. A different needle should be used if moving from biopsying the pancreatic mass to potential metastatic lesions in order to avoid contaminating benign tissue. Antibiotics are not routinely given for EUS-FNA/FNB of solid pancreatic lesions.

Summary

EUS-guided FNA/FNB is the premier method for tissue acquisition of the pancreas. FNB is superior to FNA, with increased yield of histological cores requiring fewer passes for diagnosis. However, careful attention to proper technique is important to ensure optimal and safe biopsy. This begins with detailed review of radiological imaging and includes thoughtfulness about needle selection, with smaller gauge needles favored for transduodenal approaches, use of suction, and macroscopic assessment of acquired tissue during the procedure. During biopsy, Doppler should be used to avoid blood vessels, the mass positioned as close to the transducer as possible, and fanning employed to increase diagnostic yield.

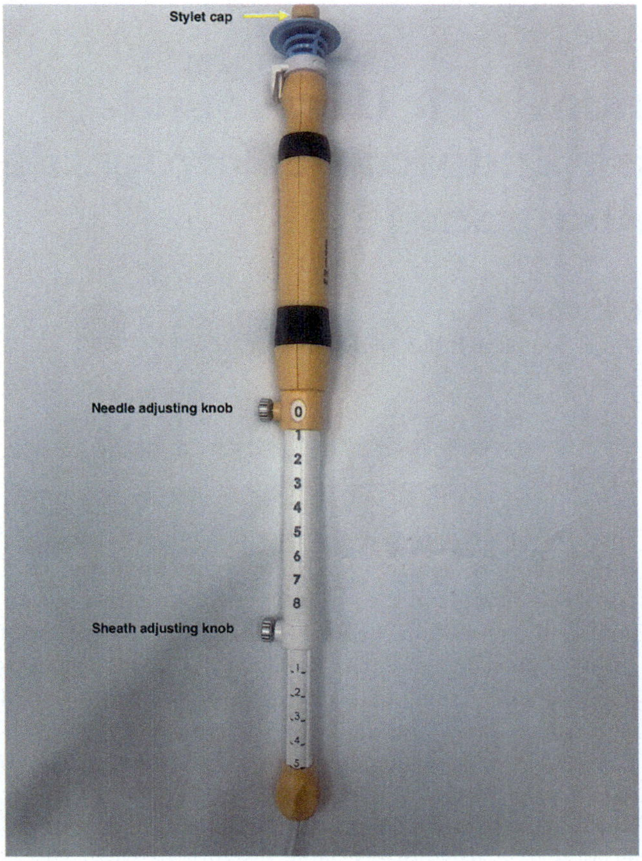

Figure 54.7 Fine needle biopsy handle. Source: Frank G. Gress.

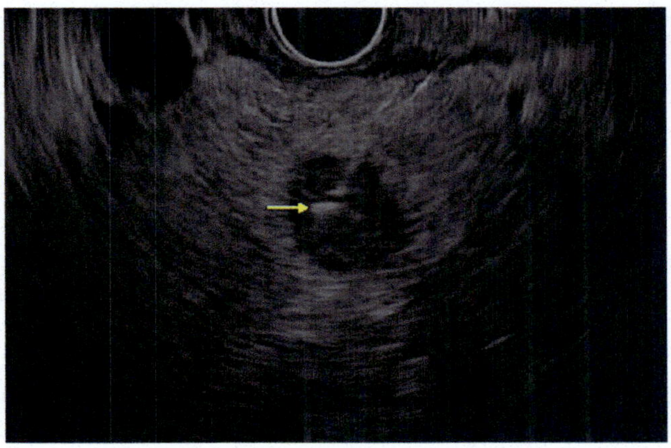

Figure 54.8 EUS-FNB of pancreatic mass. Tip of FNB needle seen within mass (yellow arrow). Source: Frank G. Gress.

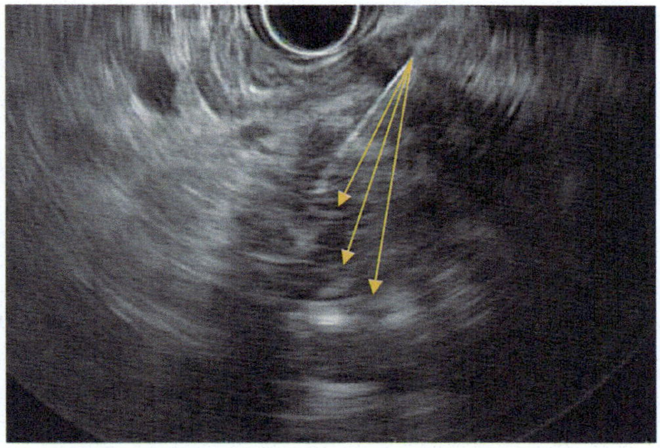

Figure 54.9 Fanning to increase tissue acquisition. Source: Frank G. Gress.

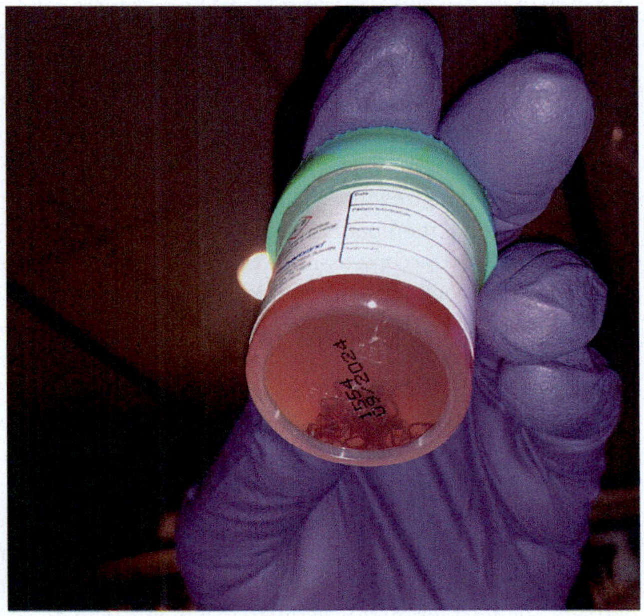

Figure 54.10 Macroscopically visible strands of fine needle biopsy tissue. Source: Frank G. Gress.

Chapter video clip

Video 54.1 Technique of pancreatic mass EUS-FNB. Source: Frank G. Gress.

55 How to Perform Endoscopic Ultrasound-directed Transgastric Endoscopic Retrograde Cholangiopancreatography (EDGE)

M. Phillip Fejleh and Wilson T. Kwong

Division of Gastroenterology, University of California San Diego Health Sciences, La Jolla, CA, USA

Introduction

Endoscopic retrograde cholangiopancreatography (ERCP) and certain endoscopic ultrasound (EUS) procedures can be challenging when managing pancreaticobiliary diseases in patients with altered gastrointestinal tract anatomy. A regularly encountered situation is the need for ERCP in a patient with prior Roux-en-Y gastric bypass (RYGB). ERCP via deep balloon-assisted enteroscopy can be considered but has limited success rates even when performed by expert endoscopists and therapeutic options and accessories are very limited. Laparoscopy-assisted ERCP is also feasible but requires laparoscopy and coordination with a surgeon.

Endoscopic ultrasound-directed transgastric ERCP or EUS (EDGE) was developed to overcome the difficulty of these situations by using a lumen-apposing metal stent (LAMS) to create a fistula tract between the gastric pouch and the excluded stomach after gastric bypass. This technique allows for standard ERCP or EUS interventions in the duodenum. EDGE can be performed in a single session for patients with urgent indications for ERCP including cholangitis, or it can be staged into two or more sessions to allow for maturation of the fistula tract for increased safety in patients who do not require urgent intervention.

Practice patterns continue to evolve but EDGE can be considered as first- or second-line management for patients with RYGB who require ERCP. Risks and benefits and all three approaches should be discussed with the patient and a bariatric surgeon for shared decision-making. The patient should also be counseled on the possible risk of weight regain and persistent fistula (though uncommon). When EDGE is undertaken, it should be performed by an endoscopist experienced in interventional EUS as well as ERCP.

Technique

The EDGE procedure can be performed on an inpatient or outpatient basis, and this will likely be determined in most cases by the nature of the patient's condition and the indication for the procedure. General anesthesia is recommended given the procedure duration and aspiration risk, and periprocedural antibiotics should be considered given the transmural nature of the procedure and biliary instrumentation.

Available cross-sectional imaging should be reviewed to assess the proximity of the excluded stomach to the gastric pouch and also assess other findings that may be a contraindication to EDGE (ascites, large distance between gastric pouch and excluded stomach, malignancy, and to verify gastric bypass anatomy vs. other bariatric surgery). An upper endoscopy should be performed to clearly define the anatomy. Next, a linear therapeutic echoendoscope is advanced to the gastric pouch to locate the excluded stomach under ultrasound imaging and to find a suitable window for gastro-gastric fistula creation (Figure 55.1). The excluded stomach can contain fluid in which case it is easy to identify but may also appear as collapsed folds of the gastric wall without a clear lumen. A site for fistula creation should be identified without intervening vessels and at a site which is ideally 10 mm or less from the gastric pouch. Once a site has been chosen on EUS, the site should be verified endoscopically to ensure the site is within the gastric pouch and not within the esophagus or jejunum as a fistula from the pouch is preferable.

If the excluded stomach is already distended with fluid, LAMS placement (15 or 20 mm) can be performed under EUS guidance. However, if the excluded stomach appears collapsed or if the operator is uncertain whether the excluded

Atlas of Endoscopic Ultrasonography, Second Edition. Edited by Frank Gress, Thomas Savides, Brenna Casey, and Everson L. A. Artifon.

Companion website: www.wiley.com/go/gress/atlas

stomach has been correctly identified, a 19-gauge needle is used to puncture the excluded stomach under direct EUS visualization (Figure 55.2) and water and/or contrast can be injected to distend the stomach for better visualization on EUS and fluoroscopy (Figure 55.3).

Cautery-enhanced LAMS delivery systems will help simplify the creation of the fistula and stent placement; however, a traditional approach with puncture using a 19-gauge fine needle aspiration (FNA) needle followed by advancement of a guidewire into the excluded stomach, tract dilation with a controlled radial expansion (CRE) balloon or bougie dilator, and then LAMS deployment is also feasible. Once the LAMS catheter has been advanced into the excluded stomach under EUS guidance, the distal flange should be deployed under EUS guidance deep within the stomach and then retracted slowly until it is snug against the excluded stomach wall. The proximal flange can then be deployed under endoscopic guidance within the gastric pouch (Figures 55.4 and 55.5).

If immediate ERCP is required, a CRE balloon should be used to dilate the stent to either 15 or 20 mm (depending on the size of the LAMS selected; Figure 55.6). Before proceeding with duodenoscope insertion through the LAMS,

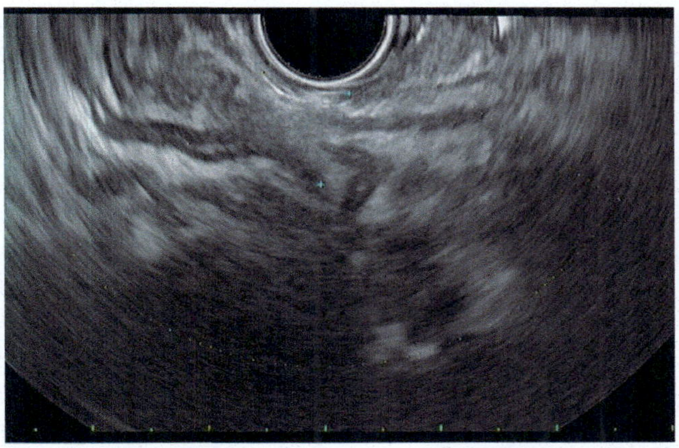

Figure 55.1 View of the excluded stomach from the gastric pouch using a linear echoendoscope. The excluded stomach can contain fluid, in which case it is easy to identify, but may also appear as collapsed folds of the gastric wall without a clear lumen.

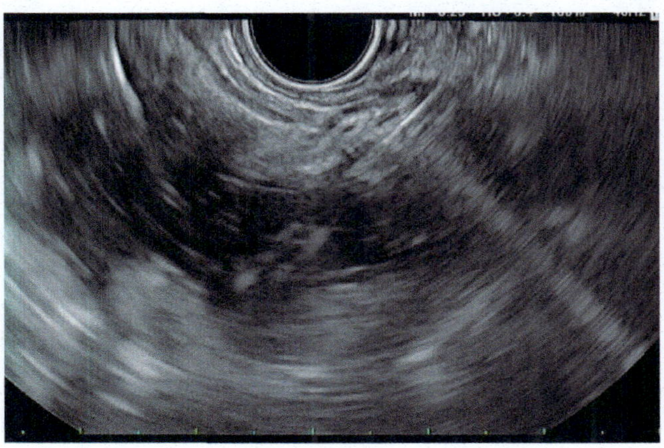

Figure 55.2 A 19-gauge needle is used to puncture the excluded stomach under direct EUS guidance. Water and/or contrast can be injected to distend the stomach for better visualization.

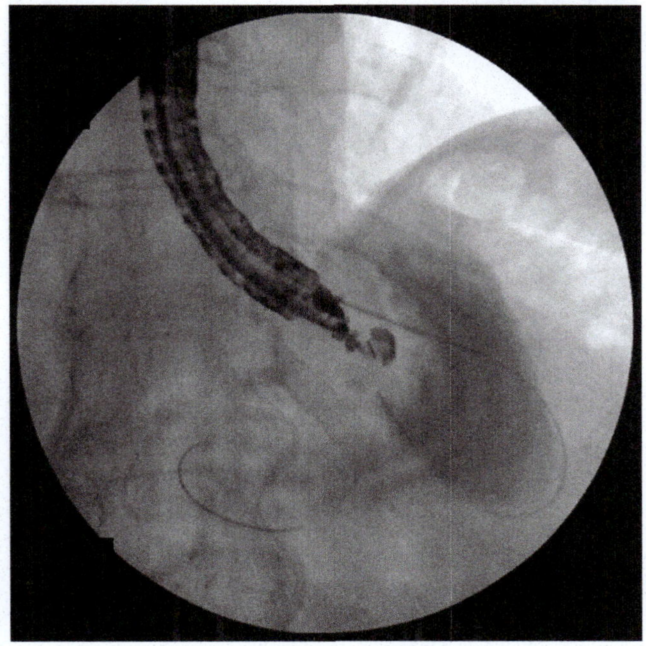

Figure 55.3 Fluoroscopic view of the excluded stomach after injection of contrast and advancement of a guidewire.

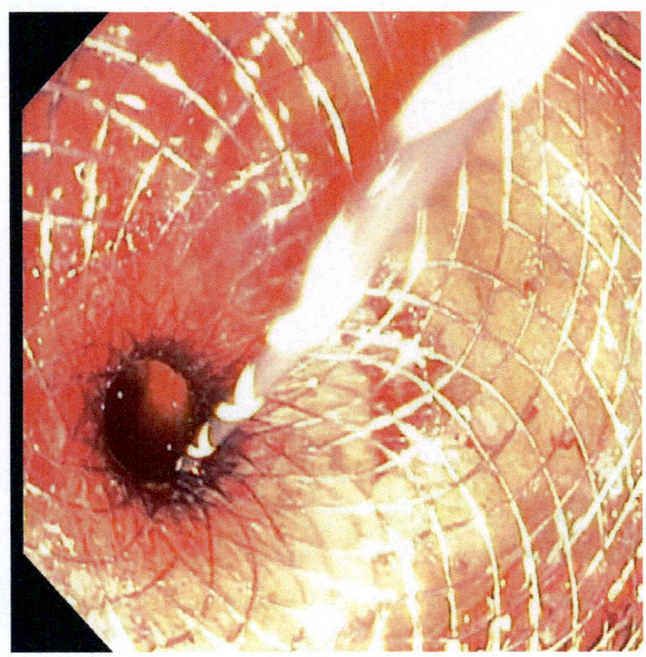

Figure 55.4 View of lumen-apposing metal stent after deploying the proximal flange under endoscopic visualization within the gastric pouch.

consideration should be given to securing the stent to the gastric pouch with either endoscopic suturing or an over-the-scope clip as stent dislodgement is a significant risk when ERCP is performed immediately. Dilation is not necessary if the plan is to allow the fistula tract to mature for two to three weeks prior to a later ERCP.

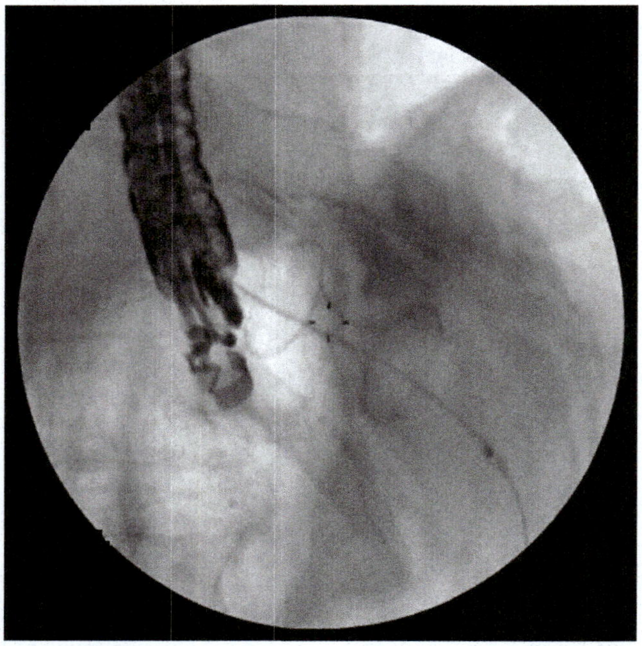

Figure 55.5 Fluoroscopic view after successful creation of a gastro-gastric fistula with a lumen-apposing metal stent.

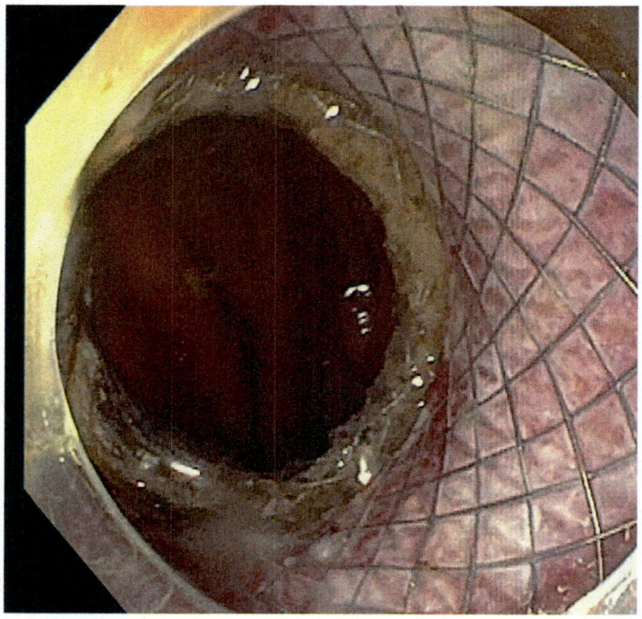

Figure 55.6 Dilation of the lumen-apposing metal stent channel during the index procedure allows for advancement of a duodenoscope or echoendoscope through the stent. Dilation is not necessary if the plan is to allow the fistula tract to mature for two to three weeks prior to a later ERCP/EUS intervention.

After creation of the gastro-gastric fistula, a duodenoscope or echoendoscope can be carefully advanced through the stent with care taken to avoid pushing forcefully or excessively contacting the stent as much as possible. This can be monitored under fluoroscopy for an extra measure of safety against stent dislodgement but is not mandatory (Figure 55.7). If ongoing management of pancreaticobiliary disease will be required, then the LAMS may be left in place. Double pigtail stents should be placed through the LAMS channel after completion of the procedure, as this may prevent LAMS migration in the interim (Figure 55.8). Potential adverse events related to EDGE include stent migration, bleeding, stent maldeployment, perforation, peritonitis, and post-ERCP pancreatitis.

Post-EDGE fistula management

If there will be no further use of the fistula, then the LAMS can be removed after three to four weeks of fistula maturation (Figure 55.9). In the majority of cases, the fistula closes spontaneously once the stent is removed. Argon plasma coagulation (APC) ablation of the tract or endoscopic closure with suturing or clipping can be done to increase the likelihood of closure. One can also perform an upper gastrointestinal series after several months to assess if there is complete closure of the fistula tract, and if the fistula remains present, an endoscopic attempt at closure can be considered at that time.

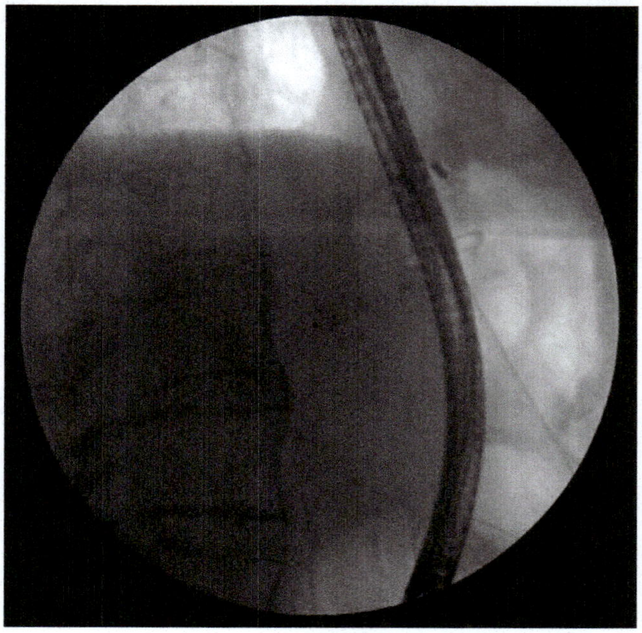

Figure 55.7 Careful advancement of a duodenoscope through a freshly placed lumen-apposing metal stent using fluoroscopic guidance to monitor for stent dislodgement.

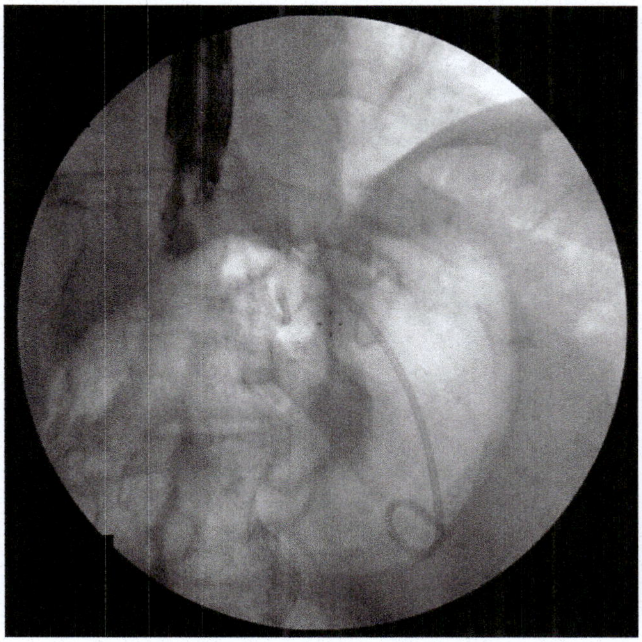

Figure 55.8 Fluoroscopic view of a double pigtail stent placed within the lumen-apposing metal stent channel, which may prevent LAMS migration.

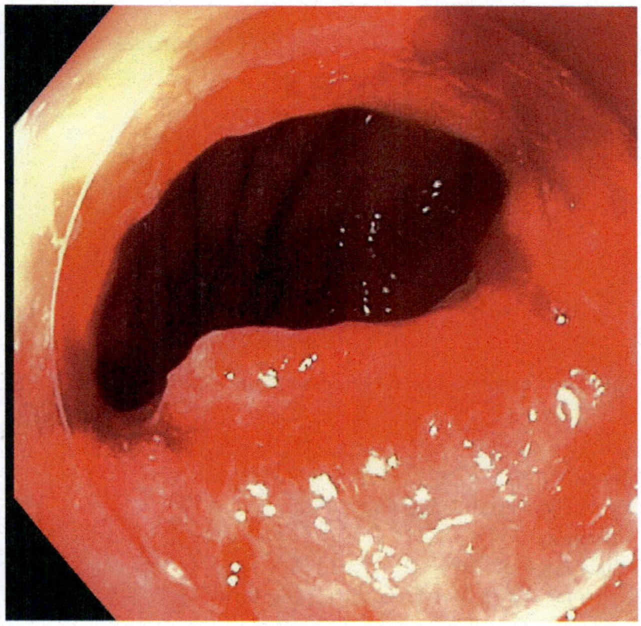

Figure 55.9 Gastro-gastric fistula seen endoscopically following removal of a lumen-apposing metal stent four weeks after placement.

Summary

EDGE has emerged as an effective and efficient means of achieving antegrade access to the duodenum/ampulla after gastric bypass. It has a higher success rate than enteroscopy-assisted ERCP and appears to have a lower complication rate than laparoscopy-assisted ERCP, making it an attractive option that allows for the full spectrum of biliary and pancreatic interventions with the usual endoscopes and accessories.

Index

Note: page numbers in italics refer to figures and those in bold refer to tables

A

abscess
- pelvic abscess drainage 182–185
- perirectal 77

achalasia 46, *47*, 48
- circular muscle wall layer thickening 46, *47*, *48*
- esophageal wall layer pattern 46, *47*
- muscularis propria 46, *47*

acinar cell carcinoma 110, 111
adrenal glands 32
alcohol free EUS-guided cyst ablation process 166, *169*
American Joint Committee on Cancer (AJCC) staging
- of esophageal cancer 39, **40**
- of gastric cancer **53**

American Thoracic Society, mediastinal staging map for lymphadenopathy 146, *148*
ampulla of Vater 95
ampullary carcinoma 96
ampullary neoplasia 95–96, *97*
anal canal 33, 35
anal sphincter disease 72–74, *75–77*
aneurysms 89
Ann Arbor staging system for gastrointestinal lymphomas **56**
anorectal neoplasia 67–71
anorectum, normal anatomy 33–35
aorta, abdominal 25, *27*
aortic arch 16
- anomalies 88

aortic pseudoaneurysm 88
aortic root dissection 89
aortopulmonary window 16, 17
arterial embolization
- gastric bleeding 205
- gastric cancer *206*
- postprocedural management 206–208, *207*
- pseudoaneurysm bleeding *207*
- technique 205–206, *207*

arteries, normal anatomy 7
ascites
- gastric cancer 57, *57*
- liver cirrhosis 130, *131*

atherosclerotic vascular disease 89
atrial myocardial metastasis 90
atrial myxoma 90
atrium, left 10, *11*
autoimmune pancreatitis (AIP) 113–116
- diagnostic features of *139*
- histologic features 115

azygos arch 13, 16
azygos vein 13

B

Barrett's esophagus 40, 42
bile duct
- malignancy 98, *99*
- normal anatomy 22–24
- staging of tumors 98
- stones 98, 100
- tumors 98

biliary stent *99*
biliary strictures 98
biliary tract
- extrahepatic 98
- pathology 98, *99*, 100

biliary tree, normal anatomy 22, 24
bilobar liver biopsy 197
Blastocystis hominis lymph node infection *52*
bleeding, Doppler probe EUS 186–188, *189*, *190*, 191, *192*, 193
breast cancer, atrial myocardial metastases 90

C

carcinoembryonic antigen (CEA) 254
- intraductal papillary mucinous neoplasm 124
- pancreatic cystic lesions 117, 155

carcinoid tumors
- gastric 58, *60*

Atlas of Endoscopic Ultrasonography, Second Edition. Edited by Frank Gress, Thomas Savides, Brenna Casey, and Everson L. A. Artifon.

Companion website: www.wiley.com/go/gress/atlas

rectum 69, *71*
carotid artery, left 12, 16
catheter probe, stomach 19
cavernous hemangiomas 132, *133*
celiac artery 27, *28*
aneurysm 89
obliteration by calcified plaque 89
pancreatic adenocarcinoma vascular invasion 104, *105*
vascular occlusion 88
celiac plexus block (CPB) neurolysis 173–175
complications 175
efficacy of 173
neurolytic agents 175
technique 173–175
celiac plexus neurolysis (CPN) 173–175
complications 175
efficacy of 173
neurolytic agents 175
technique 173–175
cervix uteri 34
CHARM trial 166
chemotherapy agent injection 179–180, *181*
response monitoring 179, 180, *181*
tumor assessment *181*
cholangiocarcinoma 98
dilated intrahepatic duct 133
cholecystitis 103
choledocholithiasis 100
chronic pancreatitis *233*
classification 126–128
diagnosis 125–126
ductal changes 126, *127*
histopathology 126, 127
pain 173
Rosemont criteria 125, 127–128, *128*
threshold criteria 126–127
tissue acquisition 129
colonic lymphangioma 69
colonic polyps 191
colorectal cancer
local recurrence 67, *70*
lymph nodes 67, *69*
restaging after chemotherapy and radiation 67
staging 67, *68*, *69*
colorectal wall
gastrointestinal stromal cell tumor 69, *70*
myogenic tumor 68–69, *71*
submucosal tumors 68–69, *70*, 71
common bile duct 28
stack sign 25, *27*
stent *152*
confocal laser endomicroscopy (CLE) 254, 255
congenital foregut cysts 51
contrast-enhanced EUS
advantages of 242–243
vs. contrast-enhanced modalities 242
vs. conventional EUS 242–243
critical points for performing 237
distinguishing a mural nodule from a mucous clot *244*
distinguishing malignant from benign lymph nodes *247*
for gastrointestinal stromal tumor (GIST) *246*
hypoechoic pancreatic solid lesions *245*
lesions
lymph node 244
pancreatic cyst 244
solid pancreatic lesions 243–244
subepithelial lesions 244
principle of 237
procedures *228–241*
contrast-enhanced harmonic (CEH)-EUS 209
contrast harmonic imaging *237*
Crohn's disease, perianal fistula 76
cryptococcal mediastinal lymph node *52*
cyanoacrylate 202, 205

D

diabetes, fatty liver disease 131
Dieulafoy lesions 90, 191, *192*
diffuse gastric cancer *55*
dilated intrahepatic ducts 133, *133*
distal esophageal adenocarcinoma 40, 41
diverticular bleeding 191
diverticular disease, anastomotic perirectal abscess *77*
Doppler flow 195, *196*
Doppler probe EUS for bleeding 186–188, *189*, *190*, 191, *192*, 193
equipment 198, 199
gastric varices 191, *192*
gastrointestinal stromal cell tumors 191, *192*
peptic ulcer 187–188, *188*, *189*, *190*
pre-procedure system check 186
Doppler ultrasound signals 186–188, 191
DopUS probe, practical application 186–191
bleeding peptic ulcer with non-bleeding visible vessel 187, *188*
Doppler ultrasound signals 186–188, 191
preprocedure system check 186
duodenum
neoplasia 95–96, *97*
normal anatomy from 5–6
duplication cysts 51, *52*, 61, *61*
dysphagia lusoria 88

E

echoendoscopes 14, *15*
echoguided treatment of gastric varices
complicatons 203–204
technique 202–203
elastography
complications 231
elastographic pattern classification **231**
indications 231
qualitative elastography 231
quantitative elastography
evaluation **234**
strain histogram 231
strain ratio 231
technique 229–231
elderly patients, ampullary neoplasms 96
electrocautery-enhanced delivery system 164

electromyography (EMG), fecal incontinence 72
endoanal ultrasound 73–74
endobronchial anatomy 7, *8*, 9
endobronchial ultrasound-guided transbronchial fine needle aspiration (EBUS-TBNA) 14
  complications 18
  equipment 14
  malignant mediastinal lesions 49
  safety 18
  technique 17
endocrine pancreatic tumors (EPTs) 108–109
Endo-Dop 186, *187*
endometriosis 78–82, *83–87*
  abdominal and pelvic magnetic resonance imaging 79
  bulging of the upper rectum wall *83*
  classification 79, *79*
  cytopathology and histopathology 82
  definition and location 78
  diagnosis 79
  endometrial gland *86*
  endometrial stroma *86*
  epidemiology and risk factors 78
  radial exploration *84, 87*
  rectosigmoid junction *80*
  sigmoid substenosis *81*
  superficial colonic mucosae *86*
  superficial mucosa *84*
  video-laparoscopy 82
endoscopic necrosectomy
  complication management
    bleeding 268
    infection 268–269
    perforation 268
  cystgastrostomy/cystenterostomy 266–267
  EUS evaluation of walled-off pancreatic necrosis 266
  preprocedure assessment 265
  tools and technique 267–268
endoscopic retrograde cholangiopancreatography (ERCP) 98, 100, 214, 274
  chronic pancreatitis 125
  fiducial placement 176–178
endoscopic retrograde pancreatography 216
endoscopic ultrasound (EUS) 229, 237
  ex vivo models 256–264
  simulation of hepatic nodules and lymph nodes *259*
  simulation of subepithelial lesions *260*
  vascular simulation of aorta *258*
endoscopic ultrasound-directed transgastric endoscopic retrograde cholangiopancreatography (EDGE) 274–277
endoscopic ultrasound-guided fine needle aspiration (EUS-FNA)
  air-dried slides 141, *142*, 143
  alcohol-fixed slides 141, 143
  aspirate biopsy 138, 139, *140*
  autoimmune pancreatitis 113, 115
  biopsy material technical quality 137–139, *140*, 141–143
  biopsy type 137–139, *138*
  brush cytology 141
  cell block 139, *140*, 141
  chemotherapeutic agent injection 179–180, *181*
  core biopsy *138*, 139, 141
  gastrointestinal stromal tumors *145*
  interpretation 135–137, *138*, 139–142, *143*
    quality 143–144, *145*
  laboratory role 144
  liquid-based cytology 143
  lymphoma *145*
  mediastinal 146, **147**, *148*, 149
  mediastinal lymph node, metastatic adenocarcinoma *145*
  metastatic renal cell carcinoma *145*
  needle preparation 142
  needle size 141–142
  pancreatic cystic lesions 155–159
  pancreatic mass 150, *151*, 152–154
  pancreatic solid pseudopapillary tumor *145*
  pathologic/clinical information integration 144
  personnel 137
  rapid cytologic evaluation 144
  rapid on-site evaluation of cytology (ROSE) 154
  slide preparation/staining 142–143
  suction 142
  technique 15–17, 155–158
  transbronchial 14
    complications 18
    equipment 14
    safety 18
  transduodenal *156*
endoscopic ultrasound-guided gallbladder drainage (EUS-GBD) 220
endoscopic ultrasound-guided gastrojejunal bypass (EUSGJ) 226
endoscopic ultrasound-guided liver biopsy (EUS-LB)
  absolute contraindications 197
  advantages 197
  adverse effects 200
  indications for 197
  post-procedure recovery after 199
  techniques 197–199, *198, 200*
    identification of liver lobes 197, *198*
    needle preparation 199, *200*
    needle selection *198*
    needle technique 199
    specimen handling 199, *200*
endoscopic ultrasound-guided pelvic abscess drainage 182–185
endoscopic ultrasound-guided portal pressure gradient measurement 194–196, *195*
endoscopic ultrasound-guided Tru-cut biopsy (EUS-TCB)
  autoimmune pancreatitis 113–115, *116*
  chronic pancreatitis 127
esophageal cancer staging 39–45
  EUS, role of 39–41
  technique 41, 45
esophageal mass, subepithelial 58–66
  extrinsic compression lesions 65, *65*, **66**
esophageal varices 191
esophageal wall, linear/radial array orientation 10, *11*
esophagogastroduodenoscopy (EGD) 270
esophagus 10, *11*, 12–13

high grade dysplasia 39
layers of wall 10, *11*
normal anatomy 3–4, 7, *8*, 9
radial 10, *11*, 12
EUS-guided and percutaneous pressure measurements 195
EUS-guided fiducial placement *177*, 177–178
EUS-guided pancreatic duct drainage (EUS-PDD) 214
EUS-guided vascular embolization 205
EUS-RFA radiofrequency system *249*
extrinsic compression lesions, of esophagus and stomach 65, *65*, **66**
ex vivo models
for dilated hepatocholedochus evaluation *263*
EASIE model 256
for EUS biliary drainage *264*
for EUS-FNA of cystic lesions *261*
for pseudocyst drainage *262*

F

fatty liver disease 130–131, *132*
alcoholic/non-alcoholic 131
fecal incontinence 72–74, *75–77*
assessment 72
diagnostic tests 72
endoanal ultrasound 73–74
etiology 72
prevalence 72
transperineal ultrasound 74, *75*
treatment 74
fiducial loading and deployment 177, *177*
fine-gauge electrocautery dilator *217*
fine needle aspiration (FNA) 198, 209, 254
fine needle biopsy (FNB) 198
foregut cysts, congenital 51

G

gallbladder
carcinoma 103
microlithiasis 101, *102*
normal anatomy 22, 23, 24
pathology 101, 102, *102*
polyps 101, *102*, 103
sludge 101, *102*
stones 101, *102*
wall thickening 103
gallbladder drainage
EUS-GBD with LAMS 221–224
EUS transmural approach 220
LAMS **221**
long-term management 224
percutaneous transhepatic gallbladder drainage (PT-GBD) 220
postprocedural management 224
stents 220–221
gastric adenocarcinoma 53
diffuse type 53, *55*
gastric bleeding 205
gastric cancer 53–57, *206*, *235*
ascites 57
malignant adenopathy 57
metastases 53, *55*
lymph nodes 57
pancreatic rest 61
signet-ring cell carcinoma *55*
staging 19, 53, **54, 56**
gastric folds, thickened 19
gastric leiomyoma 62, 64
gastric lipoma 58, *59*
gastric lymphoma 53, *56*
gastric mass, subepithelial 58–66
extrinsic compression lesions 65, *65*, **66**
gastric outlet obstruction (GOO) 226
gastric varices, bleeding 88, 191, *192*
gastric varices, EUS guided treatment of
complicatons 203–204
technique 202–203, *203*
gastric wall 19
layers 19–21
gastrinoma 108, *109*
gastritis cystica profunda (GCP) 63, *64*
gastroesophageal junction 10, *11*
gastroesophageal varices 62, *62*
gastro-gastric fistula 277
gastrointestinal stromal cell tumors (GIST) 205, *236*
colorectal wall 69, *70*
contrast-enhanced EUS for *246*
Doppler probe EUS for bleeding 191, *192*
EUS-FNA *145*
gastric 62, 64
metastases 63
gastrojejunostomy
complications 226
EUSGJ 226
gastric outlet obstruction 226
techniques 226
glomus tumors 63, *64*
glucagonoma 108
granular cell tumor 58–59, *60*

H

Habib™ EUS RFA 249
hemorrhoidal plexus 33
hepatic cysts 131–132
congenital/simple 131–132
hepatic venous pressure 194
hepatitis C, liver cirrhosis 130
hepatocellular carcinoma 132
risk with liver cirrhosis 130
heterotopic pancreas 61
hilar region 17
histoplasmosis, benign mediastinal lesions 51
hydatid cysts 132

I

image-guided radiation therapy (IGRT) systems
fiducial placement 176–178
equipment 176
needles 176

image-guided radiation therapy (IGRT) systems (*cont'd*)
peri-procedural care 178
technique 177–178
infection
pelvic abscess drainage 182–185
perianal fistula 74, *76*
perirectal abscess *77*
insulinoma 108, *109*
International Association of Pancreatology (IAP) algorithm 124
intraductal papillary mucinous neoplasm, management *123*
international normalized ratio (INR) 265
intraductal papillary mucinous neoplasms (IPMNs) 121–122, *123*, 124, 165, 254
intraductal ultrasound (IDUS) 98, 100

K
kidney
metastatic renal cell carcinoma *50*, *145*
normal anatomy 30–31
polycystic kidney disease 132

L
left carotid artery 16
radial array orientation 12
left subclavian artery 16
radial array orientation 12
leiomyomas 62, 64
leiomyosarcoma 90
lesions
lymph node 244
pancreatic cyst 244
solid pancreatic lesions 243–244
subepithelial lesions 244
linear array orientation 3–4, *4*
adrenal glands 32
aorta 12, *13*
aortic root 12–13
aortopulmonary window 13
bile duct 22–24
celiac artery 12, *13*
from duodenum 5–6
esophageal wall 10, *11*
from esophagus 3–4
kidney 30–31
liver 30
mitral valve 12–13
pancreas 26–29
from rectum 7
from stomach 5
thoracic anatomy 12–13
linear endosonography
adrenal glands 32
kidney 30–31
liver 30
linitis plastica 53
lipoma
colorectal wall 68
gastric 58, *59*
liver 130–133
cholangiocarcinoma 132
cirrhosis 130, *131*
dilated intrahepatic ducts 133, *133*
fatty liver disease 130–131, *132*
hepatic cysts 131–132
hepatocellular carcinoma 132
malignancy 132, *133*
metastases 41, 132
neoplasms 132, *133*
normal anatomy 30, *31*
polycystic liver disease 132
lumen-apposing metal stents (LAMS) 160, 220, *267*, 274
placement 164
lung cancer *236*
drainage to lymphadenopathy 50, *50*
intra-pulmonary *49*, 50
non-small cell
mediastinal lymph node metastases 14
mediastinal staging 146, **147**
primary *50*
staging 49–50, 146, **147**
lymphadenopathy
lung cancer drainage 50, *50*
mediastinal staging 146, **147**
perigastric *57*
peripancreatic 106
lymph nodes 244
colorectal cancer 67, *69*
EUS-guided elastography *230*
staging for esophageal cancer 39, **40**
lymphoma
EUS-FNA *145*
MALT 19
pancreatic 108, *109*, 110

M
magnetic resonance cholangiopancreatography (MRCP) 100, *100*
intraductal papillary mucinous neoplasms 121–122
secretin-stimulated in chronic pancreatitis 127
main pancreatic duct (MPD) strictures 214
mediastinal malignant lesions 49–50, *49–50*
mediastinal lesions
benign 51–52
FNA 49, *50*, 146, **147**, *148*, 149
malignant 49–50, *49–50*
mediastinal lymph nodes 14
anatomical correlations **15**
classification 146, *148*
metastatic adenocarcinoma *145*
stations *15*
techniques 15–17
mediastinal melanoma, metastatic *50*
mediastinum
cervical area 16
evaluation 146
inferior posterior 15, *16*
lymph node metastases 14

normal anatomy 14–18
radial array orientation 16–17
subcarinal area 16, 17
metastases
ampullary neoplasia 96
atrial myocardial 90
gastric cancer 53, *55*, 59, *61*
lymph nodes 57
gastrointestinal stromal cell tumors 63
hepatic in pancreas *153*
intraductal papillary mucinous neoplasm 124
liver malignancy 132
mediastinal lymph node adenocarcinoma *145*
mediastinal melanoma *50*
pancreatic cancer *111*, 112
renal cell cancer *50*, *145*
mitral valve
linear array orientation 12–13
radial array orientation 10, *11*
mucinous cystic neoplasms (MCNs) 118, *119*, 254
mucinous lesions 121–122, *123*, 124
mucosa-associated lymphoid tissue (MALT), lymphoma 19
multidetector CT (MDCT), intraductal papillary mucinous neoplasms 121, 122
myogenic tumor, colorectal wall 68–69, *71*

N

needle-based confocallaser endomicroscopy (nCLE) 254, *255*
neuroendocrine tumors (NETs) 209
neurolytic agents 175
non-electrocautery-enhanced delivery system 164
non-functional pancreatic neuroendocrine tumors (NF-pNETs) 248
non-Hodgkin's lymphoma 108, 110
non-small cell lung cancer *50*
mediastinal lymph node metastases 14
mediastinal staging 146, **147**
normal anatomy 3–9
adrenal glands 32
anorectum 33–35
arteries 7
bile duct 22–24
from duodenum 5–6
endobronchial 7, *8*, 9
from esophagus 3–4, 10, *11*, 12
gallbladder 22, 23, 24
kidney 30–31
liver 30, *31*
mediastinum 14–18
pancreas 25–29
rectum 7, 33–35
stomach 5–6, 19–21
thoracic linear 12–13
veins 7

O

obesity, fatty liver disease 131
ovarian endometriomas 81, *85*

P

paclitaxel, pancreatic cyst ablation 168
pain, pancreatic cancer/pancreatitis 173
pancreas
chemotherapeutic agent injection *180*, *181*
hepatic metastases *153*
heterotopic 61
linear array examination 26–29
normal anatomy 25–29
parenchyma 28, 29
invasion 96
radial array orientation 25, *26*
pancreatic adenocarcinoma 104, *105*, 106–107, *232*
EUS-FNA *151*
fiducial placement *177*
equipment 176
needles 176
peri-procedural care 178
technique 177–178
image-guided 176
peripancreatic lymphadenopathy 106
vascular invasion evaluation 104, *105*
pancreatic cancer
acinar cell carcinoma 110, 112
ampullary neoplasia 95–96, *97*
complications of EUS 106–107
cystic neoplasm *153*
diagnosis 104, *105*
endocrine tumors 108, *109*, 119, *120*
identification 104, *105*
limitations of EUS 106–107
lymphoma 108, *109*, 110
metastases *111*, 112
neuroendocrine tumors, EUS-FNA 150, *152*, 154
pain 173
peri-tumoral inflammation 115
solid pseudopapillary tumors 110, *145*
unresectable *99*
pancreatic cystic lesions 117–119, **118**, *120*, 244
ablation 165, 166, **167**, 168, 169, 171
of anechoic septated lobular cyst *157*
aspiration 156, 165, 168
benign 168
chemoablation
patient selection 166, 168
postoperative care and follow up 168, 169, *170*, 171
pretreatment evaluation 166
clinical data 154
CT 165
endocrine tumors 119, *120*
examination 155, *156*
FNA 155–159, *158*
lavage 165, 166, **167**, 168
malignant 166, 168
MRI *170*
mucinous lesions 156, 158, 168, *169*, *170*
paclitaxel ablation 168
patient preparation 168

pancreatic cystic lesions (*cont'd*)
  premalignant *170*
  serous lesions 168
  solid pseudopapillary epithelial neoplasm 119
  structural characteristics 117, **118**
  surveillance strategy 171
  wall aspiration 157
pancreatic cysts 244
  carcinoembryonic antigen (CEA) 254
  confocal laser endomicroscopy (CLE) 254
  EUS-guided needle confocal laser endomicroscopy 254–255
  fine needle aspiration (FNA) 254
  intraductal papillary mucinous neoplasms (IPMNs) 254
  mucinous cystic neoplasms (MCNs) 254
  needle-based confocal laser endomicroscopy (nCLE) 254, *255*
pancreatic duct 21, 22, 23, 24, 25, *27*, 27–28
  adenocarcinoma 119
  chronic pancreatitis 126, *127*
  storiform fibrosis 115
pancreatic duct drainage
  algorithm 218, *219*
  contraindications 214
  EUS-PDD 214
  fine-gauge electrocautery dilator *217*
  general anesthesia 214
  indications 214
  outcomes of EUS-PDD **218**
  techniques for
    access points and routes *215*
    anterograde approach 214
    anterograde or retrograde technique 216–217, *217*
    guidewire insertion and manipulation 215
    needle puncture 215
    Rendezvous technique *216*
    transmural stent 217–218
  transgastric EUS-PDD *217*
pancreatic function testing (PFT) 126
pancreatic lymphoma 108, *109*, 110
pancreatic mass
  FNA 150, *151*, 152–154
  fine needle biopsy 270–273
pancreatic NETs (pNETs) 209
pancreatic neuroendocrine tumors (pNETs)
  indications 210
  methods for EUS-guided RFA 209–210, *210*
  positron emission tomography (PET) 211
  prophylaxis 210
  results for EUS-guided radiofrequency ablation 211–211, 248, **250**
  technical aspects of EUS-guided ethanol injection 249–252, **253**
  technical aspects of EUS-guided radiofrequency system 248–249, *249*
pancreaticoduodenectomy 104, *105*
pancreatic pseudocyst 117, *118*, 168
  aspiration 160
  drainage 160–164
    accessories 160
    assessment 161
    instruments 160
    lubrication 164
    patient selection 160
    post-procedure follow-up 164
    stent deployment 163–164
  intervening vasculature 161
  lumen-apposing metal stent placement 164
  multilocular/mucinous 161
  plastic endoprosthesis placement 162–164
  puncture 162, *163*
  transmural tract dilatation 162, *163*
pancreatic rest 61, *62*
pancreatic serous cystadenoma 168
pancreatic solid pseudopapillary tumor 110, *145*
pancreatic tail symptomatic insulinoma *251*
pancreatitis
  alcohol-induced 115
  chronic 125–129
    classification 126–128
    diagnosis 125–126
    ductal changes 126, *127*
    histopathology 126, 127
    pain 173
    Rosemont criteria 125, 127–128, *128*
    threshold criteria 126–127
    tissue acquisition 129
  vascular injury 89
paratracheal region, left/right 17
pelvic abscess drainage 182–185
  accessories 182
  clinical outcomes 184–185
  devices 182
  patient preparation 182
  response to therapy 183
  stent 182–185
  technical limitations 185
  technique 182–184, *183*, *184*, *185*
  transmural tract dilation 182, 183, *184*
peptic ulcer, Doppler probe EUS for bleeding 187–188, *188*, *189*, *190*
percutaneous transhepatic gallbladder drainage (PT-GBD) 220
periampullary tumors 95
perianal fistula 74, *76*
peri-anastomotic varices 205
perigastric lymphadenopathy 57
peripancreatic lymphadenopathy 106
perirectal abscess 77
plastic endoprosthesis, placement 162–164
polidocanol 205
polycystic kidney disease 132
polycystic liver disease 132
portal hypertension (PH) 194
portal pressure gradient measurement (PPGM) 194–196
portal vein 25, *27*
  pancreatic adenocarcinoma involvement 106
  thrombosis 89
positron emission tomography (PET) 211
post-endoscopic submucosal dissection (ESD) ulcer 192
postprocedural antibiotics 195

primary pancreatic lymphoma (PPL) 109–110
primary sclerosing cholangitis, dilated intrahepatic duct 133
prostate 34
  cancer 78
proton pump inhibitor infusion 205
pseudoaneurysms 89
  bleeding *207*
pseudocyst puncture 162, *163*
pseudo-linitis plastica *55*
pudendal nerve terminal latency testing (PNTL) 72
pulmonary artery 16, 17
pulmonary embolism 205
pulmonary infection, benign mediastinal lesions 51, *52*

R
radial array orientation 3, *4*
  adrenal glands 32
  aortic arch 12, *12*
  aortic root 10, *11*
  atrium, left 10, *11*
  azygos arch 10, *12*
  bile duct 22, *23*
  from duodenum 5
  esophageal wall 10, *11*
  from esophagus 3
  gastro-esophageal junction 10, *11*
  kidney 30–31
  left carotid artery 12, *12*
  left subclavian artery 12, *12*
  liver 30
  mediastinum 14–15
  mitral valve 10, *11*
  pancreas 25, *26*
  from rectum 6–7
  from stomach 4–5
  thyroid 12, *12*
radial endosonography
  adrenal glands 32
  kidney 30–31
  liver 30
radiation therapy (RT)
  fiducial placement 176–178
    equipment 176
    needles 176
    peri-procedural care 178
    technique 177–178
  image-guided 176
radiofrequency ablation (RFA) 209, 248
rapid on-site evaluation of cytology (ROSE) 154
rectal adenocarcinoma *68*
rectum
  carcinoid tumors 69, *71*
  normal anatomy 6–7, 33–35
  wall 33–34
renal cell carcinoma, metastatic *50, 145*
rhabdomyosarcoma 90
right subclavian artery 88
Rosemont Criteria for chronic pancreatitis 125, 127–128, *128*
Roux-en-Y gastric bypass (RYGB) 274

S
sarcoid, benign mediastinal lesions 51
self-expanding metal stents (SEMS) 217
serous cystadenoma 117–118
serous lesions 117–118
sigmoidectomy, anastomotic perirectal abscess 77
single lobe liver biopsy 197
solid pancreatic lesions 243–244
solid pseudopapillary epithelial neoplasm (SPEN) 118
solid pseudopapillary tumors (SPTs) 110
somatostatinoma 108
spindle cell neoplasms 61
spleen
  extrinsic compression *65*
  normal anatomy 30
splenic artery 27, *28*
  aberrancies 90
  aneurysm 89
  pseudoaneurysm 89
splenic vein 25, *27*, 28
  thrombosis 89, 161
stack sign, common bile duct 25, *27*
stents
  AXIOS **221**, *223*, *224*
  biliary *99*
  common bile duct *152*
  deployment 163–164
  HANAROSTENT **221**
  pancreatic pseudocyst drainage 160–164
  pelvic abscess drainage 182–185
  SPAXUS **221**, *223*
stomach
  catheter probe 19
  normal anatomy 4–5, 19–21
stones
  common bile duct 98, 100
  pancreatic duct 125–129, *126*
subcarinal area 16, 17
subclavian artery
  left 12
  right 88
subepithelial lesions 244
submucosal tumors, colorectal wall 68–69, *70*, 71
superior mesenteric artery (SMA) 25, *26*, 27, *28*
  obliteration by calcified plaque 89
  pancreatic adenocarcinoma vascular invasion 104, *105*, 106
  vascular occlusion 88
superior mesenteric vein, pancreatic adenocarcinoma involvement 106

T
T4a lesion 40, 44
T4b lesion 40, 45
thyroid gland 16
  radial array orientation 12, *12*
TIGAR-O classification for chronic pancreatitis 126

Tis lesion 39
TNFerade injection 179
T3N1Mx adenocarcinoma 40, 44
T2N0Mx lesion 40, 43
T2N1Mx lesion 40, 43
T3N3Mx lesion 40, 44
trachea, normal anatomy 7, *8*, 9
transgastric EUS-PDD *217*
transmural tract dilatation 162, *163*
transperineal ultrasound 74, *75*
trauma, perianal fistula 76
tuberculosis, benign mediastinal lesions 51
tumor markers, intraductal papillary mucinous neoplasm 124
tumor necrosis factor-alpha (TNF-α) 179

V
vascular anomalies/abnormalities 88–91
  aberrancies 90, 91
  aneurysms 89
  atherosclerotic 88, 89
  calcification 88–89
  neoplasms 90
  plaques 88–89
  pseudoaneurysms 89
  venous thrombosis 89–90
veins, normal anatomy 7
venous thrombosis 89–90
VIPoma 108
VTI endoscopic Doppler system 186, *187*

Wiley The manufacturer's authorized representative according to the EU General Product Safety Regulation is Wiley-VCH GmbH, Boschstr. 12, 69469 Weinheim, Germany, e-mail: Product_Safety@wiley.com.

Printed and bound by CPI Group (UK) Ltd, Croydon, CR0 4YY
15/09/2026
02217280-0002